The GALE ENCYCLOPEDIA *of* SURGERY AND MEDICAL TESTS

SECOND EDITION

The GALE ENCYCLOPEDIA of SURGERY AND MEDICAL TESTS

SECOND EDITION

VOLUME

4

Q–Z
ORGANIZATIONS
GLOSSARY
INDEX

BRIGHAM NARINS, EDITOR

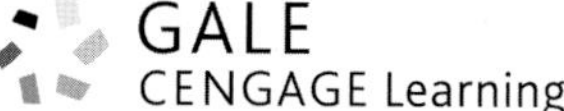

Detroit • New York • San Francisco • New Haven, Conn • Waterville, Maine • London

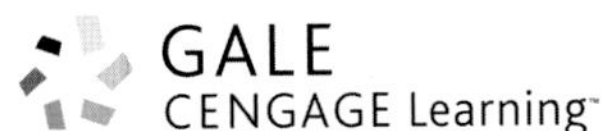

Gale Encyclopedia of Surgery and Medical Tests, Second Edition

Project Editor: Brigham Narins

Editorial: Donna Batten, Amy Kwolek, Jeffrey Wilson

Product Manager: Kate Hanley

Editorial Support Services: Andrea Lopeman

Indexing Services: Katherine Jensen, Indexes, etc.

Rights Acquisition and Management: Margaret Chamberlain-Gaston, Kelly A. Quin, and Robyn V. Young

Composition: Evi Abou-El-Seoud

Manufacturing: Wendy Blurton

Imaging: Lezlie Light

Product Design: Pam Galbreath

Library of Congress Cataloging-in-Publication Data

The Gale encyclopedia of surgery and medical tests : a guide for patients and caregivers / Brigham Narins, editor. -- 2nd ed.
p. cm.
Includes bibliographical references and index.
ISBN-13: 978-1-4144-4884-8 (set : alk. paper)
ISBN-13: 978-1-4144-4885-5 (vol. 1 : alk. paper)
ISBN-13: 978-1-4144-4886-2 (vol. 2 : alk. paper)
ISBN-13: 978-1-4144-4887-9 (vol. 3 : alk. paper)
[etc.]
1. Surgery--Encyclopedias. 2. Diagnosis--Encyclopedias. I. Narins, Brigham, 1962-.

RD17.G342 2008
617.003--dc22 2008020207

Gale
27500 Drake Rd.
Farmington Hills, MI, 48331-3535

ISBN-13: 978-1-4144-4884-8 (set) ISBN-10: 1-4144-4884-8 (set)
ISBN-13: 978-1-4144-4885-5 (vol. 1) ISBN-10: 1-4144-4885-6 (vol. 1)
ISBN-13: 978-1-4144-4886-2 (vol. 2 ISBN-10: 1-4144-4886-4 (vol. 2)
ISBN-13: 978-1-4144-4887-9 (vol. 3) ISBN-10: 1-4144-4887-2 (vol. 3)
ISBN-13: 978-1-4144-4888-6 (vol. 4) ISBN-10: 1-4144-4888-0 (vol. 4)

This title is also available as an e-book.
ISBN-13: 978-1-4144-4889-3 ISBN-10: 1-4144-4889-9
Contact your Gale, Cengage Learning sales representative for ordering information.

Printed in China
1 2 3 4 5 6 7 12 11 10 09 08

CONTENTS

LIST OF ENTRIES

A

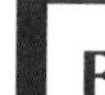

B

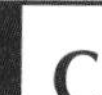

C

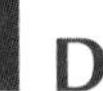

D

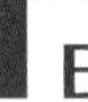

E

F

G

N

O

P

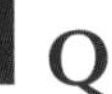

Q

R

S

T

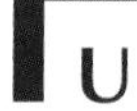

U

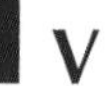

V

W

LIST OF ENTRIES BY BODY SYSTEM

Cardiovascular

Angiography
Angioplasty
Aortic aneurysm repair
Aortic valve replacement
Arteriovenous fistula
Balloon valvuloplasty
Cardiac catheterization
Cardiac event monitor
Cardiac marker tests
Cardiac monitor
Cardiopulmonary resuscitation
Cardioversion
Carotid endarterectomy
Coronary artery bypass graft surgery
Coronary stenting
Defibrillation
Echocardiography
Electrocardiogram
Electrocardiography
Electrophysiology study of the heart
Endovascular stent surgery
Femoral hernia repair
Heart surgery for congenital defects
Heart transplantation
Heart-lung machines
Heart-lung transplantation
Hemangioma excision
Implantable cardioverter-defibrillator
Magnetic resonance angiogram
Magnetic resonance venogram
Maze procedure for atrial fibrillation
Mechanical circulation support
Minimally invasive heart surgery
Mitral valve repair
Mitral valve replacement
Multiple-gated acquisition (MUGA) scan
Myocardial resection
Pacemakers
Pericardiocentesis
Peripheral endarterectomy
Peripheral vascular bypass surgery
Portal vein bypass
Sclerotherapy for varicose veins
Stress test
Vascular surgery
Vein ligation and stripping
Venous thrombosis prevention
Ventricular assist device
Ventricular shunt

Endocrine

Adenoidectomy
Adrenalectomy
Endoscopic retrograde cholangiopancreatography
Hypophysectomy
Intra-Operative Parathyroid Hormone Measurement
Islet cell transplantation
Oral glucose tolerance test
Pancreas transplantation
Pancreatectomy
Parathyroidectomy
Sestamibi scan
Thyroidectomy
Whipple procedure

Gastrointestinal

Antrectomy
Appendectomy
Artificial sphincter insertion
Barium enema
Biliary stenting
Bowel preparation
Bowel resection
Bowel resection, small intestine
Cholecystectomy
Colonic stent
Colonoscopy
Colorectal surgery
Colostomy
Defecography
Diverticulitis
Endoscopic ultrasound
Esophageal atresia repair
Esophageal function tests
Esophageal resection
Esophagogastrectomy
Esophagogastroduodenoscopy
Gastrectomy
Gastric acid inhibitors
Gastric bypass
Gastroduodenostomy

Hematological

Integumentary

Musculoskeletal

Neurological

Reproductive, Female

Reproductive, Male

Respiratory

Sensory

Urinary

Other Surgeries

Other Tests & Procedures

Drugs

Antianxiety drugs
Antibiotics
Antibiotics, topical
Antihypertensive drugs
Antinausea drugs
Antiseptics
Aspirin
Barbiturates
Cephalosporins
Corticosteroids
Diuretics
Erythromycins
Fluoroquinolones
Immunosuppressant drugs
Muscle relaxants
Nonsteroidal anti-inflammatory drugs
Prophylaxis, antibiotic
Proton pump inhibitors
Scopolamine patch
Sedation, conscious
Sulfonamides
Tetracyclines

Related Issues & Topics

Admission to the hospital
Adult day care
Ambulatory surgery centers
Anesthesiologist's role
Aseptic technique
Bandages and dressings
Body temperature
Closures: stitches, staples, and glue
Death and dying
Discharge from the hospital
Do not resuscitate (DNR) order
Drug-resistant organisms
Exercise
Fibrin sealants
Finding a surgeon
Health care proxy
Health history
Health Maintenance Organization (HMO)Home care
Hospice
Hospital services
Hospital-acquired infections
Incision care
Informed consent
Intensive care unit
Intensive care unit equipment
Length of hospital stay
Living will
Long-term care insurance
Managed care plans
Medicaid
Medical charts
Medical co-morbidities
Medical errors
Medicare
Medication Monitoring
Mental health assessment
Negative pressure rooms
Nursing homes
Operating room
Pain management
Patient confidentiality
Patient rights
Patient-controlled analgesia
Pediatric concerns
Planning a hospital stay
Postoperative care
Post-surgical infections
Post-surgical pain
Power of attorney
Preoperative care
Preparing for surgery
Presurgical testing
Private insurance plans
Recovery at home
Recovery room
Reoperation
Second opinion
Smoking cessation
Stethoscope
Surgical instruments
Surgical mesh
Surgical oncology
Surgical risk
Surgical team
Surgical training
Surgical triage
Syringe and needle
Talking to the doctor
Thermometer
Trocars
Vital signs
Wound care
Wound culture

PLEASE READ—IMPORTANT INFORMATION

The *Gale Encyclopedia of Surgery and Medical Tests, 2nd Edition* is a health reference product designed to inform and educate readers about a wide variety of surgeries, tests, diseases and conditions, treatments and drugs, equipment, and other issues associated with surgical and medical practice. Cengage Learning believes the product to be comprehensive, but not necessarily definitive. It is intended to supplement, not replace, consultation with physicians or other healthcare practitioners. While Cengage Learning has made substantial efforts to provide information that is accurate, comprehensive, and up-to-date, Cengage Learning makes no representations or warranties of any kind, including without limitation, warranties of merchantability or fitness for a particular purpose, nor does it guarantee the accuracy, comprehensiveness, or timeliness of the information contained in this product. Readers should be aware that the universe of medical knowledge is constantly growing and changing, and that differences of opinion exist among authorities. Readers are also advised to seek professional diagnosis and treatment for any medical condition, and to discuss information obtained from this book with their healthcare provider.

INTRODUCTION

The *Gale Encyclopedia of Surgery and Medical Tests, 2nd Edition* is a unique and invaluable source of information. This collection of 535 entries provides in-depth coverage of various issues related to surgery, medical tests, diseases and conditions, hospitalization, and general health care. These entries generally follow a standard format, including a definition, purpose, demographics, description, diagnosis/preparation, aftercare, precautions, risks, side effects, interactions, morbidity and mortality rates, alternatives, normal results, questions to ask your doctor, and information about who performs the procedures and where they are performed. Topics of a more general nature related to surgical hospitalization and medical testing round out the set. Examples of this coverage include entries on Adult day care, Ambulatory surgery centers, Death and dying, Discharge from the hospital, Do not resuscitate (DNR) order, Exercise, Finding a surgeon, Hospice, Hospital services, Informed consent, Living will, Long-term care insurance, Managed care plans, Medicaid, Medicare, Patient rights, Planning a hospital stay, Power of attorney, Private insurance plans, Second opinion, Talking to the doctor, and others.

Scope

The *Gale Encyclopedia of Surgery and Medical Tests, 2nd Edition* covers a wide variety of topics relevant to the user. Entries follow a standardized format that provides information at a glance. Rubrics include the following (not every entry will make use of all of them):

- Definition
- Description
- Purpose
- Demographics
- Diagnosis/preparation
- Aftercare
- Precautions
- Risks
- Side effects
- Interactions
- Morbidity and mortality rates
- Alternatives
- Normal results
- "Questions to ask the doctor"
- "Who performs the procedure and where is it performed?"
- Resources
- Key Terms

Inclusion criteria

A preliminary list of topics was compiled from a wide variety of sources, including health reference books, general medical encyclopedias, and consumer health guides. The advisory board evaluated the topics and made suggestions for inclusion. Final selection of topics to include was made by the advisory board in conjunction with the editor.

About the contributors

The essays were compiled by experienced medical writers, including medical doctors, pharmacists, and registered nurses. The advisers reviewed the completed essays to ensure that they are appropriate, up-to-date, and accurate.

How to use this book

The *Gale Encyclopedia of Surgery and Medical Tests, 2nd Edition* has been designed with ready reference in mind.

- Straight **alphabetical arrangement** of topics allows users to locate information quickly.
- **Bold-faced terms** within entries direct the reader to related articles.
- **Cross-references** placed throughout the encyclopedia direct readers from alternate names and related topics to entries.
- A list of **Key terms** is provided where appropriate to define terms or concepts that may be unfamiliar to the user. A **glossary** of key terms in the back of the fourth volume contains a concise list of terms arranged alphabetically.
- The **Resources** section directs readers to additional sources of information on a topic.
- Valuable **contact information** for health organizations is included with most entries. An Appendix of **organizations** in the back of the fourth volume contains an extensive list of organizations arranged alphabetically.
- A comprehensive **general index** guides readers to significant topics mentioned in the text.

Graphics

The *Gale Encyclopedia of Surgery and Medical Tests, 2nd Edition* is also enhanced by color photographs, illustrations, and tables.

Acknowledgements

The editor wishes to thank all of the people who contributed to this encyclopedia. There are too many names to list here, so the reader is urged to review the Advisory board and Contributors pages for the list of writers, physicians, and health-care experts to whom he is indebted. Special thanks must go to Rosalyn Carson-DeWitt for all the writing, updating, and advising she did; the project could not have been completed without her. L. Fleming Fallon provided invaluable assistance at every step of the way; his writing, advice, and good humor made this project a pleasure. Laurie Cataldo's expertise in so many areas helped make this book as good as it is. And Maria Basile provided not only many beautifully written entries, but she performed some last-minute review work for which the editor is most grateful. To all of you, my deepest thanks.

ADVISORS

A number of experts in the medical community provided invaluable assistance in the formulation of this encyclopedia. Our advisory board performed a myriad of duties, from defining the scope of coverage to reviewing individual entries for accuracy and accessibility. The editor would like to express his appreciation to them.

Rosalyn Carson-DeWitt, MD
Medical Writer
Durham, NC

Laura Jean Cataldo, RN, EdD
Nurse, Medical Consultant, Educator
Germantown, MD

L. Fleming Fallon, Jr, MD, DrPH
Professor of Public Health
Bowling Green State University
Bowling Green, OH

Chitra Venkatasubramanian, MD
Clinical Assistant Professor, Neurology and Neurological Sciences
Stanford University School of Medicine
Palo Alto, CA

CONTRIBUTORS

Laurie Barclay, MD
Neurological Consulting Services
Tampa, FL

Jeanine Barone
Nutritionist, Exercise Physiologist
New York, NY

Julia Barrett
Science Writer
Madison, WI

Donald G. Barstow, RN
Clinical Nurse Specialist
Oklahoma City, OK

Maria Basile, PhD
Neuropharmacologist
Roselle, NJ

Mary Bekker
Medical Writer
Willow Grove, PA

Mark A. Best, MD, MPH, MBA
Associate Professor of Pathology
St. Matthew's University
Grand Cayman, BWI

Randall J. Blazic, MD, DDS
Oral and Maxillofacial Surgeon
Goodyear, AZ

Robert Bockstiegel
Medical Writer
Portland, OR

Maggie Boleyn, RN, BSN
Medical Writer
Oak Park, MN

Susan Joanne Cadwallader
Medical Writer
Cedarburg, WI

Diane M. Calabrese
Medical Sciences and Technology Writer
Silver Spring, MD

Richard H. Camer
Editor
International Medical News Group
Silver Spring, MD

Rosalyn Carson-DeWitt, MD
Medical Writer
Durham, NC

Laura Jean Cataldo, RN, EdD
Nurse, Medical Consultant, Educator
Germantown, MD

Lisa Christenson, Ph.D.
Science Writer
Hamden, CT

Rhonda Cloos, RN
Medical Writer
Austin, TX

Constance Clyde
Medical Writer
Dana Point, CA

Angela M. Costello
Medical writer
Cleveland, OH

L. Lee Culvert, PhD
Health writer
Alna, ME

Tish Davidson, AM
Medical Writer
Fremont, CA

Lori De Milto
Medical Writer
Sicklerville, NJ

Victoria E. DeMoranville
Medical Writer
Lakeville, MA

Altha Roberts Edgren
Medical Writer
Medical Ink
St. Paul, MN

Lorraine K. Ehresman
Medical Writer
Northfield, Quebec, Canada

Abraham F. Ettaher, MD

L. Fleming Fallon, Jr, MD, DrPH
Professor of Public Health
Bowling Green State University
Bowling Green, OH

Paula Ford-Martin
Medical Writer
Warwick, RI

Janie F. Franz
Journalist
Grand Forks, ND

Rebecca J. Frey, PhD
Medical Writer
New Haven, CT

Debra Gordon
Medical Writer
Nazareth, PA

Jill Granger, MS
Sr. Research Associate
Dept. of Pathology
University of Michigan Medical Center
Ann Arbor, MI

Peter Gregutt
Medical Writer
Asheville, NC

Laith Farid Gulli, MD, MS
Consultant Psychotherapist in Private Practice
Lathrup Village, MI

Stephen John Hage, AAAS, RT(R), FAHRA
Medical Writer
Chatsworth, CA

Maureen Haggerty
Medical Writer
Ambler, PA

Robert Harr
Associate Professor and Chair
Department of Public and Allied Health
Bowling Green State University
Bowling Green, OH

Dan Harvey
Medical Writer
Wilmington, DE

Katherine Hauswirth, APRN
Medical Writer
Deep River, CT

Caroline A. Helwick
Medical Writer
New Orleans, LA

Lisette Hilton
Medical Writer
Boca Raton, FL

Fran Hodgkins
Medical Writer
Sparks, MD

René A. Jackson, RN
Medical Writer
Port Charlotte, FL

Nadine M. Jacobson, RN
Medical Writer
Takoma Park, MD

Randi B. Jenkins, BA
Copy Chief
Fission Communications
New York, NY

Michelle L. Johnson, MS, JD
Patent Attorney
ZymoGenetics, Inc.
Seattle, WA

Paul Johnson
Medical Writer
San Diego, CA

Cindy L. A. Jones, PhD
Biomedical Writer
Sagescript Communications
Lakewood, CO

Linda D. Jones, BA, PBT (ASCP)
Medical Writer
Asheboro, NY

Crystal H. Kaczkowski, MSc
Health writer
Chicago, IL

Beth A. Kapes
Medical Writer
Bay Village, OH

Mary Jeanne Krob, MD, FACS
Physician, writer
Pittsburgh, PA

Monique Laberge, PhD
Sr. Res. Investigator
Dept. of Biochemistry & Biophysics, School of Medicine
University of Pennsylvania
Philadelphia, PA

Richard H. Lampert
Senior Medical Editor
W.B. Saunders Co.
Philadelphia, PA

Renee Laux, MS
Medical Writer
Manlius, NY

Victor Leipzig, PhD
Biological Consultant
Huntington Beach, CA

Lorraine Lica, PhD
Medical Writer
San Diego, CA

John T. Lohr, PhD
Assistant Director, Biotechnology Center
Utah State University
Logan, UT

Jennifer Lee Losey, RN
Medical Writer
Madison Heights, MI

Nicole Mallory, MS, PA-C
Medical Student, Wayne State University
Detroit, MI

Jacqueline N. Martin, MS
Medical Writer
Albrightsville, PA

Nancy McKenzie, PhD
Public Health Consultant
Brooklyn, NY

Mercedes McLaughlin
Medical Writer
Phoenixville, CA

Miguel A. Melgar, MD, PhD
Neurosurgeon
New Orleans, LA

Christine Miner Minderovic, BS, RT, RDMS
Medical Writer
Ann Arbor, MI

Mark Mitchell, MD, MPH, MBA
Medical Writer
Bothell, WA

Alfredo Mori, MD, FACEM, FFAEM
Emergency Physician
The Alfred Hospital
Victoria, Australia

Bilal Nasser, MD, MS
Senior Medical Student, Wayne State University
Detroit, MI

Erika J. Norris
Medical Writer
Oak Harbor, WA

Teresa Norris, RN
Medical Writer
Ute Park, NM

Debra Novograd, BS, RT(R)(M)
Medical Writer
Royal Oak, MI

Jane E. Phillips, PhD
Medical Writer
Chapel Hill, NC

J. Ricker Polsdorfer, MD
Medical Writer
Phoenix, AZ

Elaine R. Proseus, MBA/TM, BSRT, RT(R)
Medical Writer
Farmington Hills, MI

Robert Ramirez, BS
Medical Student
University of Medicine & Dentistry of New Jersey
Stratford, NJ

Esther Csapo Rastegari, RN, BSN, EdM
Medical Writer
Holbrook, MA

Martha Reilly, OD
Clinical Optometrist, Medical Writer
Madison, WI

Toni Rizzo
Medical Writer
Salt Lake City, UT

Richard Robinson
Medical Writer
Sherborn, MA

Nancy Ross-Flanigan
Science Writer
Belleville, MI

Belinda Rowland, PhD
Medical Writer
Voorheesville, NY

Laura Ruth, PhD
Medical, Science, & Technology Writer
Los Angeles, CA

Uchechukwu Sampson, MD, MPH, MBA

Kausalya Santhanam, PhD
Technical Writer
Branford, CT

Joan M. Schonbeck
Medical Writer
Nursing
Massachusetts Department of Mental Health
Marlborough, MA

Stephanie Dionne Sherk
Medical Writer
University of Michigan
Ann Arbor, MI

Lee A. Shratter, MD
Consulting Radiologist
Kentfield, CA

Jennifer E. Sisk, MA
Medical Writer
Havertown, PA

Allison Joan Spiwak, MSBME
Circulation Technologist
The Ohio State University
Columbus, OH

Kurt Richard Sternlof
Science Writer
New Rochelle, NY

Margaret A Stockley, RGN
Medical Writer
Boxborough, MA

Dorothy Elinor Stonely
Medical Writer
Los Gatos, CA

Bethany Thivierge
Biotechnical Writer and Editor
Technicality Resources
Rockland, ME

Carol A. Turkington
Medical Writer
Lancaster, PA

Samuel D. Uretsky, PharmD
Medical Writer
Wantagh, NY

Chitra Venkatasubramanian, MD
Clinical Assistant Professor, Neurology and Neurological Sciences
Stanford University School of Medicine
Palo Alto, CA

Ellen S. Weber, MSN
Medical Writer
Fort Wayne, IN

Barbara Wexler
Medical Writer
Chatsworth, CA

Abby Wojahn, RN, BSN, CCRN
Medical Writer
Milwaukee, WI

Kathleen D. Wright, RN
Medical Writer
Delmar, DE

Mary Zoll, PhD
Science Writer
Newton Center, MA

Michael Zuck, PhD
Medical Writer
Boulder, CO

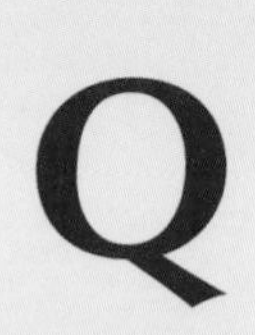

Quadrantectomy

Definition

Quadrantectomy is a surgical procedure in which a "quadrant" (approximately one-fourth) of the breast, including tissue surrounding a cancerous tumor, is removed. It is also called a partial or segmental **mastectomy**.

Purpose

Quadrantectomy is a type of breast-conserving surgery used as a treatment for breast cancer. Prior to the advent of breast-conserving surgeries, total mastectomy (complete removal of the breast) was considered the standard surgical treatment for breast cancer. Procedures such as quadrantectomy and **lumpectomy** (removing the tissue directly surrounding the tumor) have allowed doctors to treat cancer without sacrificing the entire affected breast.

Demographics

The American Cancer Society estimates that approximately 211,300 new cases of breast cancer are diagnosed annually in the United States, and 39,800 women die as a result of the disease. Approximately one in eight women will develop breast cancer at some point in her life. The risk of developing breast cancer increases with age: women ages 30–40 have a one in 252 chance; ages 40–50 have a one in 68 chance; ages 50–60 have a one in 35 chance; and ages 60–70 have a one in 27 chance.

In the 1990s, the incidence of breast cancer was higher among white women (113.1 cases per 100,000 women) than African American women (100.3 per 100,000). The **death** rate associated with breast cancer, however, was higher among African American women (29.6 per 100,000) than Caucasian women (22.2 per 100,000). Rates were lower among Hispanic women (14.2 per 100,000), Native American women (12.0), and Asian women (11.2 per 100,000).

Description

The patient is usually placed under **general anesthesia** for the duration of the procedure. In some instances, a local anesthetic may be administered with sedation to help the patient relax.

During quadrantectomy, a margin of normal breast tissue, skin, and muscle lining is removed around the periphery of the tumor. This decreases the risk of any abnormal cells being left behind and spreading locally or to other parts of the body (a process called metastasis). The amount removed is generally about one-fourth of the size of the breast (hence, the "quadrant" in quadrantectomy). The remaining tissue is then reconstructed to minimize any cosmetic defects, and then sutured closed. Temporary drains may be placed through the skin to remove excess fluid from the surgical site.

Some patients may have the lymph nodes removed from under the arm (called the axillary lymph nodes) on the same side as the tumor. Lymph nodes are small, oval- or bean-shaped masses found throughout the body that act as filters against foreign materials and cancer cells. If cancer cells break away from their primary site of growth, they can travel to and begin to grow in the lymph nodes first, before traveling to other parts of the body. Removal of the lymph nodes is therefore a method of determining if a cancer has begun to spread. To remove the nodes, a second incision is made in the area of the armpit and the fat pad that contains the lymph nodes is removed. The tissue is then sent to a pathologist, who extracts the lymph nodes from the fatty tissue and examines them for the presence of cancer cells.

Diagnosis/Preparation

Breast tumors may be found during self-examination or an examination by a health care professional. In

KEY TERMS

Mammogram—A set of x rays taken of the front and side of the breast; used to diagnose various abnormalities of the breast.

Pathologist—A medical doctor who specializes in the diagnosis of diseases from the microscopic analyses of cells and tissues.

other cases, they are visualized during a routine mammogram. Symptoms such as breast pain, changes in breast size or shape, redness, dimpling, or irritation may be an indication that medical attention is warranted.

Prior to surgery, the patient is instructed to refrain from eating or drinking after midnight on the night before the operation. The physician will tell the patient what will take place during and after surgery, as well as expected outcomes and potential complications of the procedure.

Aftercare

The patient may return home the same day or remain in the hospital for one to two days after the procedure. Discharge instructions will include how to care for the incision and drains, what activities to restrict (i.e., driving and heavy lifting), and how to manage postoperative pain. Patients are often instructed to wear a well-fitting support bra for at least a week following surgery. A follow-up appointment to remove **stitches** and drains is usually scheduled 10–14 days after surgery.

If lymph nodes are removed, specific steps should be taken to minimize the risk of developing lymphedema of the arm, a condition in which excess fluid is not properly drained from body tissues, resulting in chronic swelling. This swelling can sometimes become severe enough to interfere with daily activity. Prior to being discharged, the patient will learn how to care for the arm, and how to avoid infection. She will also be told to avoid sunburn, refrain from heavy lifting, and to be careful not to wear tight jewelry and elastic bands.

Most patients undergo radiation therapy as part of their complete treatment plan. The radiation usually begins immediately or soon after quadrantectomy, and involves a schedule of five days of treatment a week for five to six weeks. Other treatments, such as chemotherapy or hormone therapy, may also be prescribed depending on the size and stage of the patient's cancer.

WHO PERFORMS THE PROCEDURE AND WHERE IS IT PERFORMED?

Quandrantectomy is usually performed by a general surgeon, breast surgeon, or surgical oncologist. Radiation therapy is administered by a radiation oncologist, and chemotherapy by a medical oncologist. The surgical procedure is frequently done in a hospital setting (especially if lymph nodes are to be removed at the same time), but specialized outpatient facilities are sometimes preferred.

Risks

Risks associated with the surgical removal of breast tissue include bleeding, infection, breast asymmetry, changes in sensation, reaction to the anesthesia, and unexpected scarring.

Some of the risks associated with removal of the lymph nodes include excessive bleeding, infection, pain, excessive swelling, and damage to nerves during surgery. Nerve damage may be temporary or permanent, and may result in weakness, numbness, tingling, and drooping. Lymphedema is also a risk whenever lymph nodes have been removed; it may occur immediately following surgery or months to years later.

Normal results

Most patients will not experience recurrences of the cancer following a treatment plan of quadrantectomy and radiation therapy. One study followed patients for a period of 20 years after breast-conserving surgery, and found that only 9% experienced recurrence of the cancer.

Morbidity and mortality rates

Following removal of the axillary lymph nodes, there is approximately a 10% risk of lymphedema and a 20% risk of abnormal skin sensations. Approximately 17% of women undergoing breast-conserving surgery have a poor cosmetic result (e.g., asymmetry or distortion of shape). The risk of complications associated with general anesthesia is less than 1%.

Alternatives

A full mastectomy, in which the entire affected breast is removed, is one alternative to quadrantectomy. A **simple mastectomy** removes the entire breast, while a radical mastectomy removes the entire breast

QUESTIONS TO ASK THE DOCTOR

- Why is quadrantectomy recommended?
- What methods of anesthesia and pain relief will be used?
- Where will the incision be located, and how much tissue will be removed?
- Will a lymph node dissection be performed?
- Is sentinel node biopsy appropriate in this case?
- Is postsurgical radiation therapy recommended?

plus parts of the chest muscle wall and the lymph nodes. In terms of recurrence and survival rates, breast-conserving surgery has been shown to be equally effective as mastectomy in treating breast cancer.

A new technique that may eliminate the need for removing many axillary lymph nodes is called sentinel node biopsy. When lymph fluid moves out of a region, the "sentinel" lymph node is the first node it reaches. The theory behind **sentinel lymph node biopsy** is that if cancer is not present in the sentinel node, it is unlikely to have spread to other nearby nodes. This procedure may allow individuals with early stage cancers to avoid the complications associated with partial or radical removal of lymph nodes if there is little or no chance that cancer has spread to them.

Resources

BOOKS

Iglehart, J. Dirk and Carolyn M. Kaelin. "Diseases of the Breast" (Chapter 30). In *Sabiston Textbook of Surgery*. Philadelphia: W. B. Saunders Company, 2001.

PERIODICALS

Apantaku, Leila. "Breast-Conserving Surgery for Breast Cancer." *American Family Physician* 66, no. 12 (December 15, 2002): 2271-8.

Sainsbury, J. R., T. J. Anderson, and D. A. L. Morgan. "Breast Cancer." *British Medical Journal* 321 (September 23, 2000): 745-50.

Veronesi, U., N. Cascinelli, L. Mariani, et al. "More Long-Term Data for Breast-Conserving Surgery." *New England Journal of Medicine* 347, no. 16 (October 17, 2002): 1227-32.

ORGANIZATIONS

American Cancer Society. 1599 Clifton Rd. NE, Atlanta, GA 30329-4251. (800) 227-2345. http://www.cancer.org.

Society of Surgical Oncology. 85 W. Algonquin Rd., Suite 550, Arlington Heights, IL 60005. (847) 427-1400. http://www.surgonc.org.

OTHER

"All About Cancer: Detailed Guide." *American Cancer Society*. 2003 [cited April 9, 2003] http://www.cancer.org/docroot/CRI/CRI_2_3.asp.

Stephanie Dionne Sherk

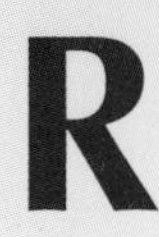

Radical neck dissection

Definition

Radical neck dissection is a surgical operation used to remove cancerous tissue in the head and neck.

Purpose

The purpose of radical neck dissection is to remove lymph nodes and other structures in the head and neck that are likely or known to be malignant. Variations on neck dissections exist, depending on the extent of the cancer. A radical neck dissection removes the most tissue. It is performed when the cancer has spread widely in the neck. A modified neck dissection removes less tissue, and a selective neck dissection even less.

Demographics

Experts estimate that there are approximately 5,000–10,000 radical neck dissections in the United States each year. Men and women undergo radical neck dissections at about the same rate.

Description

Cancers of the head and neck (sometimes inaccurately called throat cancer) often spread to nearby tissues and into the lymph nodes. Removing these structures is one way of controlling the cancer.

Of the 600 lymph nodes in the body, approximately 200 are in the neck. Only a small number of these are removed during a neck dissection. In addition, other structures such as muscles, veins, and nerves may be removed during a radical neck dissection. These include the sternocleidomastoid muscle (one of the muscles that functions to flex the head), internal jugular (neck) vein, submandibular gland (one of the salivary glands), and the spinal accessory nerve (a nerve that helps control speech, swallowing, and certain movements of the head and neck). The goal is always to remove all the cancer, but to save as many components surrounding the nodes as possible.

An incision is made in the neck, and the skin is pulled back (retracted) to reveal the muscles and lymph nodes. The surgeon is guided in what to remove by tests performed prior to surgery and by examination of the size and texture of the lymph nodes.

Diagnosis/Preparation

This operation should not be performed if cancer has metastasized (spread) beyond the head and neck, or if the cancer has invaded the bones of the cervical vertebrae (the first seven bones of the spinal column) or the skull. In these cases, the surgery will not effectively contain the cancer.

Radical neck dissection is a major operation. Extensive tests are performed before the operation to try to determine where and how far the cancer has spread. These may include lymph node biopsies, computed tomography (CT) scans, **magnetic resonance imaging** (MRI) scans, and barium swallows. In addition, standard preoperative blood and **liver function tests** are performed, and the candidate will meet with an anesthesiologist before the operation. The candidate should tell the anesthesiologist about all drug allergies and all medication (prescription, non-prescription, or herbal) that are presently being taken.

Aftercare

A person who has had a radical neck dissection will stay in the hospital several days after the operation, and sometimes longer if surgery to remove the primary tumor was performed at the same time. Drains are inserted under the skin to remove the fluid that accumulates in the neck area. Once the drains are removed

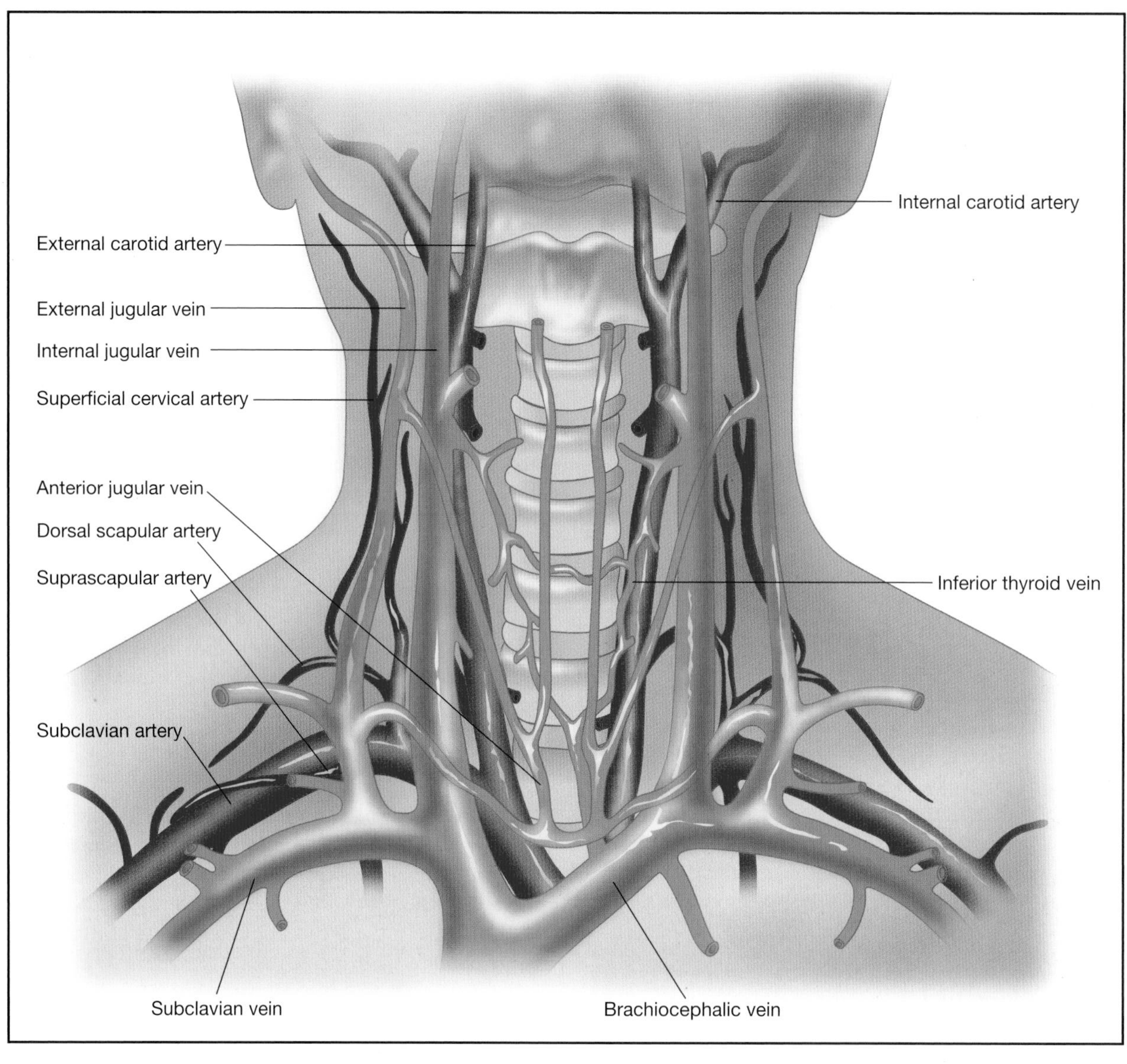

Major veins and arteries in the neck. *(Illustration by Electronic Illustrators Group.)*

and the incision appears to be healing well, people are usually discharged from the hospital, but will require follow-up doctor visits. Depending on how many structures are removed, a person who has had a radical neck dissection may require physical therapy to regain use of the arm and shoulder.

Risks

The greatest risk in a radical neck dissection is damage to the nerves, muscles, and veins in the neck. Nerve damage can result in numbness (either temporary or permanent) to different regions on the neck and loss of function (temporary or permanent) to parts of the neck, throat, and shoulder. The more extensive the neck dissection, the more function a person is likely to lose. As a result, it is common following radical neck dissection for people to have stooped shoulders, limited ability to lift one or both arms, and limited head and neck rotation and flexion due to the removal of nerves and muscles. Other risks are the same as for all major surgery: potential bleeding, infection, and allergic reaction to anesthesia.

Normal results

Normal lymph nodes are small and show no cancerous cells under a microscope. Abnormal lymph

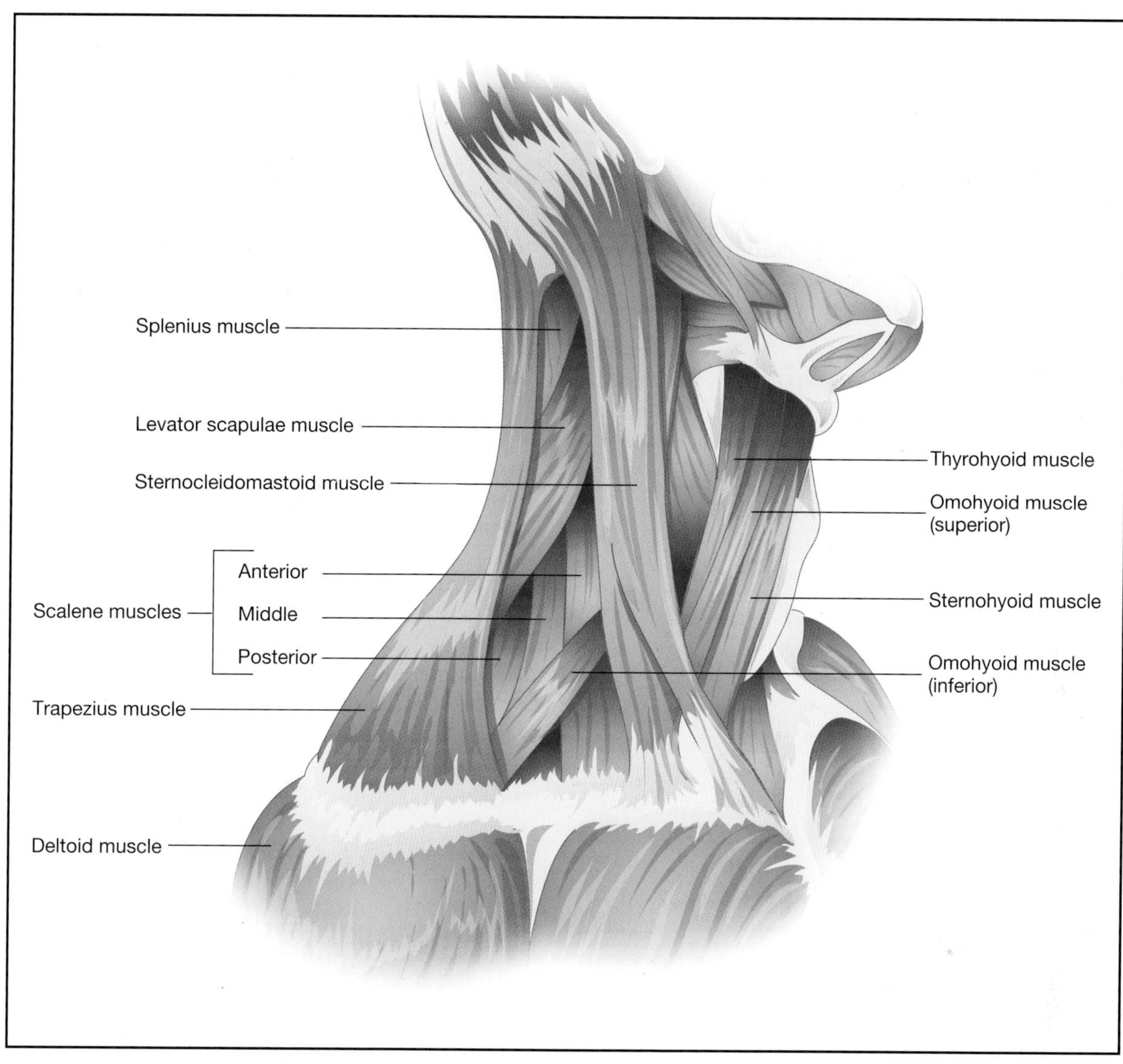

Major muscles of the neck. *(Illustration by Electronic Illustrators Group.)*

nodes may be enlarged and show malignant cells when examined under a microscope.

Morbidity and mortality rates

The mortality rate for radical neck dissection can be as high as 14%.

Morbidity rates are somewhat higher and are due to bleeding, post-surgery infection, and medicine errors.

Alternatives

Alternatives to radical neck dissection depend on the reason for the proposed surgery. Most alternatives are far less acceptable. Radiation and chemotherapy may be used instead of a radical neck dissection in the case of cancer. Alternatives for some surgical procedures may reduce scarring, but are not as effective in the removal of all pathological tissue. Chemotherapy and radiation or altered fractionated radiotherapy are reasonable alternatives.

Resources

BOOKS

Bland, K. I., W. G. Cioffi, and M. G. Sarr. *Practice of General Surgery*. Philadelphia: Saunders, 2001.

Braunwald, E., D. L. Longo, and J. L. Jameson. *Harrison's Principles of Internal Medicine,* 15th Edition. New York: McGraw-Hill, 2001.

KEY TERMS

Barium swallow—Barium is used to coat the throat to highlight the tissues lining the throat, allowing them to be visualized using x-ray pictures.

Computed tomography (CT or CAT) scan—Using x rays taken from many angles and computer modeling, CT scans help locate and estimate the size of tumors and provide information on whether they can be surgically removed.

Lymph nodes—Small, bean-shaped collections of tissue found in lymph vessels. They produce cells and proteins that fight infection and filter lymph. Nodes are sometimes called lymph glands.

Lymphatic system—Primary defense against infection in the body; the tissues, organs, and channels (similar to veins) that produce, store, and transport lymph and white blood cells to fight infection.

Magnetic resonance imaging (MRI)—Uses magnetic fields and computers to create detailed cross-sectional pictures of the interior of the body.

Malignant—Cancerous. Cells tend to reproduce without normal controls on growth and form tumors or invade other tissues.

Metastasize—Spread of cells from the original site of a cancer to other parts of the body where secondary tumors are formed.

Goldman, L., and J. C. Bennett. *Cecil Textbook of Medicine,* 21st Edition. Philadelphia: Saunders, 1999.

Schwartz, S. I., J. E. Fischer, F. C. Spencer, G. T. Shires, and J. M. Daly. *Principles of Surgery,* 7th edition. New York: McGraw Hill, 1998.

Townsend, C., K. L. Mattox, R. D. Beauchamp, B. M. Evers, and D. C. Sabiston. *Sabiston's Review of Surgery,* 3rd Edition. Philadelphia: Saunders, 2001.

PERIODICALS

Agrama, M. T., D. Reiter, M. F. Cunnane, A. Topham, and W. M. Keane. "Nodal Yield in Neck Dissection and the Likelihood of Metastases." *Otolaryngology Head and Neck Surgery* 128, no.2 (2003): 185–190.

Cmejrek, R. C., J. M. Coticchia, and J. E. Arnold. "Presentation, Diagnosis, and Management of Deep-neck Abscesses in Infants." *Archives of Otolaryngology Head and Neck Surgery* 128, no.12 (2002): 1361–1364.

Ferlito, A., et al. "Is the Standard Radical Neck Dissection No Longer Standard?" *Acta Otolaryngolica* 122, no.7 (2002): 792–795.

Kamasaki, N., H. Ikeda, Z. L. Wang, Y. Narimatsu, and T. Inokuchi. "Bilateral Chylothorax Following Radical Neck Dissection." *International Journal of Oral and Maxillofacial Surgery* 32, no.1 (2003): 91–93.

Myers, E. N., and B. R. Gastman. "Neck Dissection: An Operation in Evolution: Hayes Martin Lecture." *Archives of Otolaryngology Head And Neck Surgery* 129, no.1 (2003): 14–25.

Ohshima, A., et al. "Is a Bilateral Modified Radical Neck Dissection Beneficial for Patients with Papillary Thyroid Cancer?" *Surgery Today* 32, no.12 (2002): 1027–1030.

Wang, L. F., W. R. Kuo, C. S. Lin, K. W. Lee, and K. J. Huang. "Space Infection of the Head and Neck." *Kaohsiung Journal of Medical Sciences* 18, no.8 (2002): 386–392.

ORGANIZATIONS

American College of Surgeons. 633 North St. Clair Street, Chicago, IL 60611-32311. (312) 202-5000, Fax: (312) 202-5001. E-mail: postmaster@facs.org. http://www.facs.org.

American Academy of Otolaryngology—Head and Neck Surgery. One Prince St., Alexandria, VA 22314-3357. (703) 836-4444. http://www.entnet.org/index2.cfm.

American Cancer Society. 1599 Clifton Road NE, Atlanta, GA 30329. (800) 227-2345. http://www.cancer.org.

American Osteopathic College of Otolaryngology—Head and Neck Surgery. 405 W. Grand Avenue, Dayton, OH 45405. (937) 222-8820 or (800) 455-9404, Fax: (937) 222-8840. info@aocoohns.org.

OTHER

Amersham Health. [cited April 7, 2003] http://www.amershamhealth.com/medcyclopaedia/Volume%20VI%202/neck%20dissection.asp.

Baylor College of Medicine. [cited April 7, 2003] http://www.bcm.tmc.edu/oto/grand/120293.html.

Eastern Virginia Medical School. [cited April 7, 2003] http://www.voice-center.com.

Medical Algorithms Project. [cited April 7, 2003] http://www.medal.org/docs_ch37/doc_ch37.23.html.

Thyroid Cancer.Net. [cited April 7, 2003] http://www.thyroid-cancer.net/topics/what+is+a+neck+dissection?CMS_ Session=4ebe4755df4793bda647c0bf21fd977f.

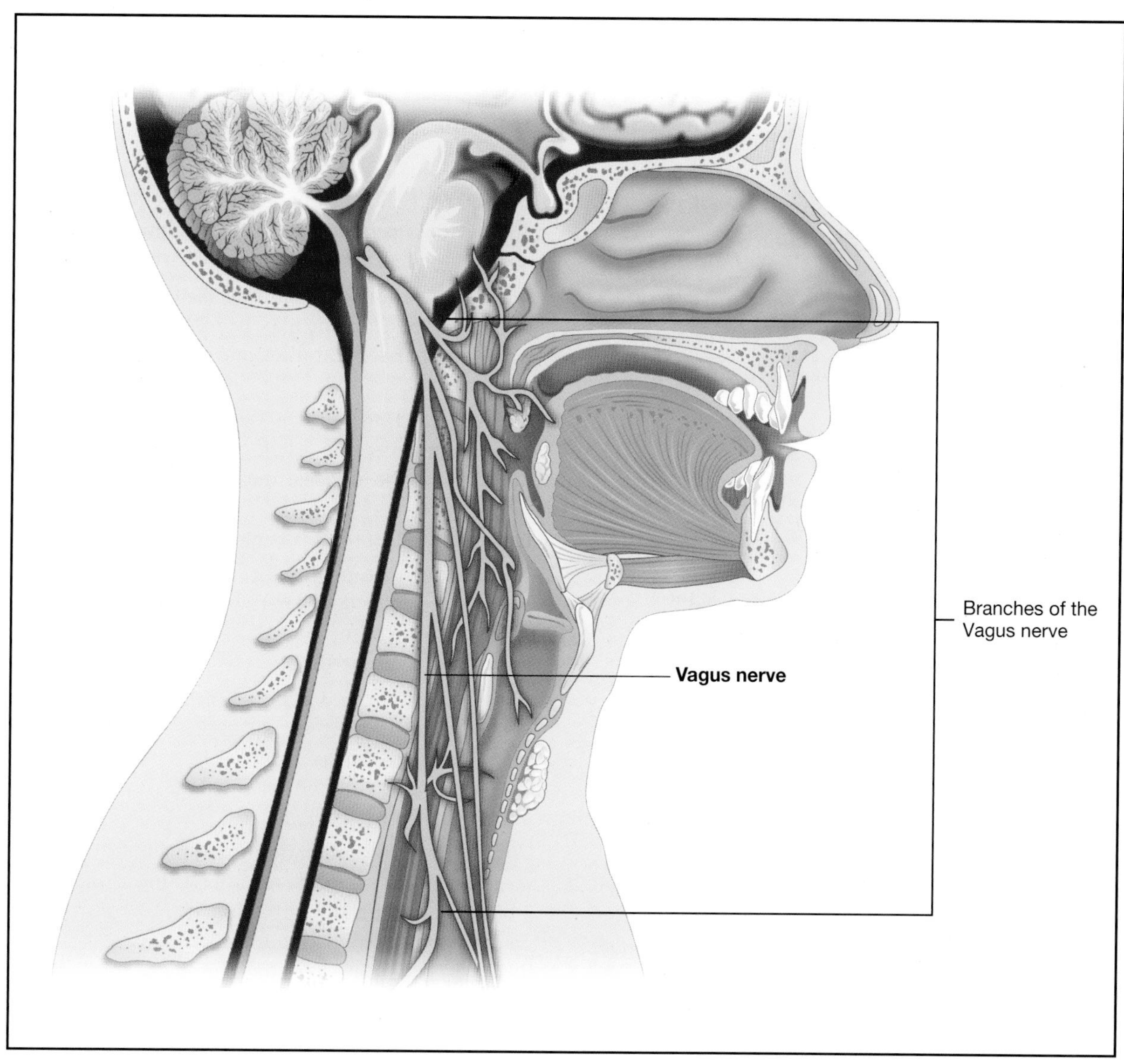

Branches of the vagus nerve. *(Illustration by Electronic Illustrators Group.)*

WHO PERFORMS THE PROCEDURE AND WHERE IS IT PERFORMED?

A radical neck dissection is usually performed by a surgeon with specialized training in otolaryngology, head and neck surgery. Occasionally, a general surgeon will perform a radical neck dissection. The procedure is performed in a hospital under general anesthesia.

University of Washington Department of Surgery. [cited April 7, 2003] <http://depts.washington.edu/soar/abstract/ab16.htm>.

L. Fleming Fallon, Jr, MD, DrPH

Radical prostatectomy *see* **Open prostatectomy**

Radioimmunoassay *see* **Immunoassay tests**

Reconstructive surgery *see* **Plastic, reconstructive, and cosmetic surgery**

QUESTIONS TO ASK THE DOCTOR

- What tests will be performed to determine if the cancer has spread?
- Which parts of the neck will be removed?
- How will a radical neck dissection affect daily activities after recovery?
- What is the likelihood that all of the cancer can be removed with a radical neck dissection?
- Are the involved lymph nodes on one or both sides of the neck?
- What will be the resulting appearance after surgery?
- How will my speech and breathing be affected?
- Is the surgeon board certified in otolaryngology head and neck surgery?
- How many radical neck procedures has the surgeon performed?
- What is the surgeon's complication rate?

Recovery at home

Definition

Recovery at home after surgery may require certain dietary and environmental restrictions, recommended rest and limitations to physical activities, and other required or restricted activities as recommended by a physician or surgeon.

Purpose

Postoperative recovery at home should promote physical healing and rest and recovery from the stress of surgery. For patients who undergo **orthopedic surgery**, the home recovery period will also involve rehabilitation to regain diminished musculoskeletal functioning. Emotional and psychological recovery from life-altering surgeries may also begin during the home recovery period.

Description

When patients are discharged from either an ambulatory surgical facility or a hospital, they will receive written instructions from their physician containing restrictions, requirements, and recommendations for their postoperative recovery at home. A nurse will usually review these instructions verbally with the patient and answer any questions and concerns. They may also call one or up to several days after a surgical discharge to follow up on how the patient is feeling and answer any questions about home recovery.

Restrictions and recommendations outlined in home recovery instructions may include:

- Driving restrictions. A patient may be prohibited from driving for a period of time due to functional limitations or to medication that impairs driving ability.
- Work restrictions. Depending on the nature of the patient's job, he or she may be required to stay home from work or request alternate duties until recovery is complete.
- Social restrictions. Patients at high risk of complications from infection, such as an organ transplant patient, may be advised to avoid anyone with a cold or flu and to stay away from crowds or social gatherings during the initial recovery period.
- Medication recommendations. Prescription and/or over the counter drugs may be recommended on an as-needed basis for pain and nausea. Other drugs may also be required.
- Dietary limitations. Certain types of gastrointestinal procedures and other surgeries may require a restricted diet during the recovery period. Alcohol may also be prohibited, particularly if pain medication has been prescribed.
- Ambulation recommendations. The doctor will note if the patient should refrain from lifting heavy objects, climbing stairs, having sex, or participating in other potentially strenuous activities.
- Exercise recommendations. If movement, stretches, or exercise is encouraged as part of recovery, that fact will also be noted.
- Incision care. Patients are instructed on how to care for their incision and educated on signs of infection (i.e., redness, warmth, swelling, fever, odor).
- Home care needs. Some patients may require a visiting nurse or live-in health aide for a period of time as they recover from surgery.
- Adaptive equipment. Assistive or adaptive devices such as crutches, a walker, prosthetics, or bed or bathroom hand rails may be necessary.
- Follow-up with physician. A patient may be instructed to call the doctor's office to schedule a follow-up appointment. The patient should also be given criteria for warning signs and symptoms that may occur with the procedure, and when to call the physician if the symptoms appear.
- Other required medical appointments. If a patient has undergone orthopedic surgery or another procedure that requires rehabilitation, he or she may need

KEY TERMS

Ambulation—To walk or move from place to place.

Ambulatory care—An outpatient facility; designed for patients who do not require inpatient hospital treatment or care.

Prosthetics—A custom-built artificial limb or other body part.

Orthopedic—Related to the musculoskeletal system, including the bones, joints, muscles, ligaments, and tendons.

to see a physical or occupational therapist to regain range of motion, strength, and mobility. Depending on the type of surgery performed, the expertise of other medical professionals may also be required.

The postoperative period is also a time of emotional healing. Patients who face a long recovery and rehabilitation may feel depressed or anxious about their situation. Providing a patient with realistic goals and expectations for recovery both before and after the surgery can help avoid feelings of failure or let down when things do not progress as quickly as the patient had hoped. Realistic recovery expectations can also prevent a patient from doing too much too early and potentially hindering the healing process.

Certain life-altering surgeries, such as an **amputation** or a **mastectomy**, carry their own set of emotional issues. Counseling, therapy, or participation in a patient support group may be an important part of postoperative recovery as a patient adjusts to the new post-surgical life.

Preparation

Discharge recommendations for home recovery are typically explained to the patient before he or she is allowed to leave the hospital or ambulatory care facility. In some cases, the patient may be required to sign paperwork indicating that he or she has both received and understood **home care** instructions.

Depending on the surgical procedure undergone, a patient may be taught some home care techniques while still in the hospital. Physical therapy exercises, **incision care**, and use of assistive devices such as crutches or splints are a few self-care skills that may be demonstrated and practiced in an inpatient environment.

A physical and emotional support system is a crucial part of a successful home recovery. Faced with restrictions to movement, driving, and possibly more, a patient needs someone at home to help with the daily tasks of independent living. If family or friends are not nearby or available, a visiting nurse or home healthcare aide should be hired before the patient is discharged to home recovery.

Normal results

Following home care instructions can help to speed a patient's recovery time and ensure the safe resumption of normal activities. In some cases, the familiar, comforting home environment may even speed the healing process or improve the degree of recovery. One study of patients 64 and older undergoing hip surgery found that patients who were allowed to undergo rehabilitation at home had significantly better outcomes than those who underwent rehabilitation as hospital inpatients. On average, the former had better physical capacity and independent living skills when assessed six months after surgery.

Some studies have also indicated that gender may have an impact on the success and speed of postoperative home recovery. Some studies have found that women recover more rapidly than men. However, animal and laboratory studies have found that progesterone and estrogen may be involved in the period immediately after surgery or injury. This would indicate that women may have a natural advantage in recovery. Scientists continue to study the recovery process to try to understand it and help patient recovery as quickly and completely as possible.

Resources

BOOKS

Brunicardi, F. Charles et al, eds. *Schwartz's Principles of Surgery*, 8th Ed. New York: McGraw-Hill, Health Pub. Division, 2005.

Hatfield, Anthea and Michael Tronson. *The Complete Recovery Room Book*, 3rd Ed. New York: Oxford University Press, 2002.

PERIODICALS

"Gym Workouts Ease Heart Patients Back Into Normal Life." *Nursing Standards* 21.30 (April 4, 2007): 10-11.

"Many Think the Worst Part of Recovering from Surgery is Getting Over the General Anaesthetic." *British Medical Journal* 328.7443 (April 3, 2004): 844-845.

Doering, Lynn V., Anthony W. McGuire and Darlene Rourke. "Recovering from Cardiac Surgery: What Patients Want You to Know." *American Journal of Critical Care* 11.4 (July 2002): 333-344.

ORGANIZATIONS

National Association for Home Care and Hospice. 228 Seventh Street SE, Washington, DC 20003. (202) 547-7424. http://www.nahc.org.

Visiting Nurses Association of America. 99 Summer Street, Suite 1700, Boston, Massachusetts 02110. (617) 737-3200. http://www.vnaa.org.

Paula Ford-Martin
Robert Bockstiegel

Recovery room

Definition

The recovery room, also called a post-anesthesia care unit (PACU), is a space a patient is taken to after surgery to safely regain consciousness from anesthesia and receive appropriate **postoperative care**.

Description

Patients who have had surgery or diagnostic procedures requiring anesthesia or sedation are taken to the recovery room, where their **vital signs** (e.g., pulse, blood pressure, temperature, blood oxygen levels) are monitored closely as the effects of anesthesia wear off. The patient may be disoriented when he or she regains consciousness, and the recovery room nursing staff will work to ease their anxiety and ensure their physical and emotional comfort.

The recovery room staff will pay particular attention to the patient's respiration, or breathing, as the patient recovers from anesthesia. A **pulse oximeter**, a clamp-like device that attaches to a patient's finger and uses infrared light to measure the oxygen saturation level of the blood, is usually used to assess respiratory stability. If the oxygen saturation level is too low, supplemental oxygen may be administered through a nasal cannula or face mask. Intravenous fluids are also frequently administered in the recovery room.

Because **general anesthesia** can cause a patient's core **body temperature** to drop several degrees, retaining body heat to prevent hypothermia and encourage good circulation is also an important part of recovery room care. Patients may be wrapped in blankets warmed in a heater or covered with a forced warm-air blanket system to bring body temperature back up to normal. They may also receive heated intravenous fluids.

The amount of time a patient requires in the recovery room will vary by surgical or diagnostic procedure and the type of anesthesia used. As the patient recovers from anesthesia, their postoperative condition is assessed by the recovery room nursing staff. A physician may order analgesic or antiemetic medication for any pain or nausea and vomiting, and the surgeon and/or anesthesiologist may come by to examine the patient.

KEY TERMS

Fast track—A protocol for postoperative patients with projected shorter recovery times. Fast-tracking a patient means that they will either bypass PACU completely, or spend a shorter time there with less intensive staff intervention and monitoring.

Hypothermia—Low core body temperature of 95°F (35°C) or less.

Nasal cannula—A piece of flexible plastic tubing with two small clamps that fit into the nostrils and provide supplemental oxygen flow.

Both hospitals and ambulatory surgical centers have recovery room facilities, which are generally located in close proximity to the **operating room**. A recovery room may be private, or it may be a large, partitioned space shared by many patients. Each patient bay, or space, is equipped with a variety of medical monitoring equipment. To keep the area sterile and prevent the spread of germs, outside visitors may be required to don a gown and cap or may be prohibited completely. Spouses or partners of women who are recovering after caesarean section and the parents of children recovering from surgery are typically excluded from any visitor prohibitions in the recovery room. In fact, parents are usually encouraged to be with their child in recovery to minimize any emotional trauma.

In some ambulatory surgery facilities, patients may have a different postoperative experience if they receive short-acting anesthetic drugs for their procedure. This protocol, known as "fast tracking," involves either shortening the time spent in the PACU or, if clinically indicated, bypassing the PACU altogether and sending the patient directly to what is known as a phase II step-down unit. A step-down unit is a transitional care area where patients can rest and recover before discharge with a lesser degree of monitoring and staff attention then in a PACU.

Normal results

After the effects of anesthesia have worn off completely and the patient's condition is considered stable, he or she will either be returned to their hospital room (for inpatient surgery) or discharged (for **outpatient surgery**). Patients who are discharged will be briefed on postoperative care instructions to follow at home before they are released.

Resources

BOOKS

Miller, R. D. *Miller's Anesthesia.* 6th ed. Philadelphia: Elsevier, 2005.

PERIODICALS

Kain, Z. N. "Family-centered preparation for surgery improves perioperative outcomes in children: a randomized controlled trial." *Anesthesiology* 106 (2007): 65.

ORGANIZATIONS

American Society of Anesthesiologists. 520 N. Northwest Highway Park Ridge, IL 60068-2573. (847) 825-5586. Fax: (847) 825-1692. http://www.asahq.org.

Paula Ford-Martin

Rectal artificial sphincter *see* **Artificial sphincter insertion**

Rectal prolapse repair

Definition

Rectal prolapse repair surgery treats a condition in which the rectum falls, or prolapses, from its normal anatomical position because of a weakening in the surrounding supporting tissues.

Purpose

A prolapse occurs when an organ falls or sinks out of its normal anatomical place. The pelvic organs normally have tissue (muscle, ligaments, etc.) holding them in place. Certain factors, however, may cause those tissues to weaken, leading to prolapse of the organs. The rectum is the last out of six divisions of the large intestine; the anus is the opening from the rectum through which stool exits the body. A complete rectal prolapse occurs when the rectum protrudes through the anus. If rectal prolapse is present, but the rectum does not protrude through the anus, it is called occult rectal prolapse, or rectal intussusception. In females, a rectocele occurs when the rectum protrudes into the posterior (back) wall of the vagina.

Factors that are linked to the development of rectal prolapse include age, repeated childbirth, constipation, ongoing physical activity, heavy lifting, prolapse of other pelvic organs, and prior **hysterectomy**. Symptoms of rectal prolapse include protrusion of the rectum during and after defecation, fecal incontinence (inadvertent leakage of feces with physical activity), constipation, and rectal bleeding. Women may experience a vaginal bulge, vaginal pressure or pain, painful sexual intercourse, and lower back pain.

> **KEY TERMS**
>
> **Perineum**—The area between the vagina and anus in females, and the scrotum and anus in males.

Demographics

The overall incidence of rectal prolapse in the United States is approximately 4.2 per 1,000 people. The incidence of the disorder increases to 10 per 1,000 among patients older than 65. Most patients with rectal prolapse are women; the ratio of male-to-female patients is one to six.

Description

Surgery is generally not performed unless the symptoms of the prolapse have begun to interfere with daily life. Because of the numerous defects that can cause rectal prolapse, there are more than 50 operations that may be used to treat the condition. A perineal or abdominal approach may be used. While abdominal surgery is associated with a higher rate of complications and a longer recovery time, the results are generally longer lasting. Perineal surgery is generally used for older patients who are unlikely to tolerate the abdominal procedure well.

Abdominal and laparoscopic approach

Rectopexy and anterior resection are the two most common abdominal surgeries used to treat rectal prolapse. The patient is usually placed under **general anesthesia** for the duration of surgery. During rectopexy, an incision into the abdomen is made, the rectum isolated from surrounding tissues, and the sides of the rectum lifted and fixed to the sacrum (lower backbone) with **stitches** or with a non-absorbable mesh. Anterior resection removes the S-shaped sigmoid colon (the portion of the large intestine just before the rectum); the two cut ends are then reattached. This straightens the lower portion of the colon and makes it easier for stool to pass. Rectopexy and anterior resection may also be performed in combination and may lead to a lower rate of prolapse recurrence.

As an alternative to the traditional laparotomy (large incision into the abdomen), laparoscopic surgery may be performed. **Laparoscopy** is a surgical procedure in which a laparoscope (a thin, lighted tube) and various instruments are inserted into the abdomen through small incisions. Rectopexy and anterior resection have been performed laparoscopically with good results. A patient's recovery time following laparoscopic surgery is shorter and less painful than following traditional abdominal surgery.

Perineal approach

Perineal repair of rectal prolapse involves a surgical approach around the anus and perineum. The patient may be placed under general or regional anesthesia for the duration of surgery.

The most common perineal repair procedures are the Altemeier and Delorme procedures. During the Altemeier procedure (also called a proctosigmoidectomy), the prolapsed portion of the rectum is resected (removed) and the cut ends reattached. The weakened structures supporting the rectum may be stitched into their anatomical position. The Delorme procedure involves the resection of only the mucosa (inner lining) of the prolapsed rectum. The exposed muscular layer is then folded and stitched up and the cut edges of mucosa stitched together.

A rarely used procedure is anal encirclement. Also called the Thiersch procedure, anal encirclement involves the insertion of a thin circular band of non-absorbable material under the skin of the anus. This narrows the anal opening and prevents the protrusion of the rectum through the opening. This procedure, however, does not address the underlying condition and therefore is generally reserved for patients who are not good candidates for more invasive surgery.

WHO PERFORMS THE PROCEDURE AND WHERE IS IT PERFORMED?

Rectal prolapse repair is usually performed in a hospital operating room. The surgery may be performed by a general surgeon, a colon and rectal surgeon (who focuses on diseases of the colon, rectum, and anus), or a gastrointestinal surgeon (who focuses on diseases of the gastrointestinal system).

Diagnosis/Preparation

Physical examination is most often used to diagnose rectal prolapse. The patient is asked to strain as if defecating; this increase in intra-abdominal pressure will maximize the degree of prolapse and aid in diagnosis. In some instances, imaging studies such as defecography (x rays taken during the process of defecation) may be administered to determine the extent of prolapse.

Before surgery, an intravenous (IV) line is placed so that fluid and/or medications may be easily administered to the patient. A Foley catheter will be placed to drain urine. **Antibiotics** are usually given to help prevent infection. The patient will be given a bowel prep to cleanse the colon and prepare it for surgery.

Aftercare

A Foley catheter may remain for one to two days after surgery. The patient will be given a liquid diet until normal bowel function returns. The recovery time following perineal repair is faster than recovery after abdominal surgery and usually involves a shorter hospital stay (one to three days following perineal surgery, three to seven days following abdominal surgery). The patient will be instructed to avoid activities for several weeks that will cause strain on the surgical site; these include lifting, coughing, long periods of standing, sneezing, straining with bowel movements, and sexual intercourse. High-fiber foods should be gradually added to the diet to avoid constipation and straining that could lead to prolapse recurrence.

Risks

Risks associated with rectal prolapse surgery include potential complications associated with anesthesia, infection, bleeding, injury to other pelvic structures, recurrent prolapse, and failure to correct the defect. Following a resection procedure, a leak may occur at the site where two cut ends of colon are reattached, requiring surgical repair.

Normal results

Most patients undergoing rectal prolapse repair will be able to return to normal activities, including work, within four to six weeks after surgery. The majority of patients will experience a significant improvement in symptoms and have a low chance of prolapse recurrence if heavy lifting and straining is avoided.

Morbidity and mortality rates

The approximate recurrence rates for the most commonly performed surgeries as reported by several studies are as follows:

- Altemeier procedure: 5–54%
- Delorme procedure: 5–26%
- anal encirclement: 25%
- rectopexy: 2–10%

QUESTIONS TO ASK THE DOCTOR

- What defect is causing the rectal prolapse?
- What surgical procedure is recommended for treatment?
- What are the risks and complications associated with the recommended procedure?
- Are any non-surgical treatment alternatives available?
- How soon after surgery may normal activities be resumed?

- anterior resection: 7–9%
- rectopexy with anterior resection: 0–4%

Abdominal surgeries are associated with a higher rate of complications than perineal repairs; rectopexy, for example, has a morbidity rate of 3–29%, and anterior resection a rate of 15–29%. The complication rate for combined rectopexy and anterior resection is slightly lower at 4–23%. Approximately 25% of patients undergoing anal encirclement will eventually require surgery to treat complications associated with the procedure.

Alternatives

There are currently no medical therapies available to treat rectal prolapse. In cases of mild prolapse where the rectum does not protrude through the anus, a high-fiber diet, stool softeners, enemas, or **laxatives** may help to avoid constipation, which may make the prolapse worse.

Resources

BOOKS

Feldman, Mark, et al. *Sleisenger & Fordtran's Gastrointestinal and Liver Disease,* 7th ed. Philadelphia: Elsevier Science, 2002.

Walsh, Patrick C., et al. *Campbell's Urology,* 8th ed. Philadelphia: Elsevier Science, 2002.

PERIODICALS

Felt-Bersma, Richelle J. F., and Miguel A. Cuesta. "Rectal Prolapse, Rectal Intussusception, Rectocele, and Solitary Rectal Ulcer Syndrome." *Gastroenterology Clinics* 30, no. 1 (March 1, 2001): 199–222.

ORGANIZATIONS

American Society of Colon and Rectal Surgeons. 85 W. Algonquin Rd., Suite 550, Arlington Heights, IL 60005. (847) 290-9184. http://www.fascrs.org.

OTHER

Flowers, Lynn K. "Rectal Prolapse." *eMedicine,* July 30, 2001. [cited April 9, 2003] http://www.emedicine.com/emerg/topic496.htm.

Poritz, Lisa S. "Rectal Prolapse." *eMedicine,* February 6, 2003. [cited April 9, 2003] http://www.emedicine.com/med/topic3533.htm.

Stephanie Dionne Sherk

Rectal resection

Definition

A rectal resection is the surgical removal of a portion of the rectum.

Purpose

Rectal resections repair damage to the rectum caused by diseases of the lower digestive tract, such as cancer, **diverticulitis**, and inflammatory bowel disease (ulcerative colitis and Crohn's disease). Injury, obstruction, and ischemia (compromised blood supply) may require rectal resection. Masses and scar tissue can grow within the rectum, causing blockages that prevent normal elimination of feces. Other diseases, such as diverticulitis and ulcerative colitis, can cause perforations in the rectum. Surgical removal of the damaged area can return normal rectal function.

Demographics

Colorectal cancer affects 140,000 people annually, causing 60,000 deaths. Incidence of the disease in 2001 differed among ethnic groups, with Hispanics having 10.2 cases per 100,000 people and African Americans having 22.8 cases per 100,000. Rectal cancer incidence is a portion of the total colorectal incidence rate. Surgery is the optimal treatment for rectal cancer, resulting in cure in 45% of patients. Recurrence due to surgical failure is low, from 4–8%, when the procedure is meticulously performed.

Crohn's disease and ulcerative colitis, both chronic inflammatory diseases of the colon, each affect approximately 500,000 young adults. Surgery is recommended when medication fails patients with ulcerative colitis. Nearly three-fourths of all Crohn's patients will require surgery to remove a diseased section of the intestine or rectum.

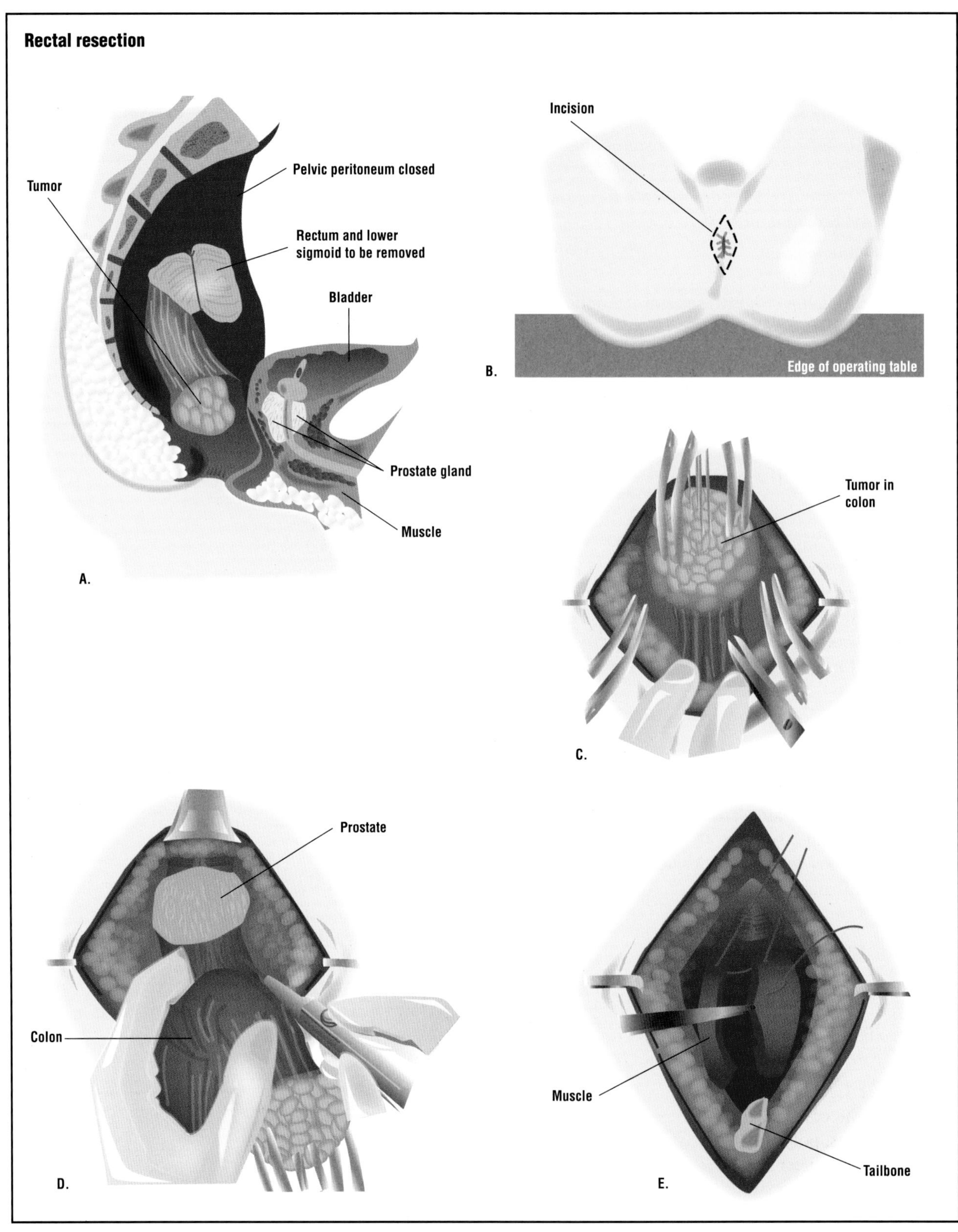

A tumor in the rectum or lower colon can be removed by a rectal resection (A). An incision is made around the patient's anus (B). The tumor is pulled down through the incision (C). An attached area of the colon is also removed (D). The area is repaired, leaving an opening for bowel functioning (E). *(Illustration by GGS Information Services. Cengage Learning, Gale.)*

KEY TERMS

Adjuvant therapy—Treatment used to increase the effectiveness of surgery, usually chemotherapy or radiation used to kill any cancer cells that might be remaining.

Anastomosis—The surgical connection of two sections of tubes, ducts, or vessels.

Diverticuli—Pouches in the intestinal wall usually created from a diet low in fiber.

Enema—Insertion of a tube into the rectum to infuse fluid into the bowel and encourage a bowel movement. Ordinary enemas contain tap water, mixtures of soap and water, glycerine and water, or other materials.

Intestine—Commonly called the bowels, divided into the small and large intestine. They extend from the stomach to the anus. The small intestine is about 20 ft (6 m) long. The large intestine is about 5 ft (1.5 m) long.

Ischemia—A compromise in blood supply delivered to body tissues that causes tissue damage or death.

Sigmoid colon—The last third of the intestinal tract that is attached to the rectum.

Description

During a rectal resection, the surgeon removes the diseased or perforated portion of the rectum. If the diseased or damaged section is not very large, the separated ends are reattached. Such a procedure is called rectal anastomosis.

Diagnosis/Preparation

Diagnostic tests

A number of tests identify masses and perforations within the intestinal tract.

- A lower GI (gastrointestinal) series is a series of x rays of the colon and rectum that can help identify ulcers, cysts, polyps, diverticuli (pouches in the intestine), and cancer. The patient is given a barium enema to coat the intestinal tract, making disease easier to see on the x rays.
- Flexible sigmoidoscopy involves insertion of a sigmoidoscope, a flexible tube with a miniature camera, into the rectum to examine the lining of the rectum and the sigmoid colon, the last third of the intestinal tract. The sigmoidoscope can also remove polyps or tissue for biopsy.
- A colonoscopy is similar to the flexible sigmoidoscopy, except the flexible tube examines the entire intestinal tract.
- Magnetic resonance imaging (MRI), used both prior to and during surgery, allows physicians to determine the precise margins for the resection, so that all of the diseased tissue can be removed. This also identifies patients who could most benefit from adjuvant therapy such as chemotherapy or radiation.

Preoperative preparation

To cleanse the bowel, the patient may be placed on a restricted diet for several days before surgery, then placed on a liquid diet the day before, with nothing by mouth after midnight. A series of enemas and/or oral preparations (GoLytely, Colyte, or senna) may be ordered to empty the bowel. Oral anti-infectives (neomycin, erythromycin, or kanamycin sulfate) may be ordered to decrease bacteria in the intestine and help prevent post-operative infection. The operation can be done with an abdominal incision (laparotomy) or using minimally invasive techniques with small tubes to allow insertion of the operating instruments (**laparoscopy**).

Aftercare

Postoperative care involves monitoring blood pressure, pulse, respiration, and temperature. Breathing tends to be shallow because of the effect of the anesthesia and the patient's reluctance to breathe deeply due to discomfort around the surgical incision. The patient is taught how to support the incision during deep breathing and coughing, and given pain medication as necessary. Fluid intake and output is measured, and the wound is observed for color and drainage.

Fluids and electrolytes are given intravenously until the patient's diet can be resumed, starting with liquids, then adding solids. The patient is helped out of bed the evening of the surgery and allowed to sit in a chair. Most patients are discharged in two to four days.

Risks

Rectal resection has potential risks similar those of other major surgeries. Complications usually occur while the patient is in the hospital and the patient's general health prior to surgery will be an indication of the risk potential. Patients with heart problems and stressed immune systems are of special concern. Both

WHO PERFORMS THE PROCEDURE AND WHERE IS IT PERFORMED?

Rectal resections are performed by general surgeons and colorectal surgeons as in-patient surgeries under general anesthesia.

during and following the procedure, the physician and nursing staff will monitor the patient for:

- excessive bleeding
- wound infection
- thrombophlebitis (inflammation and blood clot in the veins in the legs
- pneumonia
- pulmonary embolism (blood clot or air bubble in the lungs' blood supply)
- cardiac stress due to allergic reaction to the general anaesthetic

Symptoms that the patient should report, especially after discharge, include:

- increased pain, swelling, redness, drainage, or bleeding in the surgical area
- flu-like symptoms such as headache, muscle aches, dizziness, or fever
- increased abdominal pain or swelling, constipation, nausea or vomiting, or black, tarry stools

Normal results

Complete healing is expected without complications. The recovery rate varies, depending on the patient's overall health prior to surgery. Typically, full recovery takes six to eight weeks.

Morbidity and mortality rates

Mortality has decreased from nearly 28% to under 6%, through the use of prophylactic **antibiotics** before and after surgery.

Alternatives

If the section of the rectum to be removed is very large, the rectum may not be able to be reattached. Under those circumstances, a **colostomy** would be preformed. The distal end of the rectum would be closed and left to atrophy. The proximal end would be brought through an opening in the abdomen to create an opening, a stoma, for feces to be removed from the body.

QUESTIONS TO ASK THE DOCTOR

- Am I a good candidate for laparoscopic surgery?
- What kinds of preoperative tests will be required?
- What medications will be given for pain relief after the surgery?
- What will I need to do to prepare for surgery?
- What will my recovery time be and what restrictions will I have?

Resources

BOOKS

Johnston, Lorraine. *Colon & Rectal Cancer: A Comprehensive Guide for Patients and Families.* Sebastopol, CA: O'Reilly, 2000.

Levin, Bernard. *American Cancer Society Colorectal Cancer.* New York: Villard, 1999.

PERIODICALS

Beets-Tan, R. G. H., et al. "Accuracy of Maganetic Resonance Imaging in Prediction of Tumour-free Resection Margin in Rectal Cancer Surgery." *The Lancet* 357 (February 17, 2001): 497.

Walling, Anne D. "Follow-up After Resection for Colorectal Cancer Saves Lives. (Tips from Other Journals)." *American Family Physician* 66 (August 1, 2002): 485.

ORGANIZATIONS

American Board of Colon and Rectal Surgery (ABCRS). 20600 Eureka Road, Suite 713, Taylor, MI 48180. (734) 282-9400. http://www.fascrs.org.

Mayo Clinic. 200 First St. S.W., Rochester, MN 55905. (507) 284-2511. http://www.mayoclinic.org.

Janie Franz

Red blood cell indices

Definition

Red blood cell (RBC) indices are calculations derived from the **complete blood count** that aid in the diagnosis and classification of anemia.

Purpose

Red blood cell indices help classify types of anemia, a decrease in the oxygen carrying capacity of the blood. Healthy people have an adequate number of correctly sized red blood cells containing enough hemoglobin to carry sufficient oxygen to all the body's tissues. Anemia is diagnosed when either the hemoglobin or **hematocrit** of a blood sample is too low.

Description

Measurements needed to calculate RBC indices are the red blood cell count, hemoglobin, and hematocrit. The hematocrit is the percentage of blood by volume that is occupied by the red cells. The three main RBC indices are:

- Mean corpuscular volume (MCV). The average size of the red blood cells expressed in femtoliters (fl). MCV is calculated by dividing the hematocrit (as percent) by the RBC count in millions per microliter of blood, then multiplying by 10.
- Mean corpuscular hemoglobin (MCH). The average amount of hemoglobin inside an RBC expressed in picograms (pg). The MCH is calculated by dividing the hemoglobin concentration in grams per deciliter by the RBC count in millions per microliter, then multiplying by 10.
- Mean corpuscular hemoglobin concentration (MCHC). The average concentration of hemoglobin in the RBCs expressed as a percent. It is calculated by dividing the hemoglobin in grams per deciliter by the hematocrit, then multiplying by 100.

The mechanisms by which anemia occurs will alter the RBC indices in a predictable manner. Therefore, the RBC indices permit the physician to narrow down the possible causes of an anemia. The MCV is an index of the size of the RBCs. When the MCV is below normal, the RBCs will be smaller than normal and are described as microcytic. When the MCV is elevated, the RBCs will be larger than normal and are termed macrocytic. RBCs of normal size are termed normocytic.

Failure to produce hemoglobin results in smaller than normal cells. This occurs in many diseases, including iron deficiency anemia, thalassemia (an inherited disease in which globin chain production is deficient), and anemias associated with chronic infection or disease. Macrocytic cells occur when division of RBC precursor cells in the bone marrow is impaired. The most common causes of macrocytic anemia are vitamin B_{12} deficiency, folate deficiency, and liver disease. Normocytic anemia may be caused by decreased production (e.g. malignancy and other causes of bone marrow failure), increased destruction (hemolytic anemia), or blood loss. The RBC count is low, but the size and amount of hemoglobin in the cells are normal.

KEY TERMS

Anemia—A variety of conditions in which a person's blood cannot carry as much oxygen as is needed by the tissues.

Hypochromic—A descriptive term applied to a red blood cell with a decreased concentration of hemoglobin.

Macrocytic—A descriptive term applied to a larger than normal red blood cell.

Mean corpuscular hemoglobin (MCH)—A calculation of the average weight of hemoglobin in a red blood cell.

Mean corpuscular hemoglobin concentration (MCHC)—A calculation of the average concentration of hemoglobin in a red blood cell.

Mean corpuscular volume (MCV)—A measure of the average volume of a red blood cell.

Microcytic—A descriptive term applied to a smaller than normal red blood cell.

Normochromic—A descriptive term applied to a red blood cell with a normal concentration of hemoglobin.

Normocytic—A descriptive term applied to a red blood cell of normal size.

Red cell distribution width (RDW)—A measure of the variation in the size of red blood cells.

A low MCH indicates that cells have too little hemoglobin. This is caused by deficient hemoglobin production. Such cells will be pale when examined under the microscope and are termed hypochromic. Iron deficiency is the most common cause of a hypochromic anemia. The MCH is usually elevated in macrocytic anemias associated with vitamin B_{12} and folate deficiency.

The MCHC is the ratio of hemoglobin mass in the RBC to cell volume. Cells with too little hemoglobin are lighter in color and have a low MCHC. The MCHC is low in microcytic, hypochromic anemias such as iron deficiency, but is usually normal in macrocytic anemias. The MCHC is elevated in hereditary spherocytosis, a condition with decreased RBC survival caused by a structural protein defect in the RBC membrane.

Cell indices are usually calculated from tests performed on an automated electronic cell counter. However, these counters measure the MCV, which is directly proportional to the voltage pulse produced as each cell passes through the counting aperture. Electronic cell counters calculate the MCH, MCHC, hematocrit, and an additional parameter called the red cell distribution width (RDW).

The RDW is a measure of the variance in red blood cell size. It is calculated by dividing the standard deviation (a measure of variation) of RBC volume by the MCV and multiplying by 100. A large RDW indicates abnormal variation in cell size, termed anisocytosis. The RDW aids in differentiating anemias that have similar indices. For example, thalassemia minor and iron deficiency anemia are both microcytic and hypochromic anemias, and overlap in MCV and MCH. However, iron deficiency anemia has an abnormally wide RDW, but thalassemia minor does not.

Diagnosis/Preparation

RBC indices require 3–5 mL of blood collected by vein puncture with a needle. A nurse or phlebotomist usually collects the sample.

Aftercare

Discomfort or bruising may occur at the puncture site. Pressure to the puncture site until the bleeding stops reduces bruising; warm packs relieve discomfort. Some people feel dizzy or faint after blood has been drawn and should be allowed to lie down and relax until they are stable.

Risks

Other than potential bruising at the puncture site, and/or dizziness, there are no complications associated with this test. However, certain prescription medications may affect the test results. These drugs include zidovudine (Retrovir), phenytoin (Dilantin), and azathioprine (Imuran). When the hematocrit is determined by centrifugation, the MCV and MCHC may differ from those derived by an electronic cell counter, especially in anemia. Plasma trapped between the RBCs tends to cause an increase in the hematocrit, giving rise to a somewhat higher MCV and lower MCHC.

Normal results

Normal results for red blood cell indices are as follows:

- MCV: 80–96 fl
- MCH: 27–33 pg
- MCHC: 33–36%
- RDW: 12–15%

Resources

BOOKS

Hoffman, R. et al. *Hematology: Basic Principles and Practice*. 4th ed. Philadelphia: Elsevier, 2005.

McPherson, R. A. et al. *Henry's Clinical Diagnosis and Management by Laboratory Methods*. 21st ed. Philadelphia: Saunders, 2007.

OTHER

National Institutes of Health [cited April 5, 2003]. http://www.nlm.nih.gov/medlineplus/encyclopedia.html.

Victoria E. DeMoranville
Robert Harr
Mark A. Best
Rosalyn Carson-DeWitt, MD

Red blood cell test *see* **Hemoglobin test**
Regional anesthetic *see* **Anesthesia, local**
Remote surgery *see* **Telesurgery**
Renal transplant *see* **Kidney transplantation**

Reoperation

Definition

Reoperation is a term used by surgeons for the duplication of a surgical procedure. Repeating surgery may involve surgery at the same site, at another site for the same condition, or to repair a structure that was treated in a previous surgery.

Purpose

Success for most surgical procedures depends, is large part, upon the lack of a need to repeat the surgery. However, failure of some feature of a procedure may be only one of many reasons that reoperation is necessary. Reasons for repeat surgery depend upon surgical skills, as well as the reason for the primary surgery. Some diseases and conditions necessitate or make probable repeating the operation.

Cancer

Surgeries for cancer are sometimes repeated because a new tumor or more surrounding tissue has been affected by the original malignancy. This is often the case with breast surgery for cancer that involves breast conservation management. Often it is necessary to re-excise the site of the previously biopsied primary cancer. In the case of breast cancer, only 50% of re-excision specimens show residual tumor. If cancer cell

KEY TERMS

Reoperation—The repeat of a surgical procedure required for a variety of reasons, from surgical failure, replacement of failed component parts, or treatment of progressive disease.

Surgical revision—The failure of a procedure, which requires surgery be performed to improve the result.

are found with the re-excision, this may change the treatment protocol. Colon cancer sometimes involves more surgeries to resect newly affected areas beyond the previous primary site.

Coronary artery surgery

Currently, about 10% of coronary artery procedures are reoperations due to the progression of the disease into native vessels between operations, as well as to treat diseased vein grafts. The mortality associated with reoperation is significantly higher than that of the original bypass procedures. In one study, patients undergoing their first coronary artery bypass graft (CABG) had a mortality rate of 1.7% versus 5.2% for elective reoperation.

Orthropedic surgeries

Arthroplasty—the operative restoration of a joint like the elbow, knee, hip, or shoulder, often involves components that need repair. Infections of the joint may also require reoperation with the complete removal of all prostheses and cement. Re-implantation is repeated after a six-week course of **antibiotics**. Other bone surgeries that have a high reoperation rate are back surgeries, including spinal surgeries involving discectomy in which discs are fused together to reduce pain. Due to scarring or infection, there may be a need for reoperation. As the frequency of repeat back surgeries increases, the chance of a satisfactory result drops precipitously.

Gastrointestinal surgeries

Crohn's disease surgeries are often repeated. Operations that cut and stitch only the area of obstruction, called strictureplasty, often have repeat operations if the affected area is the small intestine. Another gastrointestinal surgery that often requires reoperation is fundoplication or flap wrapping of the lower part of the esophagus to prevent the reflux of acid from the stomach back into the esophagus. Folding the loose valve above the stomach in such a way as to tighten its ability to close treats the condition known as gastroesophageal reflux disease (GERD). The surgery has a high failure rate of between 30% after five years and 63% after 10 years. Reoperation may be required because of surgical failure, breakdown of tissue, injury to nearby organs, or an excessively wrapped fundus that leads to trouble swallowing.

Vasectomy and penile prostheses

These surgeries often have complications that lead to reoperation, largely due to surgical failure.

Normal results

In general, reoperation is more difficult and involves more risks that the original procedure. It requires more operative time; more blood is lost; and the incidences of infection and clots are higher. Advancements in design and improvements in cementing techniques for component failure in **arthroplasty** have improved the results of reoperation.

Resources

BOOKS

Khatri, VP and JA Asensio. *Operative Surgery Manual.* 1st ed. Philadelphia: Saunders, 2003.

Townsend, CM et al. *Sabiston Textbook of Surgery.* 17th ed. Philadelphia: Saunders, 2004.

OTHER

"Inflammatory Bowel Disease (Crohn's Disease and Ulcerative Colitis)." MDConsult. http://www.MDConsult.com.

"Gastroesophageal Reflux Disease and Heartburn." MDConsult. http://www.MDConsult.com.

"Vasectomy and Vasovasotomy: Comprehensive Version." MDConsult. http://www.MDConsult.com.

Nancy McKenzie, Ph.D.

Replantation of digits *see* **Finger reattachment**

Replantation, tooth *see* **Tooth replantation**

Retinal cryopexy

Definition

Retinal cryopexy, also called retinal **cryotherapy**, is a procedure that uses intense cold to induce a chorioretinal scar and to destroy retinal or choroidal tissue.

Purpose

The retina is the very thin membrane in the back of the eye that acts like the "film" in a camera. It is held against the inside back portion of the eye by pressure from fluid within the eye. In the front part of the eye, the retina is firmly attached at a ring just behind the lens called the pars plana. In the back part of the eye, the retina is continuous with the optic nerve. In between the pars plana and the optic nerve the retina has no fixed attachments. The retina collects information from the images projected on it from the eye lens and sends it along the optic nerve to the brain, where the information is interpreted and experienced as sight.

Several disorders can affect the retina and retinal cryopexy is used to treat the following conditions:

- retinal breaks or detachments
- retinal ischemia (retinal tissue that lacks oxygen)
- neovascularization (proliferation of blood vessels in the retina)
- Coats' disease (abnormal retinal blood vessels that cause loss of vision)
- retinoblastoma (intraocular tumors)

Demographics

Disease and disorders affecting the retina cause the majority of the visual disability and blindness in the United States. Retinal detachment occurs in one in 10,000 Americans each year, with middle-aged and older individuals being at higher risk than the younger population. Coats' disease usually affects children, especially boys, in the first 10 years of life, but it can also affect young adults. The condition affects central vision, typically in only one eye. Severity can range from mild vision loss to total retinal detachment and blindness. No cause has yet been identified for Coats' disease. According to the National Cancer Institute, retinoblastoma accounts for approximately 11% of cancers developing in the first year of life, and for 3% of the cancers developing among children younger than 15 years. In the United States, approximately 300 children and adolecents below the age of 20 are diagnosed with retinoblastoma each year. The majority of cases occur among young children, with 63% of all retinoblastoma occurring before the age of two years.

Description

Usually, retinal cryopexy is administered under **local anesthesia**. The procedure involves placing a metal probe against the eye. When a foot pedal is depressed, the tip of the cryopexy probe becomes very cold as a result of the rapid expansion of very cold gases (usually nitrous oxide) within the probe tip. When the probe is placed on the eye, the formation of water crystals followed by rapid thawing results in tissue destruction. This is followed by healing and scar tissue formation.

In the case of retinal detachment, treatment calls for irritating the tissue around each of the retinal tears. Cryopexy stimulates scar formation, sealing the edges of the tear. This is typically done by looking into the eye using the indirect ophthalmoscope while pushing gently on the outside of the eye using the cryopexy probe, producing a small area of freezing that involves the retina and the tissues immediately underneath it. Using multiple small freezes like this, each of the tears is surrounded. Irritated tissue forms a scar, which brings the retina back into contact with the tissue underneath it.

KEY TERMS

Chorioretinal—Relating to the choroid coat of the eye and retina.

Choroid—Middle layer of the eye, between the retina and sclera.

Coats' disease—Also called exudative retinitis, a chronic abnormality characterized by the deposition of cholesterol on the outer retinal layers.

Ophthalmoscope—An instrument for viewing the interior of the eye, particularly the retina. Light is thrown into the eye by a mirror (usually concave) and the interior is then examined with or without the aid of a lens.

Retina—Light-sensitive layer of the eye.

Retinoblastoma—Malignant tumor of the retina.

Sclera—The tough white outer coat of the eyeball.

Diagnosis/Preparation

The earlier the retinal disorder diagnosis is confirmed, the greater the chance of successful outcome. Diagnosis is based on symptoms and a thorough examination of the retina. An ophthalmoscope is used to examine the retina. This is a small, hand-held instrument consisting of a battery-powered light and a series of lenses that is held up to the eye. The ophthalmologist is able to see the retina and check for abnormalities by shining the light into the eye and looking through the lens. Eye drops are placed in the eyes to dilate the pupils and help visualization. Afterward, an indirect ophthalmoscope is used. This instrument is worn on the specialist's head, and a lens is held in front of the patient's eye. It allows a better view of the retina. Examination with a slit lamp microscope may also be done. This microscope enables the ophthalmologist to examine the different parts of the eye under magnification. After instilling drops to dilate the pupil, the slit lamp is used to detect retinal tears and detachment. A visual acuity test is also usually performed to assess vision loss. This test involves reading letters from a standard eye chart.

Additional diagnostic procedures are used in the case of Coats' disease and retinoblastoma. Ultrasonography helps in differentiating Coats' disease from retinoblastoma. CT scan may be used to characterize the intraocular features of Coats' disease. MRI is another very useful diagnostic tool used to distinguish retinoblastoma from Coats' disease.

Aftercare

After the procedure, patients are taken to a **recovery room**, and observed for 30–60 minutes. Tylenol or pain medication is usually given. Healing typically takes 10–14 days. Vision may be blurred briefly, and the operated eye is usually red and swollen for some time following cryopexy. Cold compresses applied to the eyelids relieve some of the discomfort. Most patients are able to walk the day after surgery and are discharged from the hospital within a week. After discharge, patients are advised to gently cleanse their eyelids every morning, and as necessary, using warm tap water and cotton balls or tissues. Day surgery patients are usually allowed to go home two hours after the surgery is complete.

Risks

Risks involved in retinal cryopexy include infection, perforation of the eye with the anesthetic needle, bleeding, double vision, and glaucoma. All of these complications however, are quite uncommon.

Normal results

If treated early, the outcome of cryopexy for Coats' disease may be successful in preventing progression and in some cases can improve vision, but this is less effective if the retina has completely detached. For retinal reattachments, the retina can be repaired in about 90% of cases. Early treatment almost always improves the vision of most patients with retinal detachment. Some patients, however, require more than one cryopexy procedure to repair the damage.

WHO PERFORMS THE PROCEDURE AND WHERE IS IT PERFORMED?

Retinal cryopexy is performed in the treating physician's office or in a hospital setting depending on the condition motivating the surgery. The physician is usually an ophtalmologist, specialized in the treatment of retinal disorders. An ophthalmologist is a physician who specializes in the medical and surgical care of the eyes and visual system and in the prevention of eye disease and injury. He has completed four or more years of college premedical education, four or more years of medical school, one year of internship, and three or more years of specialized medical and surgical and refractive training and experience in eye care.

Morbidity and mortality rates

Survival rates for children with retinoblastoma are favorable, with more than 93% alive five years after diagnosis. Males and females have similar five-year survival rates for the period 1976–1994, namely 93 and 94% respectively. African American children had slightly lower survival rates (86%) than Caucasian children (94%).

Alternatives

Several alternatives to retinal cryopexy are available, depending on the condition being treated. A few examples include:

- Laser photocoagulation. This type of surgery induces a therapeutic effect by destroying outer retinal tissue, thus reducing the oxygen requirements of the retina, and increasing oxygen delivery to the remaining retina through alterations in oxygen diffusion from the choroid. It is used for repairing retinal tears.
- Pneumatic retinopexy. This procedure is used to reattach retinas. After numbing the eye with a local anesthesia, the surgeon injects a small gas bubble into the inside of the eye. The bubble presses against the retina, flattening it against the back wall of the eye. Since the gas rises, this treatment is most effective for detachments located in the upper portion of the eye.
- Scleral buckle. With this technique, a tiny sponge or silicone band is attached to the outside of the eye, pressing inward and holding the retina in position. After removing the vitreous gel from the eye

QUESTIONS TO ASK THE DOCTOR

- How is retinal cryopexy performed?
- Why is the surgery required?
- Will my vision improve?
- What are the risks of retinal cryopexy?
- Is the procedure painful?
- How long will it take to recover from the surgery?
- How much retinal cryopexies do you perform each year?

(vitrectomy), the surgeon seals a few areas of the retina into position with laser or cryotherapy.

- Radiation therapy. For neuroblastomas, this treatment uses high-energy radiation to kill or shrink cancer cells.
- Chemotherapy. Another alternative for neuroblastoma. Chemotherapy uses drugs to kill cancer cells. The drugs are delivered through the bloodstream, and spread throughout the body to the cancer site.

Resources

BOOKS

Packer, A. J., ed. *Manual of Retinal Surgery*. Boston: Butterworth-Heinemann, 2001.

Schepens, C. L., M. E. Hartnett, and T. Hirose, eds. *Schepens's Retinal Detachment and Allied Diseases*. Boston: Butterworth-Heinemann, 2000.

Wong, D., and A. H. Chignell. *Management of Vitreo-Retinal Disease: A Surgical Approach*. New York: Springer Verlag, 1999.

PERIODICALS

Anagnoste, S. R., I. U. Scott, T. G. Murray, D. Kramer, and S. Toledano. "Rhegmatogenous retinal detachment in retinoblastoma patients undergoing chemoreduction and cryotherapy." *American Journal of Ophthalmology* 129 (June 2000): 817–819.

Palner, E. A., et al. "Cryotherapy for Retinopathy of Prematurity Cooperative Group. Multicenter trial of cryotherapy for retinopathy of prematurity: ophthalmological outcomes at 10 years." *Archives of Ophthalmology* 119 (2001): 1110–1118.

Steel, D. H., J. West, and W. G. Campbell. "A randomized controlled study of the use of transscleral diode laser and cryotherapy in the management of rhegmatogenous retinal detachment." *Retina* 20 (2000): 346–357.

Veckeneer, M., K. Van Overdam, D. Bouwens, E. Feron, D. Mertens, et al. "Randomized clinical trial of cryotherapy versus laser photocoagulation for retinopexy in conventional retinal detachment surgery." *American Journal of Ophthalmology* 132 (September 2001): 343–347.

ORGANIZATIONS

American Academy of Ophthalmology. P.O. Box 7424, San Francisco, CA 94120-7424. (415) 561-8500. http://www.aao.org/index.html.

New England Ophthalmological Society (NEOS). P.O. Box 9165, Boston, MA 02114. (617) 227-6484. http://www.neos-eyes.org/.

OTHER

University Ophthalmology Consultants. "What is cryotherapy?" http://www.umdnj.edu/eyeweb/faqs/cryo.html.

Monique Laberge, Ph.D.

Retinal detachment surgery *see* **Scleral buckling**

Retropubic suspension

Definition

Retropubic suspension refers to the surgical procedures used to correct incontinence by supporting and stabilizing the bladder and urethra. The Burch procedure, also known as retropubic urethropexy procedure or Burch colosuspension, and Marshall-Marchetti-Krantz procedure (MMK) are the two primary surgeries for treating stress incontinence. The major difference between these procedures is the method for supporting the bladder. The Burch procedure uses sutures to attach the urethra and bladder to muscle tissue in the pelvic area. MMK uses sutures to attach these organs to the pelvic cartilage. Laparoscopic retropubic surgery can be performed with a video laparoscope through small incisions in the belly button and above the pubic hairline.

Purpose

The urinary system expels a quart and a half of urine per day. The amount of urine produced depends upon diet and medications taken, as well as **exercise** and loss of water due to sweating. The ureters, two tubes connecting the kidneys and the bladder, pass urine almost continually and when the bladder is full the brain sends a signal to the bladder to relax and let urine pass from the bladder to the urethra. People who are continent control the release of urine from the urethra via the sphincter muscles. These two sets of muscles act like rubber bands to keep the bladder closed until a conscious decision is made to urinate. The intrinsic sphincter or urethral sphincter muscles

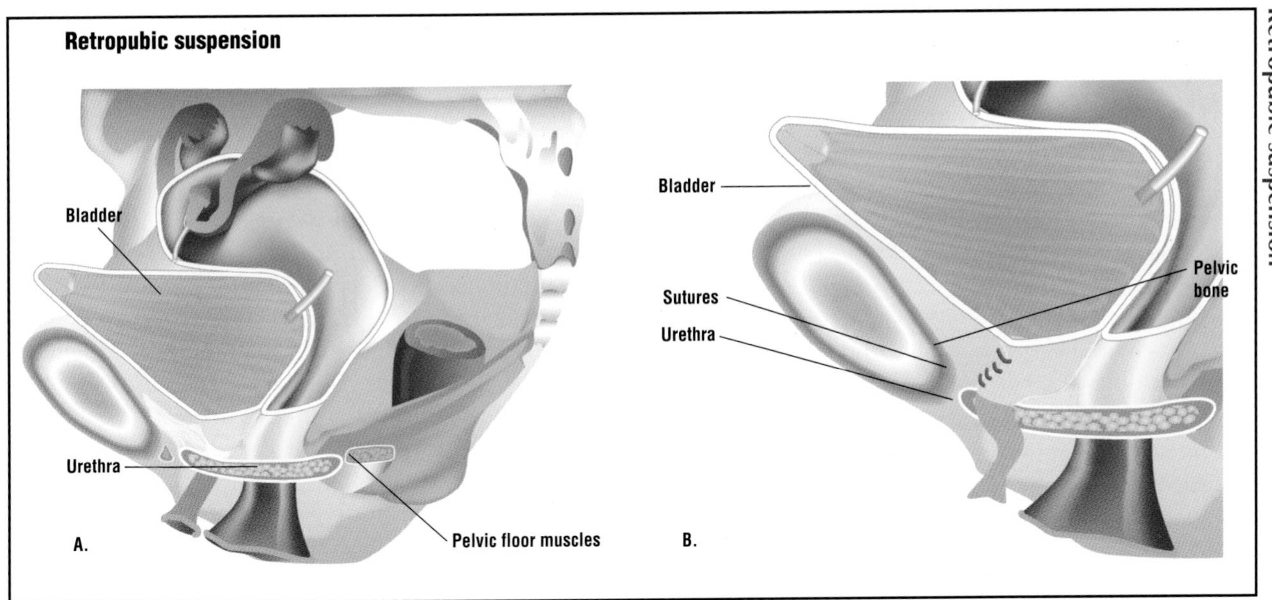

Weak pelvic floor muscles (A) can cause stress incontinence. In a retropubic suspension, the neck of the bladder is elevated and stitched to the pubic bone to hold it in place (B). *(Illustration by GGS Information Services. Cengage Learning, Gale.)*

keep the bladder closed and the extrinsic sphincter muscles surround the urethra and prevent leakage. Incontinence is common when either the urethra lacks tautness and stability (genuine stress urine incontinence, SUI) and/or the sphincter muscles are unable to keep the bladder closed (intrinsic sphincter deficiency, ISD).

Incontinence occurs in many forms with four primary types related to anatomic, neurological, and dietary causes; or disease and injury.

Stress incontinence

The most frequent form of incontinence is stress incontinence. This relates to leakage of the urethra with activity that puts stress on the abdominal muscles. The primary sign of stress incontinence is this leakage at sneezing, coughing, exercise, or other straining activities, which indicates a lack of support for the urethra due to weakened muscles, fascia, or ligaments. Pressure from the abdomen with movement, like exercising, uncompensated by tautness or stability in the urethra, causes the urethra to be displaced or mobile leading to leakage. Essentially, this hypermobility of the urethra is an indication that it is moving down or herniating through weakened pelvic structures.

To diagnose incontinence and determine treatment, three grades of severity for stress incontinence are used.

- Type I: Moderate movement of the urethra, with no hernia or cystocele.
- Type II: Severe or hypermobility in the urethra of more than 0.8 in (2 cm), with or without decent of the urethra into pelvic structures.
- Type III: Hypermobility of the urethra where the primary source of incontinence is the inability of the sphincter muscles to keep the bladder closed. This is due to weakness or deficiency in the intrinsic sphincter muscles.

Urge incontinence

Urge incontinence relates to the frequent need to urinate and may involve going to the bathroom every two hours. Accidents are common when not reaching a bathroom in time. Urge incontinence is not due to general changes in the urethra or supporting muscles. It is often linked to other disorders that produce muscle spasms in the bladder, such as infections. Urge incontinence can also be due to underlying illnesses like stroke, spinal cord injury, multiple sclerosis and Alzheimer's disease, which cause detrusor hyperflexia—the contracting of the bladder muscle responsible for sending urine from the bladder to the urethra. Urge incontinence is very common in the elderly, especially those in long term care facilities.

Mixed incontinence

Mixed incontinence is a combination of stress incontinence and urge incontinence, especially in older women. Since each form of incontinence pertains to different

KEY TERMS

Genuine urinary stress incontinence (USI)—Stress incontinence due to hypermobility of the urethra.

Intrinsic sphincter deficiency (ISD)—A factor in severe stress incontinence due to the inadequacy of the sphincter muscles to keep the bladder closed.

Retropubic urethropexy—A generic term for the Burch procedure and its variants that treat mild stress incontinence by stabilizing the urethra with retropubic surgery.

Stress incontinence—Leakage of urine upon movements that put pressure on the abdominal muscles such as coughing, sneezing, laughing, or exercise. One of four types of incontinence.

Urethra hypermobility—Main factor in stress urinary incontinence, with severity based upon how far the urethra has descended into the pelvic floor through herniation or cystocele.

functions or anatomy, it is very important to distinguish which part of the incontinence is to be treated by surgery.

Overflow incontinence

Overflow incontinence results in leakage from a bladder that never completely empties due to weakened bladder muscles. Overflow incontinence is involuntary and not accompanied by the urge to urinate. Many causes exist for overflow incontinence, including weak bladder muscles due to diabetes, nerve damage, or a blocked urethra. Men are more frequently affected than women.

Demographics

Over 15 million Americans have urinary incontinence and women comprise 85% of all cases. It affects 25% of women of reproductive age and 50% of women past menopause. Due to the female anatomy, women have twice the risk for stress incontinence compared to men. In addition, childbirth places pressure and burden on the pelvic muscles that often weaken with age, thereby weakening urethra stability. Women are more prone to surgeries for urological changes than men and severe urinary incontinence is often associated with these surgeries as well as hysterectomies. The majority of women with incontinence have stress incontinence or mixed incontinence. Male incontinence occurs primarily in response to blockage in the prostate or after prostate surgery. It is usually treated with implants and/or an artificial sphincter insert.

Description

There are a variety of retropubic suspension surgeries available to treat stress incontinence. The variations differ by the types of structures used to support the urethra and bladder. In all procedures, parts of the pelvic anatomy (pubic bone, ligaments) serve as an anchor or wall upon which the urethra is tacked for stability. The surgery is called a suspension surgery because it stabilizes the urethra from tilting by suspending it against a part of the pelvic anatomy. The Burch procedure is often performed when other surgery is needed such as repair of the urethra for cystoceles and urethral reconstruction. However, this procedure is the most difficult of the anti-incontinent surgeries and is more common in mild forms of stress incontinence where intrinsic sphincter deficiency is not present.

The Burch procedure can be done through open abdominal surgery, which requires a long incision at the bikini line, or surgery performed through the vagina. The patient, in stirrups, receives **general anesthesia**. Within the retropubic area, the anterior vaginal wall is separated from the bladder manually. The bladder neck is identified and old adhesions or fatty tissues are removed. The neck of the bladder is sutured to pubic ligaments where it will form adhesions and thereby gain stability. The surgeon examines for bladder injury and the surgery is completed. Urethral position is tested by placing a cotton-tipped swab in the urethra and measuring the angle. With abdominal surgery or vaginal surgery a catheter may be put in place by the surgeon for postoperative voiding and to decrease the risks of infection. A suction drain may be placed in the retropubic space for bleeding. The drain is removed one to three days after surgery.

Recently, laparoscopic surgery has been used to perform retropubic suspensions. Laparoscopic surgery requires only three or four 0.25-inch (0.6-cm) incisions in the belly button, pubic hairline, or groin area and uses small instruments without opening the abdominal cavity. A shorter healing time is seen with this procedure. the hospital stay is usually not more than 24 hours and recovery to normal activities takes about seven to 14 days. However, the Burch procedure performed using laparoscopic techniques requires great skill on the part of the surgeon and research indicates that the results may not be as long lasting as those developed with abdominal or vaginal surgery.

Diagnosis/Preparation

A patient with incontinence may have multiple factors that induce transient or chronic incontinence. It is crucial that the physician obtain a complete history, physical, clinical, neurological and medication evaluation of the patient, as well as a radiographic assessment before continuing urological tests aimed at a surgical solution. The specific indications for the Burch colosuspension procedure or its variants is the correction of stress urinary incontinence. This can be a patient who also requires abdominal surgery that cannot be performed vaginally, like **hysterectomy** or sigmoid surgery, as well as patients who have SUI without ISD.

A urodynamic study with a point pressure leak test will allow a diagnosis to be made that can distinguish the patient who has a hypermobile urethra from the patient who also has ISD. The point pressure leak test, also known as the Valsalva leak test, measures the amount of abdominal pressure required to induce leakage. The patient is asked to cough or strain in order to encourage leakage. The point at which the patient leaks helps determine if stress incontinence with ISD contribution is present. Obese patients and patients that engage in high impact exercise regimens are not considered good candidates for retropubic suspension.

Aftercare

Patients with open retropubic procedures are given pain medication postoperatively that is tapered down over the next two days. A suprapubic catheter stays in place for approximately five days with voiding difficulties encountered initially in many patients. Patients with laparoscopic suspensions are reported to have less blood loss during surgery, less postoperative narcotic requirements, and shorter hospital stays. Patients are expected to refrain from strenuous activity for three months and to have a follow-up visit within three weeks after surgery.

Risks

As with any major abdominal or pelvic surgical procedures, complications that may occur after a retropubic suspension include bleeding; injury to the bladder, urethra, and ureters; wound infection; and blood clots. Specific to the Burch procedure are complications that involve urethral obstruction because of urethral kinking due to elevation of the vagina or bladder base. Postoperative voiding difficulties are common and depend upon the suture tension of the urethral axis. Corrective surgery and the release of the urethra to a more anatomic position resolves voiding issues with a very high rate of success. Vaginal prolapse is also a risk of this procedure.

WHO PERFORMS THE PROCEDURE AND WHERE IS IT PERFORMED?

Retropubic suspension procedures are performed by a urological surgeon specially trained in incontinence surgeries. Surgery is performed in a general hospital.

Normal results

The patient can expect more than 80–90% cure or great improvement in their incontinence. There is a large body of literature documenting the success of the Burch procedure. Published research shows a cure rate ranging from 63% to 93%, according to the actual version of colosuspension used. Laparoscopic surgery has not produced the long term results that open surgery has and there is the possibility that the fibrosis (adhesion) necessary for a successful outcome does not occur as easily with the laparoscopic procedure. Patients not carefully screened out for ISD will not have a high level of success with the Burch procedure since the source of the incontinence will not have been treated. Sling procedures are recommended for patients with ISD instead of colosuspension surgery.

Morbidity and mortality rates

The Burch procedure may aggravate vaginal wall weakness or vaginal prolapse. This incident varies between 3% and 17%. Research on the Marshall-Marchetti-Krantz procedure pertaining to 2,712 patients found a complication rate of 21%, with wound complications and infections making up the majority, 5.5% and 3.9% respectively. Direct wound injury occurred in 1.6% and obstructions in 0.3% overall.

Alternatives

General or simple severe stress incontinence related primarily to weakening of the urethral support can be remedied with changes in diet, weight loss, and certain behavioral and rehabilitative measures. These include:

- Regular, daily exercising of the pelvic muscles called Kegel exercises, requiring 30–200 contractions a day for eight weeks.

QUESTIONS TO ASK THE DOCTOR

Which retropubic suspension procedure is recommended?

What is your cure rate with this procedure?

What is your injury rate for this procedure?

Could my incontinence be treated just as well with the sling procedure?

Do you perform laparoscopic surgeries to treat incontinence?

- Biofeedback to gain awareness and control of pelvic muscles.
- Vaginal weight training in which small weights are inserted in the vagina to tighten vaginal muscles.
- Mild electrical stimulation to increase contractions in pelvic muscles.
- Bladder retraining in which the patient is taught how to resist the urge to urinate and expand the intervals between urinations.

There are also medications that can facilitate continence for those experiencing stress or urge incontinence. These include some kinds of antidepressants, although the mechanism of action is not quite understood, as well as antispasmodic medication and estrogen therapy. Finally, should behavioral, rehabilitative, and surgical procedures fail, there remain alternatives through the use of vaginal cones and urethral plugs that can be inserted and removed by the patient.

Resources

BOOKS

Walsh, Patrick. *Campbell's Urology*. 8th ed. Elsevier Science, 2000.

PERIODICALS

Liu, C. Y. "Laparoscopic Treatment of Stress Urinary Incontinence." *Obstetrics and Gynecology Clinics of North America* 26, no. 1 (March 1999): 149-67.

Melton, Lisa. "Targeted Treatment for Incontinence Beckons." *Lancet* 359, no. 9303 (January 2002): 326.

Smoger, S. H., T. L. Felice, and G. H. Kloecker. "Urinary Incontinence Among Male Veterans Receiving Care in Primary Care Clinics." *Annals of Internal Medicine* 132, no. 7 (April 4, 2000): 547-551.

Stoffel, J. T., J. Bresette, and J. J. Smith. "Retropubic Surgery for Stress Urinary Incontinence." *Urologic Clinics of North America* 29, no. 3 (August 2002).

Weber, A. M., and M. D. Walters. "The Burch and Sling Procedures are Similarly Effective for Surgical Treatment of Genuine Stress Urinary Incontinence." *Evidence-based Obstetrics & Gynecology* 4, no. 1 (March 2002).

ORGANIZATIONS

American Foundation for Urologic Diseases. The Bladder Health Council, 1128 North Charles Street, Baltimore, MD 21201. (410) 468-1800. http://www.afud.org/education/bladder.html.

National Kidney and Urologic Diseases Information Clearinghouse. 3 Information Way, Bethesda, MD 20892-3580. (800) 891-5390 or (301) 654-4415. http://www.niddk.nih.gov.

The Simon Foundation for Continence, P.O. Box 835, Wilmette, IL 60091. (800) 23-SIMON or (847) 864-3913. http://www.simonfoundation.org.

OTHER

Bladder Control in Women. National Kidney and Urologic Disease Information Clearinghouse. NIH Publication No. 97-4195. May 2002 [cited May 12, 2003]. < http://www.niddk.nih.gov/health/urolog/uibcw/bcw/bcw.htm.

Ginsberg, David. "Trends in Surgical Therapy for Stress Urinary Incontinence." American Urological Association 97th Annual Meeting, WebMD Conference Coverage. 2002 [cited May 12, 2003]. http://www.medscape.com/viewarticle/437091.

Hendrix, Susan L., and S. Gene McNeeley. "Urinary Incontinence and Menopause: Update on Evidence-Based Treatment." Clinical Update. *Medscape*. October 28, 2002 [cited May 12, 2003]. http://www.medscape.com/viewprogram/2052.

Nancy McKenzie, PhD

Rh blood typing

Definition

Rh blood typing is performed in order to determine the Rh factor of an individual's blood. The term "Rh factor" refers to an antigen on the surface of the red blood cells. All red blood cells have certain substances on their surfaces. These substances are called "antigens," and may be molecules of protein, carbohydrate, glycolipid, or glycoprotein. Blood typing categorizes blood by identifying the presence or absence of these antigens on the surface of the red blood cell.

The Rh system identifies the presence (denoted as positive) or absence (denoted as negative) of a particular antigen termed the Rhesus antigen. Its names stems from the fact that the Rh factor was first identified on the red blood cell surfaces of Rhesus monkeys. When the Rh factor is present on the surface of the red blood cell, the blood is said to be Rh-positive; when the Rh factor is absent from the surface of the red blood cell, the blood is said to be Rh-negative.

The Rh factor status is reported in conjunction with identification of the major ABO blood group of the individual. The ABO blood group system identifies a type of protein antigen on the red blood cell surface as Type A, Type B, Type AB, or Type O. An individual's blood type, then is reported as a combination of information obtained about the ABO and RH blood group systems; for example, A-positive, or A-negative, etc.

Blood typing is particularly important when an individual needs to receive a blood **transfusion**. If the wrong blood type is given, there is a high risk of an adverse transfusion reaction. For example, the first time an Rh-negative individual is given blood from an Rh-positive donor, there will probably not be any problem. However, if the Rh-negative individual receives future transfusions of Rh-positive blood, the recipient's immune system will recognize the Rh antigen on the donor blood as foreign, and will begin to produce antibodies directed against that antigen. The antibodies will attack the donor blood, damaging and bursting the donor red blood cells. This results in high serum levels of hemoglobin spilling from the burst red blood cells (called hemoglobinemia), disseminated intravascular coagulation or DIC (a condition in which clotting factors are used up very rapidly, resulting in the potential for severe, uncontrollable bleeding), kidney failure, and eventually complete cardiovascular collapse (a combination of heart attack, shock, and lack of blood flow to all major organs and tissues).

Knowing a pregnant woman's Rh-factor is crucial because there is always a chance during pregnancy, labor, and delivery, that some of the baby's blood will get into the mother's bloodstream. If this happens in an Rh-negative mother with an Rh-positive baby, the mother's body will identify the baby's Rh-negative blood as foreign and begin producing antibodies against the Rh-factor. This is called Rh-sensitization. The first time this sensitization occurs between a mother and her baby, the baby usually doesn't suffer any ill-effects. But in subsequent pregnancies, if the mother is again carrying an Rh-positive baby, having already been exposed to the Rh-antigen previously, her body will begin to produce Rh-antibodies more quickly and in greater numbers. If these cross over into the baby's bloodstream, they can begin destroying the baby's red blood cells, resulting in severe illness. This problem is referred to as Rh disease, hemolytic disease of the newborn, or erythroblastosis fetalis. In order to avoid this problem, Rh testing is done prior to pregnancy or early in pregnancy. Rh-negative women can be given a special shot called Rh-immune globulin which can prevent Rh-sensitization.

Purpose

Blood typing is ordered prior to a blood transfusion, to make sure that the donor blood type is appropriately compatible with the recipient's blood type. It is also done on donor blood, on a donor who is giving an organ to be used for transplantation, as well as prior to surgery (so that the patient's blood type is known, should the individual needs an unexpected, emergency blood transfusion). Rh-typing is also important in pregnant women. When the mother and the baby have different Rh-types, there is a risk to the baby of illness caused by the mother's antibodies; if the mother is identified as having Rh-negative blood, a shot called Rh-immune globulin can prevent the problem from developing.

Precautions

Some situations may confuse the results of blood typing, including recent x-ray test using contrast, use of medications such as methyldopa, levodopa, and certain **antibiotics** (including cephalexin). Other factors that may confuse test results include having received a blood transfusion in the previous three months, having had a bone marrow transplant in the past, or having a history of cancer or leukemia.

Description

This test requires blood to be drawn from a vein (usually one in the forearm), generally by a nurse or phlebotomist (an individual who has been trained to draw blood). A tourniquet is applied to the arm above the area where the needle stick will be performed. The site of the needle stick is cleaned with antiseptic, and the needle is inserted. The blood is collected in vacuum tubes. After collection, the needle is withdrawn, and pressure is kept on the blood draw site to stop any bleeding and decrease bruising. A bandage is then applied.

Preparation

There are no restrictions on diet or physical activity, either before or after the blood test.

KEY TERMS

Disseminated intravascular dissemination—A condition in which the clotting factors in the blood are rapidly used up, resulting in a severe deficit in clotting factors and a very high risk of severe, uncontrollable bleeding.

Erythroblastosis fetalis—A condition in which the incompatability between a mother's Rh-negative blood type and a baby's Rh-positive blood type results in destruction of the baby's red blood cells by maternal antibodies.

Aftercare

As with any blood tests, discomfort, bruising, and/or a very small amount of bleeding is common at the puncture site. Immediately after the needle is withdrawn, it is helpful to put pressure on the puncture site until the bleeding has stopped. This decreases the chance of significant bruising. Warm packs may relieve minor discomfort. Some individuals may feel briefly woozy after a blood test, and they should be encouraged to lie down and rest until they feel better.

Risks

Basic blood tests, such as Rh blood typing, do not carry any significant risks, other than slight bruising and the chance of brief dizziness.

Results

Rh blood typing reports back whether the individual's red blood cells have the Rh antigen present on their surface (Rh-postive) or absent from their surface (Rh-negative). About 84% of all people are Rh-positive; about 16% are Rh-negative.

Resources

BOOKS

Goldman L, Ausiello D., eds. *Cecil Textbook of Internal Medicine*. 23rd ed. Philadelphia: Saunders, 2008.

Hoffman R. et al. *Hematology: Basic Principles and Practice*. 4th ed. Philadelphia: Elsevier, 2005.

McPherson RA et al. *Henry's Clinical Diagnosis and Management By Laboratory Methods*. 21st ed. Philadelphia: Saunders, 2007.

ORGANIZATIONS

American Association of Clinical Chemistry. 1850 K St., N.WSuite 625, Washington, DC 20006. http://www.aacc.org.

OTHER

National Institutes of Health. [cited February 10, 2008]. http://www.nlm.nih.gov/medlineplus/encyclopedia.html.

Rosalyn Carson-DeWitt, MD

Rh typing *see* **Type and screen**

Rheumatoid factor testing

Definition

Rheumatoid factor is a type of antibody. Antibodies, also called immunoglobulins, are proteins produced by the body. Antibodies work to clear the body of potentially threatening infections or substances, fighting off various invaders, such as virsues, bacteria, toxins, mold spores, etc.

The body's immune system is made up of lymphoid organs, including lymph nodes, the bone marrow (located within the center of long bones) and the thymus (located in the chest). These lymphoid organs produce lymphocytes, including T cells and B cells. These lymphocytes circulate within the bloodstream, within the lymph system, and are also positioned in clumps within organs and on mucosal surfaces of the body. When a B cell encounters a foreign invader, it recognized it as foreign by virtue of a chemical identifier on its surface (called an antigen). Once the B cell recognizes an antigen, the B cell gives rise to a large number of plasma cells. These plasma cells are capable of producing antibodies.

Antibodies are made up of units called "chains." All antibodies are composed of two larger chains (called heavy chains) and two smaller chains (called light chains). The tip of the antibody is referred to as the hypervariable region. This hypervariable region is responsible for unique chemical properties possessed by each antibody that allow a specific antibody to "recognize" and match up to a particular antigen. The combination of an antibody with a specific antigen, creates an antibody-antigen complex, marking the invader as foreign and in need of inactivation or destruction by other immune cells in the body.

The first time an antigen is encountered by the immune system, the body's response is slow. Time is required in order to activate the machinery necessary to produce the very specific type of antibody necessary to combat that antigen. However, if that particular antigen is encountered in the future, the needed machinery is already available, and antibody production in response to a "familiar" antigen is quite rapid.

One of the important attributes of a healthy, well-functioning immune system rests on its ability to distinguish between "self" and "other." This means that it's crucial that the antibodies don't mistakenly identify parts of the body itself as foreign invaders. When this does happen, the body's immune system attacks the body, damaging and destroying it. Conditions in which this occurs are referred to as autoimmune disorders. One example of an autoimmune disorder is the condition called rheumatoid arthritis or RA. In RA, the lining of the joints (synovium) is mis-recognized by the immune system as foreign, resulting in the immune system creating specific antibodies that repeatedly attack, damage, and destroy the joints' lining, resulting in the cluster of symptoms that accompany this disease.

Rheumatoid factor belongs to the class of antibodies known as IgM antibodies. IgM antibodies are primarily found in the blood, and comprise about 13% of all antibodies. IgM functions to kill bacteria, and is found in the earlier phases of immune response to bacterial invasion of the bloodstream (bacteremia).

In rheumatoid arthritis, rheumatoid factor is directed against IgG antibodies. IgG antibodies are very common circulating antibodies; in fact, about 80% of all circulating antibodies are IgG. IgG is found in blood and tissue fluids. IgG functions to coat invading particles, marking them so that they can more easily and rapidly be taken up by other types of immune cells. IgG is the predominant antibody cell in the later or secondary phase of the immune response.

When rheumatoid factor encounters IgG, it attaches itself to the IgG, forming an immune complex. This immune complex kicks off a complicated immune cascade, prompting the production and release of a variety of chemicals that ultimately misidentify the synovium as "non-self," attack the lining, and over time cause tremendous destruction.

KEY TERMS

Antibody—A protein that the body produces in response to exposure to a foreign invader such as a virus, bacteria, fungus, or allergen.

Antigen—The protein marker that prompts the body's immune system to produce antibodies.

Autoimmune disorder—A condition in which the body produces antibodies that serve to attack organs or tissues of the body itself.

Immune system—The collection of organs, tissues, and cells that serve to protect the body against foreign invaders, such as bacteria, viruses, and fungi.

Lymphocyte—A white blood cell; part of the immune system responsible for the production of antibodies.

Plasma cell—The specific type of white blood cell that produces antibodies.

Rheumatoid arthritis—A condition in which the immune system damages and destroys the synovial lining of the joints. Red, warm, swollen, stiff joints are a common symptom. Over time, other organ systems may also be affected, including the heart, eyes, lungs, and kidneys.

Sjögren's syndrome—A disease in which the immune system damages and destroys exocrine glands, such as those that produce tears and saliva. Dry eyes and mouth are the usual initial symptoms of this disorder, but other organ systems can also be severely affected over time, including the skin, pancreas, liver, lungs, brain, and kidneys.

Purpose

Rheumatoid factor testing is usually done when an individual is having symptoms compatible with an autoimmune disorder, particularly rheuumatoid arthritis or Sjogren's syndrome. Suspicious symptoms include joint stiffness, pain and swelling (especially in the morning), bumps (nodules) under the skin, and/or dry eyes, mouth, and skin.

Precautions

Rheumatoid factor testing is not diagnostic. This means that getting a specific result does not definitively confirm the presence of any particular disease. Instead, the test is used to correlate with the clinical picture, meaning the history and the symptoms that an individual is experiencing.

Some situations may confuse the results of testing for rheumatoid factor, including very high blood levels of triglycerides or other fats, or advanced age (people over 65 years of age have a higher chance of having a higher-than-normal rheumatoid factor that is not associated with disease).

Description

This test requires blood to be drawn from a vein (usually one in the forearm), generally by a nurse or phlebotomist (an individual who has been trained to draw blood). A tourniquet is applied to the arm above the area where the needle stick will be performed. The site of the needle stick is cleaned with antiseptic, and the needle is inserted. The blood is collected in vacuum tubes. After collection, the needle is withdrawn, and pressure is kept on the blood draw site to stop any bleeding and decrease bruising. A bandage is then applied.

Preparation

There are no restrictions on diet or physical activity, either before or after the blood test.

Aftercare

As with any blood tests, discomfort, bruising, and/or a very small amount of bleeding is common at the puncture site. Immediately after the needle is withdrawn, it is helpful to put pressure on the puncture site until the bleeding has stopped. This decreases the chance of significant bruising. Warm packs may relieve minor discomfort. Some individuals may feel briefly woozy after a blood test, and they should be encouraged to lie down and rest until they feel better.

Risks

Basic blood tests, such as rheumatoid factor testing, do not carry any significant risks, other than slight bruising and the chance of brief dizziness.

Results

Normal rheumatoid factor results would demonstrate a rheumatoid factor titer less than 1:20-1:40, or a rheumatoid factor of less than 43 nephlometry units.

The patient's, history, symptoms, and rheumatoid factor results are used together in order to arrive at a diagnosis. An elevated rheumatoid factor may indicate the possibility of rheumatoid arthritis or Sjogren's syndrome. However, some patients (about 20%) with these diseases do not have an elevated rheumatoid factor, or have the condition for several years before their rheumatoid factor becomes abnormally elevated.

Rheumatoid factor may also be elevated in a number of other autoimmune conditions, such as systemic lupus erythematosus, vasculitis, or scleroderma; in severe infections such as syphilis or tuberculosis, mononucleosis, malaria, hepatitis, or endocarditis; in certain types of cancer, including leukemia; and in a number of other conditions, such as cirrhosis of the liver, and lung or kidney disease.

Resources

BOOKS

Goldman L, Ausiello D., eds. *Cecil Textbook of Internal Medicine*. 23rd ed. Philadelphia: Saunders, 2008.

Hoffman R. et al. *Hematology: Basic Principles and Practice*. 4th ed. Philadelphia: Elsevier, 2005.

Harris ED et al. *Kelley's Textbook of Rheumatology*. 7th ed. Philadelphia: Saunders, 2005.

McPherson RA et al. *Henry's Clinical Diagnosis and Management By Laboratory Methods*. 21st ed. Philadelphia: Saunders, 2007.

ORGANIZATIONS

American Association of Clinical Chemistry. 1850 K St., N.W., Suite 625, Washington, DC 20006. http://www.aacc.org.

OTHER

National Institutes of Health. [cited February 10, 2008]. http://www.nlm.nih.gov/medlineplus/encyclopedia.html.

Rosalyn Carson-DeWitt, MD

Rhinoplasty

Definition

The term rhinoplasty means "nose molding" or "nose forming." It refers to a procedure in **plastic surgery** in which the structure of the nose is changed. The change can be made by adding or removing bone or cartilage, grafting tissue from another part of the body, or implanting synthetic material to alter the shape of the nose.

Purpose

Rhinoplasty is most often performed for cosmetic reasons. A nose that is too large, crooked, misshapen, malformed at birth, or deformed by an injury can be given a more pleasing appearance. If breathing is impaired due to the form of the nose or to an injury, it can often be improved with rhinoplasty.

Demographics

Rhinoplasty is the third most common cosmetic procedure among both men and women. Total number of rhinoplasty procedures in the United States in 1999 was 133,058. More than 13,100 of those procedures were performed on men.

Description

The external nose is composed of a series of interrelated parts that include the skin, the bony pyramid, cartilage, and the tip of the nose, which is composed of cartilage and skin. The strip of skin separating the nostrils is called the columella.

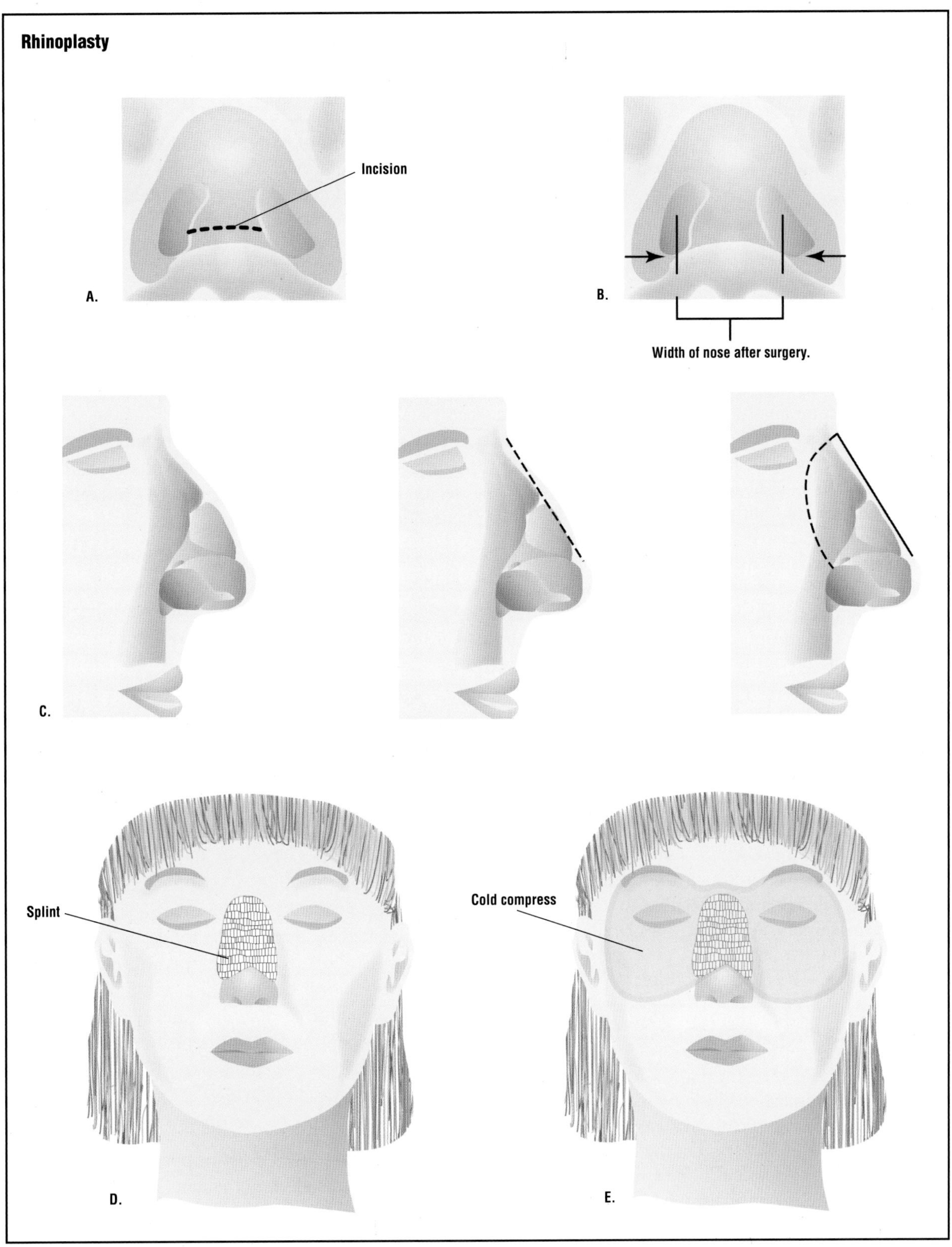

During an open rhinoplasty, an incision is made in the skin between the nostrils (A). Closed rhinoplasty involves only incisions inside the nose. Rhinoplasty may involve a change in nostril width (B) or removal of a hump on the nose (C) using bone sculpting. After surgery, a splint supports the nose (D), and a cold compress reduces swelling (E). *(Illustration by GGS Information Services. Cengage Learning, Gale.)*

KEY TERMS

Cartilage—Firm supporting tissue that does not contain blood vessels.

Columella—The strip of skin running from the tip of the nose to the upper lip, which separates the nostrils.

Septum—The dividing barrier in the center of the nose.

Surgical approaches to nasal reconstruction are varied. Internal rhinoplasty involves making all incisions from inside the nasal cavity. The external, or "open," technique involves a skin incision across the base of the nasal columella. An external incision allows the surgeon to expose the bone and cartilage more fully and is most often used for complicated procedures. During surgery, the surgeon will separate the skin from the bone and cartilage support. The framework of the nose is then reshaped in the desired form. Shape can be altered by removing or adding bone, cartilage, or skin. The remaining skin is then replaced over the new framework. If the procedure requires adding to the structure of the nose, the donated bone, cartilage, or skin can come from another location on the patient's body or from a synthetic source.

When the operation is completed, the surgeon will apply a splint to help the bones maintain their new shape. The nose may also be packed, or stuffed with a dressing, to help stabilize the septum.

When a local anesthetic is used, light sedation is usually given first, after which the operative area is numbed. It will remain insensitive to pain for the length of the surgery. A general anesthetic is used for lengthy or complex procedures, or if the doctor and patient agree that it is the best option.

Diagnosis/Preparation

The quality of the skin plays a major role in the outcome of rhinoplasty. Persons with extremely thick skin may not see a significant change in the underlying bone structure after surgery. On the other hand, thin skin provides almost no cushion to hide many minor bone irregularities or imperfections.

Rhinoplasty should not be performed until the pubertal growth spurt is complete, age 14–15 for girls and older for boys.

During the initial consultation, the candidate and surgeon will determine what changes can be made in the shape of the nose. Most doctors take photographs during that consult. The surgeon will also explain the techniques and anesthesia options available to the candidate.

The candidate and surgeon should also discuss guidelines for eating, drinking, smoking, taking or avoiding certain medications, and washing the face for the weeks immediately following surgery.

WHO PERFORMS THE PROCEDURE AND WHERE IS IT PERFORMED?

Simple rhinoplasty is usually performed in an outpatient surgery center or in the surgeon's office. Most procedures take only an hour or two, and patients go home right away. Complex procedures may be performed in a hospital and require a short stay.

Rhinoplasty is usually performed by a surgeon with advanced training in plastic and reconstructive surgery.

Aftercare

Patients usually feel fine immediately after surgery. As a precaution, most surgery centers do not allow patients to drive themselves home after an operation.

The first day after surgery, there will be some swelling of the face. Persons should stay in bed with their heads elevated for at least a day. The nose may hurt and a headache is common. The surgeon will prescribe medication to relieve these conditions. Swelling and bruising around the eyes will increase for a few days, but will begin to diminish after about the third day. Slight bleeding and stuffiness are normal, and vary according to the extent of the surgery performed. Most people are walking in two days, and back to work or school in a week. No strenuous activities are allowed for two to three weeks.

Patients are given a list of postoperative instructions, which include requirements for hygiene, **exercise**, eating, and follow-up visits to the doctor. Patients should not blow their noses for the first week to avoid disruption of healing. It is extremely important to keep the surgical dressing dry. **Dressings**, splints, and **stitches** are removed in one to two weeks. Patients should avoid excessive sun or sunburn.

QUESTIONS TO ASK THE DOCTOR

Candidates for a rhinoplasty procedure should consider asking the following questions:

- What will be the resulting appearance? (Often, computer programs are available to assist in visualizing the final result.)
- Is the surgeon board certified in plastic and reconstructive surgery?
- How many rhinoplasty procedures has the surgeon performed?
- What is the surgeon's complication rate?
- Will this surgery really make a huge difference to my life or am I trying to live up to an impossible media stereotype of beauty?

Risks

Any type of surgery carries a degree of risk. There is always the possibility of unexpected events such as an infection or a reaction to the anesthesia.

When the nose is reshaped or repaired from inside, the scars are not visible. If the surgeon needs to make the incision on the outside of the nose, there will be some slight scarring. In addition, tiny blood vessels may burst, leaving small red spots on the skin. These spots are barely visible, but may be permanent.

Normal results

The best candidates for rhinoplasty are those persons with relatively minor deformities. Nasal anatomy and proportions are quite varied and the final look of any rhinoplasty operation depends on a person's anatomy, as well as the surgeon's skill.

A cosmetic change of the nose will change a person's appearance, but it will not change self-image. A person who expects a different lifestyle after rhinoplasty is likely to be disappointed.

The cost of rhinoplasty depends on the difficulty of the work required and on the specialist chosen. If the problem was caused by an injury, insurance will usually cover the cost. A rhinoplasty done only to change a person's appearance is not usually covered by insurance.

Morbidity and mortality rates

Death from a rhinoplasty procedure is exceedingly rare. When it occurs, the cause is often due to an adverse reaction to anesthesia or postoperative medications or to an infection. About 10% of persons receiving rhinoplasty require a second procedure.

Alternatives

The alternative to cosmetic rhinoplasty is to accept oneself, literally, at face value. Persons contemplating rhinoplasty may want to question some of the conventional standards of beauty and work on their body image issues to improve their self-confidence.

Resources

BOOKS

Cummings, CW, et al. *Otolayrngology: Head and Neck Surgery*. 4th ed. St. Louis: Mosby, 2005.

PERIODICALS

Becker DG. "Reducing complications in rhinoplasty." *Otolaryngology Clinics of North America* 39, no.3 (2006): 475–492.

Citardi MJ. "Advanced Techniques in Rhinology." *Otolaryngology Clinics of North America* 39, no.3 (2006): xiii–xiv.

Romo T. "Reduction Structured Rhinoplasty." *Dermatology Clinics* 23, no.3 (2005): 529–540.

Rohrich, R. J., and A. R. Muzaffar. "Rhinoplasty in the African-American Patient." *Plastic and Reconstructive Surgery* 111, no.3 (2003): 1322–1339.

Russell, P., and C. Nduka. "Digital Photography for Rhinoplasty." *Plastic and Reconstructive Surgery* 111, no.3 (2003): 1266–1267.

ORGANIZATIONS

American Board of Plastic Surgery. Seven Penn Center, Suite 400, 1635 Market Street, Philadelphia, PA 19103-2204. (215) 587-9322. http://www.abplsurg.org/.

American College of Plastic and Reconstructive Surgery. http://www.breast-implant.org.

American College of Surgeons. 633 North Saint Claire Street, Chicago, IL 60611. (312) 202-5000. http://www.facs.org/.

American Society for Aesthetic Plastic Surgery. 11081 Winners Circle, Los Alamitos, CA 90720. (800) 364-2147 or (562) 799-2356. http://www.surgery.org/.

American Society for Dermatologic Surgery. 930 N. Meacham Road, P.O. Box 4014, Schaumburg, IL 60168-4014. (847) 330-9830. http://www.asds-net.org.

American Society of Plastic Surgeons. 444 E. Algonquin Rd., Arlington Heights, IL 60005. (847) 228-9900. http://www.plasticsurgery.org/.

OTHER

American Academy of Facial and Reconstructive Plastic Surgery. [cited April 9, 2003] http://www.facial-plastic-surgery.org/patient/procedures/rhinoplasty.html.

National Library of Medicine. [cited April 9, 2003] http://www.nlm.nih.gov/medlineplus/plasticcosmeticsurgery.html.

Restoration of Appearance Trust. [cited April 9, 2003] http://www.raft.ac.uk/plastics/rhinoplasty.html.

Revision Rhinoplasty. [cited April 9, 2003] http://www.revisionrhinoplasty.net/.

L. Fleming Fallon, Jr., MD, DrPH

Rhizotomy

Definition

Rhizotomy is the cutting of nerve roots as they enter the spinal cord.

Purpose

Rhizotomy (also called dorsal rhizotomy, selective dorsal rhizotomy, and selective posterior rhizotomy) is a treatment for spasticity that is unresponsive to less invasive procedures.

Demographics

Spasticity (involuntary muscle contractions) affects many thousands of Americans, but very few are affected seriously enough to require surgery for its treatment.

Description

Rhizotomy is performed under **general anesthesia**. The patient lies face down. An incision is made along the lower spine, exposing the sensory nerve roots at the center the spinal cord. Individual nerve rootlets are electrically stimulated. Since these are sensory nerves, they should not stimulate muscle movement. Those that do (and therefore cause spasticity) are cut. Typically, one-quarter to one-half of nerve rootlets tested are cut.

Diagnosis/Preparation

Rhizotomy is performed on patients with spasticity that is insufficiently responsive to oral medications or injectable therapies (botulinum toxin, phenol, or alcohol). It is most commonly performed for those patients with lower extremity spasticity that interferes with walking or severe spasticity that prevents hygiene or positioning of the legs. It is most commonly performed on children with cerebral palsy.

WHO PERFORMS THE PROCEDURE AND WHERE IS IT PERFORMED?

Rhizotomy is performed by a neurosurgeon in a hospital. The patient's neurologist and physical therapist may also be in attendance to help with the evaluation during surgery.

Patients undergoing rhizotomy receive a large battery of tests before the procedure, in order to document the functional effects of spasticity, and the patient's medical health and likely response to anesthesia and other operative stresses. Rhizotomy is performed as an in-patient procedure, and the patient is likely to require an overnight hospital stay before the operation.

Aftercare

After surgery, the patient will spend one to several days in the hospital. Physical therapy and strength training usually begin the next day, in order to maximize the gains expected from surgery, and to keep the limbs mobile. Medication may be given for pain.

Risks

Rhizotomy carries small but significant risks of nerve damage, permanent loss of sensation or altered sensation, weakness of the lower extremities, bowel and bladder dysfunction, increased likelihood of hip dislocation, and scoliosis progression. Anesthesia carries its own risks.

Normal results

Rhizotomy reduces spasticity, which should allow more normal gait and improve mobility. Patients may require fewer walking aids, such as walkers or crutches.

Morbidity and mortality rates

Other than the risks from anesthesia, rhizotomy does not carry a risk of **death** during surgery. Morbidity rates vary among centers performing the surgery. Persistent and significant adverse effects may occur in 1–5% of patients, including bowel or bladder changes and low back pain.

QUESTIONS TO ASK THE DOCTOR

- How many rhizotomies have you performed?
- What is your complication rate?
- Is orthopedic surgery still likely to be necessary later on?

Alternatives

Other spasticity treatments include oral medications and an implanted pump delivering baclofen to the space around the spinal cord (intrathecal baclofen). These may be appropriate alternatives for some patients. **Orthopedic surgery** can correct deformities that occur from untreated spasticity. Some controversy exists whether rhizotomy can delay or prevent the need for other spasticity procedures, especially orthopedic surgery such as **tenotomy**, with some evidence suggesting it can, and other evidence suggesting it may not.

Resources

ORGANIZATIONS

United Cerebral Palsy. 1660 L Street, NW, Suite 700, Washington, DC 20036. (800) 872-5827 or (202)776-0406. TTY: (202) 973-7197. Fax: (202) 776-0414. webmaster@ucp.org. http://www.UCP.org.

WE MOVE. http://www.wemove.org.

Richard Robinson

Rhytidoplasty *see* **Face lift**

Robot-assisted surgery

Definition

Robot-assisted surgery involves the use of a robot under the direction and guidance of a surgeon.

Purpose

Robot-assisted surgery provides many benefits in the surgical care of patients. Computer-assisted robots provide exact motion and trajectories to minimize the side effects of surgical intervention. Robot-assisted surgeries can use three-dimensional imaging and smaller surgical tools to operate in a closed environment through smaller incisions. For example, traditional methods of cardiac surgery usually required a six-to-eight inch incision in the sternum and the use of a heart-lung machine to maintain the functions of the heart and lungs while they are stopped for the surgery. Robot-assisted surgery has furthered the use of the keyhole approach, in which multiple small incisions are made between the ribs. With robot-assisted surgery, the surgeon is also able to make more precise movements using motion scaling. In this practice, an image is enlarged and the movements of the surgeon's hands are translated by the computer into smaller movements. This allows surgeons to perform more precisely, which can be especially important when the surgery is to be performed on particularly small parts of the body.

Demographics

Patients undergoing surgical procedures classified as **neurosurgery**, **orthopedic surgery**, radio surgery and radiotherapy, prostatectomy, endoscopy, **laparoscopy**, cardiac surgery and craniofacial surgery may experience robot-assisted surgical techniques.

Description

Neurosurgery

A high level of accuracy is required when operating on the brain to avoid damage to the sensitive brain tissue. Biopsies and minor interventions are best assisted by the robotic device. Interventions include drilling into the skull and making an incision through the dura mater to gain brain tissue samples, empty cysts, or eliminate hemorrhage.

Orthopedic surgery

Applications such as cementless hip-replacement, total knee arthroplasties, and pedicle screw placement can benefit from the more accurate cutting and drilling provided by a robot. Femur bone-cutting devices provide improved drilling to carve a cavity in the bone for prosthesis implant. Pins inserted into the bone before surgery are used as landmarks for computerized tomography (CT) imaging. The CT image provides the surgeon with the necessary information for choosing an implant. The surgeon removes the head from the femur bone, eliminating the joint. The leg is secured in position and the robot is brought into position. A high speed cutter is then applied to create the cavity, and then followed by a smoothing tool. The surgeon manually inserts the implant into the femur and completes the cap implant into the pelvic bone.

KEY TERMS

Arthoplastic—Manufactured replacement joint.

Cardiac surgery—Surgery performed on the heart.

Craniofacial surgery—Surgery of the facial tissue and skull.

Endoscopy—Used to visualize internal structures of the body, such as the trachea, esophagus or intestines.

Laparoscopy—Surgery on internal structures through small incisions and visualized with the laparoscope.

Neurosurgery—Surgery performed on the brain.

Orthopedic surgery—Surgery performed on the bones. May include joint replacements and surgery of the vertebrae.

Prostatectomy—Performed for the treatment of prostate disease including prostate cancer.

Radio surgery and radiotherapy—Used in the treatment of cancerous growths or kidney stones.

Radiosurgery and radiotherapy

Radiation treatment is provided by a robot. The CT image or magnetic resonance image (MRI) is used to determine where the radiation treatment should be delivered. The robot aligns with patient anatomy, delivering specific doses of radiation to the intended location.

Prostatectomy

Removal of all or part of the prostate is another robot-assisted procedure. The robot controls instruments inserted through the urethra to the prostate gland. A diathermic hot wire cutting loop is guided to remove tissue in an appropriate pattern around the urethra. Fastening the guiding frame to the upper legs of the patient secures the device for accurate guidance.

Endoscopy

Endoscopy is used to examine patient cavities for the presence of polyps, tumors, and other diseases. The endoscope can be better passed through cavities such as the colon or trachea. Three-dimensional images of the cavity are obtained and used to dictate the path taken by the endoscope. Sedation and heavy analgesia can be avoided.

THE DA VINCI SURGICAL SYSTEM

Approved by the U.S. Food and Drug Administration in 2000, the da Vinci surgical system is the most popular surgical robotic system used in hospitals as of 2008. According to the company that manufactures the system, Intuitive Surgical, over 210 are used in hospitals throughout the world. The system has four robotic arms which move the cameras and tools the surgeon controls from a consol. While the da Vinci costs over one million dollars, many surgeons who use the system say that is has become an indispensable aid to complicated surgical procedures. Moreover, it has been estimated that hospitals save money overall because the length of post-surgical hospitalization is cut in half.

Laparoscopy

In laparoscopic surgeries, three to four small incisions are made in the abdominal or thoracic cavity to insert the instruments and video equipment. The surgeon performs the operation from a remote console that provides the human-machine interface. The console provides video monitoring images that are three-dimensional. Joysticks are used to manipulate the tools within the chest cavity to complete the surgical procedure.

Cardiac surgery

Robots can be used in the coronary artery bypass grafting surgeries and cardiac valve replacement and repair surgeries. The harvesting of artery and vein grafts can also be accomplished with the aid of laparoscopic techniques.

Craniofacial surgery

Difficult bone cuts and bone tumor removals are accomplished successfully using robotic instruments. Pre-planned trajectories are programmed into the machine. Precision cuts are made in the manner desired to achieve an aesthetically satisfactory result. As the surgeon manipulates the saw, he or she is guided along the path by a predetermined trajectory determined during an initial run on a model of the surgical site.

Aftercare

The patient should expect a faster recovery then that achieved by traditional surgery procedures.

QUESTIONS TO ASK THE DOCTOR

- Is there an institution in the vicinity which uses robot-assisted surgery?
- How experienced is the surgeon with robot-assisted surgical techniques?
- What benefits would the robot-assisted surgery provide?
- What complications can be avoided and which may be encountered with robot-assisted surgery?

Risks

With some of these procedures, a longer surgical time is required to achieve the same desired outcome as the traditional surgical approach. There is an increased risk of anesthesia related complications as surgical times increase. Additionally, if the robotic procedure is not completed successfully, the surgeon may need to complete the procedure with a traditional technique.

Normal results

Results for each procedure are comparable to or better than the standard surgical procedure.

Morbidity and mortality rates

Complications should be comparable to the standard surgical procedure, and even reduced. Some complications may only be associated with the robot-assisted procedure.

Alternatives

The alternative to using robot-assisted surgery is for the surgeon to employ a traditional surgical approach.

Resources

BOOKS

DiGioia, Anthony et al, eds. *Computer and Robotic Assisted Hip and Knee Surgery*. New York: Oxford University Press, 2004.

Faust, Russel A., ed. *Robotics in Surgery: History, Current and Future Applications*. New York: Nova Science Publishers, 2007.

Stiehl, James B., Werner H. Konermann and Rolf G. Haaker, eds. *Navigation and Robotics in Total Joint and Spine Surgery*. New York: Springer, 2004.

PERIODICALS

Bates, Betsy. "Robots Can Assist in Improving Care." *Internal Medicine News* 39.17 (Sept 1, 2006): 1-3.

Diks, J., D. Nio, V. Jongkind, M. A. Cuesta, J. A. Rauwerda and W. Wisselink. "Robot-Assisted Laparoscopic Surgery of the Infrarenal Aorta; The Early Learning Curve." *Surgical Endoscopy* 21.11 (Nov 2007): 2118-2120.

Allison Joan Spiwak, MSBME
Robert Bockstiegel

Root canal treatment

Definition

Root canal treatment, also known as endodontic treatment, is a dental procedure in which the diseased or damaged pulp (central core) of a tooth is removed and the inside areas (the pulp chamber and root canals) are filled and sealed.

Purpose

An inflamed or infected pulp is called pulpitis. It is the most common cause of a toothache. To relieve the pain and prevent further complications, the tooth may be extracted (surgically removed) or saved by root canal treatment.

Demographics

Root canal treatment has become a common dental procedure. According to the American Association of Endodontists, more than 14 million root canal treatments are performed every year, with a 95% success rate.

Description

Inside the tooth, the pulp of a tooth is comprised of soft tissue that contains the blood supply, by which the tooth receives its nutrients; and the nerve, by which the tooth senses hot and cold. This tissue is vulnerable to damage from deep dental decay, accidental injury, tooth fracture, or trauma from repeated dental procedures such as multiple fillings or restorations over time. If a tooth becomes diseased or injured, bacteria may build up inside the pulp, spreading infection from the natural crown of the tooth to the root tips in the jawbone. Pus accumulating at the ends of the roots can form a painful abscess that can damage the bone supporting the teeth. Such an infection may produce pain that is severe, constant, or throbbing. It can also

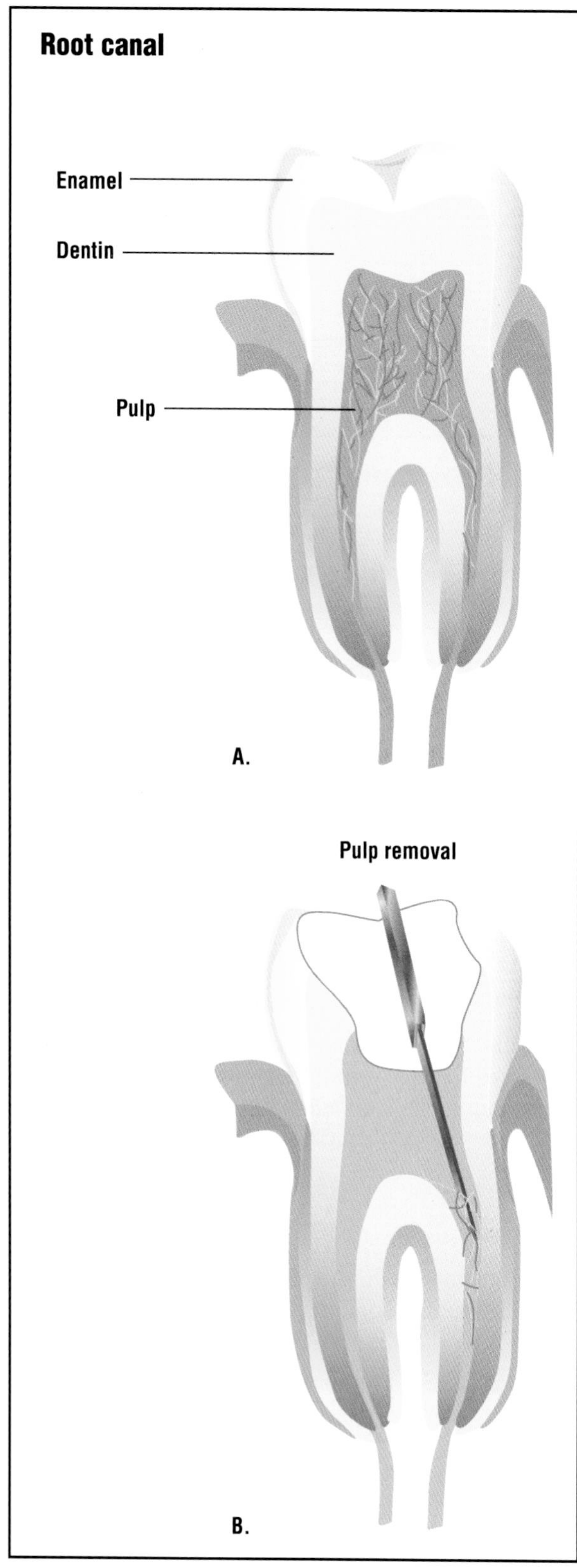

During a root canal, the diseased pulp of a tooth (A), is removed (B). The remaining empty tooth is filled and sealed with a filling or crown. *(Illustration by GGS Information Services. Cengage Learning, Gale.)*

KEY TERMS

Abscess—A cavity or space in tooth or gum tissue filled with pus as the result of infection. Its swelling exerts pressure on the surrounding tissues, causing pain.

Apicoectomy—Also called root resectioning. The root tip of a tooth is accessed in the bone and a small amount is shaved away. The diseased tissue is removed and a filling is placed to reseal the canal.

Crown—The natural crown of a tooth is that part of the tooth covered by enamel. Also, a restorative crown is a protective shell that fits over a tooth.

Endodontic—Pertaining to the inside structures of the tooth, including the dental pulp and tooth root, and the periapical tissue surrounding the root.

Endodontist—A dentist who specializes in the diagnosis and treatment of disorders affecting the inside structures of teeth.

Extraction—The surgical removal of a tooth from its socket in a bone.

Gutta percha—An inert, latex-like substance used for filling root canals.

Pulp—The soft innermost layer of a tooth, containing blood vessels and nerves.

Pulp chamber—The area within the tooth occupied by dental pulp.

Pulpitis—Inflammation of the pulp of a tooth involving the blood vessels and nerves.

Root canal—The space within a tooth that runs from the pulp chamber to the tip of the root.

Root canal treatment—The process of removing diseased or damaged pulp from a tooth, then filling and sealing the pulp chamber and root canals.

result in prolonged sensitivity to heat or cold, swelling, and tenderness in the surrounding gums, facial swelling, or discoloration of the tooth. In some cases, however, the pulp may die so gradually that there is little noticeable pain.

Root canal treatment is performed under **local anesthesia**. A thin sheet of rubber, called a rubber dam, is placed in the mouth and around the base of the tooth to isolate the tooth and help to keep the operative field dry. The dentist removes any tooth decay and makes an opening through the natural crown of the tooth into the pulp chamber. Creating this access also relieves the pressure inside the tooth and can dramatically ease pain.

The dentist determines the length of the root canals, usually with a series of x rays. Small wire-like files are then used to clean the entire canal space of diseased pulp tissue and bacteria. The debris is flushed out with large amounts of water (irrigation). The canals are also slightly enlarged and shaped to receive an inert (non-reactive) filling material called gutta percha. However, the tooth is not filled and permanently sealed until it is completely free of active infection. The dentist may place a temporary seal, or leave the tooth open to drain, and prescribe an antibiotic to counter any spread of infection from the tooth. This is why root canal treatment may require several visits to the dentist.

Once the canals are completely clean, they are filled with gutta percha and a sealer cement to prevent bacteria from entering the tooth in the future. A metal post may be placed in the pulp chamber for added structural support and better retention of the crown restoration. The tooth is protected by a temporary filling or crown until a permanent restoration may be made. This restoration is usually a gold or porcelain crown, although it may be a gold inlay, or an amalgam or composite filling (paste fillings that harden).

Diagnosis/Preparation

Signs that a root canal treatment is necessary include severe pain while chewing, prolonged sensitivity to heat or cold, or a darkening of the tooth. Swelling and tenderness of the gums or pimples appearing on the gums are also common symptoms. However, it is also possible that no symptoms will be noticed. The dentist will take an x ray of the tooth to determine if there is any sign of infection in the surrounding bone.

Aftercare

Once a root canal treatment is performed, the recipient must have a crown placed over the tooth to protect it. The cost of the treatment and the crown may be expensive. However, replacing an extracted tooth with a fixed bridge, a removable partial denture, or an implant to maintain the space and restore the chewing function is typically even more expensive.

During the time when **antibiotics** are being used, care should be taken to avoid using the tooth to chew food. The tooth has been structurally weakened and may break, or there is a possibility of the interior of the tooth becoming reinfected.

If the tooth feels sensitive following the procedure, a standard over-the-counter pain medication such as ibuprofen or naproxen may be taken. This sensitivity will fade after a few days. In most cases the patient can resume regular activity the following day.

WHO PERFORMS THE PROCEDURE AND WHERE IS IT PERFORMED?

A root canal treatment may be performed by a general dentist or by an endodontist. An endodontist is a dentist who specializes in endodontic (literally "inside of the tooth") procedures. The procedure is usually performed in a professional dental office. In rare situations, it may be performed in a hospital outpatient facility.

Risks

There is a possibility that a root canal treatment will not be successful the first time. If infection and inflammation recur and an x ray indicates a repeat treatment is feasible, the old filling material is removed and the canals are thoroughly cleaned out. The dentist will try to identify and correct problems with the first root canal treatment before filling and sealing the tooth a second time.

In cases where an x ray indicates that another root canal treatment cannot correct the problem, endodontic surgery may be performed. In a procedure called an apicoectomy, or root resectioning, the root end of the tooth is accessed in the bone, and a small amount is shaved away. The area is cleaned of diseased tissue and a filling is placed to reseal the canal.

Normal results

With successful root canal treatment, the tooth will no longer cause pain. However, because it does not contain an internal nerve, it no longer has sensitivity to hot, cold, or sweets. Because these are signs of dental decay, the root canal recipient must receive regular dental check-ups with periodic x rays to avoid further disease in the tooth. The restored tooth may last a lifetime. However, with routine wear, the filling or crown may eventually need to be replaced.

Morbidity and mortality rates

In some cases, despite proper root canal treatment and endodontic surgery, the tooth dies and must be extracted. This is relatively uncommon.

QUESTIONS TO ASK THE DOCTOR

What will be the resulting functional capacity of the tooth?

Is the oral surgeon board certified in endodontic surgery?

How many root canal procedures has the oral surgeon performed?

What is the oral surgeon's complication rate?

Alternatives

The only alternative to performing a root canal procedure is to extract the diseased tooth. After restoration or extraction, the two main goals are to allow normal chewing and to maintain proper alignment and spacing between teeth. A fixed bridge, a removable partial denture or an implant will accomplish both goals. However, these are usually more expensive than a root canal treatment.

Resources

BOOKS

Peterson, L. J., E. Ellis, J. R. Hupp, and M. R. Tucker. *Contemporary Oral and Maxillofacial Surgery,* 4th ed. Amsterdam: Elsevier, 2002.

Tronstad, L. *Clinical Endodontics: A Textbook,* 2nd ed. New York: Thieme Medical Publishers, 2003.

Walton, R. E. and M. Torabinejad. *Principles and Practice of Endodontics,* 3rd ed. Philadelphia: Saunders, 2001.

Wray, D. *Textbook of General and Oral Surgery.* Amsterdam: Elsevier, 2003.

PERIODICALS

Bader, H. I. "Treatment planning for implants versus root canal therapy: a contemporary dilemma." *Implant Dentistry* 11, no. 3 (2002): 217–223.

Buchanan, L. S. "Negotiating root canals to their termini." *Dentistry Today* 19, no. 11 (2001): 60–71.

Douglass, A. B., and J. M. Douglass. "Common dental emergencies." *American Family Physician* 67, no. 3 (2003): 511–516.

Himel, V. T., and M. E. Levitan. "Use of nickel titanium instruments for cleaning and shaping root canal systems." *Texas Dental Journal* 120, no. 3 (2003): 262–268.

ORGANIZATIONS

Academy of General Dentistry, 211 East Chicago Avenue, Chicago, IL 60611. (312) 440-4300. http://www.agd.org.

American Academy of Pediatric Dentistry, 211 East Chicago Avenue, #700, Chicago, IL 60611-2663. (312) 337-2169. Fax: (312) 337-6329. http://www.aapd.org.

American Association of Endodontists, 211 E. Chicago Ave., Suite 1100, Chicago, IL 60611-2691. (800) 872-3636 or (312) 266-7255. Fax: (866) 451-9020 or (312) 266-9867. E-mail: info@aae.org. http://www.aae.org.

American Dental Association, 211 E. Chicago Avenue, Chicago, IL 60611. (312) 440-2500. Fax: (312) 440-7494. http://www.ada.org.

OTHER

Animated-Teeth.com. [cited May 2, 2003]. http://www.animated-teeth.com/root_canal/t1_root_canal.htm.

Health Promotion Board of Singapore. [cited May 2, 2003]. http://www.hpb.gov.sg/hpb/haz/haz03029.asp.

New Zealand Dental Association. [cited May 2, 2003]. http://www.nzda.org.nz/public/rootcanals.htm.

L. Fleming Fallon, Jr., MD, DrPH

Rotator cuff repair

Definition

Rotator cuff surgery is the repair of inflammation or tears of the rotator cuff tendons in the shoulder. There are four tendons in the rotator cuff, and these tendons are attached individually to the following muscles: teres minor, subscapularis, infraspinatus, and the supraspinatus. The tears and inflammation associated with rotator cuff injury occur in the region near where these tendon/muscle complexes attach to the humerus (upper arm) bone.

Purpose

Rotator cuff surgery is necessary when chronic shoulder pain associated with rotator cuff injury does not respond to conservative therapy such as rest, heat/ice application, or the use of non-steroidal anti-inflammatory drugs (NSAIDs). Rotator cuff injuries are often lumped into the category referred to as rotator cuff syndrome. Rotator cuff syndrome describes a range of symptoms from basic sprains and tendon swelling (tendonitis) to total rupture or tearing of the tendon.

Demographics

Approximately 5–10% of the general population is believed to have rotator cuff syndrome at a given time. It is not commonly found in individuals under the age of 20 years, even though many in this population are athletically active. In general, males are more likely than females to develop rotator cuff syndrome and require surgery. Most rotator cuff injuries are

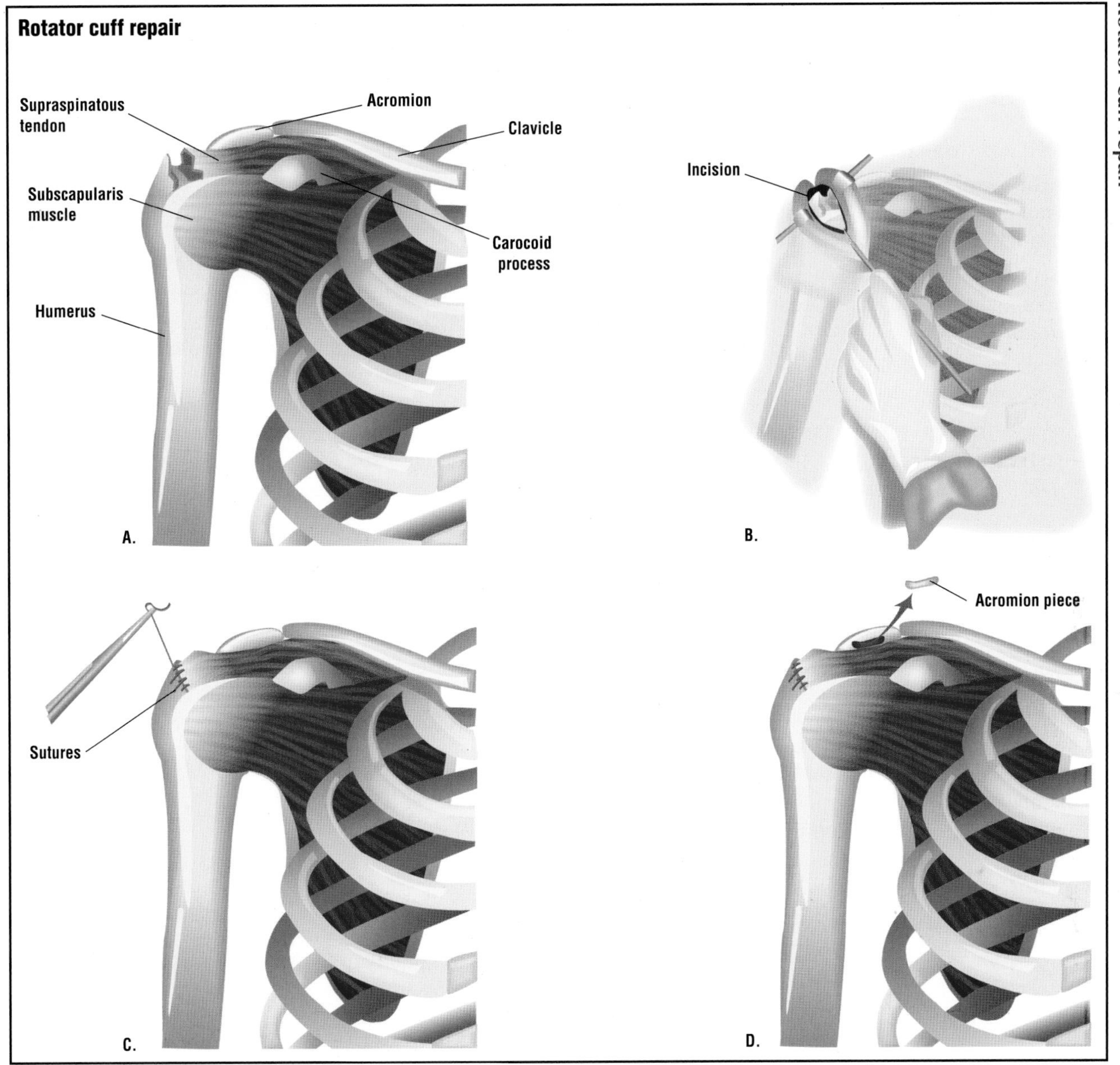

A rotator cuff injury results in a torn tendon at the top of the shoulder (A). To repair it, an incision is made over the site of the tear (B). The tendon's attachment to the bone is repaired with sutures (C), and a small piece of bone from the acromion may be removed (D) to ensure smoother movement of the tendons. *(Illustration by GGS Information Services. Cengage Learning, Gale.)*

associated with athletic activities such as baseball, tennis, weight lifting, and swimming, where the arms are repeatedly lifted over the head. Rotator cuff injuries can also occur in accidents involving falling to the ground or when the humerus is pushed into the shoulder socket. Rotator cuff injuries can also occur in older, active individuals because the rotator cuff tendons begin to deteriorate after age 40. Occupations that have been associated with rotator cuff injuries include nursing, painting, carpentry, tree pruning, fruit picking, and grocery clerking.

Description

For most patients, if the pain begins to subside, they are encouraged to undergo a period of physical therapy. If the pain does not subside after a few weeks, then the physician may suggest the use of cortisone

KEY TERMS

Adhesions—A fibrous band that holds together tissue that are usually separated and that are associated with wound healing.

Arthrography—Visualization of a joint by radiographic means following injection of a contrast dye into the joint space.

Arthroscope—An endoscope, or a tube containing an optical system, that is used to examine the interior of a joint.

Bone spurs—A sharp or pointed calcified projection.

Bursa—A sac found in connective tissue that acts to reduce friction between tendon and bone.

Deltoid muscle—Muscle that covers the prominence of the shoulder.

WHO PERFORMS THE PROCEDURE AND WHERE IS IT PERFORMED?

Rotator cuff repair is generally performed by a specialist known as an orthopedic surgeon, who has received specialized training in the diseases and injuries of the musculoskeletal system. Orthopedic surgeons who perform rotator cuff repair receive extensive training in general surgery and in the specific techniques involving the musculoskeletal system. Rotator cuff repairs are often performed in the specialized department of a general hospital, but they are also performed in specialized orthopedic surgery clinics or institutes for orthopedic conditions.

injections into the shoulder region. Rotator cuff repair is then considered if the more conservative methods are not successful.

The primary aim of rotator cuff repair is to repair the connection between the damaged tendon and the bone. Once this bridge is re-established and the connection between the tendon and the bone has thoroughly healed, the corresponding muscles can once again move the arm in a normal fashion. The goal of the surgery is to ensure the smooth movement of the rotator cuff tendons and bursa under the upper part of the shoulder blade. The surgery is also performed to improve the comfort of the patient and to normalize the function of the shoulder and arm. There are a variety of surgical approaches that can be used to accomplish rotator cuff repair. The most common approach is called the anterior acromioplasty approach. This approach allows for excellent access to the most common sites of tears—the biceps groove, anterior cuff, and the undersurface of the joint.

Three types of rotator cuff repair surgeries are performed: open incision, mini-open incision, and arthroscopic. Most rotator cuff repairs are accomplished using incisions that minimize cosmetic changes in the skin following healing. If possible, the surgery is performed with an arthroscope to minimize cosmetic damage to the skin. Typically, the incision made is about the size of a buttonhole. The arthroscope, a pencil-sized instrument, is then inserted into the joint. The surgeon usually accesses the rotator cuff by opening part of the deltoid muscle. If bone spurs, adhesions, and damaged bursa are present in the rotator cuff region, then the surgeon will generally remove these damaged structures to improve function in the joint. In cases where the arthroscopic technique is not advised or when it fails to achieve the desired results, a conversion to open surgery is made. This involves a larger incision and usually requires more extensive anesthesia and a longer recovery period.

The success of the rotator cuff repair is dependent on the following factors:

- age of the patient
- type of surgical technique employed
- degree of damage present
- patient's recovery goals
- patient's ability to follow a physical therapy program following surgery
- smoking status
- number of previous cortisone injections

Diagnosis/Preparation

The diagnosis of rotator cuff injury is based on a combination of clinical signs and symptoms, coupled with diagnostic testing. The most common clinical signs and symptoms include:

- tenderness in the rotator cuff
- pain associated with the movement of the arm above the head
- pain that is fairly constant but more intense at night
- weakness or pain with the forward movement of the arm
- muscle atrophy (wasting) in long-term injuries that involve a complete tendon tear

QUESTIONS TO ASK THE DOCTOR

- What are my alternatives?
- Is surgery the answer for me?
- Can you recommend a surgeon who performs rotator cuff repairs?
- If surgery is appropriate for me, what are the next steps?

X rays are used to rule out other types of injuries or abnormalities present in the shoulder region. While x rays are often used to help solidify the diagnosis, **arthrography**, ultrasonography, computed tomography (CT), and **magnetic resonance imaging** (MRI) are the definitive tests in the diagnosis of rotator cuff injury. Arthography and ultrasonography of the shoulder can help determine whether or not there is a full tear in the rotator cuff. A MRI can help determine whether there is a full tear, partial tear, chronic tendonitis, or other cause of the shoulder pain. The final decision to repair the tear ultimately rests on the amount of pain and restriction suffered by the patient.

Aftercare

Following the procedure, the patient will typically spend several hours in the **recovery room**. Generally, an ice pack will be applied to the affected shoulder joint for a period up to 48 hours. The patient will usually be given either prescription or non-prescription pain medication. The dressing is usually removed the day after surgery and is replaced by adhesive strips. The patient should contact a physician if there are any significant changes in the affected area once the patient goes home. These changes can include increased swelling, pain, bleeding, drainage in the affected area, nausea, vomiting, or signs of infection. Signs of infection include fever, dizziness, headache, and muscle aches.

It often takes several days for the arthroscopic puncture wounds to heal, and the joint usually takes several weeks to recover. Most patients can resume normal daily activities, with the permission of a physician, within a few days following the procedure. Most patients are advised to undergo a rehabilitation program that includes physical therapy. Such a program can facilitate recovery and improve the functioning of the joint in the future.

QUESTIONS TO ASK THE SURGEON

- How many times have you performed rotator cuff repair?
- Are you a board-certified surgeon?
- What type of outcomes have you had?
- What are the most common side effects or complications?
- What should I do to prepare for surgery?
- What should I expect following the surgery?
- Can you refer me to one of your patients who has had this procedure?
- What type of diagnostic procedures are performed to determine if patients require surgery?
- Will I need to see another specialist for the diagnostic procedures?

Risks

Complications following arthroscopic rotator cuff surgery are very rare. Such complications occur in less than 1% of cases. These complications include instrument breakage, blood vessel or nerve damage, blood vessel clots, infection, and inflammation. Complications, though still rare, are more common following open surgery. This is due to the larger incisions and more complicated anesthesia that is often necessary.

Normal results

The prognosis for the long-term relief from rotator cuff syndrome is good, especially when both conservative and surgical therapeutic approaches are used. In those patients who do require surgery, six weeks of physical therapy is typically instituted following surgery. Complete recovery following surgery may take several months. In rare cases, the rotator cuff injury is so severe that the patient may require muscle transfers and tendon grafts. Even more rarely, the injury can be so severe that the tendons are not repairable. This typically occurs when a severe rotator cuff injury is neglected for a long period of time.

Morbidity and mortality rates

Morbidity is rare in both the arthroscopic and open procedures. Mortality is exceedingly rare in patients undergoing rotator cuff repair.

Alternatives

Conservative approaches are typically used before surgery is considered in patients with rotator cuff injury. This is true even in cases where there is evidence of a full tendon tear. Some patients with a full or partial tear do not suffer a significant amount of pain and retain normal or nearly normal range of motion in shoulder movement. A majority of those with rotator cuff syndrome respond to conservative non-surgical approaches. Conservative therapies include the following:

- heat or ice to reduce pain and swelling
- cessation or reduction of activities that involve the movement of the arms overhead
- medication such as non-steroidal anti-inflammatory agents to reduce pain and inflammation
- cortisone injections to reduce pain and inflammation
- rest

Once the pain begins to subside, the patient usually is encouraged to begin a program of physical therapy to help re-institute normal motion and function to the shoulder.

Resources

BOOKS

Browner BD et al. *Skeletal Trauma: Basic science, management, and reconstruction*. 3rd ed. Philadelphia: Elsevier, 2003.

Canale, ST, ed. *Campbell's Operative Orthopaedics*. 10th ed. St. Louis: Mosby, 2003.

DeLee, JC and D. Drez. *DeLee and Drez's Orthopaedic Sports Medicine*. 2nd ed. Philadelphia: Saunders, 2005.

PERIODICALS

Welling, Ken R. "Rotator Cuff Surgery." *Surgical Technologist* 31 (1999): 4.

Mark Mitchell

Routine urinalysis *see* **Urinalysis**

S

Sacral nerve stimulation

Definition

Sacral nerve stimulation, also known as sacral neuromodulation, is a procedure in which the sacral nerve at the base of the spine is stimulated by a mild electrical current from an implanted device. It is done to improve functioning of the urinary tract, to relieve pain related to urination, and to control fecal incontinence.

Purpose

As a proven treatment for urinary incontinence, sacral nerve stimulation (SNS) has recently been found effective in the treatment of interstitial cystitis, a disorder that involves hyperreflexia of the urinary sphincter. SNS is also used to treat pelvic or urinary pain as well as fecal incontinence.

A person's ability to hold urine or feces depends on three body functions:

- a reservoir function represented by the urethra/bladder or colon
- a gatekeeping function represented by the urethral or anal sphincter and
- the brain's ability to control urination, defecation, and nerve sensitivity

A dysfunction or deficiency in any of these components can result in incontinence. The most common forms of incontinence are stress urinary incontinence and urge incontinence. Stress incontinence is related to an unstable detrusor muscle that controls the urinary sphincter. When the detrusor muscle is weak, urine can leak out of the bladder from pressure on the abdomen caused by sneezing, coughing, and other movements. Urge incontinence is characterized by a sudden strong need to urinate and inability to hold urine until an appropriate time; it is also associated with hyperactivity of the urinary sphincter. Both conditions can be treated by SNS. SNS requires an implanted device that sends continuous stimulation to the sacral nerve that controls the urinary sphincter. This treatment has been used with over 1500 patients with a high rate of success. It was approved in Europe in 1994. The Food and Drug Administration (FDA) approved SNS for the treatment of urinary urge incontinence in 1997 and for urinary frequency in 1999.

Interstitial cystitis (IC) is a chronic condition of unknown origin that causes pain in the bladder and lower abdomen, urinary urgency, a frequent need to urinate at night, and pain during intercourse. IC has no known cause; it is diagnosed by the level of reported discomfort and by excluding other sources of urinary pain, frequency and urgency. SNS has only recently been used to treat IC. According to three studies presented to the American Urological Association in 2001, SNS significantly reduced urinary urgency and frequency, with some relief of pain, in patients who had not responded to other treatments. The use of SNS in treating IC is still considered experimental, however.

Treatment of fecal incontinence with SNS is very recent; it is also considered experimental. Newer research from Italy, however, indicates that patients with anorectal disturbances that are usually treated by augmentation of the sphincter muscle or implanting an artificial sphincter can benefit from electrical stimulation of the sacral nerve. Although the mechanism of SNS is not completely clear, researchers believe that the patient's control of the pelvic region is restored by the stimulation or activation of afferent fibers in the muscles of the pelvic floor.

Demographics

Urinary incontinence affects between 15% and 30% of American adults living in the community, and as many as 50% of people confined to **nursing homes**. It is a disorder that affects women far more frequently than men; 85% of people suffering from urinary incontinence are women. According to the chief of geriatrics

KEY TERMS

Afferent fibers—Nerve fibers that conduct nerve impulses from tissues and organs toward the central nervous system.

Detrusor muscle—The medical name for the layer of muscle tissue covering the urinary bladder. When the detrusor muscle contracts, the bladder expels urine.

Fecal incontinence—Inability to control bowel movements.

Hyperreflexia—A condition in which the detrusor muscle of the bladder contracts too frequently, leading to inability to hold one's urine.

Interstitial cystitis—A condition of unknown origin that causes urinary urgency, pain in the bladder and abdomen, and pain during sexual intercourse.

Neuromodulation—Electrical stimulation of a nerve for relief of pain.

Sacral nerve—The nerve in the lower back region of the spine that controls the need to urinate.

Sphincter—A ringlike band of muscle that tightens or closes the opening to a body organ.

Urgency—A sudden compelling need to urinate.

Urinary incontinence—Inability to control urination.

at a Boston hospital, 25 million Americans suffer each year from occasional episodes of urinary or fecal incontinence.

Interstitial cystitis is less common than urinary or fecal incontinence but still affects about 12% of women in the United States each year. The average age of IC patients is 40; 25% of patients are younger than 30. Although 90% of patients diagnosed with IC are women, it is thought that the disorder may be underdiagnosed in men.

Description

Sacral nerve stimulation (SNS) is conducted through an implanted device that includes a thin insulated wire called a lead and a neurostimulator much like a cardiac pacemaker. The device is inserted in a pocket in the patient's lower abdomen. SNS is first tried on an outpatient basis in the doctor's office with the implantation of a test lead. If the trial treatment is successful, the patient is scheduled for inpatient surgery.

Permanent surgical implantation is done under **general anesthesia** and requires a one-night stay in the hospital. After the patient has been anesthetized, the surgeon implants the neurostimulator, which is about the size of a pocket stopwatch, under the skin of the patient's abdomen. Thin wires, or leads, running from the stimulator carry electrical pulses from the stimulator to the sacral nerves located in the lower back. After the stimulator and leads have been implanted, the surgeon closes the incision in the abdomen.

Diagnosis/Preparation

Incontinence significantly affects a patient's quality of life; thus patients usually consult a doctor when their urinary problems begin to cause difficulties in the workplace or on social occasions. A family care practitioner will usually refer the patient to a urologist for diagnosis of the cause(s) of the incontinence. Patients with urinary and fecal incontinence are evaluated carefully through the taking of a complete patient history and a **physical examination**. The doctor will use special techniques to assess the capacity of the bladder or rectum as well as the functioning of the urethral or anal sphincter in order to determine the cause or location of the incontinence. **Cystoscopy**, which is the examination of the full bladder with a scope attached to a small tube, allows the physician to rule out certain disorders as well as plan the most effective treatment. These extensive tests are especially important in diagnosing interstitial cystitis because all other causes of urinary urgency, frequency, and pain must be ruled out before surgery can be suggested. Cystoscopy is done under anesthesia and often works as a treatment for IC. Once the doctor has made the diagnosis of urinary incontinence due to sphincter insufficiency, he or she will explain and discuss the surgical implant with the patient. SNS may be tried out on a temporary basis. The same pattern of diagnosis and treatment is used for patients with IC and fecal incontinence. Temporary implants can help eliminate those patients who will not benefit from a permanent implant.

Aftercare

Following surgery, the patient remains overnight in the hospital. **Antibiotics** may be given to reduce the risk of infection and pain medications to relieve discomfort. The patient will be given instructions on **incision care** and follow-up appointments before he or she leaves the hospital.

Aftercare includes fine-tuning of the SNS stimulator. The doctor can adjust the strength of the electrical

WHO PERFORMS THE PROCEDURE AND WHERE IS IT PERFORMED?

SNS devices are implanted under general anesthesia by urologists, who are physicians specializing in treating disorders of the urinary tract. The procedure is usually performed in a hospital.

QUESTIONS TO ASK THE DOCTOR

- Am I likely to benefit from SNS?
- How many stimulators have you implanted?
- How many of your patients consider SNS a successful treatment?
- What side effects have your patients reported?

impulses in his or her office with a handheld programmer. The stimulator runs for about five to 10 years and can be replaced during an outpatient procedure. About a third of patients require a second operation to adjust or replace various elements of the stimulator device.

Risks

In addition to the risks of bleeding and infection that are common to surgical procedures, implanting an SNS device carries the risks of pain at the insertion site, discomfort when urinating, mild electrical shocks, and displacement or dislocation of the leads.

Normal results

Patients report improvement in the number of urinations, the volume of urine produced, lessened urgency, and higher overall quality of life after treatment with SNS. Twenty-two patients undergoing a three- to seven-day test of sacral nerve stimulation on an outpatient basis reported significant reduction in urgency and frequency, according to the American Urological Association. Studies have indicated complete success in about 50% of patients. Sacral nerve stimulation is being used to treat fecal incontinence in the United States and Europe, with promising early reports. As of 2003, SNS is the least invasive of the recognized surgical treatments for fecal incontinence.

Morbidity and mortality rates

Sacral nerve stimulation has been shown to be a safe and effective procedure for the treatment of both urinary and fecal incontinence. Two groups of researchers, in Spain and the United Kingdom respectively, have reported that "The effects of neuromodulation are long-lasting and associated morbidity is low." The most commonly reported complications of SNS are pain at the site of the implant (15.3% of patients); pain on urination (9%); and displacement of the leads (8.4%).

Alternatives

There are three types of nonsurgical treatments that benefit some patients with IC:

- Behavioral approaches. These include biofeedback, diet modifications, bladder retraining, and pelvic muscle exercises.
- Medications. These include antispasmodic drugs, tricyclic antidepressants, and pentosan polysulfate sodium, which is sold under the trade name Elmiron. Elmiron appears to work by protecting the lining of the bladder from bacteria and other irritating substances in urine.
- Intravesical medications. These are medications that affect the muscular tissues of the bladder. Oxybutynin is a drug that is prescribed for patients who are incontinent because their bladders fail to store urine properly. Capsaicin and resiniferatoxin are used to treat hyperreflexia of the detrusor muscle.

Surgical alternatives to SNS are considered treatments of last resort for IC because they are invasive, irreversible, and benefit only 30–40% of patients. In addition, some studies indicate that these surgeries can lead to long-term kidney damage. They include the following procedures:

- Augmentation cystoplasty. In this procedure, the surgeon removes the patient's bladder and replaces it with a section of the bowel—in effect creating a new bladder. The patient passes urine through the urethra in the normal fashion.
- Urinary diversion. The surgeon creates a tube from a section of the patient's bowel and places the ureters (tubes that carry urine from the kidneys to the bladder) in this tube. The tube is then attached to a stoma, or opening in the abdomen. Urine is carried into an external collection bag that the patient must empty several times daily.
- Internal pouch. The surgeon creates a new bladder from a section of the bowel and attaches it inside the abdomen. The patient empties the pouch by self-catheterization four to six times daily.

Resources

BOOKS

Feldman, M, et al.. *Sleisenger & Fordtran's Gastrointestinal and Liver Disease*. 8th ed. St. Louis: Mosby, 2005.

Katz VL et al. *Comprehensive Gynecology*. 5th ed. St. Louis: Mosby, 2007.

Wein, AJ et al. *Campbell-Walsh Urology*. 9th ed. Philadelphia: Saunders, 2007.

PERIODICALS

Leng WW. "Sacral Nerve Stimulation for the Overactive Bladder." *Urology Clinics of North America* 33 (November 2006): 494-501.

Siegel SW. "Selecting Patients for Sacral Nerve Stimulation." *Urology Clinics of North America* 32 (February 2005): 19-26.

ORGANIZATIONS

American Urological Association (AUA). 1120 North Charles Street, Baltimore, MD 21201. (410) 727-1100. www.auanet.org.

National Association for Continence (NAFC). P. O. Box 1019, Charleston, SC 29402-1019. (843) 377-0900. www. nafc.org.

National Kidney Foundation. 30 East 33rd Street, Suite 1100, New York, NY 10016. (800) 622-9010 or (212) 889-2210. www.kidney.org.

National Kidney and Urologic Diseases Information Clearinghouse (NKUDIC). 3 Information Way, Bethesda, MD 20892-3580.

OTHER

"Sacral Nerve Stimulation." Mayo Clinic. www.mayoclinic.org/incontinence-jax/sacralstim.html.

"Sacral Nerve Stimulation Can Relieve Interstitial Cystitis, Studies Suggest." Interstitial Cystitis Association. www.ichelp.com/research/SacralNerveStimulationCanRelieveIC.html.

Nancy McKenzie, PhD

Salpingo-oophorectomy

Definition

Unilateral salpingo-oophorectomy is the surgical removal of a fallopian tube and an ovary. If both sets of fallopian tubes and ovaries are removed, the procedure is called a bilateral salpingo-oophorectomy.

Purpose

This surgery is performed to treat ovarian or other gynecological cancers, or infections caused by pelvic inflammatory disease. Occasionally, removal of one or both ovaries may be done to treat endometriosis, a condition in which the lining of the uterus (the endometrium) grows outside of the uterus (usually on and around the pelvic organs). The procedure may also be performed if a woman has been diagnosed with an ectopic pregnancy in a fallopian tube and a **salpingostomy** (an incision into the fallopian tube to remove the pregnancy) cannot be done. If only one fallopian tube and ovary are removed, the woman may still be able to conceive and carry a pregnancy to term. If both are removed, however, the woman is rendered permanently infertile. This procedure is commonly combined with a **hysterectomy** (surgical removal of the uterus); the ovaries and fallopian tubes are removed in about one-third of hysterectomies.

Until the 1980s, women over age 40 having hysterectomies routinely had healthy ovaries and fallopian tubes removed at the same time. Many physicians reasoned that a woman over 40 was approaching menopause and soon her ovaries would stop secreting estrogen and releasing eggs. Removing the ovaries would eliminate the risk of ovarian cancer and only accelerate menopause by a few years.

In the 1990s, the thinking about routine salpingo-oophorectomy began to change. The risk of ovarian cancer in women who have no family history of the disease is less than 1%. Moreover, removing the ovaries increases the risk of cardiovascular disease and accelerates osteoporosis unless a woman takes prescribed hormone replacements.

Demographics

Overall, ovarian cancer accounts for only 4% of all cancers in women. For women at increased risk, **oophorectomy** may be considered after the age of 35 if childbearing is complete. Factors that increase a woman's risk of developing ovarian cancer include age (most ovarian cancers occur after menopause), the presence of a mutation in the BRCA1 or BRCA2 gene, the number of menstrual periods a woman has had (affected by age of onset, pregnancy, breastfeeding, and oral contraceptive use), history of breast cancer, diet, and family history. The incidence of ovarian cancer is highest among Native American (17.5 cases per 100,000 population), Caucasian (15.8 per 100,000), Vietnamese (13.8 per 100,000), Hispanic (12.1 per 100,000), and Hawaiian (11.8 per 100,000) women; it is lowest among Korean (7.0 per 100,000) and Chinese (9.3 per 100,000) women. African American women have an ovarian cancer incidence of 10.2 per 100,000 population.

Endometriosis, another reason why salpingo-oophorectomy may be performed, has been estimated

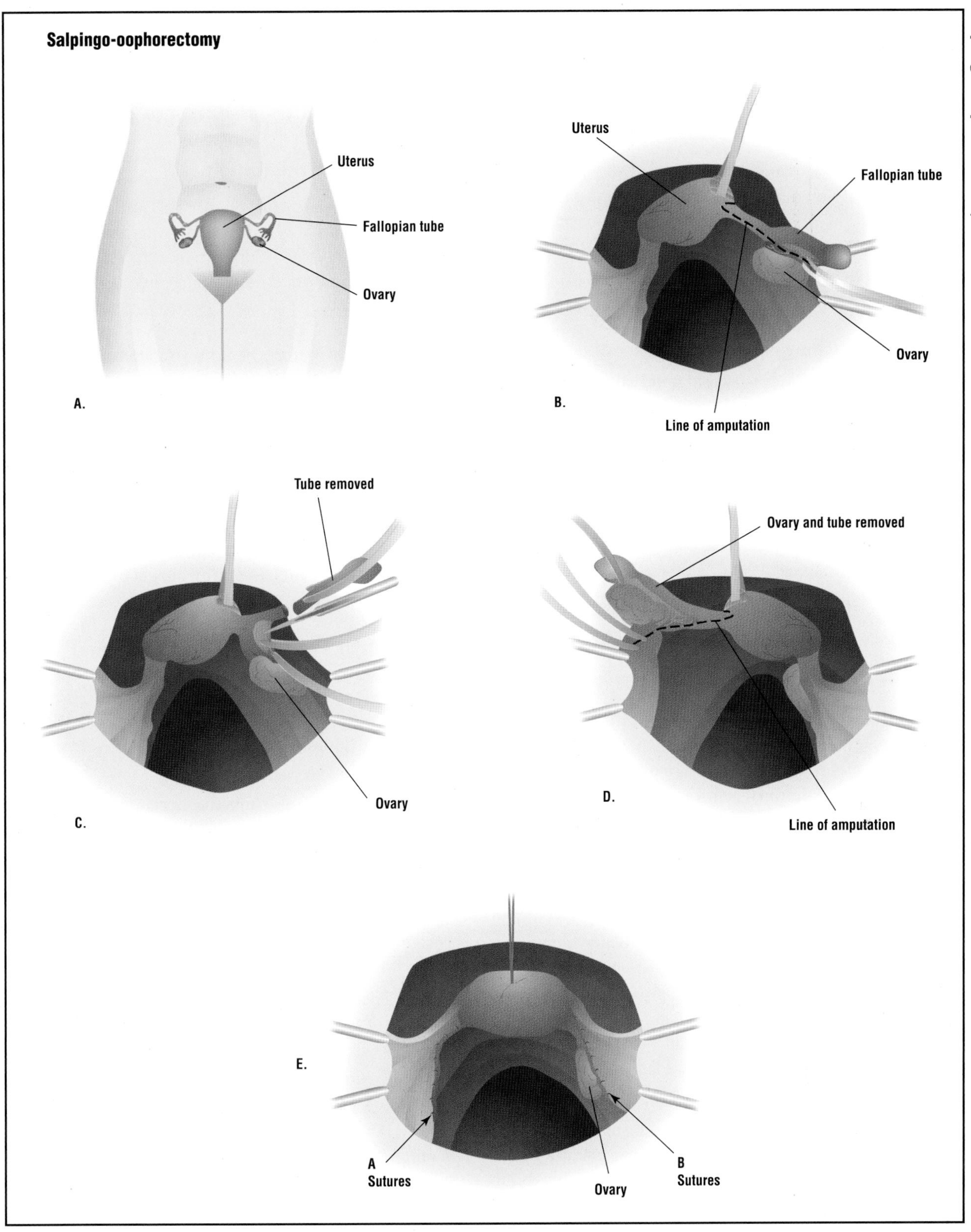

In a salpingo-oophorectomy, a woman's reproductive organs are accessed through an incision in the lower abdomen, or laparoscopically (A). Once the area is visualized, a diseased fallopian tube can be severed from the uterus and removed (B and C). The ovary can also be removed with the tube (D). The remaining structures are stitched (E), and the wound is closed. *(Illustration by GGS Information Services. Cengage Learning, Gale.)*

KEY TERMS

BRCA1 or BRCA2 genetic mutation—A genetic mutation that predisposes otherwise healthy women to breast cancer.

Endometriosis—A painful disease in which cells from the lining of the uterus (endometrium) become attached to other organs in the pelvic cavity. The condition is hard to diagnose and often causes severe pain as well as infertility.

Fallopian tubes—Tubes that extend from either end of the uterus that convey the egg from the ovary to the uterus during each monthly cycle.

Hysterectomy—The surgical removal of the uterus.

Ureter—The tube that carries urine from the bladder to the kidneys.

to affect up to 10% of women. Approximately four out of every 1,000 women are hospitalized as a result of endometriosis each year. Women 25–35 years of age are affected most, with 27 being the average age of diagnosis.

Description

General or regional anesthesia will be given to the patient before the procedure begins. If the procedure is performed through a laparoscope, the surgeon can avoid a large abdominal incision and can shorten recovery. With this technique, the surgeon makes a small cut through the abdominal wall just below the navel. A tube containing a tiny lens and light source (a laparoscope) is then inserted through the incision. A camera can be attached that allows the surgeon to see the abdominal cavity on a video monitor. When the ovaries and fallopian tubes are detached, they are removed though a small incision at the top of the vagina. The organs can also be cut into smaller sections and removed. When the laparoscope is used, the patient can be given either regional or **general anesthesia**; if there are no complications, the patient can leave the hospital in a day or two.

If a laparoscope is not used, the surgery involves an incision 4–6 in (10–15 cm) long into the abdomen extending either vertically up from the pubic bone toward the navel, or horizontally (the "bikini incision") across the pubic hairline. The scar from a bikini incision is less noticeable, but some surgeons prefer the vertical incision because it provides greater visibility while operating. A disadvantage to abdominal salpingo-oophorectomy is that bleeding is more likely to be a complication of this type of operation. The procedure is more painful than a laparoscopic operation and the recovery period is longer. A woman can expect to be in the hospital two to five days and will need three to six weeks to return to normal activities.

Diagnosis/Preparation

Before surgery, the doctor will order blood and urine tests, and any additional tests such as **ultrasound** or x rays to help the surgeon visualize the woman's condition. The woman may also meet with the anesthesiologist to evaluate any special conditions that might affect the administration of anesthesia. A colon preparation may be done, if extensive surgery is anticipated.

On the evening before the operation, the woman should eat a light dinner, then take nothing by mouth, including water or other liquids, after midnight.

Aftercare

If performed through an abdominal incision, salpingo-oophorectomy is major surgery that requires three to six weeks for full recovery. However, if performed laparoscopically, the recovery time can be much shorter. There may be some discomfort around the incision for the first few days after surgery, but most women are walking around by the third day. Within a month or so, patients can gradually resume normal activities such as driving, exercising, and working.

Immediately following the operation, the patient should avoid sharply flexing the thighs or the knees. Persistent back pain or bloody or scanty urine indicates that a ureter may have been injured during surgery.

If both ovaries are removed in a premenopausal woman as part of the operation, the sudden loss of estrogen will trigger an abrupt premature menopause that may involve severe symptoms of hot flashes, vaginal dryness, painful intercourse, and loss of sex drive. (This is also called "surgical menopause.") In addition to these symptoms, women who lose both ovaries also lose the protection these hormones provide against heart disease and osteoporosis many years earlier than if they had experienced natural menopause. Women who have had their ovaries removed are seven times more likely to develop coronary heart disease and much more likely to develop bone problems at an early age than are premenopausal women whose ovaries are intact. For these reasons, some form of hormone replacement therapy (HRT) may be prescribed to relieve the symptoms of surgical menopause and to help prevent heart and bone disease.

WHO PERFORMS THE PROCEDURE AND WHERE IS IT PERFORMED?

Salpingo-oophorectomies are usually performed in a hospital operating room by a gynecologist, a medical doctor who has completed specialized training in the areas of women's general health, pregnancy, labor and childbirth, prenatal testing, and genetics.

QUESTIONS TO ASK THE DOCTOR

- Why is a salpingo-oophorectomy being recommended?
- How will the procedure be performed?
- Will one or both sets of ovaries/fallopian tubes be removed?
- What alternatives to salpingo-oophorectomy are available to me?

Reaction to the removal of fallopian tubes and ovaries depends on a wide variety of factors, including the woman's age, the condition that required the surgery, her reproductive history, how much social support she has, and any previous history of depression. Women who have had many gynecological surgeries or chronic pelvic pain seem to have a higher tendency to develop psychological problems after the surgery.

Risks

Major surgery always involves some risk, including infection, reactions to the anesthesia, hemorrhage, and scars at the incision site. Almost all pelvic surgery causes some internal scars, which in some cases can cause discomfort years after surgery.

Potential complications after a salpingo-oophorectomy include changes in sex drive, hot flashes, and other symptoms of menopause if both ovaries are removed. Women who have both ovaries removed and who do not take estrogen replacement therapy run an increased risk for cardiovascular disease and osteoporosis. Women with a history of psychological and emotional problems before an oophorectomy are more likely to experience psychological difficulties after the operation.

Normal results

If the surgery is successful, the fallopian tubes and ovaries will be removed without complication, and the underlying problem resolved. In the case of cancer, all the cancer will be removed. A woman will become infertile following a bilateral salpingo-oophorectomy.

Morbidity and mortality rates

Studies have shown that the complication rate following salpingo-oophorectomy is essentially the same as that following hysterectomy. The rate of complications differs by the type of hysterectomy performed. Abdominal hysterectomy is associated with a higher rate of complications (9.3%), while the overall complication rate for vaginal hysterectomy is 5.3%, and 3.6% for laparoscopic vaginal hysterectomy. The risk of **death** is about one in every 1,000 (1/1,000) women having a hysterectomy. The rates of some of the more commonly reported complications are:

- excessive bleeding (hemorrhaging): 1.8–3.4%
- fever or infection: 0.8–4.0%
- accidental injury to another organ or structure: 1.5–1.8%

Because of the cessation of hormone production that occurs with a bilateral oophorectomy, women who lose both ovaries also prematurely lose the protection these hormones provide against heart disease and osteoporosis. Women who have undergone bilateral oophorectomy are seven times more likely to develop coronary heart disease and much more likely to develop bone problems at an early age than are premenopausal women whose ovaries are intact.

Alternatives

Depending on the specific condition that warrants an oophorectomy, it may be possible to modify the surgery so at least a portion of one ovary remains, allowing the woman to avoid early menopause. In the case of endometriosis, there are a number of alternative treatments that are usually pursued before a salpingo-oophorectomy (with or without hysterectomy) is performed. These include excising the growths without removing any organs, blocking or destroying the nerves that provide sensation to some of the pelvic structures, or prescribing drugs that decrease estrogen levels.

Resources

PERIODICALS

Kauff, N. D., J. M. Satagopan, M. E. Robson, et al. "Risk-Reducing Salpingo-oophorectomy in Women with a BRC1 or BRC2 Mutation." *New England Journal of Medicine* 346 (May 23, 2002): 1609–15.

ORGANIZATIONS

American Cancer Society. 1599 Clifton Road NE, Atlanta, GA 30329. (800) ACS-2345. http://www.cancer.org.

American College of Obstetricians and Gynecologists. 409 12th St., SW, PO Box 96920, Washington, DC 20090-6920. http://www.acog.org.

Midlife Women's Network. 5129 Logan Ave. S., Minneapolis, MN 55419. (800) 886-4354.

OTHER

Hernandez, Manuel, and Robert McNamara. "Endometriosis." *eMedicine*. December 23, 2002 [cited March 15, 2003]. http://www.emedicine.com/aaem/topic181.htm.

Kapoor, Dharmesh. "Endometriosis." *eMedicine*. September 17, 2002 [cited March 15, 2003]. http://www.emedicine.com/med/topic3419.htm.

Surveillance, Epidemiology, and End Results. "Racial/Ethnic Patterns of Cancer in the United States: Ovary." *National Cancer Institute*. 1996 [cited March 14, 2003]. <http://seer.cancer.gov/publications/ethnicity/ovary.pdf>.

"What Is Endometriosis?" *Endo-Online*. 2002 [cited March 15, 2003]. http://www.endometriosisassn.org/endo.html.

Carol A. Turkington
Stephanie Dionne Sherk

Salpingostomy

Definition

A salpingostomy is a surgical incision into a fallopian tube. This procedure may be done to repair a damaged tube or to remove an ectopic pregnancy (one that occurs outside of the uterus).

Purpose

The fallopian tubes are the structures that carry a mature egg from the ovaries to the uterus. These tubes, which are about 4 inches (10 cm) long and 0.2 inches (0.5 cm) in diameter, are found on the upper outer sides of the uterus, and open into the uterus through small channels. It is within the fallopian tubes that fertilization, the joining of an egg and a sperm, takes place.

During a normal pregnancy, the fertilized egg passes from the fallopian tubes into the uterus and then implants into the lining of the uterus. If the fertilized egg implants anywhere outside of the uterus, it is called an ectopic (or tubal) pregnancy. The majority of ectopic pregnancies occur in the fallopian tubes (95%); they may also occur in the uterine muscle (1–2%), the abdomen (1–2%), the ovaries (less than 1%), and the cervix (less than 1%).

As an ectopic pregnancy progresses, the fallopian tubes are unable to contain the growing embryo and may rupture. A ruptured ectopic pregnancy is considered a medical emergency as it can cause significant hemorrhaging (excessive bleeding). If an ectopic pregnancy is diagnosed early (i.e., before rupture has occurred), it may be possible to manage medicinally; the drug methotrexate targets rapidly dividing fetal cells, preventing the fetus from developing further. If medicinal management is not possible or has failed, surgical intervention may be necessary. A salpingostomy may then be performed to remove the pregnancy.

Salpingostomy may also be performed in an effort to restore fertility to a woman whose fallopian tubes have been damaged, such as by adhesions (bands of scar tissue that may form after surgery or trauma). In the case of hydrosalpinx, a condition in which a tube becomes blocked and filled with fluid, a salpingostomy may be performed to create a new tubal ostium (opening).

Demographics

Ectopic pregnancy occurs in approximately 2% of all pregnancies. Once a woman has an ectopic pregnancy, she has an increased chance (10–25%) of having another. Women between the ages of 25 and 34 have a higher incidence of ectopic pregnancy, although the mortality rate among women over the age of 35 is 2.5–5.9 times higher. Minority women are also at an increased risk of ectopic pregnancy-related **death**.

Description

Salpingostomy may be performed via laparotomy or **laparoscopy**, under general or regional anesthesia. A laparotomy is an incision made in the abdominal wall through which the fallopian tubes are visualized. If the tube has already ruptured as a result of an ectopic pregnancy, a salpingectomy will be performed

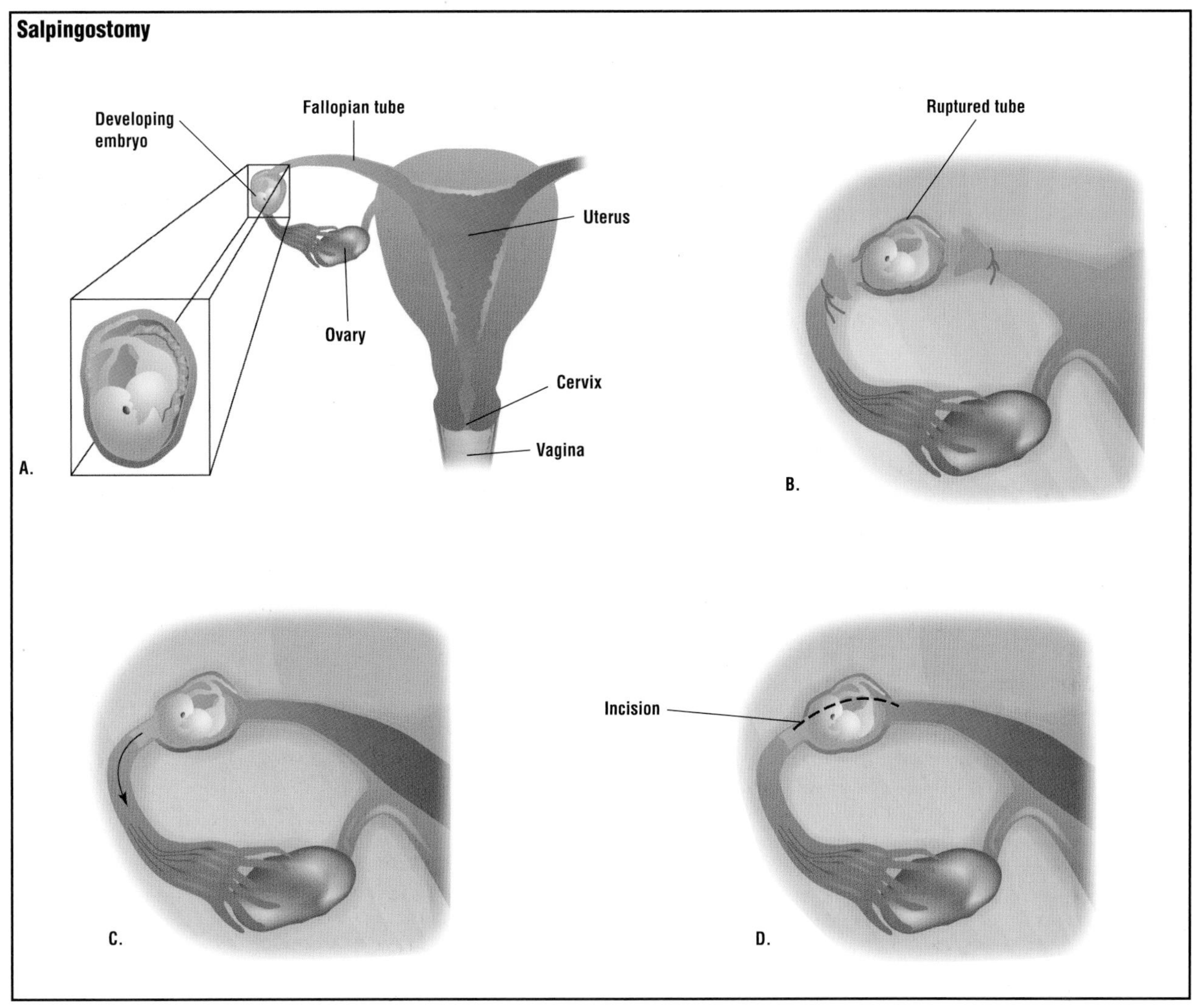

A tubal or ectopic pregnancy can be removed in several ways. If the Fallopian tube is ruptured (A), the tube is tied off on both sides, and the embryo removed. If the tube is intact, the embryo can be pulled out the end of the tube (C), or tube can be cut open and the contents removed (D). *(Illustration by GGS Information Services. Cengage Learning, Gale.)*

to remove the damaged fallopian tube. If rupture has not occurred, a drug called vasopressin is injected into the fallopian tube to minimize the amount of bleeding. An incision (called a linear salpingostomy) is made through the wall of the tube in the area of the ectopic pregnancy. The products of conception are then flushed out of the tube with an instrument called a suction-irrigator. Any bleeding sites are treated by suturing or by applying pressure with forceps. The incision is not sutured but instead left to heal on its own (called closure by secondary intent). The abdominal wall is then closed.

A neosalpingostomy is similar to a linear salpingostomy but is performed to treat a tubal blockage (e.g., hydrosalpinx). An incision is made to create a new opening in the fallopian tube; the tissue is folded over and stitched into place. The new hole, or ostium, replaces the normal opening of the fallopian tube through which the egg released by an ovary each menstrual cycle is collected.

Salpingostomy may also be performed laparoscopically. With this surgery, a tube (called a laparoscope) containing a tiny lens and light source is inserted through a small incision in the navel. A camera can be attached that allows the surgeon to see the abdominal cavity on a video monitor. The salpingostomy is then performed with instruments inserted through **trocars**, small incisions of 0.2–0.8 in (0.5–2 cm) made through the abdominal wall.

An advantage of laparoscopic salpingostomy is that the operation is less invasive, thus recovery time is quicker and less painful as compared to a

KEY TERMS

Adhesions—Bands of scar tissue that may form after surgery or trauma.

Hydrosalpinx—A condition in which a fallopian tube becomes blocked and filled with fluid.

Methotrexate—A drug that targets rapidly dividing fetal cells, preventing a fetus from developing further.

Salpingectomy—The surgical removal of a fallopian tube.

laparotomy; the average duration of recovery following laparoscopy is 2.4 weeks, compared to 4.6 weeks for laparotomy. An abdominal incision, on the other hand, allows the surgeon a better view of and easier access to the pelvic organs. Several studies have indicated a reduced rate of normal pregnancy after salpingostomy by laparoscopy versus laparotomy.

Diagnosis/Preparation

It has been estimated that 40–50% of ectopic pregnancies are incorrectly diagnosed when first presenting to emergency room medical personnel. Often the symptoms of ectopic pregnancy are confused with other conditions such as miscarriage or pelvic inflammatory disease. Diagnosis is usually based on presentation of symptoms, a positive pregnancy test, and detection of a pregnancy outside of the uterus by means of ultrasonography (using a machine that transmits high frequency sound waves to visualize structures in the body).

Diagnosis of hydrosalpinx or other defects of the fallopian tubes may be done surgically, using a laparoscope to visualize the fallopian tubes. Alternatively, a hysterosalpingogram may be performed, in which the uterus is filled with a dye and an x ray is taken to see if the dye flows through the fallopian tubes.

Aftercare

If performed through an abdominal incision, a salpingostomy requires three to six weeks for full recovery. If salpingostomy is performed laparoscopically, the recovery time can be much shorter (an average of 2.4 weeks). There may be some discomfort around the incision for the first few days after surgery, but most women are walking by the third day. Within a month or so, patients can gradually resume normal activities such as driving, exercising, and working.

WHO PERFORMS THE PROCEDURE AND WHERE IS IT PERFORMED?

Salpingostomies are usually performed in a hospital operating room by a surgeon or gynecologist, a medical doctor who has completed specialized training in the areas of women's general health, pregnancy, labor and childbirth, prenatal testing, and genetics.

Risks

Complications associated with the surgical procedure include reaction to anesthesia, excessive bleeding, injury to other organs, and infection. With an ectopic pregnancy, there is a chance that not all of the products of conception will be removed and that the persistent tissue will continue growing. If this is the case, further treatment will be necessary.

Normal results

In the case of ectopic pregnancy, the products of conception will be removed without significantly impairing fertility. If salpingostomy is being performed to restore fertility, the procedure will increase a woman's chance of conceiving without resorting to artificial reproductive techniques.

Morbidity and mortality rates

Abdominal pain occurs in 97% of women with an ectopic pregnancy, vaginal bleeding in 79%, abdominal tenderness in 91%, and infertility in 15%. Persistent ectopic pregnancy after surgical treatment occurs in 5–10% of cases. Ectopic pregnancy accounts for 10–15% of all maternal deaths; the mortality rate for ectopic pregnancy is approximately one in 2,500 cases.

Alternatives

Some ectopic pregnancies may be managed expectantly (allowing the pregnancy to progress to see if it will resolve on its own). This may occur in up to 25% of ectopic pregnancies. There is, of course, a chance that the fallopian tube will rupture during the period of observation. Treatment with methotrexate is gaining popularity and has been shown to have success rates similar to laparoscopic salpingostomy if multiple doses are given and the patient is in stable condition. Salpingectomy is another surgical option and is indicated if a tube has ruptured or is seriously damaged.

QUESTIONS TO ASK THE DOCTOR

- Why is a salpingostomy being recommended?
- How will the procedure be performed?
- If an ectopic pregnancy is suspected, how will the diagnosis be confirmed?
- What alternatives to salpingostomy are available to me?

Resources

PERIODICALS

Hajenius, P. J., B. Mol, P. Bossuyt, W. Ankum, and F. Van der Veen. "Interventions for tubal ectopic pregnancy (Cochrane Review)." *The Cochrane Library* 1 (January 20, 2003).

Tay, J. I., J. Moore, and J. J. Walker. "Ectopic Pregnancy." *British Medical Journal* 320 (April 1, 2000): 916–19.

Tenore, Josie L. "Ectopic Pregnancy." *American Family Physician* (February 15, 2000): 1073–79.

Watson, A., P. Vandekerckhove, and R. Lilford. "Techniques for pelvic surgery in subfertility (Cochrane Review)." *The Cochrane Library* 1 (January 20, 2003).

ORGANIZATIONS

American College of Obstetricians and Gynecologists. 409 12th St., SW, PO Box 96920, Washington, DC 20090-6920. http://www.acog.org.

OTHER

Daiter, Eric. "Ectopic Pregnancy." *OBGYN.net* [accessed April 22, 2008]. http://www.obgyn.net/women/women.asp?page=/pb/cotm/9902/9902.

"Early Diagnosis and Management of Ectopic Pregnancy." *American Society for Reproductive Medicine (Technical Bulletin)*. March 2001 [cited March 16, 2003]. http://www.asrm.org/Media/Practice/ectopicpregnancy.PDF.

"Hysterosalpingogram." *The Harvard Medical School Family Health Guide*.http://www.health.harvard.edu/fhg/diagnostics/hystero/hystero.shtml [accessed April 22, 2008].

Jazayeri, Allahyar. "Surgical Management of Ectopic Pregnancy." *eMedicine*, January 7, 2008 [cited April 22, 2008]. http://www.emedicine.com/med/topic3316.htm.

"Salpingostomy." *The McGill Gynecology Page*. August 27, 2002 [cited March 16, 2003]. <http://sprojects.mmip.mcgill.ca/gynecology/lapmain.html>.

Stephanie Dionne Sherk

Saphenous vein bypass *see* **Peripheral vascular bypass surgery**

Scar revision surgery

Definition

Scar revision surgery refers to a group of procedures that are done to partially remove scar tissue following surgery or injury, or to make the scar(s) less noticeable. The specific procedure that is performed depends on the type of scar; its cause, location, and size; and the characteristics of the patient's skin.

Purpose

Scar revision surgery is performed to improve the appearance of the patient's face or other body part, but it is also done to restore or improve functioning when the formation of a scar interferes with the movement of muscles and joints. The shortening or tightening of the skin and underlying muscles that may accompany scar formation is known as contracture. Contractures may interfere with range of motion and other aspects of joint functioning, as well as deform the shape of the hand or other body part. Contractures in the face often affect the muscles that control facial expressions.

Scar revision surgery may be considered as either a cosmetic procedure or a **reconstructive surgery**, depending on whether the patient's concern is primarily related to appearance or whether contractures have also affected functioning. Some insurance companies will cover the cost of scar revision surgery if the scarring resulted from injury. Patients who are considering scar revision surgery should consult their insurance carriers to learn whether their condition may be covered. According to the American Academy of Facial Plastic and Reconstructive Surgery (AAFPRS), the average cost for scar revision surgery on the face is $1,135, compared to $1,376 for **dermabrasion**, $149 for microdermabrasion and $2,484 for **laser skin resurfacing**.

Demographics

The demographics of scar revision are difficult to establish precisely because of the number of different procedures that are grouped under this heading and the different types of scars that they are intended to treat. In addition, although dermabrasion and laser resurfacing of the skin are often described as surgical methods of scar treatment to distinguish them from medical modalities, they are usually listed separately in statistical tables. According to the American Society of Plastic Surgeons (ASPS), in 2006 the number of procedures, by type, were as follows: 164,684 for scar

KEY TERMS

Collagen—A type of protein found in connective tissue that gives it strength and flexibility.

Contracture—A condition in which the skin and underlying muscles shorten and tighten as the result of the formation of scar tissue or a disorder of the muscle fibers.

Dermabrasion—Planing of the skin done by a mechanical device, most commonly fine sandpaper or a wire brush.

Epidermis—The outermost layer of the skin.

Flap—A piece of tissue used for grafting that has kept its own blood supply.

Hypertrophic—A type of thick scar that is raised above the surface of the skin, usually caused by increasing or prolonging the inflammation stage of wound healing.

Keloid—A raised, irregularly shaped scar that gradually increases in size due to the overproduction of collagen during the healing process. The name comes from a Greek word that means "crablike."

Microdermabrasion—A technique for skin resurfacing that uses abrasive crystals passed through a hand piece to even out skin irregularities.

Nonablative—Not requiring removal or destruction of the epidermis. Some techniques for minimizing scars are nonablative.

revision; 69,300 for dermabrasion; 262,926 for laser resurfacing; and 816,774 for microdermabrasion.

The female to male ratio for scar revision surgery is about four to three, whereas women are almost five times as likely as men to have laser skin resurfacing and almost 13 times as likely to have a microdermabrasion procedure. Most patients who have scar revision surgery are between 15 and 39, although a significant number choose to undergo this type of surgery in their 40s and 50s.

It is difficult to compare scar revision surgery with other treatments across ethnic and racial groups because skin color is a factor in the effectiveness of some forms of therapy. In addition, some types of scars—particularly keloids—are more likely to form in darker skin. On the whole, it is estimated that between 4.5% and 16% of the United States population is affected by keloids and hypertrophic scars. These are the most difficult scars to treat, and are discussed in further detail below.

Description

Scar formation

A description of the process of scar formation may be helpful in understanding scar revision surgery and other procedures intended to improve the appearance of scarred skin. There are three phases in the formation of a scar:

- Inflammation. This phase begins right after the injury and lasts until the wound is closed. It is the body's way of preventing infection, because a wound is not sterile until it is covered by a new outer layer of skin.
- Transitional repair. Scar tissue is formed during this phase to hold the wound together. The length of this phase depends on the severity of the injury.
- Maturation. This phase usually begins about seven to 12 weeks after the injury occurs. It is also the phase in which problem scars appear. Under normal conditions, a repair process takes place in which the development of new skin is combined with breaking down the scar tissue that was formed in the second phase of healing. A problem scar is likely to develop when the repair process is interrupted or disturbed.

Causes and types of problem scars

Problem scars may result from inflammatory diseases—particularly acne; trauma, including cuts and burns; previous surgery; and a genetic predisposition for the skin to overreact to injury. Tension on the skin around the wound, foreign material in the wound, infection, or anything that delays closure of the wound may also contribute to scar formation.

The most difficult types of scars to treat are characterized by overproduction of collagen, which is the extracellular protein found in connective tissue that gives it strength and flexibility. The two types of scars that are most often considered for treatment are keloids and hypertrophic scars. Keloids are shiny, smooth benign tumors that arise in areas of damaged skin and look like irregular growths in the wound area. Hypertrophic scars, on the other hand, are thick, ropy-textured scars that are often associated with contractures.

Keloids can be distinguished from hypertrophic scars by the following characteristics:

- Timing. Hypertrophic scars usually begin to form within weeks of the injury, whereas keloids may not appear until a year later.
- Growth pattern. Hypertrophic scars do not continue to grow after they form, and remain within the original area of injury. Keloids continue to grow and spread outward into normal tissue.

- Role of genetic factors. Keloids tend to run in families, whereas hypertrophic scars do not.
- Racial and age distribution. Keloids occur more frequently in persons with darker skin than in fair-skinned persons. They are also more likely to develop during adolescence and pregnancy, which are periods of high hormone production.
- Recurrence. Hypertrophic scars may fade with time and do not recur. Keloids, on the other hand, may recur even after surgical removal.
- Collagen structure. The collagen fibers in a hypertrophic scar are shorter and generally arranged in a wavelike pattern, whereas the collagen fibers in keloids tend to be randomly arranged.

Surgical approaches to scar revision

The treatment of scars is highly individualized. Most plastic surgeons use a variety of nonsurgical and surgical approaches to improve the appearance of scars. In addition, patients might need several different surgical procedures if their scar revisions require a series of operations at different stages of the healing process.

SURGICAL EXCISION. Surgical excision is a procedure in which the surgeon shaves down and cuts out scar tissue to reduce the size of the scar. This technique is most commonly used on large scars that cannot be treated adequately with medications or other nonsurgical means. When excision is done in stages, it is referred to as "serial excision." This is performed if the area of the scar is too large to remove at one time without distorting nearby skin.

FLAPS, GRAFTS, AND ARTIFICIAL SKIN. Flaps, grafts, and artificial skin are used to treat contractures and large areas of scarring resulting from burns and other traumatic injuries. When there is not enough skin at the site of the injury to cover an incision made to remove scar tissue, the surgeon implants a skin graft or flap after cutting out the scar tissue itself. Skin grafts are thin layers of skin that are removed from another part of the patient's body and carefully matched to the color and texture of the face or other area where the graft is to be placed. A skin flap is a full-thickness piece of tissue with its own blood supply that is taken from a site as close as possible to the scarred area.

Dermal regeneration templates, often called "artificial skin," are used to treat people with contracture scars or severe burns. These devices were approved by the Food and Drug Administration (FDA) in April 2002. The templates are made of two layers of material, a bottom layer composed of collagen derived from cows and a top layer made of silicone. To use the artificial skin, the surgeon first removes all the burned skin or scar tissue from the patient's wound. The collagen layer, which is eventually absorbed, allows the patient's body to start growing new skin while the silicone layer closes and protects the wound. After 14–21 days, the silicone layer can be removed and a very thin graft of the patient's own skin is applied to the surface of the wound. The advantages of using a dermal regeneration template are that it lowers the risk of infection and minimizes the amount of tissue that must be removed from the patient's other body sites.

Z-PLASTY AND W-PLASTY. Z-plasty and W-plasty are surgical techniques used to treat contractures and to minimize the visibility of scars by repositioning them along the natural lines and creases in the patient's skin. They are not usually used to treat keloids or hypertrophic scars. In Z-plasty, the surgeon makes a Z-shaped incision with the middle line of the Z running along the scar tissue. The flaps of skin formed by the other lines of the Z are rotated and sewn into a new position that reorients the scar about 90 degrees. In effect, the Z-plasty minimizes the appearance of the scar by breaking up the straight line of the scar into smaller units.

A W-plasty is similar to a Z-plasty in that the goal of the procedure is to minimize the visibility of a scar by turning a straight line into an irregular one. The surgeon makes a series of short incisions to form a zigzag pattern to replace the straight line of the scar. The primary difference between a Z-plasty and a W-plasty is that a W-plasty does not involve the formation and repositioning of skin flaps. A variation on the W-plasty is known as the geometric broken line closure, or GBLC.

LASER SKIN RESURFACING AND DERMABRASION. Skin resurfacing and dermabrasion are techniques used to treat acne scars or to smooth down scars with raised or uneven surfaces. They are known as ablative skin treatments because they remove the top layer of skin, or the epidermis. In dermabrasion, the surgeon moves an instrument with a high-speed rotating wheel over the scar tissue and surrounding skin several times in order to smooth the skin surface down to the lowest level of scarring. Laser skin resurfacing involves the use of a carbon dioxide or Er:YAG laser to evaporate the top layer of skin and tighten the underlying layer. Keloid or hypertrophic scars are treated with a pulsed dye laser. Dermabrasion or laser resurfacing can be used about five weeks after a scar excision to make the remaining scar less noticeable.

Laser skin resurfacing, however, is less popular than it was in the late 1990s because of increasing awareness of its potential complications. The skin of patients who have undergone laser skin resurfacing takes several months to heal, often with considerable discomfort as well as swelling and reddish discoloration of the skin. In addition, there is a 33–85% chance that changes in the color of the skin will be permanent; the risk of permanent discoloration is higher for patients with darker skin. As of 2003, some plastic surgeons are recommending laser resurfacing only for patients with deep wrinkles or extensive sun damage who are willing to accept the pain and permanent change in skin color.

Diagnosis/Preparation

Preparation for scar revision surgery includes the surgeon's assessment of the patient's psychological stability as well as the type and extent of potential scar tissue. Many patients respond to scarring following trauma with intense anger, particularly if the face is disfigured or their livelihood is related to their appearance. Some people are impatient to have the scars treated as quickly as possible, and may have the idea that revision surgery will restore their skin to its original condition. During the initial interview, the surgeon must explain that scar revision may take months or years to complete; that some techniques essentially replace one scar with another, rather than remove all scar tissue; and that it is difficult to predict the final results in advance. Most plastic surgeons recommend waiting at least six months, preferably a full year, for a new scar to complete the maturation phase of development. Many scars will begin to fade during this period of time, and others may respond to more conservative forms of treatment.

Good candidates for scar revision surgery are people who have a realistic understanding of its risks as well as its benefits, and equally realistic expectations of its potential outcomes. On the other hand, the following are considered psychological warning signs:

- The patient is considering scar revision surgery to please someone else—most often a spouse or partner.
- The patient has a history of multiple cosmetic procedures and/or complaints about previous surgeons.
- The patient has an unrealistic notion of what scar revision surgery will accomplish.
- The patient seems otherwise emotionally unstable.

In addition to discussing the timing and nature of treatments, the surgeon will take a careful medical history, noting whether the patient is a heavy smoker or has a family history of keloids, as well as other disorders that may influence the healing of scar tissue. These disorders include diabetes, lupus, scleroderma, and other disorders that compromise body's immune system.

Aftercare

Aftercare following Z-plasty or surgical removal of a scar is relatively uncomplicated. The patient is given pain medication, told to rest for a day or two at home, and advised to avoid any activities that might put tension or pressure on the new incision(s). Most patients can return to work on the third day after surgery. The most important aspect of long-term aftercare is protecting the affected area from the sun because the surgical scar will take about a year to mature and is only about 80% as strong as undamaged skin. Sunlight can cause burns, permanent redness, loss of pigment in the skin, and breakdown of the collagen that maintains the elasticity of the skin.

Aftercare following the use of skin grafts, flaps, or dermal regeneration templates begins in the hospital with standard postoperative patients care. If sutures have been used, they are usually removed three to four days after surgery on the face and five to seven days after surgery for incisions elsewhere on the body. Patients are usually asked to return to the hospital at regular intervals so that the graft sites can be monitored. If artificial skin has been used, the patients must keep the site absolutely dry, which may require special precautions or restrictions on bathing or showering.

Aftercare for some patients includes going for psychotherapy or joining a support group to deal with emotions related to disfigurement and scar treatment.

Risks

Scar revision surgery carries the same risks as other surgical procedures under anesthesia, such as bleeding, infection at the incision site, and an adverse reaction to the anesthetic. The chief risk specific to this type of surgery is that the scar may grow, change color, or otherwise become more noticeable. Some plastic surgeons use the "90–10 rule," which means that there is a 90% chance that the scar will look better after surgery; a 9% chance that it will look about the same; and a 1% chance that it will look significantly worse.

Normal results

Normal results of scar revision surgery and associated nonsurgical treatments are a less noticeable scar.

WHO PERFORMS THE PROCEDURE AND WHERE IS IT PERFORMED?

Scar revision surgery is a specialized procedure performed only by a qualified plastic surgeon. Plastic surgeons are physicians (with M.D. or D.O. [doctors of osteopathy]) who have completed three years of general surgical training, followed by two to three years of specialized training in plastic surgery.

Scar revision may be conducted either in a hospital or in an outpatient clinic that specializes in plastic surgery. Scar revision surgery that involves skin grafts and flaps, however, is usually done in a hospital as an inpatient procedure. Microdermabrasion, chemical peels, steroid injections, pressure wraps, and silicone treatments may be performed in the surgeon's office.

QUESTIONS TO ASK THE DOCTOR

- Am I a candidate for treatment by a nonsurgical method of scar revision?
- What treatment technique(s) would be best for my scar?
- How long should I wait before scar revision surgery?
- What are the risks of the specific procedures you are recommending in my case?

Morbidity and mortality rates

Mortality rates for scar revision surgery are very low. Rates of complications depend on the specific technique that was used, the condition of the patient's general health, and genetic factors affecting the condition of the patient's skin.

Alternatives

There are a number of nonsurgical treatments that can be used before, after, or in place of scar revision surgery.

Drugs

Medications may be used during the initial inflammatory phase of scar formation, as well as therapy for such specific skin disorders as acne. Keloids are often treated by direct injections of **corticosteroids** to reduce itching, redness, and burning; steroid treatment may also cause the keloid to shrink. Corticosteroid injections, gels, or tapes impregnated with medication are also used after scar excisions and Z-plasty to prevent recurrence or formation of hypertrophic scars. Acne scars are treated with oral **antibiotics** or isotretinoin.

Massage, wraps, radiation, and nonablative treatments

The most conservative treatments of scar tissue include several techniques that help to minimize scar formation and improve the appearance of scars that existing already. The simplest approach is repeated massage of the scarred area with cocoa butter or vitamin E preparations. Burn scars are treated typically with the application of pressure **dressings**, which restrict movement of the affected area and provide insulation. Another technique that is often used is silicone gel sheeting. The sheeting is applied to the scarred area, and remains for a minimum of 12 hours a day over a period of three to six months. It is effective in improving the appearance of keloids in about 85% of cases.

Keloids that do not respond to any other form of treatment may be treated with low-dose radiation therapy.

Nonablative treatments, which do not remove the epidermal layer of skin, include microdermabrasion and superficial chemical peels. Microdermabrasion, the use of which has increased widely since 2000, is a technique for smoothing the skin. During this procedure, the physician uses a handheld instrument that buffs the skin with aluminum oxide crystals; skin flakes are removed through a vacuum tube. Microdermabrasion does not remove deep wrinkles or extensive scar tissue, but can make scars somewhat less noticeable without the risk of serious side effects. Mild chemical peels, such as those made with alphahydroxy acid (AHA), are used sometimes to treat acne scars or uneven skin pigmentation resulting from other types of scar revision treatment.

Camouflage

Scars on the face and legs can often be covered with specially formulated cosmetics that even out the color of the surrounding skin and help to make the scar less noticeable. Some of these preparations are available in waterproof formulations for use during swimming and other athletic activities during which one perspires.

Resources

BOOKS

Canale, ST, ed. *Campbell's Operative Orthopaedics*. 10th ed. St. Louis: Mosby, 2003.

Cummings, CW, et al. *Otolayrngology: Head and Neck Surgery*. 4th ed. St. Louis: Mosby, 2005.

Wein, AJ et al. *Campbell-Walsh Urology*. 9th ed. Philadelphia: Saunders, 2007.

PERIODICALS

Lee KK. "Surgical Revision." *Dermatologic Clinics* 23 (January 2005): 141-50.

ORGANIZATIONS

American Academy of Facial Plastic and Reconstructive Surgery (AAFPRS). 310 South Henry Street, Alexandria, VA 22314. (703) 299-9291. www.facemd.org.

American Burn Association. 625 North Michigan Avenue, Suite 1530, Chicago, IL 60611. (312) 642-9260. www.ameriburn.org.

American Society of Plastic Surgeons (ASPS). 444 East Algonquin Road, Arlington Heights, IL 60005. (847) 228-9900. www.plasticsurgery.org.

FACES: The National Craniofacial Association. P. O. Box 11082, Chattanooga, TN 37401. (800) 332-2373. www.faces-cranio.org.

OTHER

American Academy of Facial Plastic and Reconstructive Surgery. 2001 Membership Survey: Trends in Facial Plastic Surgery. Alexandria, VA: AAFPRS, 2002.

American Academy of Facial Plastic and Reconstructive Surgery. Procedures: Understanding Facial Scar Treatment. [April 8, 2003]. www.facial-plastic-surgery.org/patients/procedures/facial_scar.html.

American Society of Plastic Surgeons. Procedures: Scar Revision. [April 7, 2003] www.plasticsurgery.org/public_education/procedures/ScarRevision.cfm.

Rebecca Frey, Ph. D.

Scleral buckling

Definition

Scleral buckling is a surgical procedure in which a piece of silicone plastic or sponge is sewn onto the sclera at the site of a retinal tear to push the sclera toward the retinal tear. The buckle holds the retina against the sclera until scarring seals the tear. It also prevents fluid leakage which could cause further retinal detachment.

Purpose

Scleral buckling is used to reattach the retina if the break is very large or if the tear is in one location. It is also used to seal breaks in the retina.

Demographics

Retinal detachment occurs in 25,000 Americans each year. Patients suffering from retinal detachments are commonly nearsighted, have had eye surgery, experienced ocular trauma, or have a family history of retinal detachments. Retinal detachments also are common after cataract removal. White males are at a higher risk, as are people who are middle-aged or older. Patients who already have had a retinal detachment also have a greater chance for another detachment.

Some conditions, such as diabetes or Coats's disease in children, make people more susceptible to retinal detachments.

Description

Scleral buckling is performed in an **operating room** under general or local anesthetic. Immediately before the procedure, patients are given eye drops to dilate the pupil to allow better access to the eye. The patient is given a local anesthetic. After the eye is numbed, the surgeon cuts the eye membrane, exposing the sclera. If bleeding or inflammation blocks the surgeon's view of the retinal detachment or hole, he or she may perform a vitrectomy before scleral buckling.

Vitrectomy is necessary only in cases in which the surgeon's view of the damage is hindered. The surgeon makes two incisions into the sclera, one for a light probe and the other for instruments to cut and aspirate. The surgeon uses a tiny, guillotine-like device to remove the vitreous, which he or she then replaces with saline. After the removal, the surgeon may inject air or gas to hold the retina in place.

After the surgeon is able to see the retina, he or she will perform one of two companion procedures.

- Laser photocoagulation. The laser is used when the retinal tear is small or the detachment is slight. The surgeon points the laser beam through a contact lens to burn the area around the retinal tear. The laser creates scar tissue that will seal the hole and prevent leakage. It requires no incision.
- Cryopexy. Using a freezing probe, the surgeon freezes the outer surface of the eye over the tear or detachment. The inflammation caused by the freezing leads to scar formation that seals the hole and prevents leakage. Cryopexy is used for larger holes or detachments, and for areas that may be hard to reach with a laser.

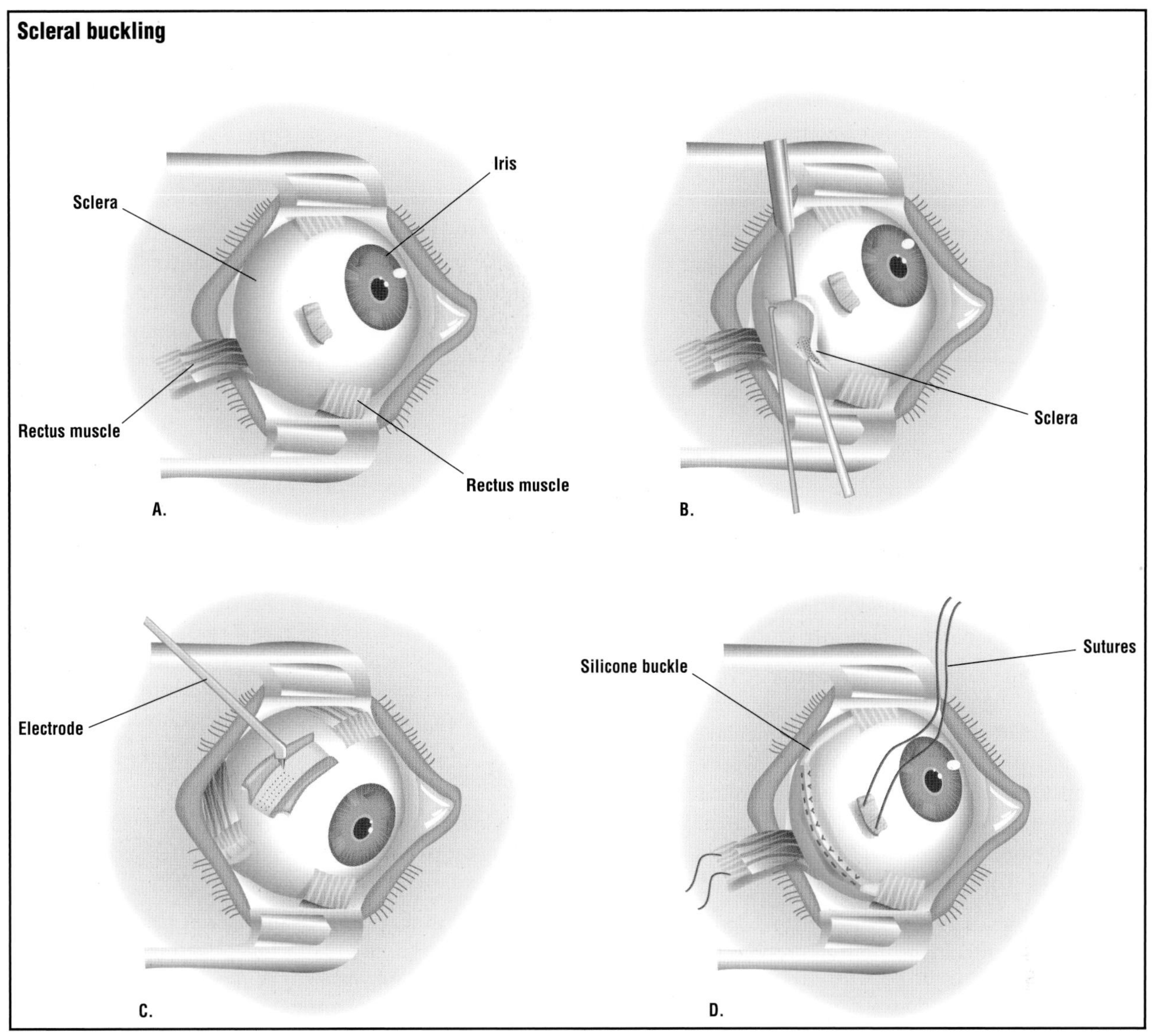

In a scleral buckling procedure, one of the eye's rectus muscles are severed to gain access to the sclera (A). The sclera is cut open (B), and an electrode is applied to the area of retinal detachment (C). A silicone buckle is threaded into place beneath the rectus muscles (D), and the severed muscle is repaired. *(Illustration by GGS Information Services. Cengage Learning, Gale.)*

After the surgeon has performed laser photocoagulation or cryopexy, he or she indents the affected area of the sclera with silicone. The silicone, either in the form of a sponge or buckle, closes the tear and reduces the eyeball's circumference. This reduction prevents further pulling and separation of the vitreous. Depending on the severity of the detachment or hole, a buckle may be placed around the entire eyeball.

When the buckle is in place, the surgeon may drain subretinal fluid that might interfere with the retina's reattachment. After the fluid is drained, the surgeon will suture the buckle into place and then cover it with the conjunctiva. The surgeon then inserts an antibiotic (drops or ointment) into the affected eye and patches it.

For less severe detachments, the surgeon may choose a temporary buckle that will be removed later. Usually, however, the buckle remains in place for the patient's lifetime. It does not interfere with vision. Scleral buckles in infants, however, will need to be removed as the eyeball grows.

Diagnosis/Preparation

Retinal detachment is considered an emergency situation. In the case of acute onset detachment, the

KEY TERMS

Conjunctiva—The mucous membrane that lines the visible part of the eye and the inner eyelid.

Glaucoma—Disease of the eye characterized by increased pressure of the fluid inside the eye. Untreated, glaucoma can lead to blindness.

Sclera—The outer part of the eyeball that creates the visible white of the eye and surrounds the optic nerve at the back of the eyeball.

Vitreous—Between the lens and the retina, this area contains a clear jelly called the vitreous humor.

longer it takes to repair the detachment, the less chance of successful reattachment. Usually the patient sees floating spots and experiences peripheral visual field loss. Patients commonly describe the vision loss as having someone pull a shade over their eyes. In extreme cases, patients may lose vision completely.

An ophthalmologist or optometrist will take a complete medical history, including family history of retinal detachment and any recent ocular trauma. In addition to performing a general eye exam, which includes a slit lamp examination, examination of the macula and lens evaluation, physicians may perform the following tests to determine the extent of retinal detachment:

- echography
- 3-mirror contact lens/panfunduscopic
- scleral indentation

Small breaks in the retina will not require surgery, but patients with acute onset detachment require reattachment in 24–48 hours. Chronic retinal detachments should be repaired within one week.

Because this is usually an emergency procedure, there is no long-term preparation. Patients are required to fast for at least six hours before surgery.

Aftercare

Immediately following the surgery, patients will need help with meals and walking. Some patients must remain hospitalized for several days. However, many scleral buckling procedures are performed on an outpatient basis.

After release from the hospital, patients should avoid heavy lifting or strenuous **exercise** that could increase intraocular pressure. Rapid eye movements should also be avoided; reading may be prohibited until the surgeon gives permission. Sunglasses should be worn during the day and an eye patch at night. Pain, redness, and a scratchy sensation in the eyes also may occur after surgery. Ice packs may be applied if the conjunctiva swells. Patients may take pain medication, but should check with their physician before taking any over-the-counter medication.

Excessive pain, swelling, bleeding, discharge from the eye or decreased vision is not normal, and should immediately be reported to the physician.

If a vitrectomy was performed in conjunction with the scleral buckling, patients must sleep with their heads elevated. They also must avoid air travel until the air bubble is absorbed.

After scleral buckling, patients will use dilating, antibiotic, or corticosteroid eye drops for up to six weeks to decrease inflammation and the chance of infection. Best visual acuity cannot be determined for at least six to eight weeks after surgery. Driving may be prohibited or restricted while vision stabilizes. At the six-to-eight week postoperative visit, physicians determine if the patient needs corrective lenses or stronger prescription lenses. Full vision restoration depends on the location and severity of the detachment.

Risks

Complications are rare but may be severe. In some instances, patients lose sight in the affected eye or lose the entire eye.

Scar tissue, even pre-existing scar tissue, may interfere with the retina's reattachment and the scleral buckling procedure may have to be repeated. Scarring, along with infection, is the most common complication.

Other possible but infrequent complications include:

- bleeding under the retina
- cataract formation
- double vision
- glaucoma
- vitreous hemorrhage

Patients may also become more nearsighted after the procedure. In some instances, although the retina reattaches, vision is not restored.

Normal results

The National Institutes of Health reports that scleral buckling has a success rate of 85–90%. Restored vision depends largely on the location and extent of the detachment, and the length of time before the detachment was repaired. Patients with a

WHO PERFORMS THE PROCEDURE AND WHERE IS IT PERFORMED?

Scleral buckling can be performed by a general ophthalmologist, an M.D. who specializes in treatment of the eye. Even more specialized ophthalmologists, vitreo-retinal surgeons who specialize in diseases of the retina, may be called upon for serious cases.

The surgery is usually performed in hospital settings. Because of the delicacy of the procedure, sometimes an overnight hospital stay is required. Less severe retinal detachments can be treated on an outpatient basis at surgery centers.

QUESTIONS TO ASK THE DOCTOR

How many scleral buckling procedures have you performed?

Could other treatments be an option?

Will I have to stay in the hospital?

Will my sight be completely restored?

What is the probability of having another retinal detachment in the same eye?

Am I likely to have a retinal detachment in my unaffected eye?

peripheral detachment have a quicker recovery then those patients whose detachment was located in the macula. The longer the patient waits to have the detachment repaired, the worse the prognosis.

Morbidity and mortality rates

The danger of mortality and loss of vision depends on the cause of the retinal detachment. Patients with Marfan syndrome, pre-eclampsia, and diabetes, for example, are more at risk during the scleral buckling procedure than a patient in relatively good health. The risk of surgery also rises with the use of **general anesthesia**. Scleral buckling, however, is considered a safe, successful procedure.

Severe infections that are left untreated can cause vision loss, but following the prescribed regimen of eye drops and follow-up treatment by the physician greatly minimizes this risk.

Alternatives

Vitrectomy is sometimes performed alone to treat retinal detachments. Laser photocoagulation and cryopexy also may be used to treat less serious tears. The more common alternative, however, is pneumatic retinopexy, which is used when the tear is located in the upper portion of the eye. The surgeon uses cryopexy to freeze the area around the tear, then removes a small amount of fluid. When the fluid is drained and the eye softened, the surgeon injects a gas bubble into the vitreous cavity. As the gas bubble expands, it seals the retinal tear by pushing the retina against the choroid. Eventually, the bubble will be absorbed.

The patient is required to remain in a certain position for at least a few days after surgery while the bubble helps seal the hole. Pneumatic retinopexy also is not as successful as scleral buckling. Complications include recurrent retinal detachments and the chance of gas getting under the retina.

Resources

BOOKS

Buettner, Helmut, M.D., ed. *Mayo Clinic on Vision and Eye Health.* Rochester, MN: Mayo Clinic Health Information, 2002.

Cassel, Gary H., M.D., Michael D. Billig, O.D., and Harry G. Randall, M.D. *The Eye Book: A Complete Guide to Eye Disorders and Health.* Baltimore, MD: Johns Hopkins University Press, 1998.

Everything You Need to Know About Medical Treatments, edited by Stephen Daly. Springhouse, PA: Springhouse Corp., 1996.

Sardgena, Jill, et al. *The Encyclopedia of Blindness and Vision Impairment*, 2nd ed. New York, NY: Facts on File, Inc. 2002.

ORGANIZATIONS

American Academy of Ophthalmology. PO Box 7424, San Francisco, CA 94120-7424. (415) 561-8500. http://www.aao.org.

American Board of Ophthalmology. 111 Presidential Boulevard, Suite 241, Bala Cynwyd, PA 19004-1075. (610) 664-1175. info@abop.org. http://www.abop.org.

National Eye Institute. 2020 Vision Place Bethesda, MD 20892-3655. (301) 496-5248. http://www.nei.nih.gov.

OTHER

Handbook of Ocular Disease Management: Retinal Detachment. *Review of Ophthalmology*. [cited April 21, 2003]. http://www.revoptom.com/handbook/SECT5R.HTM.

"Retinal Detachment." VisionChannel.net. [cited April 12, 2003]. http://www.visionchannel.net/retinaldetachment/treatment.shtml.

"Retinal Detachment Repair." EyeMdLink.com. [cited May 1, 2003]. http://www.eyemdlink.com/EyeProcedure.asp?EyeProcedureID = 52.

Wu, Lihteh, M.D. "Retinal Detachment, Exudative." emedicine.com. June 28, 2001 [cited May 1, 2003]. http://www.emedicine.com/oph/topic407htm.

Mary Bekker

Sclerostomy

Definition

A sclerostomy is a procedure in which the surgeon makes a small opening in the outer covering of the eyeball to reduce intraocular pressure (IOP) in patients with open-angle glaucoma. It is classified as a type of glaucoma filtering surgery. The name of the surgery comes from the Greek word for "hard," which describes the tough white outer coat of the eyeball, and the Greek word for "cutting" or "incision."

Purpose

Sclerostomies are usually performed to reduce IOP in open-angle glaucoma patients who have not been helped by less invasive forms of treatment, specifically medications and **laser surgery**. In some cases—most commonly patients who are rapidly losing their vision or who cannot tolerate glaucoma medications—an ophthalmologist (eye specialist) may recommend a sclerostomy without trying other forms of treatment first.

As of 2003, glaucoma is not considered a single disease but rather a group of diseases characterized by three major characteristics: elevated intraocular pressure (IOP) caused by an overproduction of aqueous humor in the eye or by resistance to the normal outflow of fluid; atrophy of the optic nerve; and a resultant loss of visual field. A sclerostomy works to reduce the IOP by improving the outflow of aqueous humor. Between 80% and 90% of aqueous humor leaves the eye through the trabecular meshwork while the remaining 10–20% passes through the ciliary muscle bundles. A sclerostomy allows the fluid to collect under the conjunctiva, which is the thin membrane lining the eyelids, to form a filtration bleb.

Demographics

In 1995, the World Health Organization (WHO) reported that over five million people around the world have lost their sight due to complications of glaucoma; about 120,000 Americans are blind as a result of glaucoma. According to the National Eye Institute (NEI), nearly three million people in the United States have the disorder; however, nearly half are unaware that they have it. Primary open-angle glaucoma (POAG) accounts for 60–70% of cases. "Primary" means that the glaucoma is not associated with a tumor, injury to the eye, or other eye disorder.

Although glaucoma can occur at any age, it is most common in adults over 35. One major study reported that less than 1% of the United States population between 60 and 64 suffer from POAG. The rate rises to 1.3% for persons between 70 and 74, however, and rises again to 3% for persons between 80 and 84.

With regard to race, African-Americans are four times as likely to develop glaucoma as Caucasians, and six to eight times more likely to lose their sight to the disease. African Americans also develop glaucoma at earlier ages; while everyone over age 60 is at increased risk for POAG, the risk for African Americans rises sharply after age 40. A 2001 study reported that the rate for Mexican Americans lies between the rate of POAG in African Americans and that in Caucasians. Mexican Americans, however, are more likely to suffer from undiagnosed glaucoma—62% as compared to 50% for other races and ethnic groups in the United States. In addition, the rate of POAG in Mexican Americans was found to rise rapidly after age 65; in the older age groups, it approaches the rates reported for African Americans. Among Caucasians, people of Scandinavian, Irish, or Russian ancestry are at higher risk of glaucoma than people from other ethnic groups.

The question of a sex ratio in open-angle glaucoma is debated. Three studies done in the United States between 1991 and 1996 reported that the male to female ratio for open-angle glaucoma is about one to one. Three other studies carried out in the United States, Barbados, and the Netherlands, however, found that the male to female ratio was almost two to one. A 2002 study from western Africa reported a male to female ratio of 2.26 to one. It appears that further research is needed in this area.

Description

Most sclerostomies are performed as outpatient procedures under **local anesthesia**. In some cases the

KEY TERMS

Angle—The open point in the anterior chamber of the eye at which the iris meets the cornea.

Aqueous humor—The watery fluid produced in the eye that ordinarily leaves the eye through the angle of the anterior chamber and Schlemm's canal.

Atrophy—Wasting away or degeneration. Atrophy of the optic nerve is one of the defining characteristics of glaucoma.

Bleb—A thin-walled auxiliary drain created on the outside of the eyeball during filtering surgery for glaucoma. It is sometimes called a filtering bleb.

Conjunctiva—The thin membrane that lines the eyelids and covers the visible surface of the sclera.

Cornea—The transparent front portion of the exterior cover of the eye.

Endophthalmitis—An infection on the inside of the eye, which may result from an infected bleb. Endophthalmitis can result in vision loss.

Glaucoma—A group of eye disorders characterized by increased fluid pressure inside the eye that eventually damages the optic nerve. As the cells in the optic nerve die, the patient gradually loses vision.

Gonioscopy—A technique for examining the angle between the iris and the cornea with the use of a special mirrored lens applied to the cornea.

Hyphema—Blood inside the anterior chamber of the eye. Hyphema is one of the risks associated with sclerostomies.

Hypotony—Intraocular fluid pressure that is too low.

Insidious—Developing in a stealthy and inconspicuous way. Open-angle glaucoma is an insidious disorder.

Ocular hypertension—A condition in which fluid pressure inside the eye is higher than normal but the optic nerve and visual fields are normal.

Open-angle glaucoma—A form of glaucoma in which fluid pressure builds up inside the eye even though the angle of the anterior chamber is open and looks normal when the eye is examined with a gonioscope. Most cases of glaucoma are open-angle.

Ophthalmology—The branch of medicine that deals with the diagnosis and treatment of eye disorders.

Peripheral vision—The outer portion of the visual field.

Schlemm's canal—A circular channel located at the point where the sclera of the eye meets the cornea. Schlemm's canal is the primary pathway for aqueous humor to leave the eye.

Sclera—The tough white fibrous membrane that forms the outermost covering of the eyeball.

Tonometry—Measurement of the fluid pressure inside the eye.

Trabecular meshwork—The main drainage passageway for fluid to leave the anterior chamber of the eye.

Visual field—The total area in which one can see objects in one's peripheral vision while the eyes are focused on a central point.

patient may be given an intravenous sedative to help him or her relax before the procedure.

Conventional sclerostomy

After the patient has been sedated, the surgeon injects a local anesthetic into the area around the eye as well as a medication to prevent eye movement. Using very small instruments with the help of a microscope, the surgeon makes a tiny hole in the sclera as a passageway for aqueous humor. Some surgeons use an erbium YAG laser to create the hole. Most surgeons apply an antimetabolite drug during the procedure to minimize the risk that the new drainage channel will be closed by tissue regrowth. The most common antimetabolites that are used are mitomycin and 5-fluouracil.

After the surgery, the aqueous humor begins to flow through the sclerostomy hole and forms a small blister-like structure on the upper surface of the eye. This structure is known as a bleb or filtration bleb, and is covered by the eyelid. The bleb allows the aqueous humor to leave the eye in a controlled fashion.

Enzymatic sclerostomy

A newer technique that was first described in 2002 is enzymatic sclerostomy, which was developed at the Weizmann Institute of Science in Israel. In enzymatic sclerostomy, the surgeon applies an enzyme called collagenase to the eye to increase the release of aqueous humor. The collagenase is applied through an applicator that is attached to the eye with tissue **glue** for 22–24 hours and then removed.

According to the researchers, the procedure reduced the intraocular pressure in all patients immediately following the procedure and in 80% of the subjects at one-year follow-up. None of the patients developed systemic complications. Enzymatic sclerostomy is considered experimental as of mid-2003.

Diagnosis/Preparation

Diagnosis

Open-angle glaucoma is not always diagnosed promptly because it is insidious in onset, which means that it develops slowly and gradually. Unlike closed-angle glaucoma, open-angle glaucoma rarely has early symptoms. It is usually diagnosed either in the course of an eye examination or because the patient has noticed that they are having problems with their peripheral vision—that is, they are having trouble seeing objects at the side or out of the corner of the eye. In some cases the patient notices that he or she is missing words while reading; having trouble seeing stairs or other objects at the bottom of the visual field; or having trouble seeing clearly when driving. Other symptoms of open-angle glaucoma may include headaches, seeing haloes around lights, or difficulty adjusting to darkness. It is important to diagnose open-angle glaucoma as soon as possible because the vision that has been already lost cannot be recovered. Although open-angle glaucoma cannot be cured, it can be stabilized and controlled in almost all patients. Because of the importance of catching open-angle glaucoma as early as possible, adults should have their eyes examined every two years at least.

HIGH-RISK GROUPS. Not everyone is at equal risk for glaucoma. People with any of the risk factors listed below should consult their doctor for advice about the frequency of eye checkups:

- Age over 40 (African Americans) or over 60 (other races and ethnic groups).
- Ocular hypertension. The normal level of IOP is between 11 mm Hg and 21 mm Hg. It is possible for people to have an IOP above 21 mm Hg without signs of damage to the optic nerve or loss of visual field; this condition is referred to as ocular hypertension. Conversely, about one out of six of patients diagnosed with open-angle glaucoma have so-called normal-tension glaucoma, which means that their optic nerve is being damaged even though their IOP is within the "normal" range. Ocular hypertension does, however, increase a person's risk of developing glaucoma in the future.
- Family history of glaucoma in a first-degree relative. As of 2003, at least six different genes related to glaucoma have been identified.
- An unusually thin cornea (the clear front portion of the outer cover of the eye). A recent National Eye Institute (NEI) study found that patients whose corneas are thinner than 555 microns are three times as likely to develop glaucoma as those whose corneas are thicker than 588 microns.
- Extreme nearsightedness. People who are very nearsighted are two to three times more likely to develop glaucoma than those who are not nearsighted.
- Diabetes.
- History of traumatic injury to the eye or surgery for other eye disorders.
- Use of steroid medications.
- Migraine headaches or sleep-related breathing disorder.
- Male sex.

Some patients should not be treated with filtration surgery. Contraindications for a sclerostomy include cardiovascular disorders and other severe systemic medical problems; eyes that are already blind; or the presence of an intraocular tumor or bleeding in the eye.

DIAGNOSTIC TESTS. Ophthalmologists use the following tests to screen patients for open-angle glaucoma:

- Tonometry. Tonometry is a painless procedure for measuring IOP. One type of tonometer blows a puff of pressurized air toward the patient's eye as the patient sits near a lamp; it measures the changes in the light reflections on the patient's corneas. Another method of tonometry involves the application of a local anesthetic to the outside of the eye and touching the cornea briefly with an instrument that measures the fluid pressure directly.
- Visual field test. This test measures loss of peripheral vision. In the simplest version of this test, the patient sits directly in front of the examiner with one eye covered. The patient looks at the examiner's eye and indicates when he or she can see the examiner's hand. In the automated version, the patient sits in front of a hollow dome and looks at a central target inside the dome. A computer program flashes lights at intervals at different locations inside the dome, and the patient presses a button whenever he or she sees a light. At the end of the test, the computer prints an assessment of the patient's responses.
- Gonioscopy. Gonioscopy measures the size of the angle in the anterior chamber of the eye with the use of a special mirrored contact lens. The examiner numbs the outside of the eye with a local anesthetic and touches the outside of the cornea with the gonioscopic lens. He or she can use a slit lamp to magnify

what appears on the lens. Gonioscopy is necessary in order to distinguish between open- and closed-angle glaucoma; it can also distinguish between primary and many secondary glaucomas.

- Ophthalmoscopic examination of the optic nerve. An ophthalmoscope is an instrument that contains a perforated mirror as well as magnifying lenses. It allows the examiner to view the interior of the eye. If the patient has open-angle glaucoma, the examiner can see a cup-shaped depression in the optic disk.

Newer diagnostic devices include a laser-scanning microscope known as the Heidelberg retinal tomograph (HRT) and **ultrasound** biomicroscopy (UBM). UBM has proved to be a useful method of long-term follow-up of sclerostomies.

Preparation

Preparation for a sclerostomy begins with the patient's decision to undergo incisional surgery rather than continuing to take medications or having repeated laser procedures. Three factors commonly influence the decision: the present extent of the patient's visual loss; the speed of visual deterioration; and the patient's life expectancy.

With regard to the procedure itself, patients may be asked to take oral antibiotic and anti-inflammatory medications for several days prior to surgery.

Aftercare

Patients can use their eyes after filtering surgery, although they should have a friend or relative to drive them home after the procedure. They can go to work the next day, although they will probably notice some blurring of vision in the operated eye for about a month. Patients can carry out their normal activities with the exception of heavy lifting, although they should not drive until their vision has completely cleared. Most ophthalmologists recommend that patients wear their eyeglasses during the day and tape an eye shield over the operated eye at night. They should apply eye drops prescribed by the ophthalmologist to prevent infection, manage pain, and reduce swelling. They should also avoid rubbing, bumping, or getting water into the operated eye. Complete recovery after filtering surgery usually takes about six weeks. Long-term aftercare includes avoiding damage to or infection of the bleb.

It is important for patients recovering from filtering surgery to see their doctor for frequent checkups in the first few weeks following surgery. In most cases the ophthalmologist will check the patient's eye the day after surgery and about once a week for the next several weeks.

Risks

The risks of a sclerostomy include the following:

- Infection. Infections may develop in the bleb (blebitis), but may spread to the interior of the eye (endophthalmitis). The symptoms of an infection include pain and redness in the eye, blurred vision, teariness, and a discharge. Infections must be treated promptly, as they can lead to loss of vision.
- Hyphema. Hyphema refers to the presence of blood inside the anterior chamber of the eye. Hyphemas are most common within the first two to three days after surgery and are usually treated with corticosteroid medications to reduce inflammation.
- Suprachoroidal hemorrhage. A suprachoroidal hemorrhage, or massive bleeding behind the retina, is a serious complication that can occur during as well as after eye surgery.
- Cataract formation.
- Hypotony (low IOP). If hypotony is not corrected, it can lead to failure of the bleb and eventual cataract formation.
- Loss of central vision. This is a very rare complication.
- Bleb leak or failure. Blebs can develop leaks at any time from several days after surgery to years later. Bleb failure usually results from inadequate control of the intraocular pressure and a new obstruction of aqueous humor outflow.
- Closing of the opening in the sclera by new tissue growth. A sclerostomy can be repeated if necessary.

Normal results

According to the National Eye Institute, sclerostomy is 80–90% effective in lowering intraocular pressure. The success rate is highest in patients who have not had previous eye surgery.

Morbidity and mortality rates

Mortality following a sclerostomy is very low because the majority of procedures are performed under local anesthesia. The most common complications of filtering surgery are cataract formation (30% of patients develop cataracts within five years of a sclerostomy) and closure of the drainage opening requiring additional surgery (10–15% of patients). Bleeding or infection occur in less than 1% of patients.

Alternatives

Nonpenetrating deep sclerectomy

There are two surgical alternatives to sclerostomy that are called nonpenetrating deep sclerectomies

WHO PERFORMS THE PROCEDURE AND WHERE IS IT PERFORMED?

Sclerostomies are performed by ophthalmologists, who are physicians who have completed four to five years of specialized training following medical school in the medical and surgical treatment of eye disorders. Ophthalmology is one of 24 specialties recognized by the American Board of Medical Specialties.

Sclerostomies are usually done as outpatient procedures, either in the ophthalmologist's office or in an ambulatory surgery center; however, they may also be performed in a hospital with sedation as well as local anesthesia.

because they do not involve entering the anterior chamber of the eye. The first alternative, viscocanalostomy, is a procedure that involves creating a window in Descemet's membrane (a layer of tissue in the cornea) to allow aqueous humor to leave the anterior chamber; and injecting a viscoelastic substance into Schlemm's canal, which is the main pathway for aqueous humor to leave the eye. The viscoelastic helps to keep the canal from scarring shut following surgery.

The second type of nonpenetrating surgery involves implanting a device called the Aquaflow® collagen wick about 0.8 in (2 cm) long under the sclera. The wick keeps open a space created by the surgeon to allow drainage of the aqueous humor. The wick is made of a material that is absorbed by the body within six to nine months, but the drainage pathway remains open after the wick is absorbed. The Aquaflow wick was approved by the Food and Drug Administration (FDA) in July 2001.

Both types of nonpenetrating deep sclerectomies allow patients to recover faster, with fewer complications than traditional sclerostomies. Their drawbacks include a lower success rate and the need for additional procedures to control the patient's IOP. Viscocanalostomy in particular is not as effective in reducing IOP levels as traditional filtering surgery.

Complementary and alternative (CAM) approaches

Bilberry (European blueberry) extract has been recommended as improving night vision; it was given to pilots during World War II for this reason. There is evidence that 80–160 mg of bilberry extract taken three times a day does improve night vision temporarily. The plant does not have any serious side effects, but it should not be used in place of regular eye examinations or other treatments for glaucoma.

QUESTIONS TO ASK THE DOCTOR

- How many sclerostomies have you performed?
- Do you prefer using miniature instruments or a laser, and why?
- What are my chances of developing a cataract if I have this procedure?
- Would you recommend nonpenetrating surgery? Why or why not?

People who support the medicinal use of marijuana have argued that cannabinoids, the active chemical compounds found in the plant, lower intraocular pressure in patients with glaucoma. According to the Glaucoma Research Foundation, however, very high doses of marijuana are required to produce any significant effect on IOP. A Canadian researcher has concluded that the effects of cannabinoids on IOP "...are not sufficiently strong, long lasting or reliable to provide a valid basis for therapeutic use [of marijuana]."

Resources

BOOKS

Pelletier, Kenneth R., MD. "CAM Therapies for Specific Conditions: Eye Disorders." In *The Best Alternative Medicine*. New York: Simon & Schuster, 2002.

"Primary Open-Angle Glaucoma." In *The Merck Manual of Diagnosis and Therapy*, edited by Mark H. Beers, MD, and Robert Berkow, MD. Whitehouse Station, NJ: Merck Research Laboratories, 1999.

PERIODICALS

Daboue, A., N. D. Meda, and A. Ahnoux-Zabsonre. "Eye Tension and Open-Angle Glaucoma in a Burkina Faso Hospital." [in French] *Journal français d'ophtalmologie* 25 (January 2002): 39–41.

Dan, J. A., S. G. Honavar, D. A. Belyea, et al. "Enzymatic Sclerostomy: Pilot Human Study." *Archives of Ophthalmology* 120 (May 2002): 548–553.

Kalant, H. "Medicinal Use of Cannabis: History and Current Status." *Pain Research and Management* 6 (Summer 2001): 80–91.

Kazakova, D., S. Roters, C. C. Schnyder, et al. "Ultrasound Biomicroscopy Images: Long-Term Results After Deep Sclerectomy with Collagen Implant." *Graefe's Archive for Clinical and Experimental Ophthalmology* 240 (November 2002): 918–923.

Lachkar, Y., and P. Hamard. "Nonpenetrating Filtering Surgery." *Current Opinion in Ophthalmology* 13 (April 2002): 110–115.

Luke, C., T. S. Dietlin, P. C. Jacobi, et al. "A Prospective Randomized Trial of Viscocanalostomy Versus Trabeculectomy in Open-Angle Glaucoma: A 1-Year Follow-Up Study." *Journal of Glaucoma* 11 (August 2002): 294–99.

Mizota, A., M. Takasoh, K. Kobayashi, et al. "Internal Sclerostomy with the Er:YAG Laser Using a Gradient-Index (GRIN) Endoscope." *Ophthalmic Surgery and Lasers* 33 (May-June 2002): 214–220.

Mizota, A., M. Takasoh, Y. Tsuyama, et al. "Sclerostomy with an Erbium YAG Laser. The Relationship with Pulse Energy." *Japanese Journal of Ophthalmology* 45 (January 2001): 111.

Pascotto, Antonio, MD, Giorgio Cusati, MD, Elena Soreca, MD, and Sergio Saccà, MD. "Glaucoma, Complications and Management of Glaucoma Filtering." *eMedicine*, November 15, 2002 [cited May 17, 2003]. http://www.emedicine.com/oph/topic720.htm.

Rastogi, Shobit, MD, Enrique Garcia-Valenzuela, MD, and Monica Allen, MD. "Hyphema, Postoperative." *eMedicine*, October 26, 2001 [cited May 18, 2003]. http://www.emedicine.com/oph/topic68.htm.

Shaarawy, T., C. Nguyen, C. Schnyder, and A. Mermoud. "Five-Year Results of Viscoanalostomy." *British Journal of Ophthalmology* 87 (April 2003): 441–445.

ORGANIZATIONS

American Academy of Ophthalmology. P.O. Box 7424, San Francisco, CA 94120-7424. (415) 561-8500. http://www.aao.org.

American Optometric Association. 243 North Lindbergh Blvd., St. Louis, MO 63141. (314) 991-4100.

Canadian Ophthalmological Society (COS). 610-1525 Carling Avenue, Ottawa ON K1Z 8R9. http://www.eyesite.ca.

(The) Glaucoma Foundation. 116 John Street, Suite 1605, New York, NY 10038. (212) 285-0080 or (800) 452-8266. http://www.glaucoma-foundation.org.

Glaucoma Research Foundation. 490 Post Street, Suite 1427, SanFrancisco, CA 94102. (415) 986-3162 or (800) 826-6693. http://www.glaucoma.org.

National Eye Institute. 2020 Vision Place, Bethesda, MD 20892-3655. (301) 496-5248. http://www.nei.nih.gov.

Prevent Blindness America. 500 East Remington Road, Schaumburg, IL 60173. (800) 331-2020. http://www.prevent-blindness.org.

Wills Eye Hospital. 840 Walnut Street, Philadelphia, PA 19107. (215) 928-3000. http://www.willseye.org.

OTHER

Lewis, Thomas L., O. D., Ph.D. *Optometric Clinical Practice Guideline: Care of the Patient with Open Angle Glaucoma.* 2nd ed. St. Louis, MO: American Optometric Association, 2002.

National Eye Institute (NEI). *Facts About Glaucoma.* Bethesda, MD: NEI, 2001. NIH Publication No. 99–651.

NEI Statement. *Prevalence of Glaucoma in Mexican-Americans.* Bethesda, MD: NEI, December 2001 [cited May 18, 2003]. http://www.nei.nih.gov/news/statements/glauc-mexamer.htm.

Prevent Blindness America. *Vision Problems in the U.S.: Prevalence of Adult Vision Impairment and Age-Related Eye Disease in America.* Schaumburg, IL: Prevent Blindness America, 2002.

Rebecca Frey, Ph.D.

Sclerotherapy for esophageal varices

Definition

Sclerotherapy for esophageal varices, also called endoscopic sclerotherapy, is a treatment for esophageal bleeding that involves the use of an endoscope and the injection of a sclerosing solution into veins.

Purpose

Esophageal varices are enlarged or swollen veins on the lining of the esophagus which are prone to bleeding. They are life-threatening; each episode of bleeding carries a 20-30% risk of **death**. 70% of patients who do not receive treatment for their varices die of bleeding within a year of their first episode of bleeding. Esophageal varices are a complication of portal hypertension, a condition characterized by increased blood pressure in the portal vein resulting from liver disease, such as cirrhosis. Increased pressure causes the veins to balloon outward. The vessels may rupture, causing vomiting of blood and bloody stools.

In most hospitals, sclerotherapy for esophageal varices is the treatment of choice to stop esophageal bleeding during acute episodes, and to prevent further incidences of bleeding. Emergency sclerotherapy is often followed by preventive treatments to eradicate distended esophageal veins.

Demographics

Bleeding esophageal varices are a serious complication of liver disease. In the United States, at least 50% of people who survive bleeding esophageal varices are at risk of recurrent bleeding during the next one to two years.

KEY TERMS

Cirrhosis—A chronic degenerative liver disease causing irreversible scarring of the liver.

Endoscope—An instrument used to examine the inside of a canal or hollow organ. Endoscopic surgery is less invasive than traditional surgery.

Esophagus—The part of the digestive canal located between the pharynx (part of the digestive tube) and the stomach. Also called the food pipe.

Portal hypertension—Abnormally high pressure within the veins draining into the liver.

Sclerosant—An irritating solution that stops bleeding by hardening the blood or vein it is injected into.

Varices—Swollen or enlarged veins, in this case on the lining of the esophagus.

Description

Sclerotherapy for esophageal varices involves injecting a strong and irritating solution (a sclerosant) into the veins and/or the area beside the distended vein. Sclerosant injected directly into the vein causes blood clots to form and stops the bleeding, while sclerosant injected into the area beside the distended vein stops the bleeding by thickening and swelling the vein to compress the blood vessel. Most physicians inject the sclerosant directly into the vein, although injections into the vein and the surrounding area are both effective. Once bleeding has been stopped, the treatment can be used to significantly reduce or destroy the varices.

Sclerotherapy for esophageal varices is performed with the patient awake but sedated. Hyoscine butylbromide (Buscopan) may be administered to freeze the esophagus, making injection of the sclerosant easier. During the procedure, an endoscope is passed through the patient's mouth to the esophagus to allow the surgeon to view the inside. The branches of the blood vessels at or just above where the stomach and esophagus come together, the usual site of variceal bleeding, are located. After the bleeding vein is identified, a long, flexible sclerotherapy needle is passed through the endoscope. When the tip of the needle's sheath is in place, the needle is advanced, and the sclerosant is injected into the vein or the surrounding area. The most commonly used sclerosants are ethanolamine and sodium tetradecyl sulfate. The needle is withdrawn. The procedure is repeated as many times as necessary to eradicate all distended veins.

Diagnosis/Preparation

A radiologist assesses patients for sclerotherapy based on blood work and liver imaging studies performed using **CT scans**, **ultrasound**, or MRI scans, and in consultation with the treating gastroenterologist, hepatologist, or surgeon. Tests to localize bleeding and detect active bleeding are also performed.

Before a sclerotherapy procedure, the patient's **vital signs** and other pertinent data are recorded, an intravenous line is inserted to administer fluid or blood, and a sedative is prescribed.

Aftercare

After sclerotherapy for esophageal varices, the patient will be observed for signs of blood loss, lung complications, fever, a perforated esophagus, or other complications. Vital signs are monitored, and the intravenous line maintained. Pain medication is usually prescribed. After leaving the hospital, the patient follows a diet prescribed by the physician, and, if appropriate, can take mild pain relievers.

Risks

Risks associated with sclerotherapy include complications that can arise from use of the sclerosant or from the endoscopic procedure. Minor complications, which cause discomfort but do not require active treatment or prolonged hospitalization, include transient chest pain, difficulty swallowing, and fever, which usually go away after a few days. Some patients may have allergic reactions to the sclerosant solution. Infection occurs in up to 50% of cases. In 2-10% of patients, the esophagus tightens, but this can usually be treated with dilatation. More serious complications may occur in 10-15% of patients. These include perforation or bleeding of the esophaggus and lung problems, such as aspiration pneumonia. Long-term sclerotherapy can also damage the esophagus, and increase the patient's risk of developing cancer.

Patients with advanced liver disease complicated by bleeding are very poor risks for this procedure. The surgery, premedications, and anesthesia may be sufficient to tip the patient into protein intoxication and hepatic coma. The blood in the bowels acts like a high-protein meal and may induce protein intoxication.

Normal results

Normal sclerotherapy results include the control of acute bleeding if present and the shrinking of the esophageal varices.

WHO PERFORMS THE PROCEDURE AND WHERE IS IT PERFORMED?

Sclerotherapy for esophageal varices is performed by a surgeon specialized in gastroenterology or hepatology in a hospital setting, very often as an emergency procedure.

Morbidity and mortality rates

Sclerotherapy for esophageal varices has a 20-40% incidence of complications and a 1–2% mortality rate. The procedure controls acute bleeding in about 90% of patients, but it may have to be repeated within the first 48 hours to achieve this success rate. During the initial hospitalization, sclerotherapy is usually performed two or three times. Preventive treatments are scheduled every few weeks or so, depending on the patient's risk level and healing rate. Several studies have shown that the risk of recurrent bleeding is much lower in patients treated with sclerotherapy: 30-50% as opposed to 70–80% for patients not treated with sclerotherapy.

Alternatives

Pharmacological agents are also used in the treatment of esophageal varices. Drugs such as vasopressin and somatostatin are administered to actively bleeding patients on admission, while propranolol, nadolol or subcutaneous octreotide are used to prevent subsequent bleeding after successful endoscopic variceal eradication. Vasopressin or vasopressin with nitroglycerin has been proven effective in the acute control of variceal hemorrhage. Somatostatin is more effective in the control of active bleeding when compared to vasopressin, glypressin, endoscopic sclerotherapy or balloon tamponade. Octreotide has comparable outcomes to vasopressin, terlipressin or endoscopic sclerotherapy. **Liver transplantation** should be considered as an alternative for patients with bleeding varices from liver disease.

Another alternative treatment is provided by Transjugular intrahepatic portal-systemic shunting (TIPS). In TIPS, a catheter fitted with a stent, a wire mesh tube used to prop open a vein or artery, is inserted through a vein in the neck into the liver. Under x ray guidance, the stent is placed in an optimal position within the liver so as to allow blood to flow more easily through the portal vein. This treatment reduces the excess pressure in the esophageal varices, and thus decreases the risk of recurrent bleeding.

QUESTIONS TO ASK THE DOCTOR

- What are esophageal varices?
- Are there alternatives to sclerotherapy?
- How do I prepare for surgery?
- What type of anesthesia will be used?
- How is the surgery performed?
- How long will I be in the hospital?
- How many sclerotherapy procedures do you perform in a year?

Resources

BOOKS

Feldman, M, et al.. *Sleisenger & Fordtran's Gastrointestinal and Liver Disease*. 8th ed. St. Louis: Mosby, 2005.

Khatri, VP and JA Asensio. *Operative Surgery Manual.* 1st ed. Philadelphia: Saunders, 2003.

Townsend, CM et al. *Sabiston Textbook of Surgery*. 17th ed. Philadelphia: Saunders, 2004.

PERIODICALS

Dhiman, R. K., and Y. K. Chawla. "A new technique of combined endoscopic sclerotherapy and ligation for variceal bleeding." *World Journal of Gastroenterology* 9 (May 2003): 1090–1093.

Mahesh, B., S. Thulkar, G. Joseph, A. Srivastava, and R. K. Khazanchi. "Colour duplex ultrasound-guided sclerotherapy. A new approach to the management of patients with peripheral vascular malformations." *Clinical Imaging* 27 (May-June 2003): 171–179.

Miyazaki, K., T. Nishibe, F. Sata, T. Imai, F. A. Kudo, J. Flores, Y. J. Miyazaki, and K. Yasuda. "Stripping Operation with Sclerotherapy for Primary Varicose Veins Due to Greater Saphenous Vein Reflux: Three-Year Results." *World Journal of Surgery* 27 (May 2003): 551–553.

ORGANIZATIONS

Society of American Gastrointestinal Endoscopic Surgeons (SAGES). 2716 Ocean Park Boulevard, Suite 3000, Santa Monica, CA 90405. (310) 314-2404. http://www.sages.org.

OTHER

SAGES: The Role of Endoscopic Sclerotherapy.http://www.sages.org/sg_asgepub1019.html.

Lori De Milto
Monique Laberge, Ph.D.

Sclerotherapy for varicose veins

Definition

Sclerotherapy, which takes its name from a Greek word meaning "hardening," is a method of treating enlarged veins by injecting an irritating chemical called a sclerosing agent into the vein. The chemical causes the vein to become inflamed, which leads to the formation of fibrous tissue and closing of the lumen, or central channel of the vein.

Purpose

Sclerotherapy in the legs is performed for several reasons. It is most often done to improve the appearance of the legs, and is accomplished by closing down spider veins—small veins in the legs that have dilated under increased venous blood pressure. A spider vein is one type of telangiectasia, which is the medical term for a reddish-colored lesion produced by the permanent enlargement of the capillaries and other small blood vessels. The word telangiectasia comes from three Greek words that mean "end," "blood vessel," and "stretch out." In a spider vein, also called a "sunburst varicosity," there is a central reddish area that is visible to the eye because it lies close to the surface of the skin; smaller veins spread outward from it in the shape of a spider's legs. Spider veins may also appear in two other common patterns—they may look like tiny tree branches or like extra-fine separate lines.

In addition to the cosmetic purposes sclerotherapy serves, it is also performed to treat the soreness, aching, muscle fatigue, and leg cramps that often accompany small- or middle-sized varicose veins in the legs. It is not, however, used by itself to treat large varicose veins.

Because sclerotherapy is usually considered a cosmetic procedure, it is usually not covered by health insurance. People who are being treated for cramps and discomfort in their legs, however, should ask their insurance companies whether they are covered for sclerotherapy. Sclerotherpy costs usually reflect the number of syringes of sclerosant required; the average cost of each syringe is $225. Many procedures will require the use of two syringes of sclerosant. The average cost is $326.

Sclerotherapy as a general treatment modality is also performed to treat hemorrhoids (swollen veins) in the esophagus.

Demographics

The American College of Phlebology (ACP), a group of dermatologists, plastic surgeons, gynecologists, and general surgeons with special training in the treatment of venous disorders, comments that about 60% of all people in the United States suffer from spider veins or varicose veins. Women are more commonly affected than men, with about half of all women experiencing some type of vein disorder. The American Society of Plastic Surgeons (ASPS) estimates that more than 40% of women over 50 in the United States have spider veins.

Women are more likely to develop spider veins than men, but the incidence among both sexes increases with age. The results of a recent survey of middle-aged and elderly people in San Diego, California, show that 80% of the women and 50% of the men had spider veins. Men are less likely to seek treatment for spider veins for cosmetic reasons, however, because the discoloration caused by spider veins is often covered by leg hair. On the other hand, men who are bothered by aching, burning sensations or leg cramps can benefit from sclerotherapy.

According to the ASPS, there were 559,285 sclerotherapy procedures performed in the United States in 2006. Most people who are treated with sclerotherapy are between the ages of 30 and 60.

Spider veins are most noticeable and common in Caucasians. Hispanics are less likely than Caucasians but more likely than either African or Asian Americans to develop spider veins.

Description

Causes of spider veins

To understand how sclerotherapy works, it is helpful to begin with a brief description of the venous system in the human body. The venous part of the circulatory system returns blood to the heart to be pumped to the lungs for oxygenation. This is in contrast to the arterial system, which carries oxygenated blood away from the heart to be distributed throughout the body. The smallest parts of the venous system are the capillaries, which feed into larger superficial veins. All superficial veins lie between the skin and a layer of fibrous connective tissue called fascia, which covers and supports the muscles and the internal organs. The deeper veins of the body lie within the muscle fascia. This distinction helps to explain why superficial veins can be treated by sclerotherapy without damage to the larger veins.

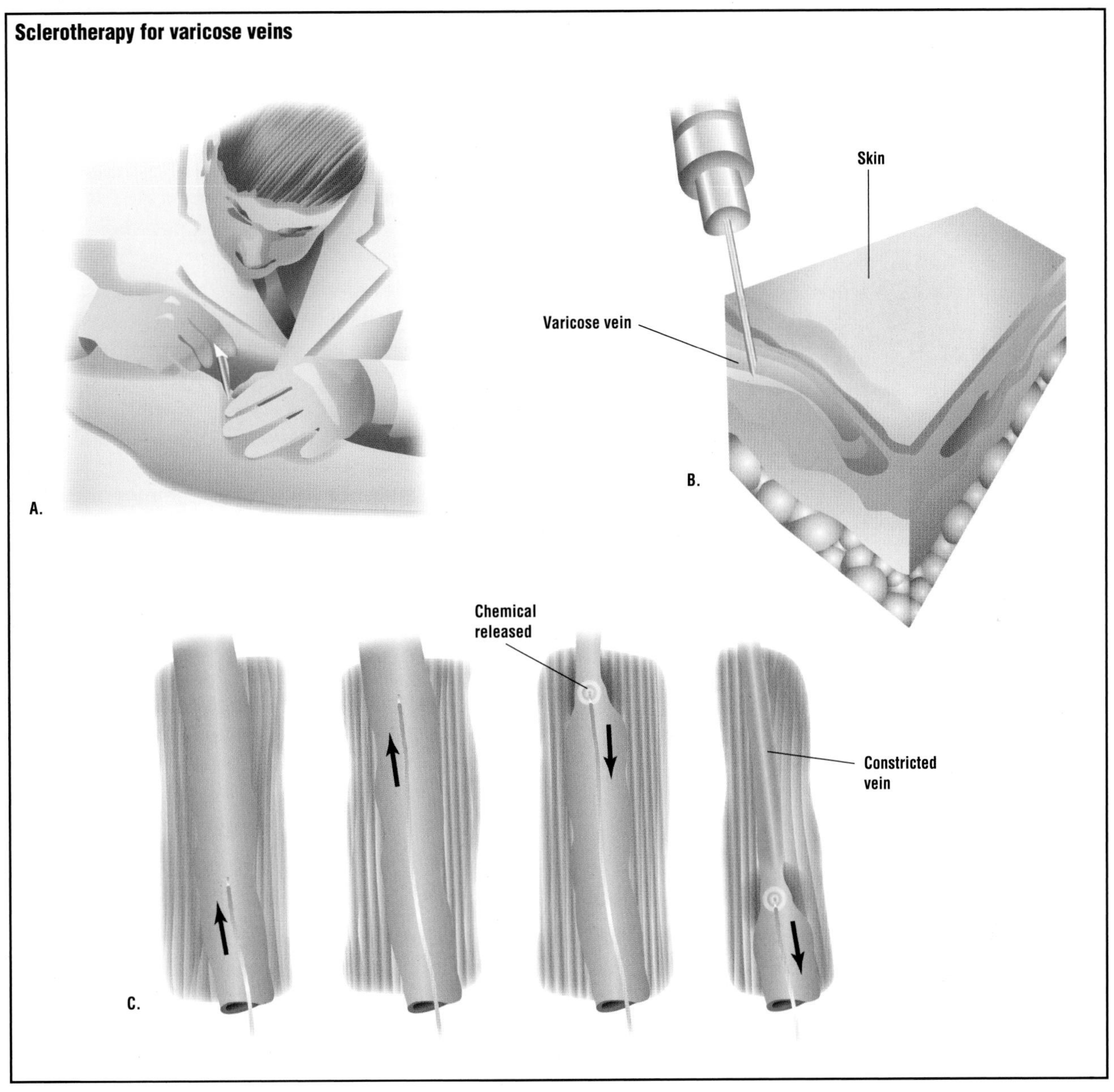

During sclerotherapy for the treatment of varicose veins, the doctor injects a chemical solution directly into the vein (A and B). The needle travels up the vein, and as it is pulled back, the chemical is released, causing the vein to form fibrous tissue that collapses the inside of it (C). *(Illustration by GGS Information Services. Cengage Learning, Gale.)*

Veins contain one-way valves that push blood inward and upward toward the heart when they are functioning normally. The blood pressure in the superficial veins is usually low, but if it rises and remains at a higher level over a period of time, the valves in the veins begin to fail and the veins dilate, or expand. Veins that are not functioning properly are said to be "incompetent." As the veins expand, they become more noticeable because they lie closer to the surface of the skin, forming the typical patterns seen in spider veins.

Some people are at greater risk for developing spider veins. These risk factors include:

- Sex. Females in any age group are more likely than males to develop spider veins.
- Genetic factors. Some people have veins with abnormally weak walls or valves. They may develop spider

KEY TERMS

Arteriole—A very small branch of an artery, usually close to a capillary network.

Edema—The presence of abnormally large amounts of fluid in the soft tissues of the body.

Electrodesiccation—A method of treating spider veins or drying up tissue by passing a small electric current through a fine needle into the affected area.

Hemosiderin—A form of iron that is stored inside tissue cells. The brownish discoloration of skin that sometimes occurs after sclerotherapy is caused by hemosiderin.

Hirsutism—Abnormal hair growth on the part of the body treated by sclerotherapy. It is also called hypertrichosis.

Incompetent—In a medical context, insufficient. An incompetent vein is one that is not performing its function of carrying blood back to the heart.

Lumen—The channel or cavity inside a tube or hollow organ of the body.

Palpation—Examining by touch as part of the process of physical diagnosis.

Percussion—Thumping or tapping a part of the body with the fingers for diagnostic purposes.

Phlebology—The study of veins, their disorders, and their treatments. A phlebologist is a doctor who specializes in treating spider veins, varicose veins, and associated disorders.

Sclerose—To harden or undergo hardening. Sclerosing agents are chemicals that are used in sclerotherapy to cause swollen veins to fill with fibrous tissue and close down.

Spider nevus (plural, nevi)—A reddish lesion that consists of a central arteriole with smaller branches radiating outward from it. Spider nevi are also called spider angiomas; they are most common in small children and pregnant women.

Spider veins—Telangiectasias that appear on the surface of the legs, characterized by a reddish central point with smaller veins branching out from it like the legs of a spider.

Telangiectasia—The medical term for the visible discolorations produced by permanently swollen capillaries and smaller veins.

Varicose—Abnormally enlarged and distended.

veins even without a rise in blood pressure in the superficial veins.

- Pregnancy. A woman's total blood volume increases during pregnancy, which increases the blood pressure in the venous system. In addition, the hormonal changes of pregnancy cause the walls and valves in the veins to soften.
- Using birth control pills.
- Obesity. Excess body weight increases pressure on the veins.
- Occupational factors. People whose jobs require standing or sitting for long periods of time without the opportunity to walk or move around are more likely to develop spider veins than people whose jobs allow more movement.
- Trauma. Falls, deep bruises, cuts, or surgical incisions may lead to the formation of spider veins in or near the affected area.

As of 2008, there is no known method to prevent the formation of spider veins.

Sclerotherapy procedures

In typical outpatient sclerotherapy treatment, the patient changes into a pair of shorts at the doctor's office and lies on an examination table. After cleansing the skin surface with an antiseptic, the doctor injects a sclerosing agent into the veins. This agent is eliminated when the skin is stretched tightly over the area with the other hand. The doctor first injects the larger veins in each area of the leg, then the smaller ones. In most cases, one injection is needed for every inch of spider vein; a typical treatment session will require five to 40 separate injections. No anesthetic is needed for sclerotherapy, although the patient may feel a mild stinging or burning sensation at the injection site.

The liquid sclerosing agents that are used most often to treat spider veins are polidocanol (aethoxysklerol), sodium tetradecyl sulfate, and saline solution at 11.7% concentration. Some practitioners prefer to use saline because it does not cause allergic reactions. The usual practice is to use the lowest concentration of the chemical that is still effective in closing the veins.

A newer type of sclerosing agent is a foam instead of a liquid chemical that is injected into the veins. The foam has several advantages: It makes better contact with the wall of the vein than a liquid sclerosing agent; it allows the use of smaller amounts of chemical; and its movement in the vein can be monitored on an **ultrasound** screen. Sclerosing foam has been shown to have a high success rate with a lower cost, and causes fewer major complications.

After all the veins in a specific area of the leg have been injected, the doctor covers the area with a cotton ball or pad and compression tape. The patient may be asked to wait in the office for 20–30 minutes after the first treatment session to ensure that there is no hypersensitivity to the sclerosing chemicals. Most sclerotherapy treatment sessions are short, lasting from 15 to 45 minutes.

It is not unusual for patients to need a second treatment to completely eliminate the spider veins; however, it is necessary to wait four to six weeks between procedures.

Diagnosis/Preparation

Diagnosis

The most important aspect of diagnosis prior to undergoing sclerotherapy is distinguishing between telangiectasias and large varicose veins, and telangiectasias and spider nevi. Because sclerotherapy is intended to treat only small superficial veins, the doctor must confirm that the patient does not have a more serious venous disorder.

Spider nevi, which are also called "spider angiomas," are small, benign reddish lesions that consist of a central arteriole, which is a very small branch of an artery with smaller vessels radiating from it. Although the names are similar, spider nevi occur in the part of the circulatory system that carries blood (away) from the heart, whereas spider veins occur in the venous system that returns blood to the heart. To distinguish between the two, the doctor will press gently on the spot in the center of the network. A spider nevus will blanch, or lose its reddish color, when the central arteriole is compressed. When the doctor releases the pressure, the color will return. Spider veins are not affected by compression in this way. In addition, spider nevi occur most frequently in children and pregnant women, rather than in older adults. They are treated by laser therapy or electrodesiccation, rather than by sclerotherapy.

After taking the patient's medical history, the doctor examines the patient from the waist down, both to note the location of spider veins and to palpate (touch with gentle pressure) them for signs of other venous disorders. Ideally, the examiner will have a small, raised platform for the patient to stand on during the examination. The doctor will ask the patient to turn slowly while standing, and will be looking for scars or other signs of trauma, bulges in the skin, areas of discolored skin, or other indications of chronic venous insufficiency. While palpating the legs, the doctor will note areas of unusual warmth or soreness, cysts, and edema (swelling of the soft tissues due to fluid retention). Next, the doctor will percuss certain parts of the legs where the larger veins lie closer to the surface. By gently tapping or thumping on the skin over these areas, the doctor can feel fluid waves in the veins and determine whether further testing for venous insufficiency is required. If the patient has problems related to large varicose veins, these must be treated before sclerotherapy can be performed to eliminate spider veins.

Some conditions and disorders are considered contraindications for sclerotherapy:

- Pregnancy and lactation. Pregnant women are advised to postpone sclerotherapy until at least three months after the baby is born, because some spider veins will fade by themselves after delivery. Nursing mothers should postpone sclerotherapy until the baby is weaned because it is not yet known whether the chemicals used in sclerotherapy may affect the mother's milk.
- Diabetes.
- A history of AIDS, hepatitis, syphilis, or other diseases that are carried in the blood.
- Heart conditions.
- High blood pressure, blood clotting disorders, and other disorders of the circulatory system.

Preparation

Patients are asked to discontinue **aspirin** or aspirin-related products for a week before sclerotherapy. Further, they are told not to apply any moisturizers, creams, tanning lotions, or sunblock to the legs on the day of the procedure. Patients should bring a pair of shorts to wear during the procedure, as well as compression stockings and a pair of slacks or a long skirt to cover the legs afterwards.

Most practitioners will take photographs of the patient's legs before sclerotherapy to evaluate the effectiveness of treatment. In addition, some insurance companies request pretreatment photographs for documentation purposes.

Aftercare

Aftercare following sclerotherapy includes wearing medical compression stockings that apply either 20–30 mmHg or 30–40 mmHg of pressure for at least seven to 10 days (preferably four to six weeks) after the procedure. Wearing compression stockings minimizes the risk of edema, discoloration, and pain. Fashion support stockings are a less acceptable alternative because they do not apply enough pressure to the legs.

The surgical tape and cotton balls used during the procedure should be left in place for 48 hours after the patient returns home.

Patients are encouraged to walk, ride a bicycle, or participate in other low-impact forms of **exercise** (examples: yoga and tai chi) to prevent the formation of blood clots in the deep veins of the legs. They should, however, avoid prolonged periods of standing or sitting, and high-impact activities, such as jogging.

Risks

Cosmetically, the chief risk of sclerotherapy is that new spider veins may develop after the procedure. New spider veins are dilated blood vessels that can form when some of the venous blood forms new pathways back to the larger veins; they are not the original blood vessels that were sclerosed. Some patients may develop telangiectatic matting, which is a network of new spider veins that surface around the treated area. Telangiectatic matting usually clears up by itself within three to 12 months after sclerotherapy, but it can also be treated with further sclerosing injections.

Other risks of sclerotherapy include:

- Venous thrombosis. A potentially serious complication, thrombosis refers to the formation of blood clots in the veins.
- Severe inflammation.
- Pain after the procedure lasting several hours or days. This discomfort can be eased by wearing medical compression stockings and by walking briskly.
- Allergic reactions to the sclerosing solution or foam.
- Permanent scarring.
- Loss of feeling resulting from damage to the nerves in the treated area.
- Edema (swelling) of the foot or ankle. This problem is most likely to occur when the foot or ankle is treated for spider veins. The edema usually resolves within a few days or weeks.
- Brownish spots or discoloration in the skin around the treated area. These changes in skin color are caused by deposits of hemosiderin, which is a form of iron that is stored within tissue cells. The spots usually fade after several months.
- Ulceration of the skin. This complication may result from reactive spasms of the blood vessels, the use of overly strong sclerosing solutions, or poor technique in administering sclerotherapy. It can be treated by diluting the sclerosing chemical with normal saline solution.
- Hirsutism. Hirsutism is the abnormal growth of hair on the area treated by sclerotherapy. It usually develops several months after treatment and goes away on its own. It is also known as hypertrichosis.

Normal results

Normal results of sclerotherapy include improvement in the external appearance of the legs and relief of aching or cramping sensations associated with spider veins. It is common for complete elimination of spider veins to require three to four sclerotherapy treatments.

Morbidity and mortality rates

Mortality associated with sclerotherapy for spider veins is almost 0% when the procedure is performed by a competent doctor. The rates of other complications vary somewhat, but have been reported as falling within the following ranges:

- Hemosiderin discoloration: 10%–80% of patients, with fewer than 1% of cases lasting longer than a year.
- Telangiectatic matting: 5%–75% of patients.
- Deep venous thrombosis: Fewer than 1%.
- Mild aching or pain: 35%–55%.
- Skin ulceration: About 4%.

Alternatives

Conservative treatments

Patients who are experiencing some discomfort from spider veins may be helped by any or several of the following approaches:

- Exercise. Walking or other forms of exercise that activate the muscles in the lower legs can relieve aching and cramping because these muscles keep the blood moving through the leg veins. One exercise that is often recommended is repeated flexing of the ankle joint. By flexing the ankles five to 10 times every few minutes and walking around for one to two minutes every half hour throughout the day, the patient can prevent the venous congestion that results from sitting or standing in one position for hours at a time.

WHO PERFORMS THE PROCEDURE AND WHERE IS IT PERFORMED?

Sclerotherapy is usually performed by general surgeons, dermatologists, or plastic surgeons, but it can also be done by family physicians or naturopaths who have been trained to do it. The American College of Phlebology holds workshops and intensive practical courses for interested practitioners. The ACP can be contacted for a list of members in each state.

Sclerotherapy is done as an outpatient procedure, most often in the doctor's office or in a plastic surgery clinic.

- Avoiding high-heeled shoes. Shoes with high heels do not allow the ankle to flex fully when the patient is walking. This limitation of the range of motion of the ankle joint makes it more difficult for the leg muscles to contract and force venous blood upwards toward the heart.
- Elevating the legs for 15–30 minutes once or twice a day. This change of position is frequently recommended for reducing edema of the feet and ankles.
- Wearing compression hosiery. Compression benefits the leg veins by reducing inflammation as well as improving venous outflow. Most manufacturers of medical compression stockings now offer some relatively sheer hosiery that is both attractive and that offers support.
- Medications. Drugs that have been used to treat the discomfort associated with spider veins include nonsteroidal anti-inflammatory drugs (NSAIDs) and preparations of vitamins C and E. One prescription medication that is sometimes given to treat circulatory problems in the legs and feet is pentoxifylline, which improves blood flow in the smaller capillaries. Pentoxifylline is sold under the brand name Trendar.

If appearance is the patient's primary concern, spider veins on the legs can often be covered with specially formulated cosmetics that come in a wide variety of skin tones. Some of these preparations are available in waterproof formulations for use during swimming and other athletic activities.

Electrodesiccation, laser therapy, and pulsed light therapy

Electrodesiccation is a treatment modality whereby the doctor seals off the small blood vessels that cause spider veins by passing a weak electric current through a fine needle to the walls of the veins. Electrodesiccation seems to be more effective in treating spider veins in the face than in treating those in the legs; it tends to leave pitted white scars when used to treat spider veins in the legs or feet.

QUESTIONS TO ASK THE DOCTOR

- How likely am I to develop new spider veins in the treated areas?
- Do you use the newer sclerosing foams when you administer sclerotherapy?
- What technique(s) do you prefer to use for sclerotherapy and why?

Laser therapy, like electrodesiccation, works better in treating facial spider veins. The sharply focused beam of intense light emitted by the laser heats the blood vessel, causing the blood in it to coagulate and close the vein. Various lasers have been used to treat spider veins, including argon, KTP 532nm, and alexandrite lasers. The choice of light wavelength and pulse duration are based on the size of the vein to be treated. Argon lasers, however, have been found to increase the patient's risk of developing hemosiderin discoloration when used on the legs. The KTP 532nm laser gives better results in treating leg spider veins, but is still not as effective as sclerotherapy.

Intense pulsed light (IPL) systems differ from lasers because the light emitted is noncoherent and not monochromatic. The IPL systems enable doctors to use a wider range of light wavelengths and pulse frequencies when treating spider veins and other skin problems, such as pigmented birthmarks. This flexibility, however, requires considerable skill and experience on the part of the doctor to remove spider veins without damaging the surrounding skin.

Complementary and alternative (CAM) treatments

According to Dr. Kenneth Pelletier, the former director of the program in complementary and alternative treatments at Stanford University School of Medicine, California, horse chestnut extract is as safe and effective as compression stockings when used as a conservative treatment for spider veins. Horse chestnut (*Aesculus hippocastanum*) has been used in Europe for some years to treat circulatory problems in the legs; most recent research has been conducted in

Great Britain and Germany. The usual dosage is 75 mg twice a day, at meals. The most common side effect of oral preparations of horse chestnut is occasional indigestion in some patients.

Resources

BOOKS

Khatri, VP and JA Asensio. *Operative Surgery Manual.* 1st ed. Philadelphia: Saunders, 2003.

Townsend, CM et al. *Sabiston Textbook of Surgery.* 17th ed. Philadelphia: Saunders, 2004.

PERIODICALS

Brunnberg, S., S. Lorenz, M. Landthaler, and U. Hohenleutner. "Evaluation of the Long Pulsed High Fluence Alexandrite Laser Therapy of Leg Telangiectasia." Lasers in Surgery and Medicine 31 (2002): 359-362.

Frullini, A., and A. Cavezzi. "Sclerosing Foam in the Treatment of Varicose Veins and Telangiectases: History and Analysis of Safety and Complications." Dermatologic Surgery 28 (January 2002): 11-15.

Goldman, M. P. "Treatment of Varicose and Telangiectatic Leg Veins: Double-Blind Prospective Comparative Trial Between Aethoxyskerol and Sotradecol." Dermatologic Surgery 28 (January 2002): 52-55.

Kern, P. "Sclerotherapy of Varicose Leg Veins. Technique, Indications, and Complications." International Angiology 21 (June 2002): 40-45.

Loo, W. J., and S. W. Lanigan. "Recent Advances in Laser Therapy for the Treatment of Cutaneous Vascular Disorders." Lasers in Medical Science 17 (2002): 9-12.

Raulin, C., B. Greve, and H. Grema. "IPL Technology: A Review." Lasers in Surgery and Medicine32 (2003): 78-87.

ORGANIZATIONS

American Academy of Dermatology. 930 East Woodfield Rd., PO Box 4014, Schaumburg, IL 60168. (847) 330-0230. www.aad.org.

American Association for Vascular Surgery (AAVS). 900 Cummings Center, #221-U, Beverly, MA 01915. www.aavs.vascularweb.org.

American College of Phlebology. 100 Webster Street, Suite 101, Oakland, CA 94607-3724. (510) 834-6500. www.phlebology.org.

American Society of Plastic Surgeons (ASPS). 444 East Algonquin Road, Arlington Heights, IL 60005. (847) 228-9900. www.plasticsurgery.org.

Peripheral Vascular Surgery Society (PVSS). 824 Munras Avenue, Suite C, Monterey, CA 93940. (831) 373-0508. www.pvss.org.

OTHER

American Society of Plastic Surgeons. Procedures: Sclerotherapy. [cited April 10, 2003]. www.plasticsurgery.org/public_education/procedures/Sclerotherapy.cfm.

Crowe, Mark A., M.D.. "Nevus Araneus (Spider Nevus)." eMedicine, April 12, 2002 [April 11, 2003]. www.emedicine.com/derm/topic293.htm.

Feied, Craig, M.D.. Venous Anatomy and Physiology. [cited April 10, 2003] www.phlebology.org/syllabus1.htm.

Fronek, Helane S., M.D.. Conservative Therapy for Venous Disease. [cited April 10, 2003] www.phlebology.org/syllabus4.htm.

Goldman, M. P., M.D.. Complications of Sclerotherapy. [cited April 10, 2003] www.phlebology.org/syllabus9.htm.

Marley, Wayne, M.D. Physical Examination of the Phlebology Patient. [cited April 10, 2003] www.phlebology.org/syllabus2.htm.

Sadick, Neil S., M.D.. Technique for Treating Telangiectasias and Reticular Veins. [cited April 10, 2003] www.phlebology.org/syllabus6.htm.

Weiss, Robert A., M.D., and Mitchel P. Goldman, M.D.. Treatment of Leg Telangiectasias with Lasers and High-Intensity Pulsed Light. [cited April 10, 2003] www.phlebology.org/syllabus10.htm.

Rebecca Frey, Ph.D.

Scoliosis surgery, Arthrodesis *see* **Spinal fusion**

Scopolamine patch

Definition

A scopolamine patch (Transdermal Scop or Transderm-V) is an adhesive medication patch that is applied to the skin behind the ear the night before surgery or a caesarean section. The patch is treated with the belladonna alkaloid scopolamine, an anticholinergic drug that is a central nervous system depressant and an antiemetic.

Purpose

Scopolamine patches are prescribed to reduce post-operative nausea and vomiting (PONV) associated with anesthesia and surgery. Scopolamine also has a mild analgesic and sedative effect, which adds to its therapeutic value for some surgical patients. In addition to PONV, scopolamine patches are also used for the treatment of motion sickness.

Demographics

Elderly patients may be more sensitive to scopolamine treatment and its use should be prescribed with caution in this group. The safety of scopolamine patches has not been determined in children; according to the Food and Drug Administration (FDA), the patch should not be used in children.

KEY TERMS

Anticholinergic—Drugs that block the action of acetylcholine, a neurotransmitter, consequently impairing the parasympathetic (involuntary) nervous system. Anticholinergic drugs inhibit secretion of bodily fluids (i.e., saliva, perspiration, stomach acid).

Antiemetic—A drug that prevents emesis, or vomiting.

Description

A potent drug derived from an alkaloid of belladonna (*Atropa belladonna*; common name deadly nightshade), scopolamine works by depressing the action of the nerve fibers near the ear and the vomiting center of the brain and central nervous system (CNS). The patch itself is designed with special layered materials that slowly release a small dose of the drug transdermally (through the skin) over a period of several days.

Patients who are instructed to apply their patch at home should wash their hands thoroughly both before and after the procedure. Scopolamine can be spread to the eyes by hand, which can cause blurred vision and pupil dilation. Patches should never be cut into pieces, as cutting destroys the time-release mechanism of the drug. The directions for use for the patch should be read thoroughly before application, and specific physician instructions should also be followed. The drug will start to work approximately four hours after the patch is applied.

Diagnosis/Preparation

The dime-sized scopolamine patch is applied just behind either the left or right ear. The area should be clean and hairless prior to the application, which should occur the evening before a scheduled surgery. For women who are prescribed a scopolamine patch to reduce nausea and vomiting related to a **cesarean section**, the patch should be applied just one hour before the procedure to minimize the baby's exposure to the drug. Scopolamine does cross the placental barrier, but as of early 2003, clinical studies have not shown any negative affects on newborn babies of mothers who used the drug in a caesarean delivery.

Patients with a history of glaucoma, prostate enlargement, kidney or liver problems, bladder obstruction, gastrointestinal obstruction, or contact dermatitis (allergic skin rash) in response to topical drugs may not be suitable candidates for scopolamine patch therapy. A physician or anesthesiologist should take a full medical history before prescribing scopolamine to determine if the medication is appropriate.

WHO PERFORMS THE PROCEDURE AND WHERE IS IT PERFORMED?

When used for surgical implications, a scopolamine patch may be ordered by a physician, surgeon, or anesthesiologist, typically in a hospital setting or an ambulatory surgery center. The patch may be applied at home by the patient, or by a nurse or physician's assistant as part of preoperative preparation.

Aftercare

Patients who receive a scopolamine patch should not drive or operate heavy machinery until the therapy is complete. Patch therapy generally lasts about three days. Patches should be disposed of according to the manufacturer's directions in a secure place to ensure that small children or pets do not get access to them. If PONV has not resolved after patch therapy has ended, patients should talk to their doctor about their treatment options.

Risks

Possible complications or side effects from transdermal scopolamine include but are not limited to: short-term memory loss, fatigue, confusion, hallucinations, difficulty urinating, and changes in heart rate. The drug can trigger seizures and psychotic delusions in patients with a history of these problems. Dizziness, nausea, headache, and hypotension (low blood pressure) have also been reported in some patients upon discontinuation of scopolamine patch therapy.

Patients who experience eye pain with redness and possible blurred vision should remove the patch immediately and call their doctor, since the symptoms could be signs of a rare but possible side effect of scopolamine called narrow-angle glaucoma. Blurriness with or without pupil dilation is also a potential but generally harmless side effect of the drug.

The FDA recommends that patients who are scheduled for a **magnetic resonance imaging** (MRI) scan remove the patch before the scan, as the patch's backing contains aluminum. The aluminum absorbs energy and heats up during the scan, which may cause a mild burn of the skin beneath the patch.

QUESTIONS TO ASK THE DOCTOR

When preparing to receive scopolamine transdermal therapy, you might ask your doctor:

- When and how do I apply the patch?
- What should I do if the patch becomes loose or falls off?
- When can I remove or replace the patch?
- Are there any warning symptoms that should signal me to remove the patch?

Normal results

When scopolamine patch therapy works, it reduces or eliminates post-surgical nausea and vomiting. Two-thirds of patients experience dry mouth, the most common side effect of the drug.

Alternatives

Intravenous or intramuscular injection of scopolamine may be used as alternatives to patch therapy for some patients. Other antiemetics that may be prescribed for PONV include anticholinergic drugs, dopaminergic drugs (i.e., promethazine, droperidol), antihistamines (i.e., diphenhydramine), and the serotonin receptor antagonists (i.e., ondansetron, granisetron, tropisetron, dolasetron). **Corticosteroids** may also be recommended for PONV in some patients.

Resources

BOOKS

Deglin, Judith Hopfer, and April Hazard Vallerand. *Davis's Drug Guide for Nurses*, 10th ed. Philadelphia: F. A. Davis, 2007.

PERIODICALS

Gan, T. J. "Postoperative nausea and vomiting—can it be eliminated?" *Journal of the American Medical Association* 287 (March 13, 2002): 1233–6.

Renner, U. D., R. Oertel, and W. Kirch. "Pharmacokinetics and Pharmacodynamics in Clinical Use of Scopolamine." *Therapeutic Drug Monitoring* 27 (October 2005): 655–665.

OTHER

Food and Drug Administration (FDA). Approved Label for Transderm. Rockville, MD: FDA, 2003.

2006 FDA Science Poster Abstract K-26. Burns in MRI Patients Wearing Transdermal Drug Delivery Systems. Rockville, MD: FDA, 2006.

Paula Ford-Martin
Rebecca Frey, Ph.D.

Secobarbital *see* **Barbiturates**

Second-look surgery

Definition

Second-look surgery is performed after a procedure or course of treatment to determine if the patient is free of disease. If disease is found, additional procedures may or may not be performed at the time of second-look surgery.

Purpose

Second-look surgery may be performed under numerous circumstances on patients with various medical conditions.

Cancer

A second-look procedure is sometimes performed to determine if a cancer patient has responded successfully to a particular treatment. Examples of cancers that are assessed during second-look surgery are ovarian cancer and colorectal cancer. In many cases, before a round of chemotherapy and/or radiation therapy is started, a patient will undergo a surgical procedure called cytoreduction to reduce the size of a tumor. This debulking increases the sensitivity of the tumor and decreases the number of necessary treatment cycles. Following cytoreduction and chemotherapy, a second-look procedure may be necessary to determine if the area is cancer-free.

An advantage to second-look surgery following cancer treatment is that if cancer is found, it may be removed during the procedure in some patients. In other cases, if a tumor cannot be entirely removed, the surgeon can debulk the tumor and improve the patient's chances of responding to another cycle of chemotherapy. However, second-look surgery cannot definitively prove that a patient is free of cancer; some microscopic cancer cells can persist and begin to grow in other areas of the body. Even if no cancer is found during second-look surgery, the rate of cancer relapse is approximately 25%.

KEY TERMS

Adhesion—A band of internal scar tissue that develops after injury or surgery.

Anastomosis (plural, anastomoses)—The surgical connection of two structures, such as blood vessels or sections of the intestine.

Cholesteatoma—A destructive and expanding sac that develops in the middle ear or mastoid process.

Debulking—The removal of part of a malignant tumor in order to make the remainder more sensitive to radiation or chemotherapy.

Endometriosis—The growth of tissue like the lining of a woman's uterus (endometrium) outside the uterus in other parts of the body.

Endoscopy—A surgical technique that uses an endoscope (a thin, lighted, telescope-like instrument) to visualize structures inside the human body.

Infertility—The inability to become pregnant or carry a pregnancy to term.

Ischemia—Inadequate blood supply to an organ or area of tissue due to obstruction of a blood vessel.

Kidney stones—Small solid masses that form in the kidney.

Pelvic disease

Second-look surgery may benefit patients suffering from a number of different conditions that affect the pelvic organs. Endometriosis is a condition in which the tissue that lines the uterus grows elsewhere in the body, usually in the abdominal cavity, leading to pain and scarring. Endometrial growths may be surgically removed or treated with medications. A second-look procedure may be performed following the initial surgery or course of medication to determine if treatment was successful in reducing the number of growths. Additional growths may be removed at this time.

Second-look surgery may also be performed following the surgical removal of adhesions (bands of scar tissue that form in the abdomen following surgery or injury) or uterine fibroids (noncancerous growths of the uterus). If the results are positive, an additional procedure may be performed to remove the adhesions or growths. Patients undergoing treatment for infertility may benefit from a second-look procedure to determine if the cause of infertility has been cured before ceasing therapy.

Abdominal disease

In patients suffering from bleeding from the gastrointestinal (GI) tract, recurrence of bleeding after attempted treatment remains a significant risk; approximately 10–25% of cases do not respond to initial treatment. Second-look surgery following treatment for GI bleeding may be beneficial in determining if bleeding has recurred and treating the cause of the bleeding before it becomes more extensive.

Patients suffering from a partial or complete blockage of the intestine are at risk of developing bowel ischemia (**death** of intestinal tissue due to a lack of oxygen). Initial surgery is most often necessary to remove the diseased segment of bowel; a second-look procedure is commonly performed to ensure that only healthy tissue remains and that the new intestinal connection (called an anastomosis) is healing properly.

Other conditions

A variety of other conditions can be assessed with second-look surgery. Patients who have undergone surgical repair of torn muscles in the knee might undergo a procedure called second-look arthroscopy to assess whether the repair is healing. A physician may use second-look mastoidoscopy to visualize the middle ear after removal of a cholesteatoma (a benign but destructive growth in the middle ear). A second endoscopic procedure may be performed on a patient who underwent endoscopic treatment for sinusitis (chronic infection of the sinuses) to evaluate the surgical site and remove debris.

Description

Second-look surgery may be performed within hours, days, weeks, or months of the initial procedure or treatment. This time interval depends on the patient's condition and the type of procedure.

Laparotomy

A laparotomy is a large incision through the abdominal wall to visualize the structures inside the abdominal cavity. After placing the patient under **general anesthesia**, the surgeon first makes a large incision through the skin, then through each layer under the skin in the region that the surgeon wishes to explore. The area will be assessed for evidence of remaining disease. For example, in the case of second-look laparotomy following treatment for endometriosis, the abdominal organs will be examined for evidence of endometrial growths. In the case of cancer, a "washing" of the abdominal cavity may be performed; sterile fluid is instilled into the abdominal cavity and washed around the organs, then extracted with a syringe. The fluid is then analyzed for the presence of cancerous cells. Biopsies may also be taken of various abdominal tissues and analyzed.

If the surgeon discovers evidence of disease or a failed surgical repair, additional procedures may be performed to remove the disease or repair the dysfunction. For example, if adhesions are encountered during a second-look procedure on an infertile female patient, the surgeon may remove the adhesions at that time. Upon completion of the procedure, the incision is closed.

Laparoscopy

Laparoscopy is a surgical technique that permits a view of the internal abdominal organs without an extensive surgical incision. During laparoscopy, a thin lighted tube called a laparoscope is inserted into the abdominal cavity through a tiny incision. Images taken by the laparoscope are seen on a video monitor connected to the scope. The surgeon may then examine the abdominal cavity, albeit with a more limited operative view than with laparotomy. Procedures such as the removal of growths or repair of deformities can be performed by instruments inserted through other small incisions in the abdominal wall. After the procedure is completed, any incisions are closed with **stitches**.

Other procedures

Depending on the area of the body in question, other procedures may be used to perform second-look surgery. These include:

- Arthroscopy. Arthroscopy uses a thin endoscope to visualize the inner space of a joint such as the knee or elbow. Second-look arthroscopy may be used to determine if previous surgery on the joint is healing properly.
- Percutaneous nephrolithotomy (PNL). This minimally invasive procedure is used to remove kidney stones. Second-look PNL may be used to remove fragments of stones that could not be removed during the initial procedure.
- Hysteroscopy. A hysteroscope is an instrument used to visualize and perform procedures on the inner cavity of the uterus. Second-look hysteroscopy may be used after surgery or medical treatment to treat adhesions or benign growths in the uterus to determine if they have been effectively removed.
- Mastoidectomy. This surgical procedure is used to treat cholesteatoma; a second-look procedure is generally performed to ensure that the entire cholesteatoma was removed during the initial procedure.

Resources

BOOKS

Cushner, Fred D., W. Norman Scott, and Giles R. Scuderi, eds. *Surgical Techniques for the Knee*. New York: Thieme, 2005.

Hatch, Kenneth D. *Laparoscopy for Gynecology and Oncology*. Philadelphia: Wolters Kluwer/Lippincott Williams and Wilkins Health, 2008.

Sabel, Michael S., Vernon K. Sondak, and Jeffrey J. Sussman, eds. *Surgical Foundations: Essentials of Surgical Oncology*. Philadelphia: Mosby Elsevier, 2007.

PERIODICALS

Ahn, J. H., J. C. Yoo, H. S. Yang, et al. "Second-Look Arthroscopic Findings of 208 Patients after ACL Reconstruction." *Knee Surgery, Sports Traumatology, Arthroscopy* 15 (March 2007): 242–248.

Barakate, M., and I. Bottrill. "Combined Approach Tympanoplasty for Cholesteatoma: Impact of Middle-Ear Endoscopy." *Journal of Laryngology and Otology*, June 7, 2007, 1–5.

Gershenson, D. M. "Management of Ovarian Germ Cell Tumors." *Journal of Clinical Oncology* 25 (July 10, 2007): 2938–2943.

Marmo, Riccardo, Gianluca Rotandano, Maria Antonia Bianca, Roberto Piscopo, Antonio Prisco, and Livio Cipolletta. "Outcome of Endoscopic Treatment for Peptic Ulcer Bleeding: Is a Second Look Necessary?" *Gastrointestinal Endoscopy* 57, no. 1 (January 2003): 62–7.

Sood, A. K. "Second-Look Laparotomy for Ovarian Germ Cell Tumors: To Do or Not to Do?" *Journal of Postgraduate Medicine* 52 (October-December 2006): 246–247.

Yanar, H., K. Taviloglu, C. Ertekin, et al. "Planned Second-Look Laparoscopy in the Management of Acute Mesenteric Ischemia." *World Journal of Gastroenterology* 13 (June 28, 2007): 3350–3353.

ORGANIZATIONS

American College of Surgeons. 633 N. Saint Clair St., Chicago, IL 60611-3211. (312) 202-5000. http://www.facs.org.

Society of Surgical Oncology. 85 W. Algonquin Rd., Suite 550, Arlington Heights, IL 60005. (847) 427-1400. http://www.surgonc.org.

OTHER

Horlbeck, Drew, and Matthew Ng. "Middle Ear Endoscopy." eMedicine. June 12, 2006. [cited January 12, 2008] http://www.emedicine.com/ENT/topic483.htm.

Johnson, Darren L., and Jeffrey B. Selby. "Meniscal Transplantation: Indications and Results." Medscape General Medicine, August 3, 2001. [cited May 20, 2003] http://www.medscape.com/viewarticle/408541_1.

Stephanie Dionne Sherk
Rebecca Frey, Ph.D.

Second opinion

Definition

A second opinion is the result of seeking an evaluation by another doctor or surgeon to confirm the diagnosis and treatment plan of a primary physician, or to offer an alternative diagnosis and/or treatment approach.

Purpose

Getting a second surgical opinion can fill an important emotional need as well as establishing medical needs and treatment goals. When a second opinion confirms initial findings, it can provide reassurance and feelings of acceptance for the patient, and may reduce anxiety and uncertainty.

From a cost-effectiveness point of view, second opinions can save health insurance providers money by establishing the certainty of a clinical need (or lack of need) for surgery, particularly when the diagnosis is life-threatening.

Patients with a diagnosis of cancer may also benefit from a second-opinion pathology review of their biopsy material. A Johns Hopkins study reported that 1.4% of patients scheduled for cancer-related surgery at their facility were found to have been misdiagnosed when their tissue samples were reevaluated by a second pathologist. Similarly, a study published in the *Annals of Surgical Oncology* in 2002 found that a pathological second opinion of breast cancers changed the initial diagnosis, prognosis, or treatment approach in 80% of the 340 study subjects.

Several clinical research studies, however, have found that patients often seek second opinions not necessarily because they doubt the diagnosis or recommendations of their first provider, but because they were dissatisfied with either the amount of information given to them or the style of communication of their doctor. A 2002 Northwestern University study found that only 46% of patients coming into a breast cancer treatment center for a second opinion had been offered a complete discussion of treatment options during their initial consultation.

Description

Doctors often have differing viewpoints as to how a particular medical problem should be managed, whether through surgery or less-invasive treatment means. One surgeon may prefer to take a "watchful waiting" approach before recommending surgery, while another may believe in performing surgery as soon as possible to avoid later complications. In some cases, several surgical techniques may be viable options for a patient. Medicine is not as black-and-white as many patients are led to believe, and physicians are not infallible. For these reasons, and because surgery is a major procedure with associated risks that should not be taken lightly, second opinions are an important part of the process of **informed consent** and decision-making.

Although a physician may strive to be objective, personal views and subjective experiences can influence their treatment recommendations. In addition, both the education and experience of a doctor in a given medical area can also influence the advice they offer a patient. For these reasons, seeking a second opinion from another physician and/or surgeon can be invaluable in making a decision on a course of treatment.

Second opinions are most frequently sought in cases of elective (nonemergency) surgery, when the patient has time to consider options and make a more informed choice about his or her course of treatment. While a second surgical opinion may be requested in some cases of **emergency surgery**, they are not as common, simply because of the logistical limitations involved with getting a qualified second opinion if a patient requires immediate care.

In some cases, a doctor or surgeon may encourage seeking a second opinion, particularly when the preferred course of treatment is not clear-cut or another surgeon with advanced training or expertise may

KEY TERMS

Informed consent—Providing a patient with complete, objective information on the risks, benefits, and potential and probable outcomes of different surgical or therapeutic options so that they may make an informed decision or consent to treatment.

Pathologist—A physician with specialized training in recognizing and identifying diseases through the analysis of abnormal bodily tissues.

Postoperative care—Medical care and support required after surgery to promote healing and recovery.

Watchful waiting—Monitoring a patient's disease state carefully to see if the condition worsens before trying surgery or another therapy. This term is often associated with prostate cancer.

provide more insights into surgical options. A doctor or surgeon may also recommend seeking a second opinion when the patient is suffering from multiple medical disorders.

Patients should remember that it is their right to seek a second opinion before committing to surgery or another treatment plan. Embarrassment or fear of disapproval from a primary care provider should not be a barrier to getting a second opinion. A competent physician will not consider the decision to seek a second opinion an insult to their ability or experience. Instead, they will consider the patient an informed individual who is proactive and responsible for his or her own health care.

Patients seeking a second-opinion consultation may ask the provider questions similar to those they asked their primary provider. Questions may include:

- Are there other options besides surgery?
- What are the risks and benefits of each treatment option?
- How might each possible treatment impact quality-of-life for the patient?
- What kind of success rate is associated with surgery and other potential therapies?
- How is the surgery performed?
- Is surgery a permanent, long-term, or temporary solution to the condition?
- What type of anesthesia will be used?
- If surgery is chosen by the patient, how soon must it be done?
- What type of aftercare and recovery time is required once the surgery is complete?
- How much pain is to be expected postoperatively, and how is it typically treated?
- What are the costs involved with surgery and other treatment options, including postoperative care?

Providing the second surgeon with appropriate background information is important, but so is refraining from detailed descriptions of what the first provider did or did not recommend before the consultation begins. Patients should allow the surgeon to draw objective conclusions based on the medical history and diagnostic data before them. If the second opinion differs from the first provider's opinion, and the patient feels comfortable doing so, he or she might then offer information on the first provider's recommendations to get further feedback and input for a final decision.

Preparation

Before seeking a second opinion, patients should contact their health insurance provider to find out if the service is covered. Some insurance companies may request that a second opinion be sought before major **elective surgery**, and may reserve the right to designate a physician or surgeon to provide the patient evaluation. As of early 2008, **Medicare** Part B covered 80% of costs for surgical second opinions after deductible, and 80% for a third opinion if the first two opinions are contradictory. Other Medicare programs may cover second opinions as well; patients should check with their Medicare carrier for details.

There are several ways to find an appropriate health care professional to provide a second opinion. Patients can:

- Ask friends and family for references.
- Ask their primary care physician or another trusted health care provider for a referral.
- Contact an appropriate specialty medical organization (e.g., American College of Surgeons) for a referral.
- Call their local medical licensing board.
- Check with their insurance provider or Medicare carrier.
- Cancer patients can consult a list of multidisciplinary institutions that will provide a second opinion on request. The list is available at < http://www.blochcancer.org/>.

When seeking a second surgical opinion, patients should find a surgeon who is board certified in the appropriate specialty by an organization that is part of the American Board of Medical Specialties (ABMS). For example, surgery of the urinary tract may be performed by a provider who is board certified by the American Board of Urology and/or the American Board of Surgery (ABS), two member organizations of the ABMS. Diplomates of ABMS member boards are surgeons who have passed rigorous written and oral testing on these specialties and have met specific accredited educational and residency requirements. In some cases, surgeons may also be certified in subspecialties within a discipline (for example, a vascular surgeon may be board certified by the **vascular surgery** board of the ABS). The ABMS provides a verification service for patients to check on the certification status of their provider.

In addition, the surgeon may also be a Fellow of the American College of Surgery (ACS), as indicated by the designation F.A.C.S. after their name. This indicates that he or she has met standards of clinical experience, education, ethical conduct, and professional expertise as prescribed by the ACS.

Once a second health care provider is selected, patients should speak with their primary doctor about providing the appropriate medical history, test results, and other pertinent information to the physician who will give the second opinion. The patient may have to sign an information release form to allow the files to be sent. If x rays, **magnetic resonance imaging** (MRI), or other radiological testing was performed, the second physician may request to see the original films, rather than the radiologist's report of the results, in order to interpret them objectively. In some cases, the office of the surgeon giving the second opinion can arrange to have these materials transferred with a patient's written approval. Patients should call ahead to ensure that all needed materials arrive at the second provider's office before the appointment, to give that physician adequate time to review them and to avoid potentially costly repeat testing.

Normal results

Second opinions that agree with the first provider's conclusions may help ease the patient's mind and provide a clearer picture of the necessary course of treatment or surgery. However, if a patient still feels uncomfortable with the treatment plan outlined by the first and second physicians, or strongly disagrees with their conclusions, a third opinion from another provider is an option.

In cases in which the second provider disagrees with the first provider on diagnosis and/or treatment, the patient has harder choices to face. Again, a third evaluation may be in order from yet another physician, and some insurance companies may actually require this step in cases of conflicting opinions. If a patient is very comfortable with and confident in their primary care provider, they may wish to revisit them to review the second opinion.

In all cases, a patient should remember that their personal preferences, beliefs, and lifestyle considerations must also be considered in their final decision on surgery or treatment, as they are the ones who will live with the results.

Resources

BOOKS

Horton, Richard C. *Second Opinion: Doctors, Diseases, and Decisions in Modern Medicine*. London: Granta Books, 2003.

Rose, Eric. *Second Opinion: The Columbia Presbyterian Guide to Surgery*. New York: St. Martin's Press, 2000.

PERIODICALS

Reichman, M. "Optimizing Referrals and Consults with a Standardized Process." *Family Practice Management* 14 (November-December 2007): 38–42.

Staradub, V. L., et al. "Changes in Breast Cancer Therapy Because of Pathology Second Opinions." *Annals of Surgical Oncology* 9, no.10 (December 2002): 982–7.

ORGANIZATIONS

American Board of Medical Specialties (ABMS). 1007 Church St., Suite 404, Evanston, IL 60201. (866) ASK-ABMS. http://www.abms.org.

American College of Surgeons (ACS). 63 N. St. Clair Drive, Chicago, IL 60611. (312) 202-5000. E-mail: postmaster @facs.org. http://www.facs.org.

OTHER

Center for Medicare and Medicaid Services (CMS). Getting a Second Opinion Before Surgery. Publication CMS-02173. Revised November 2007. http://www.medicare.gov/Publications/Pubs/pdf/02173.pdf. A Spanish version of this document is available at < http://www.medicare.gov/publications/pubs/pdf/02173_s.pdf >.

Yale-New Haven Hospital. Getting a Good Second Opinion. < http://www.ynhh.org/choice/secondopinion.html>.[cited January 12, 2008].

Paula Ford-Martin
Rebecca Frey, Ph.D.

Sedation, conscious

Definition

Conscious sedation, produced by the administration of certain medications, is an altered level of consciousness that still allows a patient to respond to physical stimulation and verbal commands, and to maintain an unassisted airway.

Purpose

The purpose of conscious sedation is to produce a state of relaxation and/or pain relief by using benzodiazepine-type and narcotic medications to facilitate a procedure such as a biopsy, radiologic imaging study, endoscopic procedure, radiation therapy, or **bone marrow aspiration**.

Description

Sedation is used inside or outside the **operating room**. Outside the operating suite, medical specialists use sedation to calm and relax their patients.

If the patient is to undergo a minor surgical procedure, screening and assessment of medical conditions that may interfere with conscious sedation must be explored. These potential risk factors include advanced age, history of adverse reactions to the proposed medications, and a past medical history of severe cardiopulmonary (heart/lung) disease. Other than those risk factors, contraindications for conscious sedation include; recent ingestion of large food or fluid volumes or a physical class IV or greater.

Once it has been established that the patient would be a good candidate for conscious sedation, just prior to the surgery or procedure, the patient will receive the sedating drug intravenously. A clip-like apparatus will be placed on the patient's finger to monitor oxygen intake during the sedation. This oxygen monitoring is called pulse oximetry and is a valuable, continuous monitor of patient oxygenation.

Dosing of medications that produce conscious sedation is individualized, and the medication is administered slowly to gauge a patient's response to the sedative. The two most common medications used to sedate patients for medical procedures are midazolam and fentanyl.

Fentanyl is a medication classified as an opioid narcotic analgesic (pain reliever) that is 50 to 100 times more potent than morphine. Given intravenously, the onset of action of fentanyl is almost immediate, and peak analgesia occurs with in 10 to 15 minutes. A single dose of fentanyl given intravenously can produce good analgesia for only 20 to 45 minutes for most patients because the drug's distribution shifts from the brain (central nervous system) to peripheral tissues. The key to correct dosage is titration, or giving the medication in small amounts until the desired patient response is achieved.

Midazolam is a medication classified as a short-acting benzodiazepine (sedative) that depresses the central nervous system. Midazolam is ineffective for pain and has no analgesic effect during conscious sedation. The drug is a primary choice for conscious sedation because midazolam causes patients to have no recollection of the medical procedure. In general, midazolam has a fast-acting, short-lived sedative effect when given intravenously, achieving sedation within one to five minutes and peaking within 30 minutes. The effects of midazolam typically last one hour but may persist for six hours (including the amnestic effect). Patients who receive midazolam for conscious sedation should not be allowed to drive home after the procedure.

WHO PERFORMS THE PROCEDURE AND WHERE IS IT PERFORMED?

Conscious sedation is administered by medical or pediatric specialists performing a procedure that may be diagnostic and/or therapeutic. It may be used in a hospital, outpatient care facility, or doctor's office.

Monitoring

Patient monitoring during conscious sedation must be performed by a trained and licensed health care professional. This clinician must not be involved in the procedure, but should have primary responsibility of monitoring and attending to the patient. Equipment must be in place and organized for monitoring the patient's blood pressure, pulse, respiratory rate, level of consciousness, and, most important, the oxygen saturation (the measure of oxygen perfusion inside the body) with a **pulse oximeter** (a machine that provides a continuous real-time recording of oxygenation). The oxygen saturation is the most sensitive parameter affected during increased levels of conscious sedation. **Vital signs** and other pertinent recordings must be monitored before the start of the administration of medications, and then at a minimum of every five minutes thereafter until the procedure is completed. After the procedure has been completed, monitoring should continue every 15 minutes for the first hour after the last dose of medication(s) was administered. After the first hour, monitoring can continue as needed. Children who receive sedative medication with a long half-life may require extended observation.

Risks and risk management

The American Academy of Pediatrics (AAP) has established safe practice guidelines to manage conscious sedation without an anesthesiologist for minor procedures. These AAP criteria include (1) a full-time licensed clinician (nurse, physician, physician assistant, surgeon assistant, respiratory therapist) who is strictly and exclusively monitoring the patient's breathing, level of consciousness, vital signs, and airway; (2) standard procedures for monitoring vital signs; and (3) immediate availability (on site) of airway equipment, resuscitative medications, suction apparatus, and supplemental oxygen delivery systems.

QUESTIONS TO ASK THE DOCTOR

When should I stop taking my regular medications? When should I begin them again?

What side effects can I expect after the procedure? Nausea? Dizziness? Drowsiness? Is there anything I can do to ward off these side effects?

What are the risks of this procedure?

Which sedative will you use?

What steps will you take if there are complications?

Will I feel any pain?

If adverse reactions occur while using fentanyl, the antidote is a drug called naloxone. It provides rapid reversal of fentanyl's narcotic effect. The incidence of oversedation or decreased respiration is low using fentanyl if the medication is carefully titrated.

Resources

BOOKS

Behrman, R. *Nelson Textbook of Pediatrics*, 16th ed. Philadelphia: W. B. Saunders Company, 2000.

PERIODICALS

U. S. Department of Health and Human Services. *Acute Pain Management: Operative or Medical Procedures and Trauma. Clinical Practice Guidelines*. Department of Health and Human Services Pub. No. AHCPR 92-0032.

The American Academy of Pediatrics and the American Academy of Pediatric Dentistry. *Guidelines for Monitoring and Management of Pediatric Patients During and After Sedation for Diagnostic and Therapeutic Procedures. Clinical Guidelines Reference Manual*. V29, no. 7 (2008). http:www.aapd.org/media/Policies_Guidelines/G_Sedation.pdf.

ORGANIZATIONS

American Association of Nurse Anesthetists. 222 South Prospect Avenue, Park Ridge, IL 60068-4001. (847) 692–7050.http://www.aana.com.

Laith Farid Gulli, M.D., M.S.
Alfredo Mori, MBBS
Renee Laux, M.S.

Sedimentation rate

Definition

The sedimentation rate (or erythrocyte sedimentation rate) is a test that measures that degree of inflammation occurring in the body. Inflammation is the sum total of the body's reaction to infection, allergy, irritation, malignancy (cancer), or injury. The test is neither specific to a particular type of disease or condition, nor does it identify what tissues or organs are inflamed. In other words, while the sedimentation rate is a useful test to verify an impression of the possible presence of a particular illness, it cannot stand alone as a definitive diagnostic tool. The patient's history and symptoms must be correlated with the sedimentation rate and other laboratory tests in order to arrive at a clinical diagnosis.

The sedimentation rate is literally a measure of the distance that red blood cells (erythrocytes) fall through a test tube filled with blood in an hour's time. This process leaves clear plasma, devoid of red blood cells, at the top of the tube. When there is an inflammatory process occurring in the body, the body produces a variety of proteins that stick to red blood cells. These protein-red blood cell complexes are heavier than unaffected red blood cells, allowing them to fall more quickly and farther through the blood in the test tube. As a result, when inflammation is present in the body, the red blood cells drop through the test tube more quickly, and more of them accumulate at a lower part of the test tube, resulting in a higher sedimentation rate.

Purpose

A sedimentation rate is usually done when an individual is having symptoms compatible with an inflammatory disorder, particularly polymyalgia rheumatica and temporal arteritis. Some symptoms that might prompt a practitioner to order a sedimentation rate include unexplained headache, joint pain or stiffness, anemia, unintentional weight loss, fevers, and severe fatigue. The sedimentation rate is also frequently used to monitor a disease process that has already been diagnosed, such as Hodgkin's lymphoma, or autoimmune disorders such as rheumatoid arthritis or systemic lupus erythematosus.

Precautions

The sedimentation rate is not diagnostic. This means that getting a specific result does not definitively confirm the presence of any particular disease.

KEY TERMS

Autoimmune disorder—A condition in which the body's immune system is accidentally attacking tissues or organs of the body, causing injury and disease.

Inflammation—Pain, swelling, redness, and heat that often occurs when tissues of the body are injured, infected, or irritated in some way.

Malignancy—Conditions that are cancerous, meaning that they produce abnormal cells capable of invading and destroying other local and distant tissues.

Polymyalgia rheumatica—A condition with symptoms of achiness and stiffness, primarily striking older adults.

Temporal arteritis—A condition in which inflammation of the blood vessels that supply the head and neck result in severe, chronic headache, particularly over one temple, as well as fever, weight loss, and severe fatigue.

Instead, the test is used to correlate with the clinical picture, meaning the history and the symptoms that an individual is experiencing.

Description

This test requires blood to be drawn from a vein (usually one in the forearm), generally by a nurse or phlebotomist (an individual who has been trained to draw blood). A tourniquet is applied to the arm above the area where the needle stick will be performed. The site of the needle stick is cleaned with antiseptic, and the needle is inserted. The blood is collected in vacuum tubes. After collection, the needle is withdrawn, and pressure is kept on the blood draw site to stop any bleeding and decrease bruising. A bandage is then applied.

Preparation

There are no restrictions on diet or physical activity, either before or after the blood test.

Aftercare

As with any blood tests, discomfort, bruising, and/or a very small amount of bleeding is common at the puncture site. Immediately after the needle is withdrawn, it is helpful to put pressure on the puncture site until the bleeding has stopped. This decreases the chance of significant bruising. Warm packs may relieve minor discomfort. Some individuals may feel briefly woozy after a blood test, and they should be encouraged to lie down and rest until they feel better.

Risks

Basic blood tests, such as sedimentation testing, do not carry any significant risks, other than slight bruising and the chance of brief dizziness.

Results

The normal sedimentation rate range in men is 0-15 mm/hour. The normal sedimentation rate range in women is 0-20 mm/hour. The normal sedimentation rate range in children is 0-10 mm/hour. The normal sedimentation rate range in newborn babies is 0-2 mm/hr. Women normally have higher sedimentation rates than men. People over the age of 50 years also have higher normal sedimentation rates than do younger individuals. Other factors that may increase the sedimentation rate without suggesting the presence of disease include obesity or pregnancy.

An elevated sedimentation rate can be caused by a number of conditions, including an episode of crisis in sickle cell disease, osteomyelitis, stroke, prostate cancer, coronary artery disease, rheumatoid arthritis, chronic infections, certain cancers (including Hodgkin's disease and renal cell carcinoma), ankylosing spondylitis, thyroid disease, temporal arteritis, scleroderma, polyarteritis nodosa, systemic lupus erythematosus, infections (appendicitis, osteomyelitis, pelvic inflammatory disease, pneumonia), and Kawasaki disease in children.

An extremely elevated sedimentation rate can be caused by multiple myeloma and polymyalgia rheumatica.

An abnormally low sedimentation rate can be caused by sickle cell anemia (not during painful crisis), use of steroid medications, polycythemia, or high serum glucose.

Resources

BOOKS

Goldman L, Ausiello D., eds. Cecil Textbook of Internal Medicine. 23rd ed. Philadelphia: Saunders, 2008.

Harris ED et al. Kelley's Textbook of Rheumatology. 7th ed. Philadelphia: Saunders, 2005.

Hoffman R. et al. Hematology: Basic Principles and Practice. 4th ed. Philadelphia: Elsevier, 2005.

McPherson RA et al. Henry's Clinical Diagnosis and Management By Laboratory Methods. 21st ed. Philadelphia: Saunders, 2007.

ORGANIZATIONS

American Association of Clinical Chemistry. 1850 K St., N.WSuite 625, Washington, DC 20006. http://www.aacc.org.

OTHER

National Institutes of Health. [cited February 10, 2008]. http://www.nlm.nih.gov/medlineplus/encyclopedia.html.

Rosalyn Carson-DeWitt, MD

Segmental resection *see* **Segmentectomy**

Segmentectomy

Definition

Segmentectomy is the excision (removal) of a portion of any organ or gland. The procedure has several variations and many names, including segmental resection, wide excision, **lumpectomy**, tumorectomy, **quadrantectomy**, and partial **mastectomy**.

Purpose

Segmentectomy is the surgical removal of a defined segment or portion of an organ or gland performed as a treatment. In this case, the purpose is the removal of a cancerous tumor. Common organs that have segments are the breasts, lungs, and liver.

Demographics

Segmentectomies are usually performed on patients with lung, liver, or breast cancer.

Lung cancer is the second most common cancer among both men and women, and is the leading cause of cancer **death** for both genders. Lung cancer kills more people (approximately 157,000 per year) than cancers of the breast, prostate, colon, and pancreas combined. Almost 90% of all lung cancers are caused by cigarette smoking. Other causes include secondhand smoke and exposure to asbestos and other occupation-related substances.

In each of the racial and ethnic groups, the rates among men are about two to three times greater than the rates among women. Among men, age-adjusted lung cancer incidence rates (per 100,000) range from a low of about 14 among Native Americans to a high of 117 among African Americans, an eight-fold difference. For women, the rates range from approximately 15 per 100,000 among Japanese to nearly 51 among Alaska natives, approximately a three-fold difference.

Excluding cancers of the skin, breast cancer is the most common form of cancer among women in the United States. The increase in incidence is primarily due to increased screening by **physical examination** and **mammography**. Although breast cancer occurs among both women and men, it is quite rare among men. Caucasian non-Hispanic women have the highest rates of breast cancer, over twice the rate for Hispanic women. There are a low number of cases for Alaska native, Native American, Korean, and Vietnamese women.

Primary cancers of the liver account for approximately 1.5% of all cancer cases in the United States. About two-thirds of liver cancers are clearly associated with hepatitis B and hepatitis C viral infections and cirrhosis. This type of liver cancer occurs more frequently in men than in women by a ratio of two to one.

Description

When cancer is confined to a segment of an organ, removal of that portion may offer cancer-control results equivalent to those of more extensive operations. This is especially true for breast and liver cancers. For breast and lung cancers, a segmentectomy is often combined with removal of some or all regional lymph nodes.

Treatment options for lung cancer depend on the stage of the cancer (whether it is in the lung only or has spread to other places in the body); tumor size; the type of lung cancer; presence (or lack) of symptoms; and the patient's general health.

A disease in which malignant (cancer) cells form in the tissues of the lung is called non-small cell lung cancer (NSCLC). There are five types of NSCLC; each consists of different types of cancer cells, which grow and spread in different ways. The types of NSCLC are named for the kinds of cells found in the cancer, and how the cells appear when viewed under a microscope.

Segmentectomy may be the treatment of choice for cancerous tumors in the occult, or hidden stage, as well as in stage 0, stage I, or stage II NSCLC. When the site and nature of the primary tumor is defined in occult stage lung cancer, it is generally removed by segmentectomy.

Segmentectomy is the usual treatment for stage 0 cancers of the lung, as they are limited to the layer of tissue that lines air passages, and have not invaded the nearby lung tissue. Chemotherapy or radiation therapy is not normally required.

Segmentectomy is recommended only for treating the smallest stage I cancers and for patients with other

KEY TERMS

Angiogram—An examination of a part of the body by injecting dye into an artery so that the blood vessels show up on an x ray.

Anterior mediastinotomy—A surgical procedure to look at the organs and tissues between the lungs and between the breastbone and spine for abnormal areas. An incision (cut) is made next to the breastbone and a thin, lighted tube is inserted into the chest. Tissue and lymph node samples may be taken for biopsy.

Biopsy—Removal and examination of tissue, cells, or fluids from the living body.

Bronchoscope—A tubular illuminated instrument used for inspecting or passing instruments into the bronchi.

Chemoprevention—The use of drugs, vitamins, or other substances to reduce the risk of developing cancer or of the cancer returning.

Chemotherapy—Cancer treatment that uses drugs to stop the growth of cancer cells, either by killing the cells or by stopping them from dividing.

Clinical breast exam—An examination of the breast and surrounding tissue by a physician, who is feeling for lumps and looking for other signs of abnormality.

Computed tomography—An x-ray machine linked to a computer that takes a series of detailed pictures of the organs and blood vessels in the body.

Conservation surgery—Surgery that preserves the aesthetics of the area undergoing an operation.

Excision—To surgically remove.

Excisional biopsy—Procedure in which a surgeon removes all of a lump or suspicious area and an area of healthy tissue around the edges. The tissue is then examined under a microscope to check for cancer cells.

Fine-needle aspiration—A procedure in which a thin needle removes fluid and cells from a breast lump to be examined.

Incisional biopsy—A procedure in which a surgeon cuts out a sample of a lump or suspicious area.

Laser therapy—A cancer treatment that uses a laser beam (a narrow beam of intense light) to kill cancer cells.

Lobectomy—Removal of a section of the lung.

Lymph node biopsy—The removal of all or part of a lymph node to view under a microscope for cancer cells.

medical conditions that make removing part or the entire lobe of the lung (lobectomy) dangerous. If the patient does not have sufficient pulmonary function to tolerate this more extensive operation, a segmentectomy will be performed. Additional chemotherapy after surgery for stage I NSCLC is not routinely recommended. If a patient has serious medical problems, radiation therapy may be the primary treatment.

A cancerous tumor will be surgically removed by segmentectomy or lobectomy in cases of stage II NSCLC. A wedge resection might be done if the patient cannot withstand lobectomy. Sometimes **pneumonectomy** (removal of the entire lung) is needed. Radiation therapy may be used to destroy cancer cells left behind after surgery, especially if malignant cells are present at the edge of the tissue removed by surgery. Some doctors may recommend additional radiation therapy even if the edges of the sample have no detectable cancer cells.

Segmentectomy is under investigation for the treatment of small-cell lung cancers.

Because of the need for radiotherapy after segmentectomy, some patients, such as pregnant women and those with syndromes not compatible with radiation treatment, may not be candidates for segmentectomy. As in any surgery, patients should alert their physician about all allergies and any medications they are taking.

Diagnosis/Preparation

The following methods may be used to help diagnose breast cancer:

- complete physical exam and family medical history
- clinical breast exam
- mammography
- biopsy (incisional, excisional, or needle)
- ultrasonography
- fine-needle aspiration

Tests help to determine whether cancer cells have spread within the lungs or to other parts of the body after a diagnosis of lung cancer. The following tests

Lymph nodes—Small, bean-shaped organs located throughout the lymphatic system. Lymph nodes store special cells that can trap cancer cells and bacteria traveling through the body.

Mammography—An x ray of the breast

Magnetic resonance imaging (MRI)—A powerful magnet linked to a computer used to make detailed images of areas inside the body. These pictures are viewed on a monitor and can also be printed.

Mediastinoscopy—A surgical procedure to look at the organs, tissues, and lymph nodes between the lungs for abnormal areas. An incision (cut) is made at the top of the breastbone and a thin, lighted tube is inserted into the chest. Tissue and lymph node samples may be taken for biopsy.

Needle biopsy—The use of a needle to remove tissue from an area that looks suspicious on a mammogram but cannot be felt. Tissue removed in a needle biopsy goes to a lab to be checked for cancer cells.

Photodynamic therapy—A cancer treatment that uses a drug that is activated by exposure to light. When the drug is exposed to light, the cancer cells are killed.

Positron emission tomography (PET) scan—A procedure to find malignant tumor cells in the body. A small amount of radionuclide glucose (sugar) is injected into a vein. The PET scanner rotates around the body and makes a picture of where the glucose is being used in the body. Malignant tumor cells show up brighter in the picture because they are more active and take up more glucose than normal cells.

Radiation therapy—A cancer treatment that uses high-energy x rays or other types of radiation to kill cancer cells.

Radiologic exams—The use of radiation or other imaging methods to find signs of cancer.

Radiosurgery—A method of delivering radiation directly to the tumor. This method does not involve surgery and causes little damage to healthy tissue.

Radiotherapy—The treatment of disease with high-energy radiation, such as x rays or gamma rays.

Ultrasonography—A proceduring using high-frequency sound waves to show whether a lump is a fluid-filled cyst (not cancer) or a solid mass (which may or may not be cancer).

Ultrasound test—A device using sound waves that produce a pattern of echoes as they bounce off internal organs. The echoes create a picture of the organs.

and procedures may be used in the staging process to diagnose lung cancer:

- complete physical exam, including personal and family medical history
- chest x-ray
- computed tomography (CT) scan
- positron emission tomography (PET) scan
- other radiologic exams
- laboratory tests (tissue, blood, urine, or other substances in the body)
- bronchoscopy
- mediastinoscopy
- anterior mediastinotomy
- lymph node biopsy

Treatment is determined when the stage of the tumor is known.

Routine preoperative preparations, such as not eating or drinking after midnight on the night before surgery are typically ordered for a segmentectomy. Information about expected outcomes and potential complications is also part of the preparation for this surgery.

Aftercare

After a segmentectomy, patients are usually cautioned against doing moderate lifting for several days. Other activities may be restricted (especially if lymph nodes were removed) according to individual needs. Pain is often enough to limit inappropriate motion, and is generally controlled with medication. If pain medications are ineffective, the patient should contact the physician, as severe pain may be a sign of a complication requiring medical attention. Women who undergo segmentectomy of the breast are often instructed to wear a well-fitting support bra both day and night for approximately one week after surgery.

The length of the hospital stay depends on the specific surgery performed and the extent of organ or tissue removed, as well as other factors.

WHO PERFORMS THE PROCEDURE AND WHERE IS IT PERFORMED?

Segmentectomies are performed in a hospital by a general surgeon, a medical doctor who specializes in surgery. If there are complicating factors, a specialized surgeon may perform the surgery.

Radiation therapy usually begins four to six weeks after surgery, and continues for four to five weeks. The timing of additional therapy is specific to each patient.

Risks

The risks for any surgical procedure requiring anesthesia include reactions to the medications and breathing problems. Bleeding and infection are risks for any surgical procedure. Infection in the area affecting a segmentectomy occurs in only 3–4% of patients. Pneumonia is also a risk.

Normal results

Successful removal of the tumor with no major bleeding or infection at the wound site after surgery is considered a normal outcome.

Morbidity and mortality rates

Although the incidence of breast cancer has been rising in the United States for the past two decades, the mortality rate has remained relatively stable since the 1950s. Mortality rates range from 15% of the incidence rate for Japanese women to 33% of the incidence rate for African American women. The highest age-adjusted mortality occurs among African American women, followed by Caucasian and Hawaiian women.

African American women have the highest mortality rates in the age groups 30–54 years and 55–69 years, followed by Hawaiian, and Caucasian non-Hispanic women. The mortality rate for Caucasian women exceeds that for African American women in the 70 year and older age group.

Five-year survival rates for liver cancer patients are usually less than 10% in the United States. The reported statistics for these cancers often include mortality rates that exceed the incidence rates. The discrepancy occurs when the cause of death is misclassified as "liver cancer" for patients whose cancer originated as a primary tumor in another organ and spread to the liver, becoming a secondary cancer.

QUESTIONS TO ASK THE DOCTOR

- Is segmentectomy an option for treatment?
- When will it be known whether or not all the cancer has been removed?
- What benefits can be expected from this operation?
- What is the risk of tumor recurrence after undergoing this procedure?
- What should be done to prepare for surgery?
- What happens if this operation does not go as planned?

For primary liver cancer, non-Hispanic Caucasian men and women have the lowest age-adjusted mortality rates in the United States, roughly one-half that of the African American and Hispanic populations.

Liver cancer mortality rates for Asian American groups are several times higher than that of the Caucasian population. The highest age-adjusted mortality rates for all groups are among the Chinese population. Alaska Native and Native American populations have a very low incidence of liver cancer.

Factors that affect the prognosis (chance of recovery) for lung cancer include:

- stage of the cancer (whether it is in the lung only or has spread to other places in the body)
- tumor size
- type of lung cancer
- presence of symptoms
- shortness of breath during activities
- shortness of breath with less and less activity
- the patient's general health

Current treatments are not a cure for most patients with non-small cell lung cancer. If it returns after treatment, it is called recurrent non-small cell lung cancer. The cancer may reappear in the brain, lung, or other parts of the body. Further treatment is then required.

Alternatives

Other cancer treatments include:

- chemotherapy
- radiation therapy
- radiosurgery
- laser therapy
- photodynamic therapy
- chemoprevention

Using a segmentectomy to remove breast cancers (as a technique that conserves the aesthetic appearance of a breast) is being investigated for large tumors after several cycles of preoperative chemotherapy.

Cancers in some locations (such as where the windpipe divides into the left and right main bronchi) are difficult to remove completely by surgery without also removing an entire lung.

Resources

BOOKS

Benedet, Rosalind Dolores, and Shannon Abbey (Illustrator). *After Mastectomy: Healing Physically and Emotionally.* Omaha, NE: Addicus Books, 2003.

Clavien, Pierre-Alain, and Nuria Roca, eds. *Malignant Liver Tumors: Current and Emerging Therapies,* 2nd edition. Sudbury, MA: Jones & Bartlett Pub., 2003.

Farrell, Susan. *Mammograms and Mastectomies: Facing Them With Humor and Prayer.* Battle Creek, MI: Acorn Publishing, 2003.

Henschke, Claudia I., Peggy McCarthy, and Sarah Wernick. *Lung Cancer: Myths, Facts, Choices—And Hope.* New York, NY: W.W. Norton & Company, 2002.

Simone, John. *The LCIS & DCIS Breast Cancer Fact Book.*Raleigh, NC: Three Pyramids Publishing, 2002.

PERIODICALS

Mahadevia, Parthiv J., Lee A. Fleisher, Kevin D. Frick, John Eng, Steven N. Goodman, and Neil R. Powe. "Lung Cancer Screening with Helical Computed Tomography in Older Adult Smokers: A Decision and Cost-Effectiveness Analysis." *Journal of the American Medical Association* 289 (2003): 313-22. http://www.atcs.jp/journal/abstract.php?ac = 3&bn = 030901& no = 10

Shimizu J. J., Y. Ishida, T. Kinoshita., T. Terada, Y. Tatsuzawa, Y. Kawaura, et al. "Left Upper Division Sleeve Segmentectomy for Early Stage Squamous Cell Carcinoma of the Segmental Bronchus: Report of Two Cases." *Annals of Thoracic Cardiovascular Surgery* 9, no.1 (2003): 62-7.

Vastag, Brian. "Consensus Panel Recommendations for Treatment of Early Breast Cancer." *Journal of American Medical Association* 284 (2002): 2707-8.

ORGANIZATIONS

American Cancer Society. 1599 Clifton Road, N.E. Atlanta, GA 30329-4251. (800) 227-2345. http://www.cancer.org.

National Alliance of Breast Cancer Organizations (NABCO). 9 East 37th Street, 10th Floor, New York, NY 10016. (888) 80-NABCO. http://www.nabco.org.

National Comprehensive Cancer Network. 50 Huntingdon Pike, Suite 200, Rockledge PA 19046. (215) 728-4788. Fax: (215) 728-3877. Email: information@nccn.org. http://www.nccn.org/ .

National Institutes of Health (NIH), Department of Health and Human Services. 9000 Rockville Pike. Bethesda, MD 20892. (800) 422-6237.

The U.S. Department of Health and Human Services. 200 Independence Avenue, S.W., Washington, D.C. 20201. (877) 696-6775.

Y-ME National Breast Cancer Organization. Suite 500-212 West Van Buren St., Chicago, IL 60607-3908. (800) 986-9505. 312-986-8338. Fax: 312-294-8597. http://www.y-me.org.

OTHER

National Cancer Institute. *Types of Cancer.* 2003. [cited April 28, 2003] http://www.nci.nih.gov/cancerinfo/types/.

Laura Ruth, Ph.D.
Crystal H. Kaczkowski, M.Sc.

Selective dorsal rhizotomy *see* **Rhizotomy**

Senna *see* **Laxatives**

Sentinel lymph node biopsy

Definition

Sentinel lymph node biopsy (SLNB) is a minimally invasive procedure in which a lymph node near the site of a cancerous tumor is first identified as a sentinel node and then removed for microscopic analysis. SLNB was developed by researchers in several different cancer centers following the discovery that the human lymphatic system can be mapped with radioactive dyes, and that the lymph node(s) closest to a tumor serve to filter and trap cancer cells. These nodes are known as sentinel nodes because they act like sentries to warn doctors that a patient's cancer is spreading.

The first descriptions of sentinel nodes come from studies of penile and testicular cancers done in the 1970s. A technique that uses blue dye to map the lymphatic system was developed in the 1980s and applied to the treatment of melanoma in 1989. The extension of sentinel lymph node biopsy to the treatment of breast cancer began at the John Wayne Cancer Institute in Santa Monica, California, in 1991. As of 2003, SLNB is used in the diagnosis and treatment of many other cancers, including cancers of the head and neck, anus, bladder, lung, and male breast.

Purpose

Sentinel lymph node biopsy has several purposes:

- Improving the accuracy of cancer staging. Cancer staging is a system that classifies malignant tumors according to the extent of their spread in the body. It is used to guide decisions about treatment.

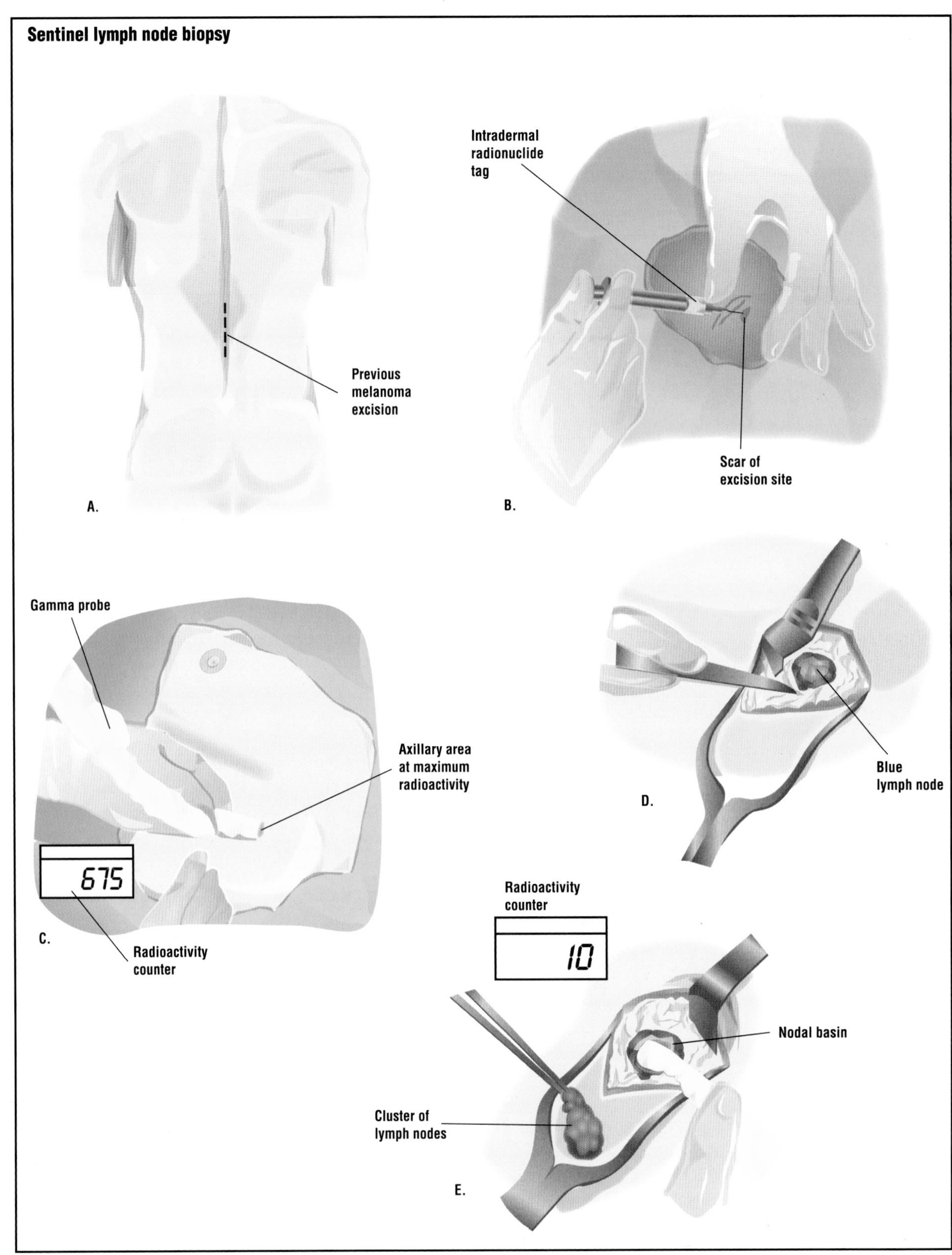

At the site of a previous cancer removal, a radionuclide dye is injected (A and B). The area of maximum radioactivity is traced to a lymph node under the arm (C). The area is cut open, and the lymph node is identified by its blue dye (D). After the lymph node is removed, the area is checked for further radioactivity (E). *(Illustration by GGS Information Services. Cengage Learning, Gale.)*

- Catching the spread of cancer to nearby lymph nodes as early as possible.
- Defining homogeneous patient populations for clinical trials of new cancer treatments.

Description

A sentinel lymph node biopsy is done in two stages. In the first part of the procedure, which takes one to two hours, the patient goes to the nuclear medicine department of the hospital for an injection of a radioactive tracer known as technetium 99. A doctor who specializes in nuclear medicine first numbs the area around the tumor with a local anesthetic and then injects the radioactive technetium. He or she usually injects a blue dye as well. The doctor will then use a gamma camera to take pictures of the lymph nodes before surgery. This type of imaging study is called lymphoscintigraphy.

After the lymphoscintigraphy, the patient must wait several hours for the dye and the radioactive material to travel from the tissues around the tumor to the sentinel lymph node. He or she is then taken to the **operating room** and put under **general anesthesia**. Next, the surgeon injects more blue dye into the area around the tumor. The surgeon then uses a hand-held probe connected to a gamma ray counter to scan the area for the radioactive technetium. The sentinel lymph node can be pinpointed by the sound made by the gamma ray counter. The surgeon makes an incision about 0.5 in long to remove the sentinel node. The blue dye that has been injected helps to verify that the surgeon is removing the right node. The incision is then closed and the tissue is sent to the hospital laboratory for examination.

Preparation

Some cancer patients should not be given an SLNB. They include women with cancer in more than one part of the breast; women who have had previous breast surgery, including **plastic surgery**; women with breast cancer in advanced stages; and women who have had radiation therapy. Melanoma patients who have undergone wide excision (removal of surrounding skin as well as the tumor) of the original skin cancer are also not candidates for an SLNB.

Apart from evaluating the patient's fitness for an SLNB, no additional preparation is necessary.

Aftercare

A sentinel lymph node biopsy does not require extensive aftercare. In most cases, the patient goes home after the procedure or after an overnight stay in the hospital.

KEY TERMS

Biopsy—The removal of a piece of living tissue from the body for diagnostic purposes.

Lymph—A clear yellowish fluid derived from tissue fluid. It is returned to the blood via the lymphatic system.

Lymph nodes—Small masses of tissue located at various points along the course of the lymphatic vessels.

Lymphedema—Swelling of the arm as a result of removal of lymphatic tissue.

Lymphoscintigraphy—A technique for detecting the presence of cancer cells in lymph nodes by using a radioactive tracer.

Prophylactic—Intended to prevent or protect against disease.

Sentinel lymph node—The lymph node(s) closest to a cancerous tumor. They are the first nodes that receive lymphatic drainage from the tissues surrounding the tumor.

Staging—The classification of cancers according to the extent of the tumor.

The surgeon will discuss the laboratory findings with the patient. If the sentinel node was found to contain cancer cells, the surgeon will usually recommend a full axillary lymph node dissection (ALND). This is a more invasive procedure in which a larger number of lymph nodes—usually 12–15—is surgically removed. A drainage tube is placed for two to three weeks, and the patient must undergo physical therapy at home.

Risks

Risks associated with an SLNB include the following:

- Mild discomfort after the procedure.
- Lymphedema (swelling of the arm due to disruption of the lymphatic system after surgery).
- Damage to the nerves in the area of the biopsy.
- Temporary discoloration of the skin in the area of the dye injection.
- False negative laboratory report. A false negative means that there is cancer in other lymph nodes in spite of the absence of cancer in the sentinel node. False negatives usually result from either poor timing of the dye injection, the way in which the pathologist

WHO PERFORMS THE PROCEDURE AND WHERE IS IT PERFORMED?

An SLNB is usually performed in a hospital that has a department of nuclear medicine, although it is sometimes done as an outpatient procedure. The radioactive material or dye is injected by a physician who specializes in nuclear medicine. The sentinel lymph node is removed by a surgeon with experience in the technique. It is then analyzed in the hospital laboratory by a pathologist, who is a doctor with special training in studying the effects of disease on body organs and tissues.

The accuracy of a sentinel lymph node biopsy depends greatly on the skill of the surgeon who removes the node. Recent studies indicate that most doctors need to perform 20–30 SLNBs before they achieve an 85% success rate in identifying the sentinel node(s) and 5% or fewer false negatives. They can gain the necessary experience through special residency programs, fellowships, or training protocols. It is vital for patients to ask their surgeon how many SLNBs he or she has performed, as those who do these biopsies on a regular basis generally have a higher degree of accuracy.

QUESTIONS TO ASK THE DOCTOR

- Am I a candidate for sentinel lymph node biopsy?
- How many SLNBs have you performed?
- Do you perform this procedure on a regular basis?
- What is your false negative rate?

prepared the tissue for examination, or the existence of previously undiscovered sentinel nodes.

Normal results

Sentinel lymph node biopsies have a high degree of accuracy, with relatively few false negatives. A negative laboratory report means that there is a greater than 95% chance that the other nearby lymph nodes are also free of cancer.

Morbidity and mortality rates

Compared to axillary lymph node dissection, sentinel lymph node biopsy has a significantly lower rate of complications, including a lower rate of post-operative pain and infection, as well as a lower long-term risk of lymphedema.

Alternatives

Breast cancer patients who should not have a sentinel lymph node biopsy usually undergo an axillary lymph node dissection to determine whether their cancer has spread. Melanoma patients who have already had a wide excision of the original melanoma may have nearby lymph nodes removed to prevent the cancer from spreading. This procedure is called a prophylactic lymph node dissection.

Resources

BOOKS

Abeloff, MD et al. *Clinical Oncology*. 3rd ed. Philadelphia: Elsevier, 2004.

Habif, TP. *Clinical Dermatology*. 4th ed. St. Louis: Mosby, 2004.

Katz, VL et al. *Comprehensive Gynecology*. 5th ed. St. Louis: Mosby, 2007.

Khatri, VP and JA Asensio. *Operative Surgery Manual*. 1st ed. Philadelphia: Saunders, 2003.

Townsend, CM et al. *Sabiston Textbook of Surgery*. 17th ed. Philadelphia: Saunders, 2004.

PERIODICALS

Burak, W. E., S. T. Hollenbeck, E. E. Zervos, et al. "Sentinel Lymph Node Biopsy Results in Less Postoperative Morbidity Compared with Axillary Lymph Node Dissection for Breast Cancer." *American Journal of Surgery* 183 (January 2002): 23-27.

Burrall, Barbara, and Vijay Khatri. "Still Debating Sentinel Lymph Node Biopsy?" *Dermatology Online Journal* 7 (2):1 [April 22, 2003].

Golshan, M., W. J. Martin, and K. Dowlatshahi. "Sentinel Lymph Node Biopsy Lowers the Rate of Lymphedema When Compared with Standard Axillary Lymph Node Dissection." *American Surgeon* 69 (March 2003): 209-211.

Peley, C., E. Farkas, I. Sinkovics, et al. "Inguinal Sentinel Lymph Node Biopsy for Staging Anal Cancer." *Scandinavian Journal of Surgery* 91 (2002): 336-338.

Pow-Sang, Julio, MD. "The Spectrum of Genitourinary Malignancies." *Cancer Control* 9 (July-August 2002): 275-276.

Schmalbach, C. E., B. Nussenbaum, R. S. Rees, et al. "Reliability of Sentinel Lymph Node Mapping with Biopsy for Head and Neck Cutaneous Melanoma." *Archives of Otolaryngology—Head and Neck Surgery* 129 (January 2003): 61-65.

Uren, R. F., R. Howman-Giles, and J. F. Thompson. "Patterns of Lymphatic Drainage from the Skin in Patients with Melanoma." *Journal of Nuclear Medicine* 44 (April 2003): 570-582.

ORGANIZATIONS

American Cancer Society (ACS). (800) ACS-2345. www. cancer.org.

National Cancer Institute (NCI). NCI Public Inquiries Office, Suite 3036A, 6116 Executive Boulevard, MSC8332, Bethesda, MD 20892-8322. (800) 4-CANCER or (800) 332-8615 (TTY). www. nci.nih.gov.

Society of Nuclear Medicine (SNM). 1850 Samuel Morse Drive, Reston, VA 20190. (703) 708-9000. www. snm.org.

Rebecca Frey, Ph. D.

Septoplasty

Definition

Septoplasty is a surgical procedure to correct the shape of the septum of the nose. The goal of this procedure is to correct defects or deformities of the septum. The nasal septum is the separation between the two nostrils. In adults, the septum is composed partly of cartilage and partly of bone. Septal deviations are either congenital (present from birth) or develop as

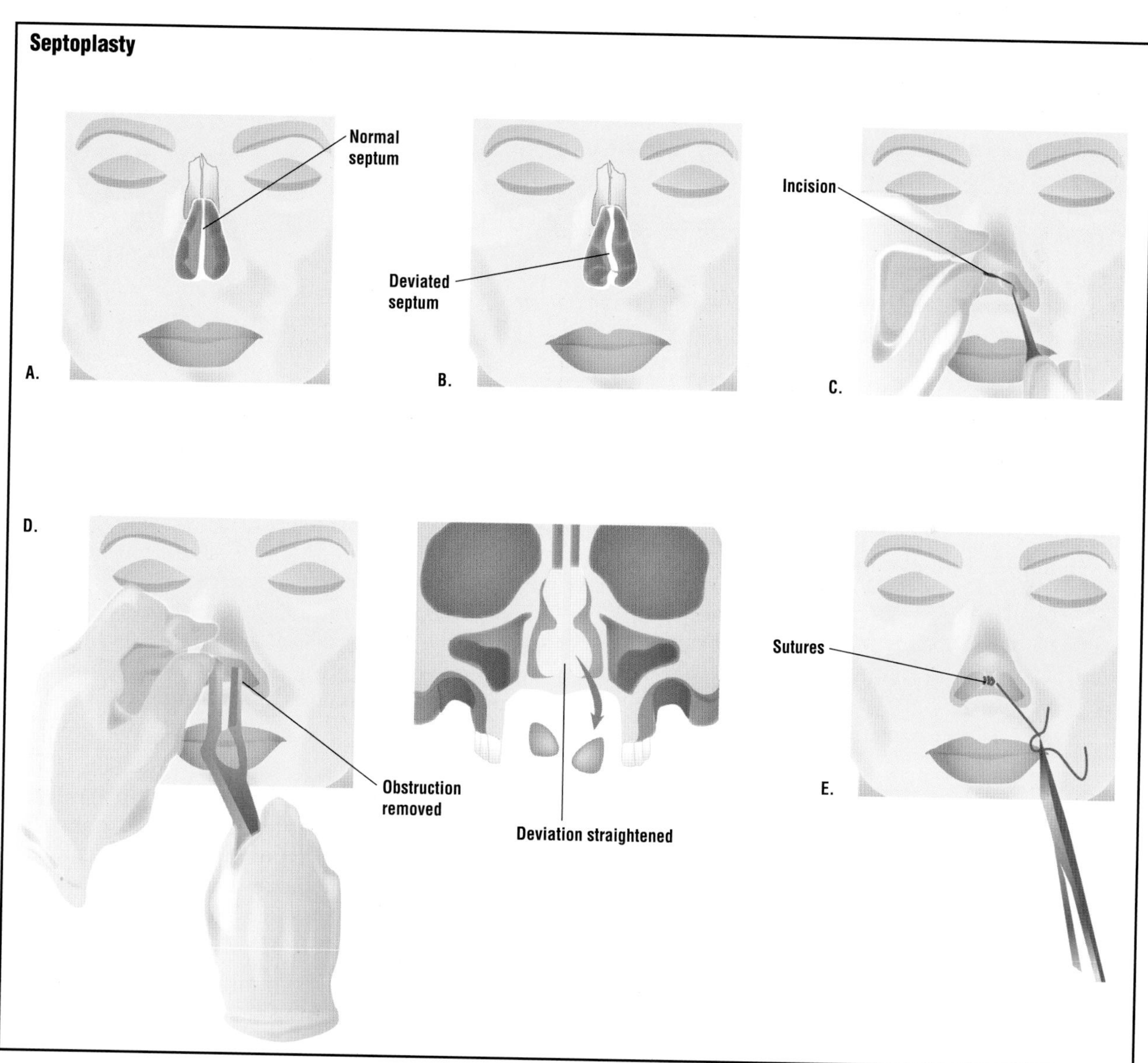

Septoplasty is used correct a deviated septum (B). First an incision is made to expose the nasal septum (C). Pieces of septum that are obstructing air flow are removed (D), and the incision is then closed (E). *(Illustration by GGS Information Services. Cengage Learning, Gale.)*

a result of an injury. Most people with deviated septa do not develop symptoms. It is typically only the most severely deformed septa that produce significant symptoms and require surgical intervention. However, many septoplasties are performed during **rhinoplasty** procedures, which are most often performed for cosmetic purposes.

Purpose

Septoplasty is performed to correct a crooked (deviated) or dislocated septum, often as part of **plastic surgery** of the nose (rhinoplasty). The nasal septum has three functions: to support the nose, to regulate air flow, and to support the mucous membranes (mucosa) of the nose. Septoplasty is done to correct the shape of the nose caused by a deformed septum or correct deregulated airflow caused by a deviated septum. Septoplasty is often needed when the patient is having an operation to reduce the size of the nose (reductive rhinoplasty), because this operation usually reduces the amount of breathing space in the nose.

During surgery, the patient's own cartilage that has been removed can be reused to provide support for the nose if needed. External septum supports are not usually needed. Splints may be needed occasionally to support cartilage when extensive cutting has been done. External splints can be used to support the cartilage for the first few days of healing. Tefla gauze is inserted in the nostril to support the flaps and cartilage and to absorb any bleeding or mucus.

Demographics

About one-third of the population may have some degree of nasal obstruction. Among those with nasal obstruction, about one-fourth have deviated septa.

Diagnosis/Preparation

The primary conditions that may suggest a need for septoplasty include:

- nasal air passage obstruction
- nasal septal deformity
- headaches caused by septal spurs
- chronic and uncontrolled nosebleeds
- chronic sinusitis associated with a deviated septum
- obstructive sleep apnea
- polypectomy (polyp removal)
- tumor excision
- turbinate surgery
- ethmoidectomy (removal of all or part of a small bone on the upper part of the nasal cavity)

KEY TERMS

Cartilage—A tough, elastic connective tissue found in the joints, outer ear, nose, larynx, and other parts of the body.

Obstructive sleep apnea—A temporary cessation of breathing that occurs during sleep and is associated with poor sleep quality.

Polyp—A tumor commonly found in vascular organs such as the nose that are often benign but can become malignant.

Rhinoplasty—Plastic surgery of the nose.

Septum (plural, septa)—The dividing partition in the nose that separates the two nostrils. It is composed of bone and cartilage.

Sinusitis—Inflammation of the sinuses.

Splint—A thin piece of rigid material that is sometimes used during nasal surgery to hold certain structures in place until healing is underway.

Spurs—A sharp horny outgrowth of the skin.

Wegener's granulomatosis—A rare condition that consists of lesions within the respiratory tract.

Septal deformities can cause nasal airway obstruction. Such airway obstruction can lead to mouth breathing, chronic nasal infections, or obstructive sleep apnea. Septal spurs can produce headaches when these growths lead to increased pressure on the nasal septum. Polypectomy, ethmoidectomy, **tumor removal**, and turbinate surgical procedures often include septoplasty. Individuals who have used significant quantities of cocaine over a long period of time often require septoplasty because of alterations in the nasal passage structures.

Septal deviation is usually diagnosed by direct observation of the nasal passages. In addition, a computed tomography (CT) scan of the entire nasal passage is often performed. This scan allows the physician to fully assess the structures and functioning of the area. Additional tests that evaluate the movement of air through the nasal passages may also be performed.

Before performing a septoplasty, the surgeon will evaluate the difference in airflow between the two nostrils. In children, this assessment can be done very simply by asking the patient to breathe out slowly on a small mirror held in front of the nose.

As with any other operation under **general anesthesia**, patients are evaluated for any physical conditions that might complicate surgery and for any medications

WHO PERFORMS THE PROCEDURE AND WHERE IS IT PERFORMED?

Septoplasty is performed by a medical doctor (M.D.) who has received additional training in surgery. Typically, septoplasty is performed by a board-certified plastic surgeon, a specialist called an otolaryngologist, or a head and neck surgeon. The procedure can be performed in a hospital or in a specialized surgical clinic.

QUESTIONS TO ASK THE PRIMARY CARE PHYSICIAN

- What are my alternatives?
- Is surgery the answer for me?
- Can you recommend a surgeon who performs septoplasty?
- If surgery is appropriate for me, what are the next steps?

that might affect blood clotting time. If a general anesthetic is used, then the patient is advised not to drink or eat after midnight the night before the surgery. In many cases, septoplasty can be performed on an outpatient basis using **local anesthesia**. Conditions that might preclude a patient from receiving a septoplasty include excessive cocaine abuse, Wegener's granulomatosis, malignant lymphomas, and an excessively large septal perforation.

Aftercare

Patients who receive septoplasty are usually sent home from the hospital later the same day or in the morning after the surgery. All **dressings** inside the nose are usually removed before the patient leaves. Aftercare includes a list of detailed instructions for the patient that focus on preventing trauma to the nose.

The head needs to be elevated while resting during the first 24-48 hours after surgery. Patients will have to breathe through the mouth while the nasal packing is still in place. A small amount of bloody discharge is normal, but excessive bleeding should be reported to the physician immediately. **Antibiotics** are usually not prescribed unless the packing is left in place more than 24 hours. Most patients do not suffer significant amounts of pain, but those who do have severe pain are sometimes given narcotic pain relievers. Patients are often advised to place an ice pack on the nose to enhance comfort during the recovery period. Patients who have splint placement usually return seven to 10 days after the surgery for examination and splint removal.

Risks

The risks from septoplasty are similar to those from other operations on the face: postoperative pain with some bleeding, swelling, bruising, or discoloration. A few patients may have allergic reactions to the anesthetics. The operation in itself, however, is relatively low-risk in that it does not involve major blood vessels or vital organs. Infection is unlikely if proper surgical technique is observed. One of the extremely rare but serious complications of septoplasty is cerebrospinal fluid leak. This complication can be treated with proper nasal packing, bed rest, and antibiotic use. Follow-up surgery may be necessary if the nasal obstruction relapses.

Normal results

Normal results include improved breathing and airflow through the nostrils, and an acceptable outward shape of the nose. Most patients have significant improvements in symptoms following surgery.

Morbidity and mortality rates

Significant morbidity associated with septoplasty is rare and is outlined in the Risks section above. Mortality is extremely rare and associated with the risks involving anesthesia. This procedure can be performed using local anesthesia on an outpatient basis or under general anesthesia during a short hospital stay. General anesthesia is associated with a greater mortality rate, but this risk is minimal.

Alternatives

In cases of sinusitis or allergic rhinitis, nasal airway breathing can be improved by using nasal sprays, such as phenylephrine (Neo-Synephrine). Patients with a history of chronic, uncontrolled nasal bleeding should receive conservative therapy that includes nasal packing to identify the source of the bleeding before surgery is contemplated. Those who have been diagnosed with obstructive sleep apnea have a variety of conservative alternatives before surgery is seriously considered. These alternatives include weight loss,

QUESTIONS TO ASK THE SURGEON

How many times have you performed septoplasty?
Are you a board-certified surgeon?
What type of outcomes have you had?
What are the most common side effects or complications?
What should I do to prepare for surgery?
What should I expect following the surgery?
Can you refer me to one of your patients who has had this procedure?
What type of diagnostic procedures are performed to determine if patients require surgery?
Will I need to see another specialist for the diagnostic procedures?

changes in sleep posture, and the use of appliances during sleep that enlarge the upper airway.

Resources

BOOKS

Muth, Annemarie S., and Karen Bellenir, eds. *Surgery Sourcebook* New York: Omnigraphics, 2002.

Schwartz, Seymour I., ed. *Principles of Surgery*. New York: McGraw-Hill, 1999.

"Septal deviation and perforation." In *The Merck Manual,* edited by Keryn A. G. Lane. West Point, PA: Merck & Co., 1999.

OTHER

"Septoplasty." *MEDLINEplus Medical Encyclopedia* [cited July 7, 2003]. http://www.nlm.nih.gov.

Mark Mitchell

Serum chloride level

Definition

Chloride is a mineral that is found throughout the body. Along with other electrolytes (such as sodium, potassium, and carbon dioxide), chloride is involved in maintaining an appropriate fluid balance throughout the body, including an appropriate blood volume; maintaining an stable blood pressure; and equilibrating the pH of the body fluids. For the body to function normally, serum chloride levels have to be maintained at a very narrow range; when chloride levels are too high or too low, it can have serious health consequences. The body keeps its chloride levels in equilibrium by prompting the kidneys to resorb more (when the body needs chloride) or excrete more (when there is excess chloride). When serum chloride levels get too high, the condition is called hyperchloremia. When serum chloride levels get too low, the condition is called hypochloremia.

Purpose

A serum chloride level is usually drawn as part of a larger panel of electrolytes. Other measurements in the electrolyte panel include sodium, potassium, and carbon dioxide. A serum chloride level is usually checked during a routine **physical examination**, as well as to evaluate patients who are experiencing prolonged or severe vomiting and/or diarrhea, fatigue, weakness, confusion, muscle spasms, or respiratory distress. Electrolyte panels are frequently used to diagnose, monitor, or otherwise evaluate patients with kidney disease, liver disease, high blood pressure, heart failure, and other chronic conditions.

Precautions

Serum chloride levels can be affected by a number of medications. Patients who are on these medications should inform their doctor, so that test results can be interpreted appropriately. Medications that may affect serum chloride levels include steroid medications, **nonsteroidal anti-inflammatory drugs** (such as ibuprofen), estrogen-containing medications, male hormones (androgens) some blood pressure medications, cholesterol-lowering agents (such as cholestyramine), and diuretic medications. Another factor that may skew the results of a serum chloride level involves the patient's level of hydration. When a patient is dehydrated, the serum chloride level will be elevated; when a patient is over-hydrated, the serum chloride level will be artificially lowered.

Patients who are taking anticoagulant medications should inform their healthcare practitioner, since this may increase their chance of bleeding or bruising after a blood test.

Description

This test requires blood to be drawn from a vein (usually one in the forearm), generally by a nurse or phlebotomist (an individual who has been trained to draw blood). A tourniquet is applied to the arm above the area where the needle stick will be performed. The site of the needle stick is cleaned with antiseptic, and the needle is inserted. The blood is collected in vacuum tubes. After collection, the needle is withdrawn, and pressure is kept on the blood draw site to stop any bleeding and decrease bruising. A bandage is then applied.

KEY TERMS

Addison's disease—A disease involving decreased functioning of the adrenal glands.

Antidiuretic hormone (ADH)—Also called vasopressin. A hormone produced by the hypothalamus and stored in and excreted by the pituitary gland. ADH acts on the kidneys to reduce the flow of urine, increasing total body fluid. When too much ADH is produced, resulting in the body retaining fluid, the sodium concentration becomes abnormally low.

Cushing's syndrome—A disorder affecting the adrenal glands and their secretion of coritsol.

Diuretic—A medication that increases the flow of urine through the kidneys and out of the body.

Hyperchloremia—Elevated serum chloride levels.

Hypochloremia—Low serum chloride levels.

Metabolic acidosis—A condition in which either too much acid or too little bicarbonate in the body results in a drop in the blood pH (towards acidity).

Metabolic alkalosis—A condition in which abnormal either too little acid or too much bicarbonate in the body results in an elevation in the blood pH (towards alkalinity).

Respiratory acidosis—A condition in which abnormal exchange of oxygen and carbon dioxide in the lungs results in too much carbon dioxide being accumulated, and a resultant drop in the blood pH (towards acidity).

Respiratory alkalosis—A condition in which abnormal exchange of oxygen and carbon dioxide in the lungs results in the exhalation of too much carbon dioxide, and a resultant rise in the blood pH (towards alkalinity).

Preparation

There are no restrictions on diet or physical activity, either before or after the blood test.

Aftercare

As with any blood tests, discomfort, bruising, and/or a very small amount of bleeding is common at the puncture site. Immediately after the needle is withdrawn, it is helpful to put pressure on the puncture site until the bleeding has stopped. This decreases the chance of significant bruising. Warm packs may relieve minor discomfort. Some individuals may feel briefly woozy after a blood test, and they should be encouraged to lie down and rest until they feel better.

Risks

Basic blood tests, such as serum chloride levels, do not carry any significant risks, other than slight bruising and the chance of brief dizziness.

Results

In adults, a normal serum chloride level is 98-106 milliequivalents per liter (mEq/L, or 98-106 millimoles per liter (mmol/L). In children, a normal serum chloride level is 90-110 milliequivalents per liter (mEq/L, or 90-110 millimoles per liter (mmol/L). In newborns, a normal serum chloride level is 96-106 milliequivalents per liter (mEq/L, or 96-106 millimoles per liter (mmol/L). In premature infants, a normal serum chloride level is 95-110 milliequivalents per liter (mEq/L, or 95-110 millimoles per liter (mmol/L).

High levels

High serum chloride levels occur whenever there is low blood sodium (hyponatremia), or may also be due to:

- Dehydration: Increased loss of body water without sufficient replacement by drinking; often occurs in febrile illnesses, with severe diarrhea and/or vomiting, or in situations involving heavy exercise in hot weather, resulting in fluid loss through heavy sweating
- Hyperventilation
- Kidney disease
- Excessive consumption of salt
- Anemia
- Use of carbonic anhydrase inhibitors (glaucoma medications)
- Hyperparathyroidism (an overactive parathyroid gland)
- Metabolic acidosis
- Respiratory alkalosis
- Excess bromide

Low levels

Low serum chloride levels may be due to any disorder that causes low blood sodium (hyponatremia) or may be due to:

- Cushing's syndrome
- Addison's disease
- Syndrome of inappropriate ADH secretion (SIADH)
- Repeated vomiting, or prolonged gastric suction
- Chronic diarrhea
- Serious burns
- Excess sweating

- Chronic lung diseases, including emphysema and chronic obstructive pulmonary disorder
- Congestive heart failure
- Kidney disease
- Cystic fibrosis
- Respiratory acidosis
- Metabolic alkalosis
- Overhydration

Resources

BOOKS

Goldman L, Ausiello D., eds. *Cecil Textbook of Internal Medicine*. 23rd ed. Philadelphia: Saunders, 2008.

McPherson RA et al. *Henry's Clinical Diagnosis and Management By Laboratory Methods*. 21st ed. Philadelphia: Saunders, 2007.

ORGANIZATIONS

American Association of Clinical Chemistry. 1850 K St., N.W Suite 625, Washington, DC 20006. http://www.aacc.org.

OTHER

National Institutes of Health. [cited February 10, 2008]. http://www.nlm.nih.gov/medlineplus/encyclopedia.html.

Rosalyn Carson-DeWitt, MD

Serum creatinine level

Definition

Creatinine is actually a chemical waste product that is produced by the muscles. The chemical "creatine" is an important chemical involved in the production of energy needed for muscle contraction. During the course of every day, about 2% of the body's creatine becomes creatinine. Creatinine enters the bloodstream and goes to the kidneys. Healthy kidneys filter out this waste material from the blood. It passes into the urine and out of the body. Unhealthy kidneys are unable to filter out the creatinine from the blood. The creatinine remains circulating in the bloodstream, and levels rise as the muscles continue to produce more and more.

The serum creatinine level is used to predict how the kidneys are functioning. In many cases, the serum creatinine level will begin to rise before a patient is even aware of any symptoms of kidney malfunction. High creatinine levels indicate the need for further investigation into the possibility that kidney failure is ensuing. If a creatinine level is elevated, then other tests such as blood urea nitrogen (BUN) or urine creatinine will be performed. Calculations involving serum and urine creatinine levels will give the creatinine clearance, a figure which reflects the capacity of the kidneys to filter small molecules out of the bloodstream. Calculations involving the serum creatinine level and the individual's gender, height, weight, and age will allow estimation of the glomerular filtration rate, which can screen for kidney damage and disease.

Serum creatinine level is tied to muscle contraction, therefore, the normal value of an individual's serum creatinine level will be dependent on the individual's size and their overall muscle mass. In general, the normal serum creatinine level for men is higher than the normal serum creatinine level in either women or children. Because athletes tend to have greater muscle mass, their normal creatinine level may be higher than that of non-athletes.

Purpose

A serum creatinine level is usually drawn as part of a larger metabolic panel or screen. Other tests performed in this panel include electrolytes (sodium, potassium, chloride, and carbon dioxide), as well as calcium, glucose, and BUN. A serum creatinine level is usually checked during a routine **physical examination**, as well as to evaluate patients for the presence of kidney disease, to monitor patients who have illnesses or who are taking medications that might affect the functioning of their kidneys, or to make sure that treatment for kidney disease is effective.

Precautions

Serum creatinine levels can be affected by a number of medications. Patients who are on these medications should inform their doctor, so that test results can be interpreted appropriately. Medications that may affect serum creatinine levels include methyldopa, trimethoprim, vitamin C, cimetidine, certain **diuretics**, and cephalosporin **antibiotics**. Additionally, if the serum creatinine level is going to be used in calculations with the urine creatinine or the BUN levels to evaluate kidney functioning, results may be skewed by the following medications: vitamin C, phenytoin, cephalosporin antibiotics, captopril, aminoglycosides, trimethoprim, cimetidine, quinine, quinidine, procainamide, amphotericin B, steroid medications, and tetracycline antibiotics.

Patients who are taking anticoagulant medications should inform their healthcare practitioner, since this may increase their chance of bleeding or bruising after a blood test.

KEY TERMS

Blood urea nitrogen (BUN)—Blood urea nitrogen is a chemical waste product of protein metabolism that circulates in the bloodstream. Healthy kidneys remove urea from the bloodstream and it leaves the body in the urine. When the kidneys are not functioning properly, they are unable to filter the urea out of the blood, and blood urea nitrogen levels become elevated.

Creatine—Creatine is a substance produced by proteins and stored in the muscles. Creatine is a source for energy, allowing muscle contraction to take place. Some creatine is converted to creatinine, and enters the bloodstream, where it is filtered out by healthy kidneys and leaves the body in the urine. When the kidneys are not functioning properly, creatinine levels in the blood become abnormally elevated.

Diabetic nephropathy—Kidney damage or disease brought on by the long-term effects of diabetes.

Glomerulonephritis—A condition in which the filtering structures within the kidneys become damaged, limiting the kidneys' ability to filter waste products from the blood.

Preeclampsia—A condition occurring in pregnancy in which high blood pressure leads to a number of complications, including a decreased ability of the kidneys to appropriately filter wastes from the blood.

Urine creatinine level—A value obtained by testing a 24–hour collection of urine for the amount of creatinine present.

Description

This test requires serum to be drawn from a vein (usually one in the forearm), generally by a nurse or phlebotomist (an individual who has been trained to draw serum). A tourniquet is applied to the arm above the area where the needle stick will be performed. The site of the needle stick is cleaned with antiseptic, and the needle is inserted. The serum is collected in vacuum tubes. After collection, the needle is withdrawn, and pressure is kept on the serum draw site to stop any bleeding and decrease bruising. A bandage is then applied.

Preparation

In the 24–48 hours prior to a serum creatinine level, patients should be advised to avoid strenuous **exercise** and to limit the amount of protein they ingest. Creatinine is a waste product of muscle contraction and, therefore, vigorous exercise in the 48 hours prior to a serum creatinine level could alter the results of the test. Similarly, ingesting more than eight ounces of meat (particularly beef) or other protein sources in the 24 hours prior to the serum creatinine level may affect the results.

Aftercare

As with any blood tests, discomfort, bruising, and/or a very small amount of bleeding is common at the puncture site. Immediately after the needle is withdrawn, it is helpful to put pressure on the puncture site until the bleeding has stopped. This decreases the chance of significant bruising. Warm packs may relieve minor discomfort. Some individuals may feel briefly woozy after a serum test, and they should be encouraged to lie down and rest until they feel better.

Risks

Basic serum tests, such as serum creatinine levels, do not carry any significant risks, other than slight bruising and the chance of brief dizziness.

Results

In adult men, a normal serum creatinine level is 0.6–1.2 milligrams per deciliter (mg/dL) or 53–106 micromoles/L (mcmol/L). In adult women, a normal serum creatinine level is 0.5–1.1 mg/dL or 44–97 mcmol/L. In teenagers, a normal serum creatinine level is 0.5–1.0 mg/dL. In children, a normal serum creatinine level is 0.3–0.7 mg/dL. In newborn babies, a normal serum creatinine level is 0.3–1.2 mg/dL.

High levels

High serum creatinine levels suggest that the kidneys are suffering from damage or disease. Kidneys can be damaged by severe infections, shock, cancer, or conditions that limit the blood flow reaching the kidneys. High serum creatinine levels can also occur when the urinary tract is blocked, or due to:

- obstruction of the urinary tract from a kidney stone or tumor;
- acute tubular necrosis;
- diabetic nephropathy;
- pre eclampsia;
- glomerulonephritis;
- dehydration;
- heart failure;
- extreme blood loss;
- gout;
- muscular dystrophy;
- rhabdomyolysis (conditions resulting in the abnormal breakdown of muscle tissue);
- myasthenia gravis;

- acromegaly; or
- gigantism.

Low levels

Low serum creatinine levels may be due to:

- abnormally low muscle mass, as may occur in muscle wasting diseases like muscular dystrophy, or due to aging;
- liver disease;
- extreme low-protein diets; or
- pregnancy

Resources

BOOKS

Brenner, B. M., and F. C. Rector, eds. *Brenner & Rector's The Kidney,* 7th ed. Philadelphia: Saunders, 2004.

Goldman L., and D. Ausiello, eds. *Cecil Textbook of Medicine,* 23rd ed. Philadelphia: Saunders, 2008.

McPherson R.A., and M. R. Pincus, eds. *Henry's Clinical Diagnosis and Management by Laboratory Methods,* 21st ed. Philadelphia: Saunders, 2006.

OTHER

Medical Encyclopedia. Medline Plus. National Institutes of Health. http://www.nlm.nih.gov/medlineplus/encyclopedia.html (February 10, 2008).

ORGANIZATIONS

American Association for Clinical Chemistry, 1850 K Street, NW, Suite 625, Washington, DC, 20006, (800) 892-1400, http://www.aacc.org.

Rosalyn Carson-DeWitt, M.D.

Serum electrolyte tests *see* **Electrolyte tests**

Serum glucose level

Definition

The serum glucose or blood sugar level is a measurement of the amount of a particular form of simple sugar in the blood. When carbohydrates are ingested, they are broken down in the intestines into component parts, including sugars such as glucose. Glucose is absorbed from the small intestine into the bloodstream. It circulates throughout the body and is used by all of the body's tissues and organs to generate the energy necessary for their normal functioning. In order for glucose to enter the body's cells, insulin must be present. Insulin is a hormone produced in and excreted by the pancreas. Insulin functions to allow the transport of glucose into the cells of the body, as well as being involved in the body's storage of excess glucose in the form of glycogen or triglycerides.

The blood levels of glucose and insulin are intimately related. When carbohydrates are metabolized after a meal, the blood glucose begins to rise. Under normal circumstances, the pancreas then secretes insulin, in an amount relative to the blood glucose elevation. Between meals, or after heavy exertion, glucose levels may begin to drop below a safe threshold for the body's cells (particular cells of the brain and nervous system). In response to this lowering of blood glucose, the pancreas secretes a different hormone, called glucagon. Glucagon prompts the liver to convert glycogen into glucose, thereby elevating the blood glucose back into a safe range.

Abnormal levels of blood glucose can be life-threatening. High blood glucose is termed hyperglycemia; low blood glucose is termed hypoglycemia. Either of these conditions can result in organ failure, severe brain damage, coma, or **death**. Diabetes occurs when the pancreas fails to produce normal amounts of insulin, or when it completely stops producing any insulin at all (this is often referred to as insulin-dependent or type I diabetes). Diabetes can also occur when cells of the body become less responsive to the effects of insulin (this is often referred to as insulin-resistance, or type II diabetes). Diabetes causes abnormal perturbations of the serum glucose level. Chronic high levels of serum glucose (which may occur in poorly controlled diabetes) can result in severe damage over time to the heart, the eyes, the kidneys, the circulatory system, and the nervous system. In diabetics, sudden, acute increases in the serum glucose level can result in the condition called diabetic ketoacidosis, in which the extremely high levels of blood glucose lead a life-threatening illness. Diabetics can also suffer from sudden drops in serum glucose levels; if untreated, glucose deprivation can affect the organs and tissues of the body and may also be life-threatening.

Purpose

A serum glucose level is usually drawn as part of a larger metabolic panel or screen. Other tests performed in this panel include electrolytes (sodium, potassium, chloride, and carbon dioxide), as well as calcium, creatinine, and BUN (blood urea nitrogen). A serum glucose level is usually checked during a routine **physical examination** or may be performed specifically to screen for diabetes, especially when there is a strong family history of diabetes, or when an individual has other specific risk factors, such as being overweight.

Serum glucose levels are also an important part of monitoring the health of pregnant women since some women develop gestational diabetes during pregnancy. Untreated, this can result in problems with the baby as well as the mother. Gestational diabetes in early pregnancy can cause birth defects (particularly of the brain and/or heart) and increase the chance of miscarriage. Gestational diabetes in the second and third trimesters can cause the baby to grow very large. The baby's size can result in problems for the mother during labor and delivery. Additionally, once the baby is born, it can suffer sudden hypoglycemia. In utero, the baby will have acclimated to its mother's high serum glucose levels by producing high levels of insulin. After birth, suddenly deprived of that glucose, the baby's relatively high insulin levels can result in severe hypoglycemia.

A serum glucose level may be ordered when there are symptoms suspicious of diabetes, such as excessive thirst and/or hunger, urinary frequency, unintentional weight loss, severe fatigue and weakness, and poor healing. The diagnosis of diabetes requires that a random high serum glucose level be confirmed by a high fasting serum glucose level or by abnormal results of an **oral glucose tolerance test**. Patients who are diabetic may also be required to check their own blood glucose one or more times a day, to make sure that their condition is under good control.

A serum glucose level may be ordered when there are symptoms suspicious of low blood sugar (hypoglycemia), such as shakiness, sweating, anxiety, confusion, dizziness, or fainting.

Precautions

The serum glucose level is highly affected by when an individual has last eaten, therefore, appropriate interpretation of the test results must take this into consideration. Serum glucose levels may be examined under random conditions, after an eight to ten hour fast (referred to as a fasting serum glucose level); two hours after a meal has been completed (referred to as a two-hour post-prandial serum glucose level); or after an individual has been given a standardized amount of a glucose-containing beverage (referred to as an oral glucose tolerance test or OGTT).

Serum glucose levels can be affected by a number of medications. Patients who are on these medications should inform their doctor, so that test results can be interpreted appropriately. Medications that may affect serum glucose levels include birth control pills, high blood pressure medications, phenytoin, furosemide, triamterene, hydrochlorothiazide, niacin, propranolol, and steroid medications. Additionally, the use of alcohol, the use of caffeine, recent illness, infection, or emotional distress may affect test results.

Patients who are taking anticoagulant medications should inform their healthcare practitioner, since this may increase their chance of bleeding or bruising after a blood test.

Description

This test requires serum to be drawn from a vein (usually one in the forearm), generally by a nurse or phlebotomist (an individual who has been trained to draw serum). A tourniquet is applied to the arm above the area where the needle stick will be performed. The site of the needle stick is cleaned with antiseptic, and the needle is inserted. The serum is collected in vacuum tubes. After collection, the needle is withdrawn, and pressure is kept on the serum draw site to stop any bleeding and decrease bruising. A bandage is then applied.

Self-glucose testing is often performed one or more times per day by diabetics themselves. This involves using a special sharp instrument, called a lancet, to prick a finger. Frequently, these lancets are placed in a spring-loaded mechanism to make it easier to accomplish the finger prick. A drop of blood from this finger prick is then put onto a special strip of paper and slipped into a machine called a blood glucose meter. The meter gives a digital readout of the serum glucose level. Alternatively, the drop of blood can be put onto a special strip of test paper which changes color based on the glucose level; this is less accurate than the blood glucose meter.

Preparation

There are no special preparations necessary prior to a random serum glucose level. For a two-hour post-prandial serum glucose level, the individual should be instructed to eat a meal exactly two hours before the blood draw. For a fasting serum glucose level, the individual should ingest nothing other than water for a minimum of eight hours prior to the blood draw. Diabetics may be asked to delay their morning dose of insulin or oral diabetes medication (oral hypoglycemic agents) prior to the blood draw.

Aftercare

As with any blood tests, discomfort, bruising, and/or a very small amount of bleeding is common at the puncture site. Immediately after the needle is withdrawn, it is helpful to put pressure on the puncture site until the bleeding has stopped. This decreases the chance of significant bruising. Warm packs may relieve minor discomfort. Some individuals may feel briefly woozy after a serum test, and they should be encouraged to lie down and rest until they feel better.

KEY TERMS

Gestational diabetes—A type of diabetes that occurs during pregnancy. Untreated, it can cause severe complications for the mother and the baby; however, it usually does not lead to long-term diabetes in either the mother or the child.

Glucose—A simple sugar that is the product of carbohydrate metabolism. It is the major source of energy for all of the organs and tissues of the body.

Glucagon—A hormone produced in the pancreas that is responsible for elevating blood glucose when it falls below a safe level for the body's organs and tissues.

Glycogen—The form in which glucose is stored in the body.

Hyperglycemia—Elevated blood glucose levels.

Hypoglycemia—Low blood glucose levels.

Insulin—A hormone produced by the pancreas that is responsible for allowing the body's cells to utilize glucose. The deficiency or absence of insulin is one of the causes of the disease diabetes.

Insulinoma—A tumor within the pancreas that produces insulin, potentially causing the serum glucose level to drop to dangerously low levels.

Ketoacidosis—A potentially life-threatening condition in which abnormally high blood glucose levels result in the blood become too acidic.

Pancreas—An organ located near the liver and stomach, responsible for various digestive functions. The pancreas produces insulin and glucagon, hormones that are responsible for maintaining safe blood levels of glucose.

Risks

Basic blood tests, such as serum glucose levels, do not carry any significant risks, other than slight bruising and the chance of brief dizziness.

Results

Normal results of a random serum glucose test range from 70–125 milligrams per deciliter (mg/dL). Normal results of a two-hour post-prandial serum glucose level range from 70–145 mg/dL. Normal results of a fasting serum glucose level range from 70–99 mg/dL.

High levels

High serum glucose levels suggest the possibility of diabetes; however, a single high, random serum glucose level is not sufficient for definitively diagnosing diabetes. The American Diabetes Association has specific criteria that must be met in order to diagnose diabetes. They require that results are verified through testing on a minimum of two different days. Levels indicative of diabetes are as follows:

- random serum glucose level of 200 mg/dL in the presence of actual symptoms of diabetes (such as increased thirst and/or hunger, urinary frequency, unintentional weight loss, weakness and fatigue, numbness/tingling in hands and feet, blurred vision, or erection problems;
- fasting serum glucose level of at least 126 mg/dL;
- two-hour oral glucose tolerance test of at least 200 mg/dL.

Individuals who don't meet the criteria for an actual diagnosis of diabetes, but who have a higher-than-normal fasting serum glucose level, also known as an impaired fasting glucose (ranging from 100 mg/dL to 125 mg/dL), have an increased risk of eventually developing diabetes, and should be followed closely. These individuals are considered to have "prediabetes."

Other causes of high serum glucose levels include:

- severe stress;
- heart attack;
- stroke;
- Cushing's syndrome;
- steroid medications; and
- acromegaly (elevated growth hormone).

Low levels

Low serum glucose levels may be due to:

- the presence of an insulinoma (a tumor that secretes insulin);
- Addison's disease;
- hypothyroidism (underactive thyroid);
- pituitary gland tumor;
- liver disease, including cirrhosis;
- kidney disease;
- malnutrition;
- eating disorders, including anorexia nervosa; and
- inappropriate doses of medicines used to treat diabetes, such as insulin or oral hypoglycemic agents.

Resources

BOOKS

Goldman L., and D. Ausiello, eds. *Cecil Textbook of Medicine,* 23rd ed. Philadelphia: Saunders, 2008.

Kronenberg H. M., S. Melmed, K. S. Polonsy, P. R. Larsen. *Williams Textbook of Endocrinology,* 11th ed. Philadelphia: Saunders Elsevier, 2007.

McPherson R.A., and M. R. Pincus, eds. *Henry's Clinical Diagnosis and Management by Laboratory Methods*, 21st ed. Philadelphia: Saunders, 2006.

OTHER

American Diabetes Association. http://www.diabetes.org (February 10, 2008).

Medical Encyclopedia. Medline Plus. National Institutes of Health. http://www.nlm.nih.gov/medlineplus/encyclopedia.html (February 10, 2008).

ORGANIZATIONS

American Association for Clinical Chemistry, 1850 K Street, NW, Suite 625, Washington, DC, 20006, (800) 892-1400, http://www.aacc.org.

Rosalyn Carson-DeWitt, M.D.

Sestamibi scan

Definition

A sestamibi scan is a highly sensitive and highly specific nuclear medicine test used to locate and image an overactive parathyroid gland in a patient with known hyperparathyroidism. Information from the test can help with planning for surgery to remove the overactive gland.

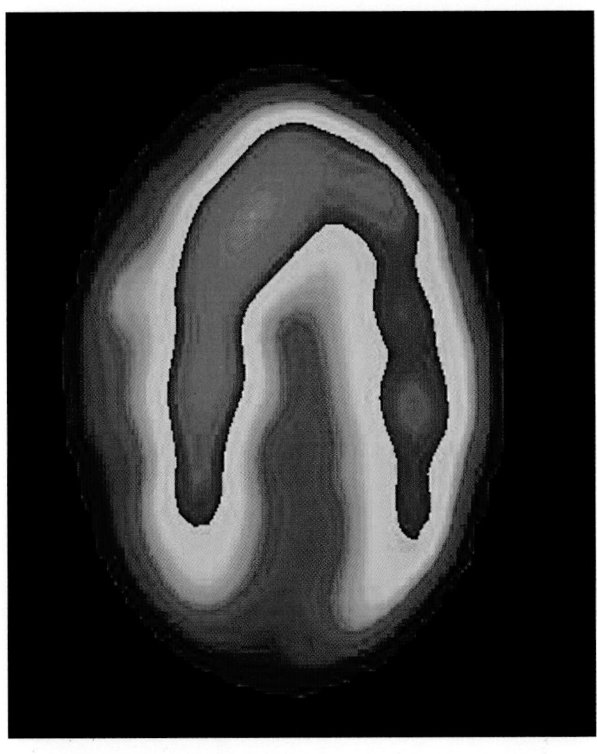

Sestamibi scan. *(ISM / Phototake. Reproduced by permission.)*

Located in the neck behind the thyroid gland, the four parathyroid glands are pea-sized endocrine glands that are responsible for the production of parthyroid hormone or PTH. PTH is important in the balance of calcium and phosphate throughout the body.

Under normal conditions, low calcium concentrations in the bloodstream prompt the parathyroid gland to put out increased amounts of PTH. PTH acts on several areas of the body. It directs the kidneys to absorb calcium back into the body, rather than flushing it out of the body in the urine. It activates osteoclasts in bone to degrade bone material, releasing calcium for use in the body. It increases the activity of vitamin D, which allows more calcium to be absorbed in the intestine.

Hyperparathyroidism is usually due to the presence of an adenoma, a benign (not cancerous) growth on one or more of the parathyroid glands. A sestamibi scan is used to generate images of the parathyroid glands prior to surgery so that the surgeon knows which of the four glands will require removal. Surgery to remove a parathyroid gland is called a **parathyroidectomy**.

During a sestamibi scan, the patient is given an injection of the radioactive material technetium-99, bound to a tiny protein called sestamibi. Unlike normal parathyroid glands, adenomatous parthyroid glands absorb the radioactive material, permitting visualization and localization of the tumor or tumors on the scan images. This test can be performed in preparation for an operation to remove the parathyroid adenoma, or during the course of such an operation (intraoperatively).

Purpose

Hyperparathyroidism is a condition in which one or more of the parathyroid glands become overactive. Too much bone is broken down, and too much calcium circulates in the bloodstream (termed hypercalcemia). The consequences of this excess bone breakdown and excess circulating calcium include:

- Weakness
- Fatigue
- Depression
- Achiness
- Decreased appetite
- Heartburn
- Nausea and vomiting
- Constipation

- High blood pressure
- Confusion
- Difficulty thinking
- Poor memory
- Excess thirst
- Frequent urination
- Thinner, weaker bones
- Increased risk of bone fracture
- Kidney stones

Hyperparathyroidism is often considered idiopathic, which means that there is no known underlying cause of the disorder. In about 5% of people with parathyroidism, there is a family tendency for the disorder, such as Familial multiple endocrine neoplasia type 1 or familial hypocalciuric hypercalcemia.

About 100,000 people in the United States are diagnosed with hyperparathyroidism annually. Women are twice as likely to get the disorder than men, and it is more common in people over the age of 60.

Description

Prior to starting the scanner for a sestamibi scan, radioactive contrast is injected through an IV in the patient's arm. The radionuclide (the technetium-99 bound to setamibi molecules) circulates in the blood stream, concentrating in diseased parathyroid glands. The patient lies on an examination table, and a gamma camera is positioned over the patient's neck. The camera consists of a crystal detector that detects emitted radiation from the radioactive contrast. A computer converts the signal into a digital image of the parathyroid glands. Scanning is done immediately after injection of the radionuclide, and 1 ½ to 2 hours after injection. Each scan takes about 10 minutes.

Preparation

There is nothing patients need to do in preparation for a sestamibi scan. To avoid confusing results, patients who have recently had another type of nuclear scan may need to wait several days to allow that radioactive tracer to leave their bodies, prior to undergoing a sestamibi scan.

Women who are pregnant or who think they may be pregnant are advised against undergoing a sestamibi scan. Women who are breastfeeding and who require a sestamibi scan should feed their baby with formula for two days following the procedure, and should pump and discard their breast milk, since it will be contaminated with the radioactive dye.

KEY TERMS

Adenoma—A benign tumor of an endocrine gland.

Hypercalcemia—Excess concentration of calcium in the blood.

Hyperparathyroidism—A condition in which the parathyroid gland is overactive; usually caused by the presence of an adenoma on one or more of the glands.

Parathyroidectomy—An operation performed in order to remove one or more parathyroid gland.

Thyroid gland—An endocrine organ in the neck which produces thyroid hormone. Thyroid hormone is involved in important growth and metabolic processes throughout the body.

Aftercare

There is no aftercare necessary following a sestamibi scan. The patient can return immediately to a normal diet and normal activities.

Risks

A sestamibi scan poses very little risk to the patient. Rarely, a patient may have an allergy to the radioactive contrast utilized.

Normal results

Normal results of a sestamibi scan would reveal no uptake of the radionuclide tracer in the neck, suggesting that no parathyroid adenoma is present.

Abnormal results

An abnormal sestamibi scan will reveal an area where the radionuclide has been absorbed by a parathyroid adenoma. Even small, single adenomas on a parathyroid gland will "light up," due to their tendency to absorb the radionuclide. This allows highly accurate localization of the exact area requiring operation. In some cases, a falsely positive sestamibi scan may occur in patients with thyroid disease.

Resources

BOOKS

Grainger, R. G., et al. *Grainger & Allison's Diagnostic Radiology: A Textbook of Medical Imaging*. 4th ed. Philadelphia: Saunders, 2001.

Kronenberg, H. M., S. Melmed, K. S. Polonsy, P. R. Larsen. *Williams Textbook of Endocrinology*. 11th ed. Philadelphia: Saunders Elsevier, 2008.

Mettler, F. A. *Essentials of Radiology*. 2nd ed. Philadelphia: Saunders, 2005.

PERIODICALS

Norton, K. S., et al. "The sestamibi scan as a preoperative screening tool." *American Surgery* 68(September 2002): 812–815.

Rosalyn Carson-DeWitt, MD

Seton glaucoma surgery *see* **Tube-shunt surgery**

Sex reassignment surgery

Definition

Also known as sex change or gender reassignment surgery, sex reassignment surgery is a procedure that changes genital organs from one gender to another.

Purpose

There are two main reasons to alter the genital organs from one sex to another.

- Newborns with intersex deformities must be assigned to one sex or the other. These deformities represent intermediate stages between the primordial female genitals and the change into male genitals caused by male hormone stimulation.
- Both men and women occasionally believe they are physically a different sex than they are mentally and emotionally. This dissonance is so profound that they are willing to be surgically altered.

In both cases, technical considerations favor successful conversion to a female rather than a male. Newborns with ambiguous organs will almost always be assigned to the female gender unless the penis is at least an inch (2.5 cm) long. Whatever their chromosomes, they are much more likely to be socially well-adjusted as females, even if they cannot have children.

Demographics

Reliable statistics are extremely difficult to obtain. Many sexual reassignment procedures are conducted in private facilities that are not subject to reporting requirements. Sexual reassignment surgery is often conducted outside of the United States. The number of gender reassignment procedures conducted in the United States each year is estimated at between 100

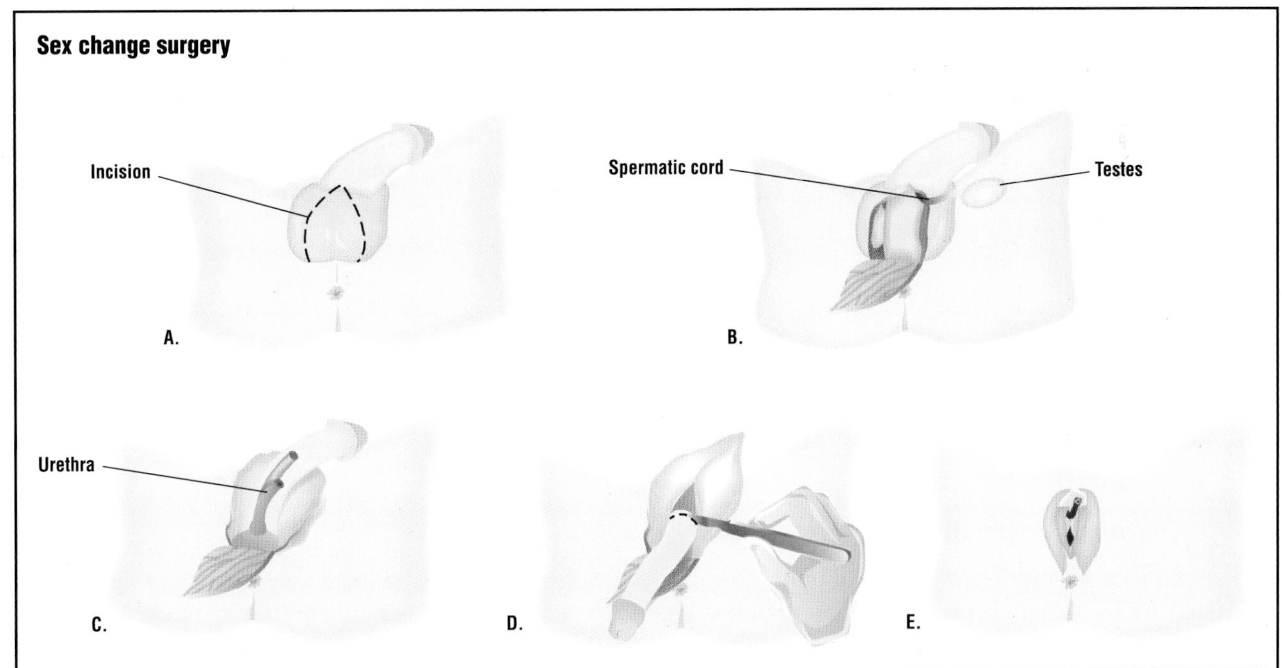

To change male genitalia to female genitalia, an incision is made into the scrotum (A). The flap of skin is pulled back, and the testes are removed (B). The skin is stripped from the penis but left attached, and a shorter urethra is cut (C). All but a stump of the penis is removed (D). The excess skin is used to create the labia (external genitalia) and vagina (E). *(Illustration by GGS Information Services. Cengage Learning, Gale.)*

KEY TERMS

Androgens—A class of chemical compounds (hormones) that stimulates the development of male secondary sexual characteristics.

Chromosomes—The carriers of genes that determine gender and other characteristics.

Estrogens—A class of chemical compounds (hormones) that stimulates the development of female secondary sexual characteristics.

Hysterectomy—Surgical removal of the uterus.

Oophorectomy—Surgical removal of the ovaries.

and 500. The number worldwide is estimated to be two to five times larger.

Description

Converting male to female anatomy requires removal of the penis, reshaping genital tissue to appear more female, and constructing a vagina. A vagina can be successfully formed from a skin graft or an isolated loop of intestine. Following the surgery, female hormones (estrogen) will reshape the body's contours and stimulate the growth of satisfactory breasts.

Female to male surgery has achieved lesser success due to the difficulty of creating a functioning penis from the much smaller clitoral tissue available in the female genitals. Penis construction is not attempted less than a year after the preliminary surgery to remove the female organs. One study in Singapore found that a third of the persons would not undergo the surgery again. Nevertheless, they were all pleased with the change of sex. Besides the genital organs, the breasts need to be surgically altered for a more male appearance. This can be successfully accomplished.

The capacity to experience an orgasm, or at least "a reasonable degree of erogenous sensitivity," can be expected by almost all persons after gender reassignment surgery.

Diagnosis/Preparation

Gender identity is an extremely important characteristic for human beings. Assigning sex must take place immediately after birth for the mental health of both children and their parents. Changing sexual identity is among the most significant changes that a human can experience. It should therefore be undertaken with extreme care and caution. By the time most adults come to surgery, they have lived for many years with a dissonant identity. The average in one study was 29 years. Nevertheless, even then they may not be fully aware of the implications of becoming a member of the opposite gender.

In-depth psychological counseling should precede and follow any gender reassignment surgical procedure.

Sex reassignment surgery is expensive. The cost for male to female reassignment is $10,000 to $20,000. The cost for female to male reassignment can exceed $50,000.

WHO PERFORMS THE PROCEDURE AND WHERE IS IT PERFORMED?

Gender reassignment surgery is performed by surgeons with specialized training in urology, gynecology, or plastic and reconstructive surgery. The surgery is performed in a hospital setting, although many procedures are completed in private clinics.

Aftercare

Social support, particularly from one's family, is important for readjustment as a member of the opposite gender. If surgical candidates are socially or emotionally unstable before the operation, over the age of 30, or have an unsuitable body build for the new gender, they tend not to fare well after gender reassignment surgery; however, in no case studied did the gender reassignment procedure diminish the ability to work.

Risks

All surgery carries the risks of infection, bleeding, and a need to return for repairs. Gender reassignment surgery is irreversible, so a candidate must have no doubts about accepting the results and outcome.

Normal results

Persons undergoing gender reassignment surgery can expect to acquire the external genitalia of a member of the opposite gender. Persons having male to female gender reassignment surgery retain a prostate. Individuals undergoing female to male gender reassignment surgery undergo a **hysterectomy** to remove the uterus and **oophorectomy** to remove their ovaries. Developing the habits and mannerisms characteristic of the patient's new gender requires many months or years.

QUESTIONS TO ASK THE DOCTOR

Candidates for gender reassignment surgery should ask the following questions.

- What will my body look like afterward?
- Is the surgeon board certified in urology, gynecology, or plastic and reconstructive surgery?
- How many gender reassignment procedures has the surgeon performed?
- How many surgeries of the type similar to the one being contemplated (i.e., male to female or female to male) has the surgeon performed?
- What is the surgeon's complication rate?

Morbidity and mortality rates

The risks that are associated with any surgical procedure are present in gender reassignment surgery. These include infection, postoperative pain, and dissatisfaction with anticipated results. Accurate statistics are extremely difficult to find. Intraoperative **death** has not been reported.

The most common complication of male to female surgery is narrowing of the new vagina. This can be corrected by dilation or using a portion of colon to form a vagina.

A relatively common complication of female to male surgery is dysfunction of the penis. Implanting a penile prosthesis is technically difficult and does not have uniformly acceptable results.

Psychiatric care may be required for many years after sex-reassignment surgery.

The number of deaths in male-to-female transsexuals was five times the number expected, due to increased numbers of suicide and death from an unknown cause.

Alternatives

There is no alternative to surgical reassignment to alter one's external genitalia. The majority of persons who experience gender disorder problems never surgically alter their appearance. They dress as members of the desired gender, rather than gender of birth. Many use creams or pills that contain hormones appropriate to the desired gender to alter their bodily appearance. Estrogens (female hormones) will stimulate breast development, widening of the hips, loss of facial hair and a slight increase in voice pitch. Androgens (male hormones) will stimulate the development of facial and chest hair and cause the voice to deepen. Most individuals who undergo gender reassignment surgery lead happy and productive lives.

Resources

BOOKS

Wein, A. J., L. R. Kavoussi, A. C. Novick, A. W. Partin, and C. A. Peters. *Campbell-Walsh Urology*, 9th ed. Philadelphia: Saunders, 2006.

PERIODICALS

Lawrence A. "Patient-reported complications and functional outcomes of male-to-female sex reassignment surgery." *Archives of Sexual Behavior* 35, no. 6 (December 2006): 717–727.

Liguori G., et al. "Laparoscopic mobilization of neovagina to assist secondary ileal vaginoplasty in male-to-female transsexuals." *Urology* 66, no. 2 (2005): 293–298.

Maharaj N. R., A. Dhai, R. Wiersma, and J. Moodley. "Intersex conditions in children and adolescents: surgical, ethical, and legal considerations." *Journal of Pediatric and Adolescent Gynecology* 18, no. 6 (December 2005): 399–402.

Stanojevics D. S., et al. "Sacrospinous ligament fixation for neovaginal prolapse prevention in male-to-female surgery." *Urology* 70, no. 4 (October 2007): 767–71.

OTHER

Intersex Society of North America. http://www.isna.org/ [Accessed April 9, 2008].

"Sex change surgery." Health A to Z. August 14, 2006. http://www.healthatoz.com/healthatoz/Atoz/common/standard/transform.jsp?requestURI = /healthatoz/Atoz/ency/sex_change_surgery.jsp [Accessed April 9, 2008).

ORGANIZATIONS

American Medical Association, 515 N. State Street, Chicago, IL, 60610, (800) 621-8335, http://www.ama-assn.org/.

American Psychiatric Association, 1000 Wilson Boulevard, Suite 1825, Arlington, VA, 22209-3901, (703) 907-7300, apa@psych.org, http://www.psych.org/.

American Psychological Association, 750 First Street, NE, Washington, DC, 20002-4242, (202) 336-5500, (800) 374-2721, http://www.apa.org/.

American Urological Association, 1000 Corporate Boulevard, Linthicum, MD, 21090, (410) 689-3700, (866) 746-4282, http://www.auanet.org/.

L. Fleming Fallon, Jr., M.D., Dr.P.H.

Shoulder arthroscopic surgery *see* **Rotator cuff repair; Bankart procedure**

Shoulder joint replacement

Definition

Shoulder joint replacement surgery is performed to replace a shoulder joint with artificial components (prostheses) when the joint is severely damaged by degenerative joint diseases such as arthritis, or in complex cases of upper arm bone fracture.

Purpose

The shoulder is a ball-and-socket joint that allows the arms to be raised, twisted, bent, and moved forward, to the side and backward. The head of the upper arm bone (humerus) is the ball, and a circular cavity (glenoid) in the shoulder blade (scapula) is the socket. A soft-tissue rim (labrum) surrounds and deepens the socket. The head of the humerus is also covered with a smooth, tough tissue (articular cartilage), and the joint, also called the acromioclavicular (AC) joint, has a thin inner lining (synovium) that facilitates movement, while surrounding muscles and tendons provide stability and support.

The AC joint can be damaged by the following conditions to such an extent as to require replacement by artificial components:

- Osteoarthritis. This is a degenerative joint disease characterized by degeneration of the articular cartilage. When nonsurgical treatment is no longer effective and shoulder resection not possible, joint replacement surgery is usually indicated.
- Rheumatoid arthritis. Shoulder replacement surgery is the most commonly performed procedure for the arthritic shoulder with severe inflammatory or rheumatoid arthritis.
- Severe fracture of the humerus. A fracture of the upper arm bone can be so severe as to require replacement of the AC joint.
- Osteonecrosis. This condition usually follows a three- or four-part fracture of the humeral head that disrupts the blood supply, resulting in bone death and disruption of the AC joint.
- Charcot's arthropathy. Also called neuropathic arthropathy or arthritis, Charcot's arthropathy is a condition in which the shoulder joint is destroyed following loss of its nerve supply.

Demographics

Shoulder arthritis is among the most prevalent causes of shoulder pain and loss of function. In the United States, arthritis of the shoulder joint is less common than arthritis of the hip or knee. Individuals with arthritis in one joint are more likely to get it in another joint. Overall, arthritis is quite common in the United States, affecting about 21% of adult Americans, and 50% of American adults over the age of 65. Projections suggest that, by the year 2030, there will be 67 million Americans who have received the diagnosis of arthritis from their doctor. Osteoarthritis is also the most common joint disorder, extremely common by age 70. Men and women are equally affected, but onset is earlier in men.

Description

Shoulder joint replacement surgery can either replace the entire AC joint, in which case it is referred to as total shoulder joint replacement or total shoulder **arthroplasty**; or replace only the head of the humerus, in which case the procedure is called a hemiarthroplasty.

Implants

The two artificial components that can be implanted in the shoulder during shoulder joint replacment surgery are:

- The humeral component. This part replaces the head of the humerus. It is usually made of cobalt or chromium-based alloys and has a rounded ball attached to a stem that can be inserted into the bone. It comes in various sizes and may consist of a single piece or a modular unit.
- The glenoid component. This component replaces the glenoid cavity. It is made of very high-density polyethelene. Some models feature a metal tray, but the 100% polyethylene type is more common.

Shoulder joint replacement surgery is performed under either regional or **general anesthesia**, depending on the specifics of the case. The surgeon makes a 3–4 in (7.6–10.2 cm) incision on the front of the shoulder from the collarbone to the point where the shoulder muscle (deltoid) attaches to the humerus. The surgeon also inspects the muscles to see if any are damaged. He or she then proceeds to dislocate the humerus from the socket-like glenoid cavity to expose the head of the humerus. Only the portion of the head covered with articular cartilage is removed. The center cavity of the humerus (humeral shaft) is then cleaned and enlarged with reamers of gradually increasing size to create a cavity matching the shape of the implant stem. The top end of the bone is smoothed so that the stem can be inserted flush with the bone surface.

If the glenoid cavity of the AC joint is not damaged and the surrounding muscles are intact, the surgeon does not replace it, thus performing a simple hemiarthroplasty; however, if the glenoid cavity is

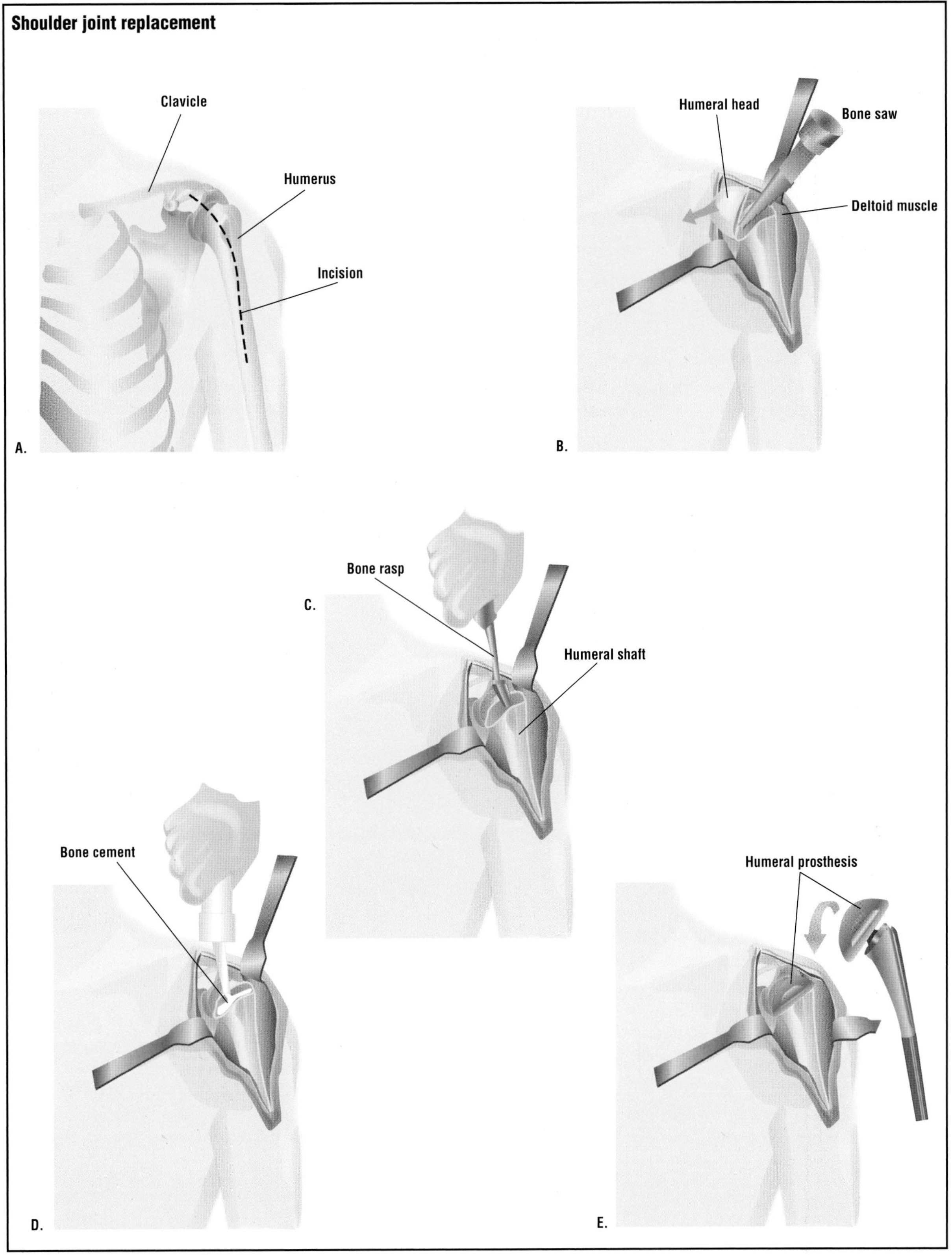

During a total shoulder joint replacement, an incision is first made in the shoulder and upper arm (A). The head of humerus is removed with a bone saw (B). The shaft of the humerus is reamed with a bone rasp to ready it for the prosthesis (C). After the shoulder joint, or glenoid cavity, is similarly prepared, bone cement is applied to areas to receive prostheses (D). The ball and socket prostheses are put in place, and the incision is closed (E). *(Illustration by GGS Information Services. Cengage Learning, Gale.)*

KEY TERMS

Acromioclavicular (AC) joint—The shoulder joint. Articulation and ligaments between the collarbone and the acromion of the shoulder blade.

Acromion—The triangular projection of the spine of the shoulder blade that forms the point of the shoulder and articulates with the collarbone.

Arthroplasty—The surgical repair of a joint.

Charcot's arthropathy—Also called neuropathic arthropathy, a condition in which the shoulder joint is destroyed following loss of its nerve supply.

Glenoid cavity—The hollow cavity in the head of the shoulder blade that receives the head of the humerus to make the glenohumeral or shoulder joint.

Humerus—The bone of the upper part of the arm.

Inflammatory arthritis—An inflammatory condition that affects joints.

Osteoarthritis—Non-inflammatory degenerative joint disease occurring chiefly in older persons, characterized by degeneration of the articular cartilage.

Osteonecrosis—Condition resulting from poor blood supply to an area of a bone and causing bone death.

Rheumatoid arthritis—Chronic inflammatory disease that destroys joints.

Shoulder resection arthroplasty—Surgery performed to repair a shoulder acromioclavicular (AC) joint. The procedure is most commonly recommended for AC joint problems resulting from osteoarthritis or injury.

damaged or diseased, the surgeon moves the humerus to the back and implants the artificial glenoid component as well. The surgeon prepares the surface by removing the cartilage and equalizes the glenoid bone to match the implant. Protrusions on the polyethylene glenoid implant are then fitted into holes drilled in the bone surface. Once a precise fit is achieved, the implant is cemented into position. The humerus, with its new implanted artificial head, is replaced in the glenoid socket. The surgeon reattaches the supporting tendons and closes the incision.

Diagnosis/Preparation

Damage to the AC joint is usually assessed using X-rays of the joint and humerus. They provide information on the state of the joint space, the position of the humeral head in relation to the glenoid, the presence of bony defects or deformity, and the quality of the bone. If glenoid wear is observed, a computed tomography (CT) scan is usually performed to evaluate the degree of bone loss.

The treating physician usually performs a general medical evaluation several weeks before shoulder joint replacement surgery to assess the patient's general health condition and risk for anesthesia. The results of this examination are forwarded to the orthopedic surgeon, along with a surgical clearance. Patients are advised to eat properly and take a daily iron supplement some weeks before surgery. Several types of tests are usually required, including blood tests, a cardiogram, a urine sample, and a chest X-ray. Patients may be required to stop taking certain medications until surgery is over.

WHO PERFORMS THE PROCEDURE AND WHERE IS IT PERFORMED?

Shoulder replacement surgery is performed in a hospital by orthopedic surgeons with specialized training in shoulder joint replacement surgery.

Aftercare

Following surgery, the operated arm is placed in a sling, and a support pillow is placed under the elbow to protect the repair. A drainage tube is used to remove excess fluid and is usually removed on the day after surgery.

A careful and well-planned rehabilitation program is very important for the successful outcome of a shoulder joint replacement. It should start no later than the first postoperative day. A physical therapist usually starts the patient with gentle, passive-assisted range of motion exercises. Before the patient leaves the hospital (usually two or three days after surgery), the therapist provides instruction on using a pulley device to help bend and extend the operated arm.

Risks

Complications after shoulder replacement surgery occur less frequently than with other joint replacement surgeries; however, there are risks associated with the surgery, including infection, intra-operative fracture of the humerus or postoperative fractures, biceps tendon rupture, and postoperative instability and loosening of the glenoid implant. Advances in surgical

QUESTIONS TO ASK THE DOCTOR

- What type of joint replacement surgery does my shoulder require?
- What are the risks associated with the surgery?
- How long will it take for my shoulder to recover from the surgery?
- How long will the artificial components last?
- Is there a risk of implant infection?
- How many shoulder joint replacement surgeries do you perform in a year?

techniques and prosthetic innovations are helping to significantly lower the occurrence of complications.

Normal results

Pain relief is expected after shoulder joint replacement because the diseased joint surfaces have been replaced with smooth gliding surfaces. Improved motion, however, is variable and depends on the following:

- the surgeon's ability to reconstruct the shoulder's supporting tissues, namely the shoulder ligaments, capsule, and muscle attachments;
- the patient's preoperative muscle strength; and
- the patient's motivation and compliance in participating in postoperative rehabilitation therapy.

Morbidity and mortality rates

Good to excellent outcomes usually follow shoulder joint replacement surgery, including pain relief and a functional range of motion that provides the ability to dress and perform the normal activities of daily living. In the hands of experienced orthopedic surgeons, such outcomes occur 90% of the time. Shoulders with artificial joints are reported to function well for more than 20 years. No **death** has ever been reported for shoulder joint replacement procedures.

Alternatives

Arthritis treatment is very complex, as it depends on the type of arthritis and the severity of symptoms. Alternatives to joint replacement may include medications and therapy. It is known that arthritis is characterized by an increased rate of cartilage degradation and a decreased rate of cartilage production. An experimental therapy featuring the use of joint supplements such as glucosamine and chondroitin is being investigated for its effectiveness to repair cartilage. The pain and inflammation resulting from arthritis are also commonly treated with nonsteroidal anti-inflammatory pain medication (NSAIDs) or cortisone injections (steroidal).

Resources

BOOKS

Browner, B., J. Jupiter, A. Levine, and P. Trafton. *Skeletal Trauma: Fractures, Dislocations, Ligamentous Injuries,* 3rd ed. Philadelphia: Saunders, 2002.

Canale, S. T. *Campbell's Operative Orthopedics,* 10th ed. St. Louis, MO: Mosby, 2002.

DeLee, J. C., D. Drez, and M. D. Miller.*DeLee and Drez's Orthopaedic Sports Medicine,* 2nd ed. Philadelphia: Saunders, 2002.

PERIODICALS

Miller, S. L., Y. Hazrati, S. Klepps, A. Chiang, and E. L. Flatow. "Loss of Subscapularis Function after Total Shoulder Replacement: A Seldom Recognized Problem." *Journal of Shoulder and Elbow Surgery* 12, no. 1 (January–February 2003): 29–34.

Roos, E. M. "Effectiveness and Practice Variation of Rehabilitation after Joint Replacement." *Current Opinions in Rheumatology* 15, no. 2 (March 2003): 160–162.

ORGANIZATIONS

American Academy of Orthopaedic Surgeons, 6300 N. River Road, Rosemont, IL, 60018-4262, (847) 823-7186, (800) 346-AAOS, (847) 823-8125, http://www.aaos.org.

American Shoulder and Elbow Surgeons, 6300 N. River Road, Suite 727, Rosemont, IL, 60018, (847) 698-1629, http://www.ases-assn.org.

Monique Laberge, Ph.D.

Shoulder resection arthroplasty

Definition

Shoulder resection **arthroplasty** is surgery performed to repair a shoulder acromioclavicular (AC) joint. The procedure is most commonly recommended for AC joint problems resulting from osteoarthritis or injury.

Purpose

The shoulder consists of three bones: the shoulder blade, the upper arm bone (humerus), and the collarbone (clavicle). The part of the shoulder blade that makes up the roof of the shoulder is called the acromion and the joint where the acromion and the collarbone join is called the acromioclavicular (AC) joint.

KEY TERMS

Acromioclavicular dislocation—Disruption of the normal articulation between the acromion and the collarbone. The acromioclavicular joint (AC joint) is normally stabilized by several ligaments that can be torn in the process of dislocating the AC joint.

Acromioclavicular (AC) joint—Articulation and ligaments between the collarbone and the acromion of the shoulder blade.

Acromion—The triangular projection of the spine of the shoulder blade that forms the point of the shoulder and articulates with the collarbone.

Arthroplasty—The surgical repair of a joint.

Arthrosis—A disease of a joint.

Glenoid cavity—The hollow cavity in the head of the shoulder blade that receives the head of the humerus to make the glenohumeral or shoulder joint.

Osteoarthritis—Non-inflammatory degenerative joint disease occurring chiefly in older persons, characterized by degeneration of the articular cartilage.

Some joints in the body are more likely to develop problems due to normal wear and tear, or degeneration resulting from osteoarthritis, a progressive and degenerative joint disease. The AC joint is a common target for developing osteoarthritis in middle age. This condition can lead to pain and difficulty using the shoulder for everyday activities. Besides osteoarthritis, AC joint disease (arthrosis) may develop from an old injury to the joint such as an acromioclavicular dislocation, which is the disruption of the normal articulation between the acromion and the collarbone. This type of injury is quite common in competitive sports, but can also result from a simple fall on the shoulder.

The goal of shoulder resection arthroplasty is to restore function to an impaired shoulder, with its required motion range, stability, strength, and smoothness.

Demographics

According to the National Ambulatory Medical Care Survey, osteoarthritis is one of the most common confirmed diagnoses in individuals over the age of 65, with the condition starting to develop in middle age.

As for AC joint injuries, they are seen especially in high-level athletes such as football or hockey players, and occur most frequently in the second decade of life. Males are more commonly affected than females, with a male-to-female ratio of approximately five to one.

Description

A resection arthroplasty involves the surgical removal of the last 0.5 in (1.3 cm) of the collarbone. This removal leaves a space between the acromion and the cut end of the collarbone where the AC joint used to be. The joint is replaced by scar tissue, which allows movement to occur, but prevents the rubbing of the bone ends. The end result of the surgery is that the flexible connection between the acromion and the collarbone is restored. The procedure is usually performed by making a small 2 in (5 cm) incision in the skin over the AC joint. In some cases, the surgery can be done arthroscopically. In this approach, the surgeon uses an endoscope to look through a small hole into the shoulder joint. The endoscope is an instrument of the size of a pen, consisting of a tube fitted with a light and a miniature video camera, which transmits an image of the joint interior to a television monitor. The surgeon proceeds to remove the segment of collarbone through a small incision with little disruption of the other shoulder structures.

Diagnosis/Preparation

The diagnosis is made by physical exam. Tenderness over the AC joint is usually present, with pain upon compression of the joint. X-rays of the AC joint may show narrowing of the joint and bone spurs around the joint. A **magnetic resonance imaging** (MRI) scan may also be performed. An MRI scan is a special imaging test that uses magnetic waves to create pictures that show the tissues of the shoulder in slices and has the advantage of showing tendons as well as bones. In some cases, an **ultrasound** test may be also be performed to inspect the soft tissues of the joint.

Prior to arthroplasty surgery, all the standard preoperative blood and urine tests are performed. The patient also meets with the anesthesiologist to discuss any special conditions that may affect the administration of anesthesia.

Aftercare

The rehabilitation following surgery for a simple resection arthroplasty is usually fairly rapid. Patients should expect the soreness to last for three to six weeks. Postoperatively, patients usually have the affected arm in a sling for two weeks. Thereafter, a progressive passive range of shoulder motion **exercise** is started, usually with range-of-motion exercises that gradually evolve into active stretching and strengthening. The patient's arm

WHO PERFORMS THE PROCEDURE AND WHERE IS IT PERFORMED?

Shoulder resection arthroplasty is performed in a hospital. It is performed by experienced orthopedic surgeons who are specialists in AC joint problems. Some medical centers specialize in joint surgery and tend to have higher success rates than less specialized centers.

QUESTIONS TO ASK THE DOCTOR

- How can I regain the use of my shoulder?
- What will it take to make my shoulder healthy again?
- Why do I have problems with my shoulder?
- What surgical procedures do you follow?
- How many shoulder resection arthroplasties do you perform each year?
- Will surgery on my shoulder condition allow me to resume my activities?

remains in the sling between sessions. At six weeks, healing is sufficient to encourage progressive functional use. Physiotherapy usually continues until range of motion and strength are maximized. The therapist may also use massage and other types of hands-on treatments to ease muscle spasm and pain. Heavy physical use of the shoulder is prohibited for an additional six weeks.

Risks

Patients who undergo shoulder resection arthroplasty are susceptible to the same complications associated with any such surgery. These include wound infection, osteomyelitis, soft tissue ossification, and failure of fixation (remaining in place), with recurrent deformity. Symptomatic AC joint arthritis may develop in patients who undergo the surgery as a result of injury.

Specific risks associated with shoulder resection arthroplasty include:

- Fractures. Fractures of the humerus may occur after surgery, although the risk is considered low.
- Shoulder instability. Shoulder dislocations may occur during the early postoperative period due to soft tissue imbalance or to inadequate postoperative protection; late dislocation may result from glenoid cavity wear.
- Degenerative changes. Progressive degeneration of the AC joint is a common late complication.

Normal results

Shoulder resection arthroplasty is generally very effective in reducing pain and restoring motion of the shoulder.

Morbidity and mortality rates

In a four-year follow-up study on shoulder arthroplasty patients, all patients experienced pain relief. Functional improvement was good in 77% of patients. Average shoulder abduction improved from 37–79° and forward flexion from 52–93°. No deaths resulting from shoulder resection arthroplasty have ever been reported.

Alternatives

Non-surgical treatments

Doctors commonly attempt to treat AC joint problems using conservative treatments. Patients may be prescribed anti-inflammatory medications such as **aspirin** or ibuprofen. Treatment also may include disease-modifying drugs such as methotrexate and sulfasalazine, as well as gold injections. Researchers are also working on biologic agents that can interrupt the progress of osteoarthritis. These agents target specific chemicals in the body to prevent them from acting on the joints. Resting the sore joint and applying ice to it can also ease pain and inflammation. Injections of cortisone into the joint may also be prescribed. Cortisone is a strong steroidal medication that decreases inflammation and reduces pain. The effects of the drug are temporary, but it provides effective relief in the short term. Physicians may also prescribe sessions with a physical or occupational therapist, who may use various treatments to relieve inflammation of the AC joint, including heat and ice.

Surgical alternatives

Alternative surgical approaches include replacing the entire shoulder joint with a prosthesis (total shoulder arthroplasty) or replacing the head of the humerus (hemiarthroplasty).

Resources

BOOKS

Browner, B., J. Jupiter, A. Levine, and P. Trafton. *Skeletal Trauma: Fractures, Dislocations, Ligamentous Injuries*, 3rd ed. Philadelphia: Saunders, 2002.

Canale, S. T. *Campbell's Operative Orthopedics,* 10th ed. St. Louis, MO: Mosby, 2002.

DeLee, J. C., D. Drez, and M. D. Miller. *DeLee and Drez's Orthopaedic Sports Medicine,* 2nd ed. Philadelphia: Saunders, 2002.

PERIODICALS

Iannotti, J. P., and T. R. Norris. "Influence of Preoperative Factors on Outcome of Shoulder Arthroplasty for Glenohumeral Osteoarthritis." *Journal of Bone and Joint Surgery* 85 (February 2003): 251–258.

Mileti, J., J. W. Sperling, and R. H. Cofield. "Shoulder Arthroplasty for the Treatment of Postinfectious Glenohumeral Arthritis." *Journal of Bone and Joint Surgery* 85 (April 2003): 609–614.

Nagels, J., M. Stokdijk, and P. M. Rozing. "Stress Shielding and Bone Resorption in Shoulder Arthroplasty." *Journal of Shoulder and Elbow Surgery* 12, no. 1 (January–February 2003): 35–39.

Sanchez-Sotelo, J., J. W. Sperling, C. M. Rowland, and R. H. Cofield. "Instability after Shoulder Arthroplasty: Results of Surgical Treatment." *Journal of Bone and Joint Surgery* 85 (April 2003): 622–631.

Sofka, C. M., and R. S. Adler. "Sonographic Evaluation of Shoulder Arthroplasty." *American Journal of Roentgenology* 180 (April 2003): 1117–1120.

Woodruff, M., A. Cohen, and J. Bradley. "Arthroplasty of the Shoulder in Rheumatoid Arthritis with Rotator Cuff Dysfunction." *International Orthopaedics* 27, no. 1 (February 2003): 7–10.

OTHER

Wheeless, Clifford R. III. "Arthroplasty of the Shoulder." Wheeless' Textbook of Orthopaedics. http://www.wheelessonline.com/ortho/arthroplasty_of_the_shoulder (April 5, 2008).

ORGANIZATIONS

American Academy of Orthopaedic Surgeons, 6300 N. River Road, Rosemont, IL, 60018-4262, (847) 823-7186, (800) 346-AAOS, (847) 823-8125, http://www.aaos.org.

American Shoulder and Elbow Surgeons, 6300 N. River Road, Suite 727, Rosemont, IL, 60018, (847) 698-1629, http://www.ases-assn.org.

Monique Laberge, Ph.D.

Sigmoidoscopy

Definition

Sigmoidoscopy is a diagnostic and screening procedure in which a rigid or flexible tube with a camera on the end (a sigmoidoscope) is inserted into the anus to examine the rectum and lower colon (bowel) for bowel disease, cancer, precancerous conditions, or causes of bleeding or pain.

Purpose

Sigmoidoscopy is used most often in screening for colorectal cancer or to determine the cause of rectal bleeding. It is also used in diagnosis of inflammatory bowel disease, microscopic and ulcerative colitis, and Crohn's disease.

Cancer of the rectum and colon is the second most common cancer in the United States. About 148,300 new cases are diagnosed annually. Between 55,000 and 60,000 Americans die each year of cancer in the colon or rectum.

After reviewing a number of studies, experts recommend that people over 50 be screened for colorectal cancer using sigmoidoscopy every three to five years. Individuals with inflammatory bowel conditions such as Crohn's disease or ulcerative colitis, and thus at increased risk for colorectal cancer, may begin their screenings at a younger age, depending on when their disease was diagnosed. Many physicians screen such persons more often than every three to five years. Screening should also be performed in people who have a family history of colon or rectal cancer, or small growths in the colon (polyps).

Some physicians do this screening with a colonoscope, which allows them to see the entire colon. Most physicians prefer sigmoidoscopy, which is less time-consuming, less uncomfortable, and less costly.

Studies have shown that one-quarter to one-third of all precancerous or small cancerous growths can be seen with a sigmoidoscope. About one-half are found with a 1 ft (30 cm) scope, and two-thirds to three-quarters can be seen using a 2 ft (60 cm) scope.

In some cases, the sigmoidoscope can be used therapeutically in conjunction with other equipment such as electrosurgical devices to remove polyps and other lesions found during the sigmoidoscopy.

Demographics

Experts estimate that in excess of 525,000 sigmoidoscopy procedures are performed each year. This number includes most of the persons who are diagnosed with colon cancer each year, a greater number who are screened and receive negative results, persons who have been treated for colon conditions and receive a sigmoidoscopy as a follow-up procedure, and individuals who are diagnosed with other diseases of the large colon.

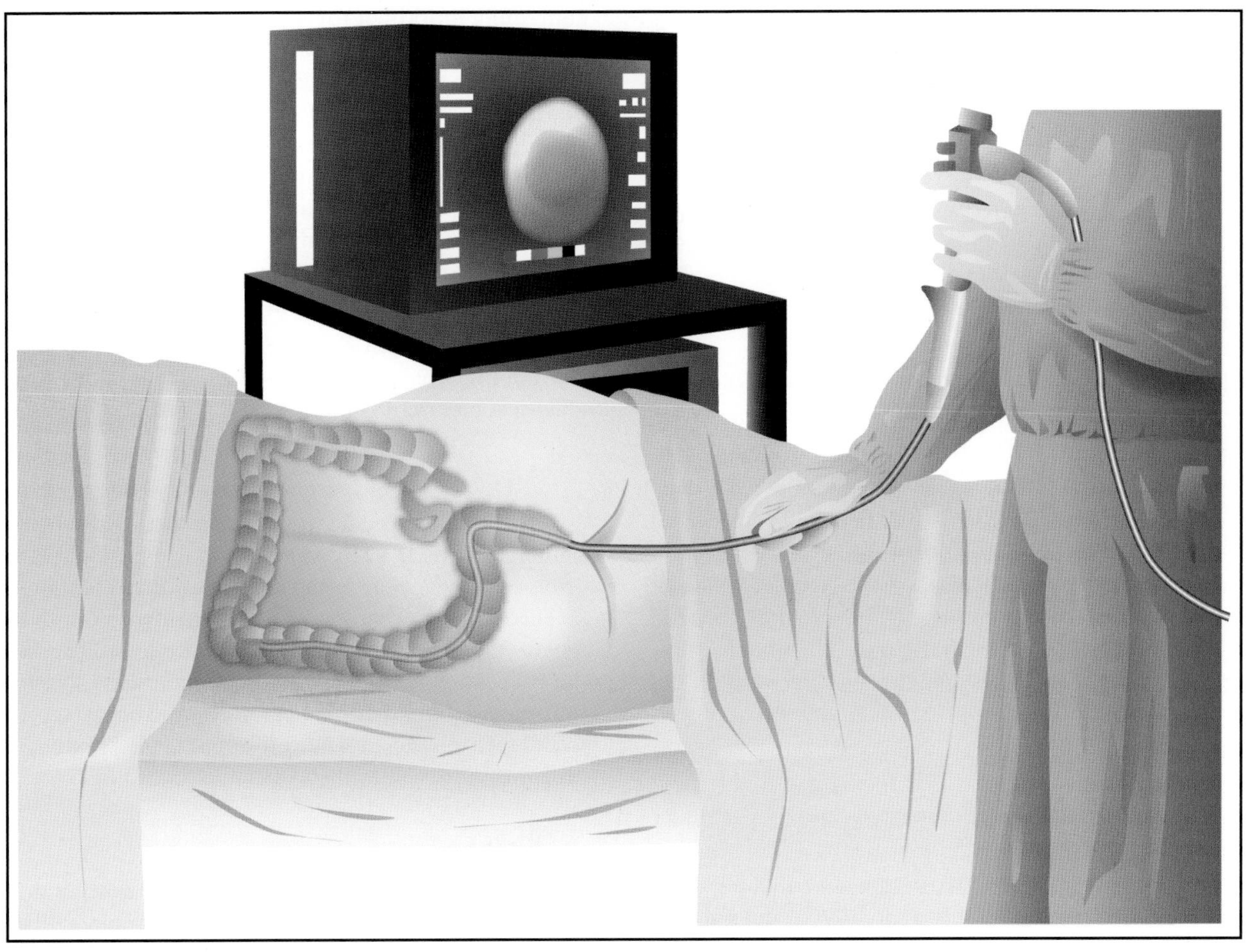

(Illustration by GGS Information Services. Cengage Learning, Gale.)

Description

Sigmoidoscopy may be performed using either a rigid or flexible sigmoidoscope. A sigmoidoscope is a thin tube with fiberoptics, electronics, a light source, and camera. A physician inserts the sigmoidoscope into the anus to examine the rectum (the first 1 ft [30 cm] of the colon) and its interior walls. If a 2 ft (60 cm) scope is used, the next portion of the colon can also be examined for any irregularities. The camera of the sigmoidoscope is connected to a viewing monitor, allowing the interior of the rectum and colon to be enlarged and viewed on the monitor. Images can then be recorded as still pictures or the entire procedure can be videotaped. The still pictures are useful for comparison purposes with the results of future sigmoidoscopic examinations.

If polyps, lesions, or other suspicious areas are found, the physician biopsies them for analysis. During the sigmoidoscopy, the physician may also use forceps, graspers, snares, or electrosurgical devices to remove polyps, lesions, or tumors.

A typical sigmoidoscopy procedure requires 15 to 20 minutes to perform. Preparation begins one day before the procedure. There is some discomfort when the scope is inserted and throughout the procedure, similar to that experienced when a physician performs a rectal exam using a finger to test for occult blood in the stool (another important screening test for colorectal cancer). Individuals may also feel some minor cramping pain. There is rarely severe pain, except for persons with active inflammatory bowel disease.

Private insurance plans almost always cover the cost of sigmoidoscopy examinations for screening in healthy individuals over 50, or for diagnostic purposes. **Medicare** covers the cost for diagnostic exams, and may cover the costs for screening exams. **Medicaid** benefits vary by state, but sigmoidoscopy is not a covered procedure in many states. Some community health clinics offer the

KEY TERMS

Biopsy—The removal of a small portion of tissue during sigmoidoscopy to perform laboratory tests to determine if the tissue is cancerous.

Colonoscopy—A diagnostic endoscopic procedure that uses a long flexible tube called a colonoscope to examine the inner lining of the entire colon; may be used for colorectal cancer screening or for a more thorough examination of the colon.

Colorectal cancer—Cancer of the large intestine, or colon, including the rectum.

Electrosurgical device—A medical device that uses electrical current to cauterize or coagulate tissue during surgical procedures, often used in conjunction with laparoscopy, colonoscopy, or sigmoidoscopy.

Inflammatory bowel diseases—Ulcerative colitis or Crohn's disease: chronic conditions characterized by periods of diarrhea, bloating, abdominal cramps, and pain, sometimes accompanied by weight loss and malnutrition because of the inability to absorb nutrients.

Pathologist—A doctor who specializes in the diagnosis of disease by studying cells and tissues under a microscope.

Polyp—A small growth, usually not cancerous, but often precancerous when it appears in the colon.

procedure at reduced cost, but this can only be done if a local gastroenterologist (a physician who specializes in treating stomach and intestinal disorders) is willing to donate personal time to perform the procedure.

Diagnosis/Preparation

The purpose of preparation for sigmoidoscopy is to cleanse the lower bowel of fecal material or stool so the physician can see the lining. Preparation begins 24 hours before the procedure, when an individual must begin a clear liquid diet. Preparation kits are available in drug stores. In normal preparation, about 20 hours before the exam, a person begins taking a series of **laxatives**, which may be oral tablets or liquid. The individual must stop drinking any liquid four hours before the exam. An hour or two prior to the examination, the person uses an enema or laxative suppository to finish cleansing the lower bowel.

Individuals need to be careful about medications before having sigmoidoscopy. They should not take **aspirin**, products containing aspirin, or products containing ibuprofen for one week prior to the exam, because these medications can exacerbate bleeding during the procedure. They should not take any iron or vitamins with iron for one week prior to the exam, since iron can cause color changes in the bowel lining that interfere with the examination. They should take any routine prescription medications, but may need to stop certain medications. Prescribing physicians should be consulted regarding routine prescriptions and their possible effect(s) on sigmoidoscopy.

Individuals with renal insufficiency or congestive heart failure need to be prepared in an alternative way, and must be carefully monitored during the procedure.

Aftercare

There is no specific aftercare necessary following sigmoidoscopy. If a biopsy was taken, a small amount of blood may appear in the next stool. Persons should be encouraged to pass gas following the procedure to relieve any bloating or cramping that may occur after the procedure. In addition, an infection may develop following sigmoidoscopy. Persons should be instructed to call their physician if a fever or pain in the abdomen develops over the few days after the procedure.

Risks

There is a slight risk of bleeding from the procedure. This risk is heightened in individuals whose blood does not clot well, either due to disease or medication, and in those with active inflammatory bowel disease. Rarely, trauma to the bowel or other organs can occur, resulting in an injury (perforation) that must be repaired, or peritonitis, which must be treated with medication.

Sigmoidoscopy may be contraindicated in persons with severe active colitis or toxic megacolon (an extremely dilated colon). In general, people experiencing continuous ambulatory peritoneal dialysis are not candidates due to a high risk of developing intraperitoneal bleeding.

Normal results

The results of a normal examination reveal a smooth colon wall, with sufficient blood vessels for good blood flow.

Morbidity and mortality rates

For a cancer screening sigmoidoscopy, an abnormal result is one or more noncancerous or precancerous polyps, or clearly cancerous polyps. People with polyps have an increased risk of developing colorectal cancer in the future and may be required to undergo

WHO PERFORMS THE PROCEDURE AND WHERE IS IT PERFORMED?

A colonoscopy procedure is usually performed by a gastroenterologist, a physician with specialized training in diseases of the colon. Alternatively, general surgeons or experienced family physicians perform sigmoidoscopic examinations. In the United States, the procedure is usually performed in an outpatient facility of a hospital or in a physician's professional office.

Persons with rectal bleeding may need full colonoscopy in a hospital setting. Individuals whose blood does not clot well (possibly as a result of blood-thinning medications) may require the procedure to be performed in a hospital setting.

additional procedures such as **colonoscopy** or more frequent sigmoidoscopic examinations.

Small polyps can be completely removed. Larger polyps may require the physician to remove a portion of the growth for laboratory biopsy. Depending on the laboratory results, a person is then scheduled to have the polyp removed surgically, either as an urgent matter if it is cancerous, or as an elective procedure within a few months if it is noncancerous.

In a diagnostic sigmoidoscopy, an abnormal result shows signs of active inflammatory bowel disease, either a thickening of the intestinal lining consistent with ulcerative colitis, or ulcerations or fissures consistent with Crohn's disease.

Mortality from a sigmoidoscopy examination is rare and is usually due to uncontrolled bleeding or perforation of the colon.

Alternatives

A screening examination for colorectal cancer is a test for fecal occult blood. A dab of fecal material from toilet tissue is smeared onto a card. The card is treated in a laboratory to reveal the presence of bleeding. This test is normally performed prior to a sigmoidoscopic examination.

A less invasive alternative to a sigmoidoscopic examination is an X-ray of the colon and rectum. Barium is used to coat the inner walls of the colon. This lower GI (gastrointestinal) X-ray may reveal the outlines of suspicious or abnormal structures. It has the disadvantage of not allowing direct visualization of the colon. It is less costly than a sigmoidoscopic examination.

QUESTIONS TO ASK THE DOCTOR

- Is the supervising physician appropriately certified to conduct a sigmoidoscopy?
- How many sigmoidoscopy procedures has the doctor performed?
- What other steps will be taken as a result of my test findings?

A more invasive procedure is direct visualization of the colon during surgery. This procedure is rarely performed in the United States.

Resources

BOOKS

Balakrishnan, V., ed. *Practical Gastroenterology,* 3rd ed. Tunbridge Wells, Kent, UK: Anshan Ltd., 2007.

Gershman, G., and M. Ament. *Practical Pediatric Gastrointestinal Endoscopy.* New York: Wiley, 2007.

Gillison, W., and H. Buchwald. *Pioneers in Surgical Gastroenterology.* Shrewsbury, Shropshire, UK: TFM Publishing, 2006.

Johns Hopkins Medical Guide to Health After 50. New York: Black Dog and Leventhal Publishers, 2006.

PERIODICALS

Kronborg, O., and J. Regula. "Population screening for colorectal cancer: advantages and drawbacks." *Digestive Diseases* 25, no. 3 (2007): 270–273.

Levy, B. T., T. Nordin, S. Sinift, M. Rosenbaum, and P. A. James. "Why hasn't this patient been screened for colon cancer? An Iowa Research Network study." *Journal of the American Board of Family Medicine* 20, no. 5 (September–October 2007): 458–468.

Mandel, J. S. "Which colorectal cancer screening test is best?" *Journal of the National Cancer Institute* 99, no. 19 (October 2007): 1424–1425.

O'Mahony, S. "Endoscopy in pregnancy." *Best Practice and Research in Clinical Gastroenterology* 21, no. 5 (2007): 893–899.

Winawer, S. J. "The multidisciplinary management of gastrointestinal cancer; colorectal cancer screening." *Best Practice and Research in Clinical Gastroenterology* 21, no. 6 (2007): 1031–1048.

OTHER

"Flexible Sigmoidoscopy." National Digestive Diseases Information Clearinghouse. November 2004. http://www.niddk.nih.gov/health/digest/pubs/diagtest/sigmo.htm (December 31, 2007).

"Frequently Asked Questions about Colonscopy and Sigmoidoscopy," American Cancer Society. February 7, 2008. http://search.cancer.org/search?client=amcancer &site=amcancer&output=xml_no_dtd&proxy stylesheet=amcancer&restrict=cancer&q= sigmoidoscopy (April 6, 2008).

Information about Sigmoidoscopy. Center of Excellence for Medical Multimedia. Video. http://www.colonscope.org/ (December 31, 2007).

Johnson, B. A. "Flexible Sigmoidoscopy: Screening for Colorectal Cancer." *American Family Physician*. January 15, 1999. http://www.aafp.org/afp/990115ap/313.html (December 31, 2007).

"Sigmoidoscopy." Medical Encyclopedia. Medline Plus. May 8, 2006. http://www.nlm.nih.gov/medlineplus/ency/article/003885.htm (December 31, 2007).

"Six Questions that Could Save Your Life (Or the Life of Someone You Love): What Women Need to Know about Colon Cancer Screening." American Society for Gastrointestinal Endoscopy. 2007. http://www.asge.org/PatientInfoIndex.aspx?id=374 (April 6, 2008).

ORGANIZATIONS

American Academy of Family Physicians, 11400 Tomahawk Creek Parkway, Leawood, KS, 66211-2672, (913) 906-6000, (800) 274-2237, http://www.aafp.org.

American College of Surgeons, 633 North Saint Claire Street, Chicago, IL, 60611, (312) 202-5000, http://www.facs.org/.

American Society for Gastrointestinal Endoscopy, 1520 Kensington Road, Suite 202, Oak Brook, IL, 60523, (630) 573-0600 , http://www.asge.org.

Society of American Gastrointestinal Endoscopic Surgeons, 11300 West Olympic Boulevard, Suite 600, Los Angeles, CA, 90064, (310) 437-0544, (310) 437-0585, http://www.sages.org.

L. Fleming Fallon, Jr., M.D., Dr.P.H.

Simple mastectomy

Definition

Simple **mastectomy** is the surgical removal of one or both breasts. The adjacent lymph nodes and chest muscles are left intact. If a few lymph nodes are removed, the procedure is called an extended simple mastectomy. Breast-sparing techniques may be used to preserve the patient's breast skin and nipple, which is helpful in cosmetic **breast reconstruction**.

Purpose

Removal of a patient's breast is usually recommended when cancer is present in the breast or as a prophylactic when the patient has severe fibrocystic disease and a family history of breast cancer. The choice of a simple mastectomy may be determined by evaluating the size of the breast, the size of the cancerous mass, where the cancer is located, and whether any cancer cells have spread to adjacent lymph nodes or other parts of the body. If the cancer has not been contained within the breast, it calls for a **modified radical mastectomy**, which removes the entire breast and all of the adjacent lymph nodes. Only in extreme circumstances is a radical mastectomy, which also removes part of the chest wall, indicated.

A larger tumor usually is an indication of more advanced disease and will require more extensive surgery such as a simple mastectomy. In addition, if a woman has small breasts, the tumor may occupy more area within the contours of the breast, necessitating a simple mastectomy in order to remove all of the cancer.

Very rapidly growing tumors usually require the removal of all breast tissue. Cancers that have spread to adjacent tissues such as the chest wall or skin make simple mastectomy a good choice. Similarly, multiple sites of cancer within a breast require that the entire breast be removed. In addition, simple mastectomy is also recommended when cancer recurs in a breast that has already undergone a **lumpectomy**, which is a less invasive procedure that just removes the tumor and some surrounding tissue without removing the entire breast.

Sometimes, surgeons recommend simple mastectomy for women who are unable to undergo the adjuvant radiation therapy required after a lumpectomy. Radiation treatment is not indicated for pregnant women, those who have had previous therapeutic radiation in the chest area, and patients with collagen vascular diseases such as scleroderma or lupus. In these cases, simple mastectomy is the treatment of choice.

Some women with family histories of breast cancer and who test positive for a cancer-causing gene choose to have one or both of their breasts removed as a preventative for future breast cancer. This procedure is highly controversial. Though prophylactic mastectomy reduces the occurrence of breast cancer by 90% in high-risk patients, it is not a foolproof method. There has been some incidence of cancer occurring after both breasts were removed.

Demographics

According to the American Cancer Society in 2003, it was estimated that more than 260,000 new cases of breast cancer in women would occur that year. New cases of breast cancer in men were expected to reach

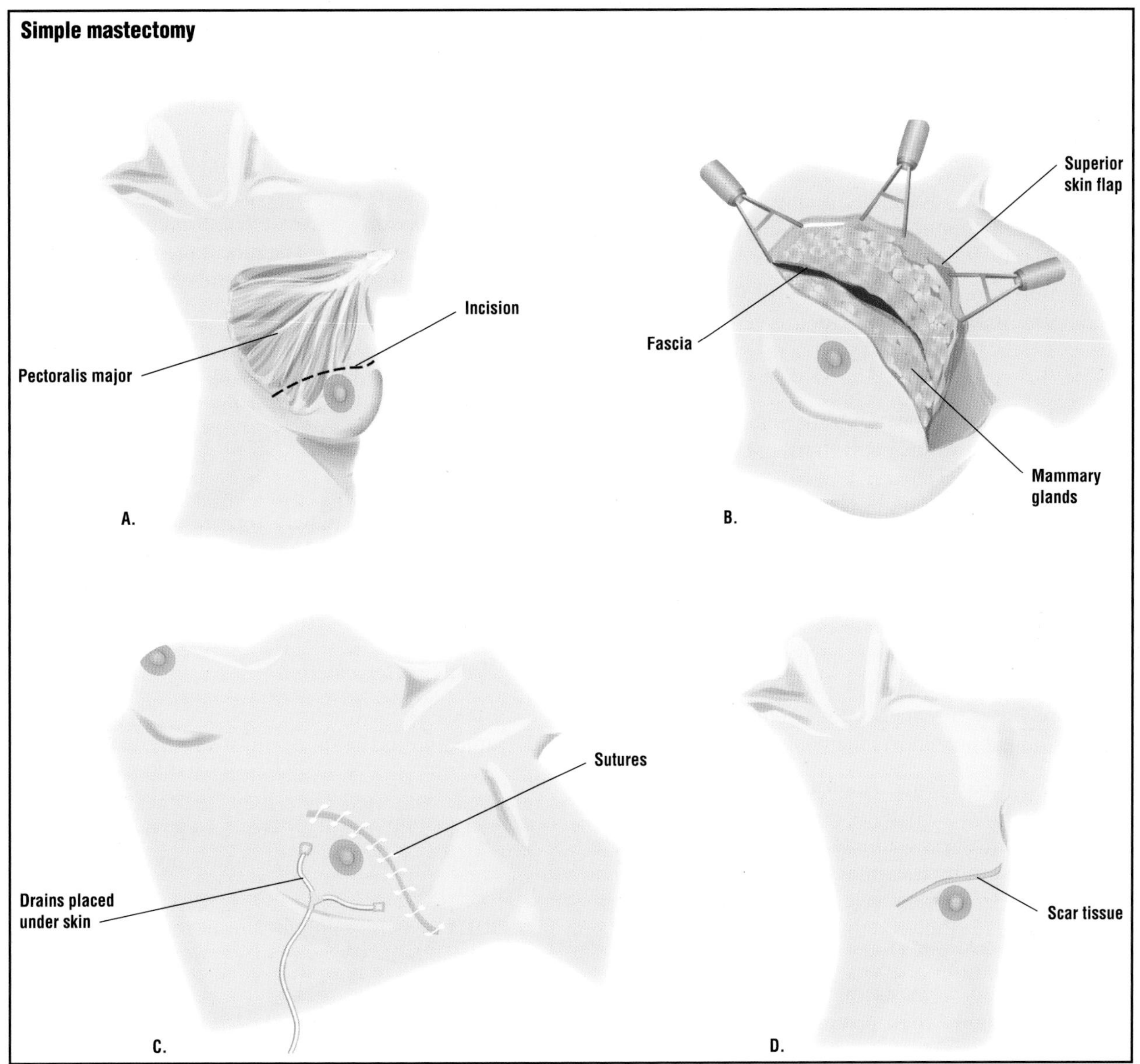

In a simple mastectomy, the skin over the tumor is cut open (A). The tumor and tissue surrounding it is removed (B), and the wound is closed (C). *(Illustration by GGS Information Services. Cengage Learning, Gale.)*

1,300. Rates of incidence have increased since 1980, due in part to the aging of the population. During the 1990s, breast cancer incidence increased only in women age 50 and over.

For approximately 80% of women, the first indication of cancer is the discovery of a lump in the breast, found either by themselves in a monthly self-exam or by a partner or by a mammogram, a special X-ray of the breast that looks for anomalies. Early detection of breast cancer means that smaller tumors are found, which require less intensive surgery and have better treatment outcomes. Simple mastectomy has been the standard treatment of choice for breast cancer for the past 60 years. Newer breast-conserving surgery techniques have gained acceptance since the mid-1980s. For larger hospitals, facilities in urban areas, and health care institutions with a cancer center or high cancer patient volume, these newer techniques are being utilized at a more rapid rate, especially on the East Coast.

In 2003, the National Cancer Institute found that American women were 21% more likely to have a mastectomy than their counterparts in the United Kingdom. Though breast-conserving procedures are

KEY TERMS

Lumpectomy—A less-invasive procedure that just removes the tumor and some surrounding tissue, without removing the entire breast.

Lymphedema—Swelling, usually of the arm after a mastectomy, caused by the accumulation of fluid from faulty drainage in the lymph system.

Mammogram—A special X-ray of the breast that looks for anomalies in the breast.

available and have proven to be viable options, some physicians and women still think breast removal will also remove all of their risk of cancer recurrence. It is clear that treatment options for cancer are highly individual and often emotionally charged.

Description

Simple mastectomy is one of several types of surgical treatments for breast cancer. Some techniques are rarely used; others are quite common. These common surgical procedures include:

- Radical mastectomy. Radical mastectomy is rarely used, and then only in cases where cancer cells have invaded the chest wall and the tumor is very large. The breast, muscles under the breast, and all of the lymph nodes are removed. This produces a large scar and severe disability to the arm nearest the removed breast.
- Modified radical mastectomy. Modified radical mastectomy was the most common form of mastectomy until the 1980s. The breast is removed along with the lining over the chest muscle and all of the lymph nodes.
- Simple mastectomy. Simple, sometimes called total, mastectomy has been the treatment of choice in the late 1980s and 1990s. Generally, only the breast is removed; though, sometimes, one or two lymph nodes may be removed as well.
- Partial mastectomy. Partial mastectomy is used to remove the tumor, the lining over the chest muscle underneath the tumor, and a good portion of breast tissue, but not the entire breast. This is a good treatment choice for early stage cancers.
- Lumpectomy. Lumpectomy or breast-conserving surgery just removes the tumor and a small amount of tissue surrounding it. Some lymph nodes may be removed as well. This is the most commonly used surgical procedure for the treatment of breast cancer in the early twenty-first century.

Two other surgical procedures are variations on the simple mastectomy. The skin-sparing mastectomy is a new surgical procedure in which the surgeon makes an incision, sometimes called a keyhole incision, around the areola. The tumor and all breast tissue are removed, but the incision is smaller and scarring is minimal. About 90% of the skin is preserved and allows a cosmetic surgeon to perform breast reconstruction at the same time as the mastectomy. The subcutaneous mastectomy, or nipple-sparing mastectomy, preserves the skin and the nipple over the breast.

During a simple mastectomy, the surgeon makes a curved incision along one side of the breast and removes the tumor and all of the breast tissue. A few lymph nodes may be removed. The tumor, breast tissue, and any lymph nodes will be sent to the pathology lab for analysis. If the skin is cancer-free, it is sutured in place or used immediately for breast reconstruction. One or two drains will be put in place to remove fluid from the surgical area. Surgery takes from two to five hours; it is longer with breast reconstruction.

Breast reconstruction

Breast reconstruction, especially if it is begun at the same time as the simple mastectomy, can minimize the sense of loss that women feel when having a breast removed. Although there may be other smaller surgeries later to complete the breast reconstruction, there will not be a second major operation nor an additional scar.

If there is not enough skin left after the mastectomy, a balloon-type expander is put in place. In subsequent weeks, the expander is filled with larger amounts of saline (salt water) solution. When it has reached the appropriate size, the expander is removed and a permanent breast implant is installed.

If there is enough skin, an implant is installed immediately. In other instances, skin, fat, and muscle are removed from the patient's back or abdomen and repositioned on the chest wall to form a breast.

None of these reconstructions have nipples at first. Nipples are later reconstructed in a separate surgery. Finally, the areola is tattooed in to make the reconstructed breast look natural.

Breast reconstruction does not prevent a potential recurrence of breast cancer.

Diagnosis/Preparation

If a mammogram has not been performed, it is usually ordered to verify the size of the lump the patient has reported. A biopsy of the suspicious lump and/or lymph nodes is usually ordered and sent to the pathology lab before surgery is discussed.

When a simple mastectomy has been determined, preoperative tests such as blood work, a chest X-ray, and an **electrocardiogram** may be ordered. Blood-thinning medications such as **aspirin** should be stopped several days before the surgery date. The patient is also asked to refrain from eating or drinking the night before the operation.

At the hospital, the patient will sign a consent form, verifying that the surgeon has explained what the surgery is and what it is for. The patient will also meet with the anesthesiologist to discuss the patient's medical history and determine the choice of anesthesia.

WHO PERFORMS THE PROCEDURE AND WHERE IS IT PERFORMED?

Simple mastectomy is performed by a general surgeon or a gynecological surgeon. If reconstructive breast surgery is to be done, a cosmetic surgeon performs it. Patients undergo simple mastectomies under general anesthesia as an inpatient in a hospital. There is a growing trend, due to reductions in insurance coverage and patient preference, to perform simple mastectomies without reconstructive breast surgery as outpatient procedures.

Aftercare

If the procedure is performed as an **outpatient surgery**, the patient may go home the same day of the surgery. The length of the hospital stay for inpatient mastectomies ranges from one to two days. If breast reconstruction has taken place, the hospital stay may be longer.

The surgical drains will remain in place for five to seven days. Sponge baths will be necessary until the **stitches** are removed, usually in a week to 10 days. It is important to avoid overhead lifting, strenuous sports, and sexual intercourse for three to six weeks. After the surgical drains are removed, stretching exercises may be begun, though some physical therapists may start a patient on shoulder and arm mobility exercises while in the hospital.

Since breast removal is often emotionally traumatic for women, seeking out a support group is often helpful. Women in these groups offer practical advice about matters such as finding well-fitting bras and swimwear, and emotional support because they have been through the same experience.

For women who chose not to have breast reconstruction, it may be necessary to find the proper fitting breast prosthesis. Some are made of cloth, and others are made of silicone, which are created from a mold from the patient's other breast.

In some case, the patient may be required to undergo additional treatments such as radiation, chemotheraphy, or hormone therapy.

Risks

The risks involved with simple mastectomy are the same for any major surgery; however, there may be a need for more extensive surgery once the surgeon examines the tumor, the tissues surrounding it, and the lymph nodes nearby. A biopsy of the lymph nodes is usually performed during surgery and a determination is made whether to remove them. Simple mastectomy usually has limited impact on range of motion of the arm nearest the breast that is removed, but physical therapy may still be necessary to restore complete movement.

There is also the risk of infection around the incision. When the lymph nodes are removed, lymphedema may also occur. This condition is a result of damage to the lymph system. The arm on the side nearest the affected breast may become swollen. It can either resolve itself or worsen.

As in any surgery, the risk of developing a blood clot after a mastectomy is a serious matter. All hospitals use a variety of techniques to prevent blood clots from forming. It is important for the patient to walk daily when at home.

Finally, there is the risk that not all cancer cells were removed. Further treatment may be necessary.

Normal results

The breast area will fully heal in three to four weeks. If the patient had breast reconstruction, it may take up to six weeks to recover fully. The patient should be able to participate in all of the activities she has engaged in before surgery. If breast reconstruction is done, the patient should realize that the new breast will not have the sensitivity of a normal breast. In addition, dealing with cancer emotionally may take time, especially if additional treatment is necessary.

Morbidity and mortality rates

Deaths due to breast cancer have declined by 1.4% each year between 1989 and 1995, and by 3.2% each year thereafter. The largest decreases have been

QUESTIONS TO ASK THE DOCTOR

- Why is this procedure necessary?
- How big is my tumor?
- Are there other breast-saving or less-invasive procedures for which I might be a candidate?
- What can I expect after surgery?
- Do you work with a cosmetic surgeon?
- Will I have to undergo radiation or chemotherapy after surgery?

among younger women, as a result of cancer education campaigns and early screening, which encourages more women to go to their physicians to be checked.

Research performed between 2000 and 2004 demonstrated that the five-year survival rate for cancers confined to the breast is 98%. For cancers that had spread to areas within the chest region, the rate was 83.5%, and it is only 26.7% for cancers occurring in other parts of the body after breast cancer treatment. The best survival rates were for early-stage tumors.

Two 20-year longitudinal studies concluded in 2002 indicated that the survival rate for patients with modified radical mastectomy (the removal of the entire breast and all lymph nodes) was no different from that of breast-conserving lumpectomy (the removal of the tumor alone). These studies suggest that the removal of the entire breast may not afford greater protection against future cancer than breast-conserving techniques; however, the majority of cancer recurrences happen within the first five years for both those with mastectomies and those with lumpectomies.

Alternatives

Skin-sparing mastectomy, also called nipple-sparing mastectomy, is becoming a treatment of choice for women undergoing simple mastectomy. In this procedure, the skin of the breast, the areola, and the nipple are peeled back to remove the breast and its inherent tumor. Biopsies of the skin and nipple areas are performed immediately to assure that they do not have cancer cells in them. Then, a cosmetic surgeon performs a breast reconstruction at the same time as the mastectomy. The breast regains its normal contours once prostheses are inserted. Unfortunately, the nipple will lose its sensitivity and, of course, its function, since all underlying tissue has been removed. If cancer is found near the nipple, this procedure cannot be done.

Resources

BOOKS

Abeloff, M. D., J. Armitage, J. Niederhuber, M. Kastan, and W. G. McKenna. *Clinical Oncology*, 3rd ed. Philadelphia: Elsevier, 2004.

Katz V. L., G. Lentz, R. A. Lobo, and D. Gershenson. *Comprehensive Gynecology*, 5th ed. St. Louis: Mosby, 2007.

Khatri, V. P., and J. A. Asensio. *Operative Surgery Manual*, 1st ed. Philadelphia: Saunders, 2002.

Townsend, C.M., R. D. Beauchamp, B. M. Evers, and K. Mattox. *Sabiston Textbook of Surgery*, 17th ed. Philadelphia: Saunders, 2004.

PERIODICALS

"American Women Still Having Too Many Mastectomies." *Women's Health Weekly* (February 6, 2003): 20.

Jancin, Bruce. "High U.S. Mastectomy Rate Is Cause for Concern." *Family Practice News* 33, no.2 (January 15, 2003): 31.

"Procedure Preserves Natural Appearance after Mastectomy." *AORN Journal* 77, no.1 (January 2003): 213.

Zepf, Bill. "Mastectomy vs. Less Invasive Surgery for Breast Cancer." *American Family Physician* 67, no.3 (February 1, 2003): 587.

ORGANIZATIONS

American Cancer Society, 1875 Connecticut Avenue, NW, Suite 730, Washington, DC, 20009, (800) ACS-2345, http://www.cancer.org.

American Society of Plastic Surgeons, 444 E. Algonquin Rd., Arlington Heights, IL, 60005, (847) 228-9900, http://www.plasticsurgery.org.

National Cancer Institute, 6116 Executive Boulevard, MSC8322, Suite 3036A, Bethesda, MD, 20892-8322, (800) 422-6237, http://www.cancer.gov.

Janie Franz

Sinus x ray *see* **Skull x rays**

Skeletal traction *see* **Traction**

Skin grafting

Definition

Skin grafting is a surgical procedure in which skin or a skin substitute is placed over a burn or non-healing wound.

Purpose

A skin graft is used to permanently replace damaged or missing skin or to provide a temporary wound covering. This covering is necessary because the skin

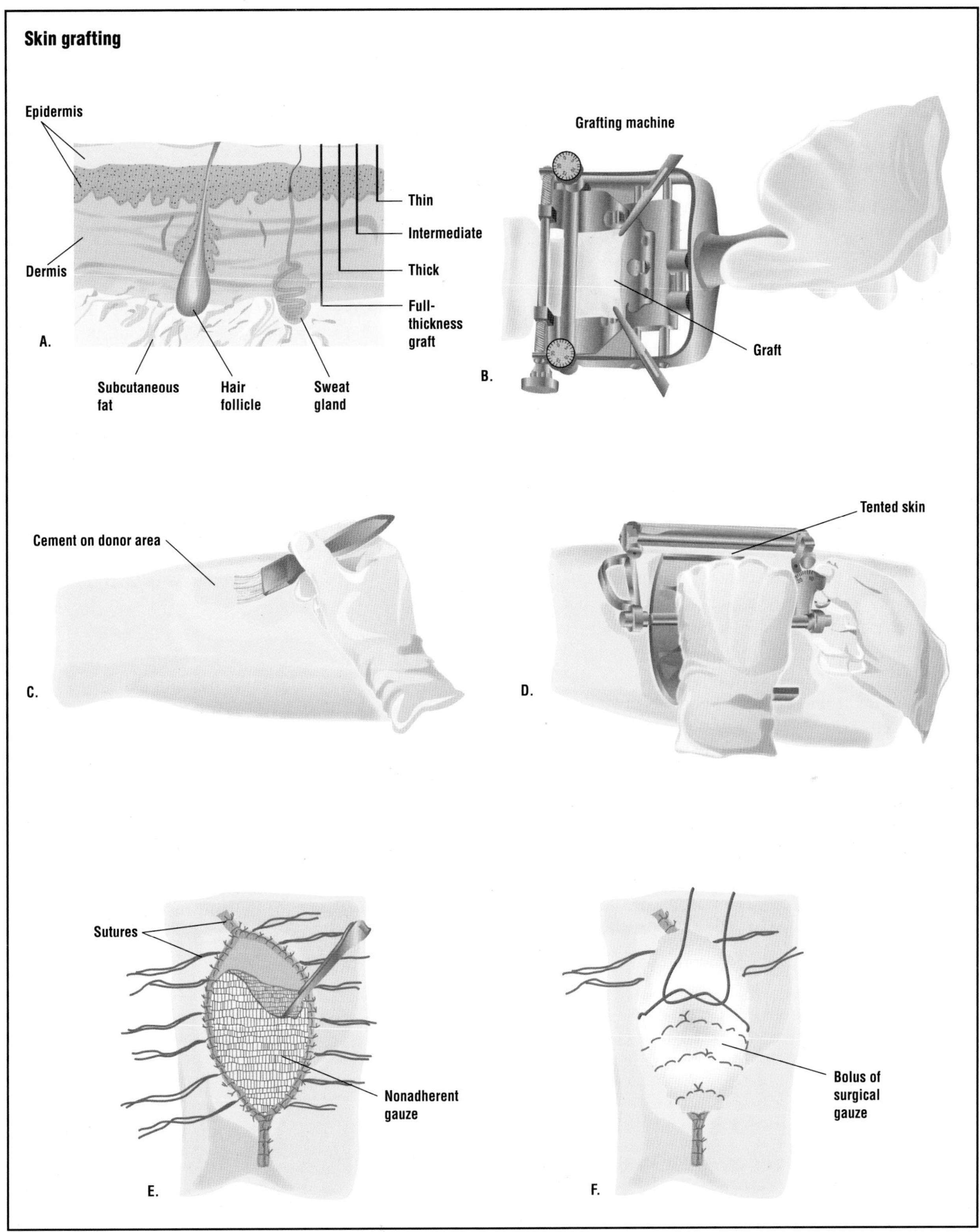

Skin grafts may be used in several thicknesses (A). To begin the procedure, a special cement is used on the donor skin area (C). The grafting machine is applied to the area, and sample taken (D). After the graft is stitched to the recipient area, it is covered with nonadherent gauze (E) and a layer of fluffy surgical gauze held in place with sutures (F). *(Illustration by GGS Information Services. Cengage Learning, Gale.)*

protects the body from fluid loss, aids in temperature regulation, and helps prevent disease-causing bacteria or viruses from entering the body. Skin that is damaged extensively by burns or non-healing wounds can compromise the health and well-being of the patient.

Demographics

Although anyone can be involved in a fire and need a skin graft, the population groups with a higher risk of fire-related injuries and deaths include:

- children four years old and younger;
- adults 65 years and older;
- African Americans and Native Americans;
- low-income Americans;
- persons living in rural areas; and
- persons living in manufactured homes (trailers) or substandard housing.

Description

The skin is the largest organ of the human body. It is also known as the integument or integumentary system because it covers the entire outside of the body. The skin consists of two main layers: the outer layer, or epidermis, which lies on and is nourished by the thicker dermis. These two layers are approximately 0.04–0.08 in (1–2 mm) thick. The epidermis consists of an outer layer of dead cells called keratinocytes, which provide a tough protective coating, and several layers of rapidly dividing cells just beneath the keratinocytes. The dermis contains the blood vessels, nerves, sweat glands, hair follicles, and oil glands. The dermis consists mainly of connective tissue, which is largely made up of a protein called collagen. Collagen gives the skin its flexibility and provides structural support. The fibroblasts that make collagen are the main type of cell in the dermis.

Skin varies in thickness in different parts of the body; it is thickest on the palms and soles of the feet, and thinnest on the eyelids. In general, men have thicker skin than women, and adults have thicker skin than children. After age 50, however, the skin begins to grow thinner again as it loses its elastic fibers and some of its fluid content.

Injuries treated with skin grafts

Skin grafting is sometimes done as part of elective **plastic surgery** procedures, but its most extensive use is in the treatment of burns. For first or second-degree burns, skin grafting is generally not required, as these burns usually heal with little or no scarring. With third-degree burns, however, the skin is destroyed to its full depth, in addition to damage done to underlying tissues. People who suffer third-degree burns often require skin grafting.

Wounds such as third-degree burns must be covered as quickly as possible to prevent infection or loss of fluid. Wounds that are left to heal on their own can contract, often resulting in serious scarring; if the wound is large enough, the scar can actually prevent movement of limbs. Non-healing wounds, such as diabetic ulcers, venous ulcers, or pressure sores, can be

KEY TERMS

Allograft—Tissue that is taken from one person's body and grafted to another person.

Autograft—Tissue that is taken from one part of a person's body and transplanted to a different part of the same person.

Collagen—A protein that provides structural support for the skin. Collagen is the main component of connective tissue.

Contracture—An abnormal persistent shortening of a muscle or the overlying skin at a joint, usually caused by the formation of scar tissue following an injury.

Débridement—The removal of foreign matter and dead or damaged tissue from a traumatic or infected wound until healthy tissue is reached.

Dermatome—A surgical instrument used to cut thin slices of skin for grafts.

Dermis—The underlayer of skin, containing blood vessels, nerves, hair follicles, and oil and sweat glands.

Epidermis—The outer layer of skin, consisting of a layer of dead cells that perform a protective function and a second layer of dividing cells.

Fibroblasts—A type of cell found in connective tissue; produces collagen.

Hematoma—A localized collection of blood in an organ or tissue due to broken blood vessels.

Integument—A covering; in medicine, the skin as a covering for the body. The skin is also called the integumentary system.

Keratinocytes—Dead cells at the outer surface of the epidermis that form a tough protective layer for the skin. The cells underneath divide to replenish the supply.

Xenograft—Tissue that is transplanted from one species to another (e.g., pigs to humans).

treated with skin grafts to prevent infection and further progression of the wounded area.

Types of skin grafts

The term "graft" by itself commonly refers to either an allograft or an autograft. An autograft is a type of graft that uses skin from another area of the patient's own body if there is enough undamaged skin available, and if the patient is healthy enough to undergo the additional surgery required. An allograft uses skin obtained from another human being. Donor skin from cadavers is frozen, stored, and available for use as allografts. Skin taken from an animal (usually a pig) is called a xenograft because it comes from a nonhuman species. Allografts and xenografts provide only temporary covering because they are rejected by the patient's immune system within seven to 10 days. They must then be replaced with an autograft.

SPLIT-THICKNESS GRAFTS. The most important part of any skin graft procedure is proper preparation of the wound. Skin grafts will not survive on tissue with a limited blood supply (cartilage or tendons) or tissue that has been damaged by radiation treatment. The patient's wound must be free of any dead tissue, foreign matter, or bacterial contamination. After the patient has been anesthetized, the surgeon prepares the wound by rinsing it with saline solution or a diluted antiseptic (Betadine) and removes any dead tissue by débridement. In addition, the surgeon stops the flow of blood into the wound by applying pressure, tying off blood vessels, or administering a medication (epinephrine) that causes the blood vessels to constrict.

Following preparation of the wound, the surgeon then harvests the tissue for grafting. A split-thickness skin graft involves the epidermis and a little of the underlying dermis; the donor site usually heals within several days. The surgeon first marks the outline of the wound on the skin of the donor site, enlarging it by 3–5% to allow for tissue shrinkage. The surgeon uses a dermatome (a special instrument for cutting thin slices of tissue) to remove a split-thickness graft from the donor site. The wound must not be too deep if a split-thickness graft is going to be successful, since the blood vessels that will nourish the grafted tissue must come from the dermis of the wound itself. The graft is usually taken from an area that is ordinarily hidden by clothes, such as the buttock or inner thigh, and spread on the bare area to be covered. Gentle pressure from a well-padded dressing is then applied, or a few small sutures used to hold the graft in place. A sterile non-adherent dressing is then applied to the raw donor area for approximately three to five days to protect it from infection.

FULL-THICKNESS GRAFTS. Full-thickness skin grafts may be necessary for more severe burn injuries. These grafts involve both layers of the skin. Full-thickness autografts are more complicated than partial-thickness grafts, but provide better contour, more natural color, and less contraction at the grafted site. A flap of skin with underlying muscle and blood supply is transplanted to the area to be grafted. This procedure is used when tissue loss is extensive, such as after open fractures of the lower leg, with significant skin loss and underlying infection. The back and the abdomen are common donor sites for full-thickness grafts. The main disadvantage of full-thickness skin grafts is that the wound at the donor site is larger and requires more careful management. Often, a split-thickness graft must be used to cover the donor site.

A composite skin graft is sometimes used, which consists of combinations of skin and fat, skin and cartilage, or dermis and fat. Composite grafts are used in patients whose injuries require three-dimensional reconstruction. For example, a wedge of ear containing skin and cartilage can be used to repair the nose.

A full-thickness graft is removed from the donor site with a scalpel rather than a dermatome. After the surgeon has cut around the edges of the pattern used to determine the size of the graft, he or she lifts the skin with a special hook and trims off any fatty tissue. The graft is then placed on the wound and secured in place with absorbable sutures.

Aftercare

Once a skin graft has been put in place, it must be maintained carefully even after it has healed. Patients who have grafts on their legs should remain in bed for seven to 10 days with their legs elevated. For several months, the patient should support the graft with an Ace bandage or Jobst stocking. Grafts on other areas of the body should be similarly supported after healing to decrease the amount of contracture.

Grafted skin does not contain sweat or oil glands, and should be lubricated daily for two to three months with mineral oil or another bland oil to prevent drying and cracking.

Aftercare of patients with severe burns typically includes psychological or psychiatric counseling as well as **wound care** and physical rehabilitation, particularly if the patient's face has been disfigured. The severe pain and lengthy period of recovery involved in burn treatment are often accompanied by anxiety and depression. If the patient's burns occurred in combat, a transportation disaster, terrorist attack, or other fire involving large numbers of people, he or she is at high risk of developing post-traumatic stress disorder (PTSD). Anti-anxiety medication may be a helpful adjunct to treatment in these patients. Additionally, because burn patients are at high risk of developing stress ulcers in their gastrointestinal system, with a high rate of bleeding, GI medications that prevent stress ulcers are often given to burn patients.

Risks

The risks of skin grafting include those inherent in any surgical procedure that involves anesthesia. These include reactions to the medications, breathing problems, bleeding, and infection. In addition, the risks of an allograft procedure include transmission of an infectious disease from the donor.

The tissue for grafting and the recipient site must be as sterile as possible to prevent later infection that could result in failure of the graft. Failure of a graft can result from inadequate preparation of the wound, poor blood flow to the injured area, swelling, or infection. The most common reason for graft failure is the formation of a hematoma, or collection of blood in the injured tissues.

Normal results

A skin graft should provide significant improvement in the quality of the wound site, and may prevent the serious complications associated with burns or non-healing wounds. Normally, new blood vessels begin growing from the donor area into the transplanted skin within 36 hours. Occasionally, skin grafts are unsuccessful or don't heal well. In these cases, repeat grafting is necessary. Even though the skin graft must be protected from trauma or significant stretching for two to three weeks following split-thickness skin grafting, recovery from surgery is usually rapid. A dressing may be necessary for one to two weeks, depending on the location of the graft. Any **exercise** or activity that stretches the graft or puts it at risk for trauma should be avoided for three to four weeks. A one to two-week hospital stay is most often required in cases of full-thickness grafts, as the recovery period is longer.

Morbidity and mortality rates

According to the American Burn Association, there are more than 1 million burn injuries in the United States each year that require medical attention. Approximately one-half of these require hospitalization, and roughly 25,000 of those burn patients are admitted to a specialized burn unit. About 4,500 people die from burns each year in the United States.

WHO PERFORMS THE PROCEDURE AND WHERE IS IT PERFORMED?

Patients with less severe burns are usually treated in a doctor's office or a hospital emergency room. Patients with any of the following conditions, however, are usually transferred to hospitals with specialized burn units: third-degree burns; partial-thickness burns over 10% of their total body area; electrical or chemical burns; smoke inhalation injuries; or preexisting medical disorders that could complicate management, prolong recovery, or affect mortality. In addition, burned children in hospitals without qualified personnel should be admitted to a hospital with a burn unit. A surgical team that specializes in burn treatment and skin grafts will perform the necessary procedures. The team may include neurosurgeons, ophthalmologists, oral surgeons, thoracic surgeons, psychiatrists, and trauma specialists as well as plastic surgeons and dermatologists.

In the United States, about 500,000 people seek medical treatment for burns every year. About 4,000 people die of their burn injury yearly (including 3,500 due to injuries from residential fires, and 500 due to injuries from fires resulting from a car or airplane crash, and chemical and electrical burns). 40,000 people are admitted to hospitals annually for burn treatment; 25,000 of these are admitted to specialized burn center.

About 38% of all burn unit admissions are for burns covering more than 10% of the patient's total body surface area. 10% of these admissions are for burns exceeding 30% of the patient's total body surface area. 70% of all burn unit admissions are for male patients, and 30% are for female patients. The source of burns breaks down as follows: 46% from fire or flame, 32% from hot water scalding, 8% from hot object contact, 4% from electrical burns, 3% from chemical burns, and 6% other source of burn. The survival rate for patients admitted to specialized burn centers is about 94.4%.

Treatment for severe burns has improved dramatically in the past 20 years. In the early twenty-first century, patients can survive with burns covering up to about 90% of the body, although they often face permanent physical impairment.

Alternatives

There has been great progress in the development of artificial skin replacement products in the early twenty-first century. Although nothing works as well as the patient's own skin, artificial skin products are important

QUESTIONS TO ASK THE DOCTOR

- Can you explain the process of skin grafting to me?
- Will I be sent to a hospital with a special burn unit?
- How long will I have to stay in the hospital?
- How long will recovery take?
- When will I be able to resume normal activities?
- What will the injured area look like after grafting?

due to the limitation of available skin for allografting in severely burned patients. Unlike allographs and xenographs, artificial skin replacements are not rejected by the patient's body and actually encourage the generation of new tissue. Artificial skin usually consists of a synthetic epidermis and a collagen-based dermis. The artificial dermis consists of fibers arranged in a lattice that acts as a template for the formation of new tissue. Fibroblasts, blood vessels, nerve fibers, and lymph vessels from surrounding healthy tissue grow into the collagen lattice, which eventually dissolves as these cells and structures build a new dermis. The synthetic epidermis, which acts as a temporary barrier during this process, is eventually replaced with a split-thickness autograft or with an epidermis cultured in the laboratory from the patient's own epithelial cells.

Several artificial skin products are available for burns or non-healing wounds, including Integra ®, Dermal Regeneration Template ® (from Integra Life Sciences Technology), Apligraft ® (Novartis), Transcyte ® (Advance Tissue Science), and Dermagraft ®. Researchers have also obtained promising results growing or cultivating the patient's own skin cells in the laboratory. These cultured skin substitutes reduce the need for autografts and can reduce the complications of burn injuries. Laboratory cultivation of skin cells may improve the prognosis for severely burned patients with third-degree burns over 50% of their body. The recovery of these patients has been hindered by the limited availability of uninjured skin from their own bodies for grafting. Skin substitutes may also reduce treatment costs and the length of hospital stays. In addition, other research has demonstrated the possibility of using stem cells collected from bone marrow or blood for use in growing skin grafts.

Resources

BOOKS

Browner, B., J. Jupiter, A. Levine, and P. Trafton. *Skeletal Trauma: Fractures, Dislocations, Ligamentous Injuries,* 3rd ed. Philadelphia: Saunders, 2002.

Canale, S. T. *Campbell's Operative Orthopedics,* 10th ed. St. Louis, MO: Mosby, 2002.

Khatri, V. P. and J. A. Asensio. *Operative Surgery Manual,* 1st ed. Philadelphia: Saunders, 2002.

Townsend, Courtney M., Daniel R. Beauchamp, Mark B. Evers, Kenneth L. Mattox, and David C. Sabiston, eds. *Sabiston Textbook of Surgery: The Biological Basis of Modern Surgical Practice,* 16th ed. London: W. B. Saunders Co., 2001.

PERIODICALS

Duenwald, Mary. "Tales from a Burn Unit: Agony, Friendship, Healing." *New York Times* (March 18, 2003).

Eto, M., H. Hackstein, K. Kaneko, et al. "Promotion of Skin Graft Tolerance Across MHC Barriers by Mobilization of Dendritic Cells in Donor Hemopoietic Cell Infusions." *Journal of Immunology* 169 (September 2002): 2390–2396.

Miraliakbari R. "Skin Grafts." *Operative Techniques in General Surgery* 8, no. 4 (December 2006): 197–206.

Revis, D. R. Jr., and M. B. Seagal. "Skin Grafts, Split-Thickness." *eMedicine* (July 20, 2001). www.emedicine.com/ent/topic47.htm (June 25, 2003).

Snyder, R. J., H. Doyle, and T. Delbridge. "Applying Split-Thickness Skin Grafts: A Step-by-Step Clinical Guide and Nursing Implications." *Ostomy Wound Management* 47, no. 11 (November 2001): 20–26.

ORGANIZATIONS

American Burn Association, 625 N. Michigan Avenue, Suite 2550, Chicago, IL, 60611, (312) 642-9260, (312) 642-9130, info@ameriburn.org, http://www.ameriburn.org.

American Diabetes Association, 1701 North Beauregard Street, Alexandria, VA, 22311, (800) 342-2383, AskADA@diabetes.org, http://www.diabetes.org.

American Society of Plastic Surgeons, 444 E. Algonquin Road, Arlington Heights, IL, 60005, (847) 228-9900, http://www.plasticsurgery.org.

National Institutes of Health, 9000 Rockville Pike, Bethesda, MD, 20892, (301) 496-4000, NIHinfo@od.nih.gov, http://www.nih.gov/.

Lisa Christenson, Ph.D.
Crystal H. Kaczkowski, M.Sc.
Rosalyn Carson-DeWitt, M.D.

Skin smoothing *see* **Dermabrasion**

Skull x rays

Definition

Skull X-rays are performed to examine the nose, sinuses, and facial bones. These studies may also be referred to as sinus X-rays. X-ray studies produce films, also known as radiographs, by aiming X-rays

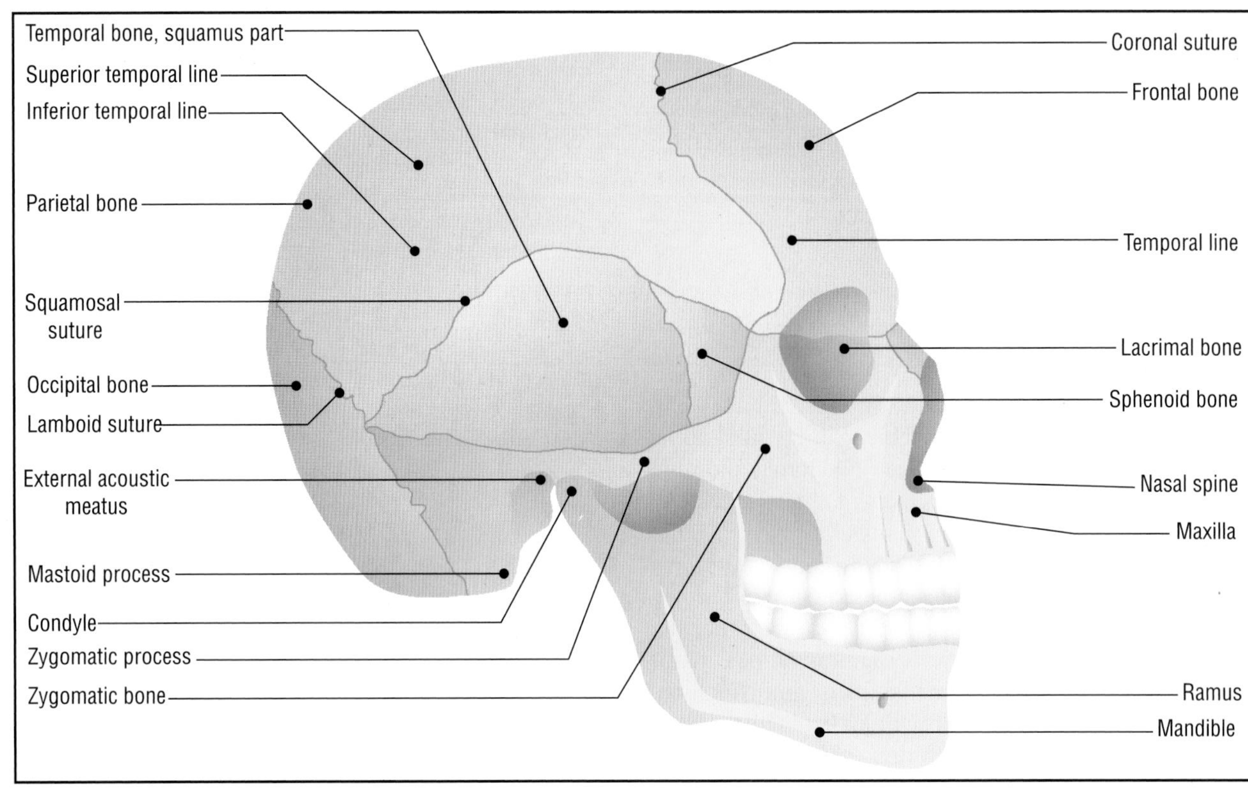

(Illustration by GGS Information Services. Cengage Learning, Gale.)

at soft bones and tissues of the body. X-ray beams are similar to light waves, except their shorter wavelength allows them to penetrate dense substances, producing images and shadows on film.

Purpose

Doctors may order skull X-rays to aid in the diagnosis of a variety of diseases or injuries.

Sinusitis

Sinus X-rays may be ordered to confirm a diagnosis of sinusitis, or sinus infection.

Fractures

A skull X-ray may detect bone fractures resulting from injury or disease. The skull X-ray should clearly show the entire skull, jaw bones, and facial bones.

Tumors

Skull radiographs may indicate tumors in facial bones, tissues, or sinuses. Tumors may be benign (not cancerous) or malignant (cancerous).

Other

Birth defects (referred to as congenital anomalies) may be detected on a skull X-ray by changes in bone structure. Abnormal tissues or glands resulting from various conditions or diseases may also be shown on a skull radiograph.

Description

Skull or sinus X-rays may be performed in a doctor's office that has X-ray equipment and a technologist available. The exam may also be performed in an outpatient radiology facility or a hospital radiology department.

In many instances, particularly for sinus views, the patient will sit upright in a chair, perhaps with the head held stable by a foam vise. A film cassette is located behind the patient. The X-ray tube is in front of the patient and may be moved to allow for different positions and views. A patient may also be asked to move his or her head at various angles and positions.

In some cases, technologists will ask the patient to lie on a table and will place the head and neck at various angles. In routine skull X-rays, as many as five different

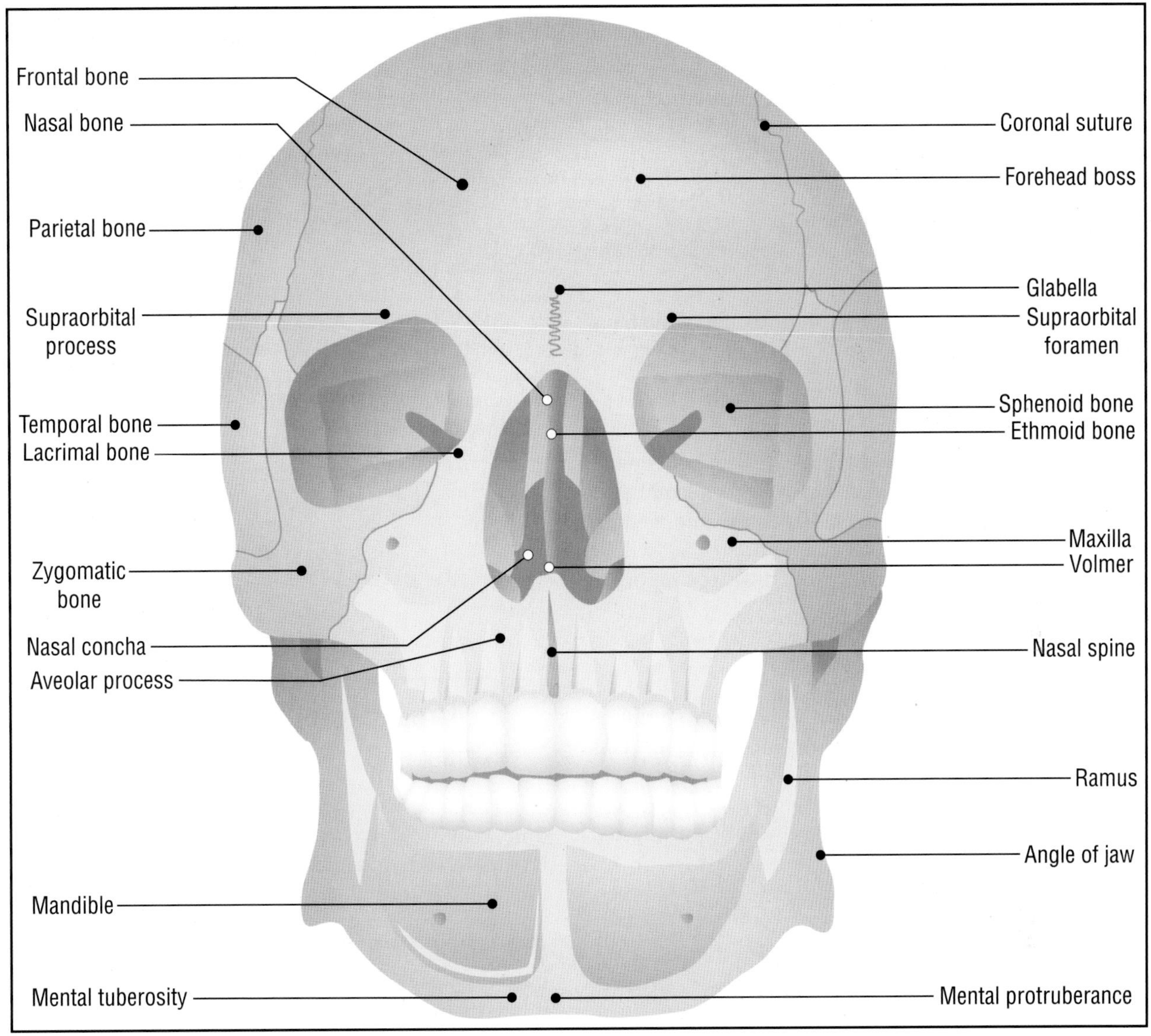

(Illustration by GGS Information Services. Cengage Learning, Gale.)

views may be taken to allow a clear picture of various bones and tissues. The length of the test will vary depending on the number of views taken, but in general, it should last about 10 minutes. The technologist will usually ask a patient to wait while the films are being developed to ensure that they are adequate before going to the radiologist.

Preparation

There is no preparation for the patient prior to arriving at the radiology facility. Patients will be asked to remove jewelry, dentures, or other metal objects that may produce artifacts on the film. The referring doctor or X-ray technologist can answer any questions regarding the procedure. Any woman who is or may be pregnant should tell the technologist.

Aftercare

There is no aftercare required following skull or sinus X-ray procedures.

Risks

There are no common side effects from skull or sinus X-ray. The patient may feel some discomfort in the positioning of the head and neck, but will have no complications. Any X-ray procedure carries minimal radiation risk; and children and pregnant women should

KEY TERMS

Radiograph—The actual picture or film produced by an X-ray study.

X-ray—A form of electromagnetic radiation with shorter wavelengths than normal light. X-rays can penetrate most structures.

be protected from radiation exposure to the abdominal or genital areas.

Normal results

Normal results should indicate sinuses, bones, tissues, and other observed areas are of normal size, shape, and thickness for the patient's age and medical history. Results, whether normal or abnormal, will be provided to the referring doctor in a written report.

Abnormal results may include:

Sinusitis

Air in sinuses will show up on a radiograph as black, but fluid will be cloudy or white (opaque). This helps the radiologist to identify fluid in the sinuses. In chronic sinusitis, the radiologist may also note thickening or destruction of the bony wall of an infected sinus.

Fractures

Radiologists may recognize even tiny facial bone fractures as a line of defect.

Tumors

Tumors may be visible if the bony sinus wall is distorted or destroyed. Abnormal findings may result in follow-up imaging studies.

Other

Skull X-rays may also detect disorders that show up as changes in bone structure, such as Paget's disease of the bone or acromegaly (a disorder associated with excess growth hormones from the pituitary gland). Areas of calcification, or gathering of calcium deposits, or destruction may indicate a condition such as an infection of bone or bone marrow (osteomyelitis).

Resources

BOOKS

Cummings, C. W., et al. *Otolaryngology: Head and Neck Surgery,* 4th ed. St. Louis: Mosby, 2004.

Grainger R. G., D. J. Allison, and A. K. Dixon. *Grainger & Allison's Diagnostic Radiology: A Textbook of Medical Imaging,* 4th ed. Philadelphia: Churchill Livingstone, 2001.

Mettler, F. A. *Essentials of Radiology,* 2nd ed. Philadelphia: Saunders, 2004.

ORGANIZATIONS

Brain Injury Association, 1608 Spring Hill Road, Suite 110, Vienna, VA, 22182, (703) 761-0750, http://www.biausa.org/.

National Cancer Institute, 6116 Executive Boulevard, MSC8322, Suite 3036A, Bethesda, MD, 20892-8322, (800) 422-6237, http://www.cancer.gov.

Radiological Society of North America, 820 Jorie Boulevard, Oak Brook, IL, 60523-2251, (630) 571-2670, http://www.rsna.org.

Teresa Norris, R.N.
Lee A. Shratter, M.D.

Sling procedure

Definition

The sling procedure, or suburethral sling procedure, refers to a particular kind of surgery using ancillary material to aid in closure of the urethral sphincter function of the bladder. It is performed as a treatment of severe urinary incontinence. The sling procedure, also known as the suburethral fascial sling or the pubovaginal sling, has many forms due to advances in the types of material used for the sling. Some popular types of sling material are teflon (polytetrafluoroethylene), Gore-Tex®, and rectus fascia (fibrous tissue of the rectum). The surgery can be done through the vagina or the abdomen and some clinicians perform the procedure using a laparoscope—a small instrument that allows surgery through very small incisions in the belly button and above the pubic hairline. The long-term efficacy and durability of the laparoscopic suburethral sling procedure for management of stress incontinence are undetermined. A new technique, the tension-free vaginal tape sling procedure (TVT), has gained popularity in recent years and early research indicates high success rates and few postoperative complications. This procedure is done under local anesthetic and offers new opportunities for treatment of stress incontinence. However, TVT has not been researched for its long-term effects. Finally, there are many surgeons who use the sling procedure for all forms of incontinence.

Purpose

Incontinence is very common and not fully understood. Generally defined as the involuntary loss of urine, incontinence comes in many forms and has many etiologies. Four established types of incontinence, according to the Agency for Health Care Policy and Research, affect approximately 13 million adults—most of them older women. Actual prevalence may be higher because incontinence is widely under reported and under diagnosed. The four types of incontinence are: stress incontinence, urge incontinence (detrusor overactivity or instability), mixed incontinence, and overflow incontinence. There are also other types of incontinence tied to specific conditions, such as neurogenic bladder in which neurological signals to the bladder are impaired.

Stress incontinence is the most frequently diagnosed form of incontinence and occurs largely with physical activity, laughter and coughing, and sneezing. The inability to hold urine can be due to weakness in the internal and external urinary sphincter or due to a weakened urethra. These two conditions, intrinsic sphincter deficiency (ISD) and urethral hypermobility or genuine stress incontinence (GSI), pertain to the inability of the "gatekeeper" sphincter muscles to stay taut and/or the urethra failing to hold urine under pressure from the abdomen. In women, as the pelvic structures relax due to age, injury, or illness, the uterus prolapses and the urethra becomes hypermobile. This allows the urethra to descend at an angle that permits loss of urine and puts pressure upon the sphincter muscles, both internal and external, allowing the mouth of the bladder to stay open.

Urge incontinence, the other frequent type of incontinence, pertains to overactivity of the sphincter in which the muscle contracts frequently, causing the need to urinate. Stress incontinence is often allied with sphincter overactivity and is often accompanied by urge incontinence.

Severe stress incontinence occurs most frequently in women younger than 60 years old. It is thought to be due to the relaxation of the supporting structures of the pelvis that results from childbirth, obesity, or lack of **exercise**. Some researchers believe that aging, perhaps due to estrogen deficiency, is a major cause of severe urinary incontinence in women, but no link has been found between incontinence and estrogen deficiency. Surgery for stress or mixed incontinence is primarily offered to patients who have failed, are not satisfied with, or are unable to comply with more conservative approaches. It is often performed during other surgeries such as urethra prolapse, cystocele surgery, urethral reconstruction, and **hysterectomy**.

KEY TERMS

Intrinsic sphincter deficiency (ISD)—One of the major factors in stress incontinence. Loss of support of the urethra causes the internal sphincter muscles to be unable to keep the bladder neck closed due to lack of contractive ability.

Pubovaginal sling—A general term for a procedure that places a sling around the urethra without the use of tension between the sling and the urethra. The is often referred to as the Tension-Free Vaginal Tape (TVT) procedure.

Stress incontinence—Incontinence that occurs when abdominal pressure is placed upon the urethra from movements such as coughing, sneezing, laughter, and exercise.

Urethral fascial sling—A support and compression aid to urethral function using auxillary material made of patient or donor tissue to undergird the urethra.

The sling procedure gets its name from the tissue attached under the mid- or proximal urethra and sutured at its ends onto a solid structure like the rectus sheath, pubic bone, or pelvic side walls. The procedure is used in the severest cases of stress incontinence, particularly those that have a concomitant sphincter inadequacy (ISD). The sling supports the urethra as it receives pressure from the abdomen and helps the internal sphincter muscles to keep the urethral opening closed. The procedure is the most popular because it has the highest success rate of all surgical remedies for severe stress incontinence related to sphincter inadequacies in both men and women.

Demographics

Urinary incontinence (UI) plagues 10–35% of adults and at least half of the million nursing home residents in the United States. Other studies indicate that between 10% and 30% of women experience incontinence during their lifetimes, compared to about 5% of men. One reason that more women than men have incontinent episodes is the relatively shorter urethras of women. Women have urethras of about 2 in (5 cm) and men have urethras of 10 in (25.4 cm). Studies have documented that about 50% of all women have occasional urinary incontinence, and as many as 10% have regular incontinence. Nearly 20% of women over age 75 experience daily urinary incontinence. Incontinence is a major factor in individuals entering long term care facilities. Women at highest risk are those who have given birth to more than three children and women who were given oxytocin to induce labor. Oxytocin puts more pressure on the pelvic muscles than does ordinary labor. Women who smoke have twice the rate of incontinence, according to one study of 600 women. Those women who do high-impact exercises are at much higher risk for incontinence. According to the medical literature, those at highest risk for urinary leakage are gymnasts, followed by softball, volleyball, and basketball players. Finally, women who have diabetes or are obese have higher rates of incontinence. Women who require sling procedures have often had other surgeries for incontinence, necessitating sling procedure to treat intrinsic sphincter deficiency caused by operative trauma. A rarer cause of stress incontinence in older women is urethral instability. In men, stress incontinence is usually caused by sphincter damage after surgery on the prostate.

Description

Anti-incontinence surgery is used to address the failure of two parts of female urinary continence: loss of support to the bladder neck or central urethra and intrinsic sphincter deficiency (ISD). The surgery does not restore function to the urethra or to the ability for closure to the sphincter. It replaces the mechanism for continence with supporting and compressive aids. Stabilizing the supporting elements of the urethra (ligaments, fascia, and muscles) was thought for many years to be the most important factor in curing incontinence. Called anatomic or genuine stress urinary incontinence (SUI), retropublic procedures, like the Burch procedure, sought only to restore the urethra to a fixed position. However, it became clear with the high failure rate of these procedures that ISD was present and unless surgery could confer some added compressive ability to the closure of the bladder, SUI would persist.

The urethral sling procedure is effective in the treatment of the severest types of incontinence (Types II and III) by re-establishing the "hammock effect" of the proximal or central point of the urethra during abdominal straining. The surgery involves the placement of a piece of material under the urethra at its arterial or vesical juncture and anchoring it on either side of the pubic bone or to the abdominal wall or vaginal wall. This technique involves the creation of a sling from a strip of tissue from the patient's own abdominal fascia (fibrous tissue) or from a cadaver. Synthetic slings also are used, but some are prone to break down over time.

The urethral sling procedure is most often performed as open surgery, which involves entering the pelvic area from the abdomen or from the vagina while the patient is under general or regional anesthesia. Broad-spectrum **antibiotics** are offered intravenously. If the patient is fitted with a urethral catheter, ampicillin and gentamicin are administered instead. The patient is placed in stirrups. Surgery takes place as a 6-to-9-cm by 1.5-cm sling is harvested from rectal tissue and sutured under the urethra at each end within the retropubic space (the area that undergirds the urethra). Synthetic tissue or fascia from a donor may also be used.

The goal of the surgery is to create a compression aid to the urethra. This involves an individualized approach to the tension needed on the sling. While the sling procedure is relatively easy to complete, the issue of tension on the sling is hard to determine and involves the use of tests during surgery for determining the compression effect of the sling on the urethra. Some manual tests are performed or a more sophisticated urodynamic test, like cystourethrography, may determine tension. It is important for the surgeon to test tension during surgery because of the high rate of retention of urine (inability to void) after surgery associated with this procedure and the miscalculation of the required tension.

Diagnosis/Preparation

Candidates for surgical treatment of incontinence must undergo a full clinical, neurological, and radiographic evaluation before there can be direct analysis of the condition to be treated and the desired outcome. Both urethral and bladder functions are evaluated and there is an attempt to determine the conditions associated with stress incontinence. In many women, incontinence may be due to vaginal prolapse. Stress incontinence can be identified by observation of urine during pelvic examination or by a sitting or standing **stress test** where patients are asked to cough or strain and evidence of leakage is obtained. Gynecologists often use a Q-tip test to determine the angle and change in the position of the urethra during straining. Other tests include subtracted cystometry to measure how much the bladder can hold, how much pressure builds up inside the bladder as it stores urine, and how full it is when the patients feels the urge to urinate.

The frequency of stress incontinence as measured by typical symptoms ranges between 33% and 65%. The frequency of stress incontinence is around 12% when measured or defined by cystometric findings. The ability to distinguish SUI as the cause of incontinence, as opposed to ISD, becomes more complicated; but it is a very important factor in the decision to have surgery. A combination of pelvic examination for urethral hypermoblity and leak point pressure as measured by coughing or other abdominal straining has been shown to be very effective in distinguishing ISD, and identifying the patient who needs surgery.

Aftercare

IV ketorolac and oral and intravenous pain medication are administered, as are postoperative antibiotics. A general diet is available usually on the evening of surgery. When the patient is able to walk, usually the same day, the urethral catheter is removed. The patient must perform self-catheterization to check urine volume every four hours to protect the urethral wall. If the patient is unwilling to perform catheterization, a tube can be placed suprapubically (in the back of the pubis) for voiding. Catheterization lasts about eight days, with about 98% of patients able to void at three months. Patients are discharged on the second day postoperatively, unless they have had other procedures and need additional recovery time. Patients may not lift heavy objects or engage in strenuous activity for approximately six weeks. Sexual intercourse may be resumed in the fourth week following surgery. Follow-up visits are scheduled for three to four weeks after surgery

Risks

Although the sling treatment has a very high success rate, it is also associated with a prolonged period of voiding difficulties, intraoperative bladder or urethra injury, infections associated with screw or staple points, and rejection of sling material from a donor or erosion of synthetic sling material. Patients should not be encouraged to undergo a sling procedure unless the risk of long-term voiding difficulty and the need for intermittent self-catheterization are understood. Fascial slings seem to be associated with the fewest complications for sling procedure treatment. Synthetic slings have a greater risk of having to be removed due to erosion and inflammation.

Normal results

Regardless of the procedure used, a proportion of patients will remain incontinent. Results vary according to the type of sling procedure used, the type of attachment used for the sling, and the type of material used for the sling. Normal results for the sling procedure overall are recurrent stress incontinence of 3–12% after bladder sling procedures. In general, reported cure rates are lower for second and subsequent surgical procedures. A recent qualitative study published in the *American Journal of Obstetrics and Gynecology* of 57 patients who underwent patient-contributed fascial sling procedures indicates good success with fascial sling procedures. At a median of 42 months after the procedure, the postoperative objective cure rate for stress urinary incontinence was 97%, with 88% of patients indicating that the sling had improved the quality of their lives. Eighty-four percent of patients indicated that the sling relieved their incontinence long term, and 82% of patients stated that they would undergo the surgery again. The study also found that voiding function was a common side effect in 41% of the patients.

WHO PERFORMS THE PROCEDURE AND WHERE IS IT PERFORMED?

The surgery is performed by a urological surgeon who has trained specifically for this procedure. The surgery takes place in a general hospital.

Morbidity and mortality rates

The most common complications of sling procedures are voiding problems (10.4%), new detrusor instability (7–27%), and lower urinary tract damage (3%). Some of the complications depend upon tension issues as well as on the materials used for the sling. There are recent and well designed studies of patient fascia and donor fascia used for slings in five centers with follow-up from 30 to 51 months that report no erosions or vaginal wall complications in any patients. Prolonged retention or voiding issues occurred in 2.3% of patients and de novo or spontaneous urge incontinence developed in 6%. These figures relate only to a large study utilizing patient or donor fascia and one that did not control for other factors like techniques of anchoring. In general, studies of the sling procedure are small and have many variables. There are no long-term studies (over five years) of this most popular procedure.

Alternatives

Alternatives to anti-incontinent sling procedure surgery depend upon the severity of the incontinence and the type. Severe stress incontinence with intrinsic sphincter deficiency can benefit from bulking agents for the urethra to increase compression, as well as external devices like a pessary that is placed in the vagina and holds up the bladder to prevent leakage. Urethral inserts can be placed in the urethra until it is time to use the bathroom. The patient learns to put the insertion in and take it out as needed. There are also

QUESTIONS TO ASK THE DOCTOR

- Do I have a urethral closure problem as a part of my incontinence?
- How many sling procedures have you performed?
- How soon will I be able to tell if I am going to have urine retention difficulties?
- If this surgery does not work, are there other procedures that will allow me a better quality of life?
- Is patient satisfaction a formal part of your evaluation of the success of the procedure you use?
- What type of material do you use for the sling and why do you choose this material?

urine seals that are small foam pads inserted in garments. Milder forms of incontinence can benefit from an assessment of medication usage, pelvic muscle exercises, bladder retraining, weight loss, and certain devices that stimulate the muscles around the urethra to strengthen them. For mild urethral mobility, procedures for tacking or stabilizing the urethra at the neck called Needle Neck Suspension, as well as procedures to hold the urethra in place with sutures, like the Burch method, are alternative forms of surgery.

Resources

BOOKS

"Urologic Surgery." In *Campbell's Urology*, 8th ed. Edited by M. F. Campbell, et al. Philadelphia: W. B. Saunders, 2002..

PERIODICALS

Lobel, B., A. Manunta, and A. Rodriguez. "The Management of Female Stress Urinary Incontinence Using the Sling Procedure." *British International Journal of Urology* 88, no. 8 (November 2001): 832.

Melton, Lisa. *"Targeted Treatment for Incontinence Beckons."* Lancet 359, no. 9303, (January 2002): 326.

Richter, H. R. "Effects of Pubovaginal Sling Procedure on Patients with Urethral Hypermobility and Intrinsic Sphincteric Deficiency: Would They Do it Again?" *American Journal of Obstetrics and Gynecology* 184, no. 2 (January 2001): 14–19.

ORGANIZATIONS

American Foundation for Urologic Disease/The Bladder Health Council. 1128 North Charles St., Baltimore, MD 21201. (410) 468-1800. Fax: (410) 468-1808. admin @afud.org. http://www.afud.org.

The Simon Foundation for Continence. P.O. Box 835, Wilmette, IL 60091. (800) 23-simon or (847) 864-3913. http://www.simonfoundation.org/html/.

OTHER

National Kidney and Urological Diseases Information Clearinghouse. *Bladder Control in Women*. Intelihealth. April 17, 2003 [cited June 25, 2003]. http://www.intelihealth.com/IH/ihtIH/WSIHW000/9103/24149/35872.html?d=dmtContent.

"Urinary Incontinence." MD Consult Patient Handout. [cited June 25, 2003]. www.MDConsult.com.

Nancy McKenzie, Ph.D.

Small bowel follow-through (SBFT): Small intestine radiography and fluoroscopy *see* **Upper GI exam**

Smoking cessation

Definition

Smoking cessation means "quitting smoking," or "withdrawal from nicotine." Tobacco is highly addictive, therefore, quitting the habit often involves irritability, headache, mood swings, and cravings associated with the sudden cessation or reduction of tobacco use by a nicotine-dependent individual.

Purpose

There are many good reasons to stop smoking; one of them is that smoking cessation may speed postsurgery recovery. Smoking cessation helps a person heal and recover faster, especially in the incision area, or if the surgery involved any bones. Research shows that patients who underwent hip and knee replacements, or surgery on other bone joints, healed better and recovered more quickly if they had quit or cut down their tobacco intake several weeks before the operation. Smoking weakens the bone mineral that keeps the skeleton strong and undermines tissue and vessel health. One study suggested that even quitting tobacco for a few days could improve tissue blood flow and oxygenation, and might have a positive effect on wound healing. If a patient has had a history of heart problems, his chances of having a second heart attack will be lowered. Quitting may also reduce wound complications, and lower the risk of cardiovascular trouble after surgery. If surgery was performed to remove cancerous tumors, quitting will reduce the

KEY TERMS

Addiction—Compulsive, overwhelming involvement with a specific activity. The activity may be smoking, gambling, alcohol, or may involve the use of almost any substance, such as a drug.

Appetite suppressant—To decrease the appetite.

Constrict—To squeeze tightly, compress, draw together.

Convulsion—To shake or effect with spasms; to agitate or disturb violently.

Depressant—A drug or other substance that soothes or lessens tension of the muscles or nerves.

Detoxification—To remove a poison or toxin or the effect of such a harmful substance; to free from an intoxicating or addictive substance in the body or from dependence on or addiction to a harmful substance.

Endorphins—Any of a group of proteins with analgesic properties that occur naturally in the brain.

Gestational age—The length of time of growth and development of the young in the mother's womb.

Metabolism—The sum of all the chemical processes that occur in living organisms; the rate at which the body consumes energy.

Nicotine—A poisonous, oily alkaloid in tobacco.

Oxygenation—To supply with oxygen.

Paraphernalia—Articles of equipment or accessory items.

Premature—Happening early or occurring before the usual time.

Psychoactive—Affecting the mind or behavior.

Respiratory infections—Infections that relate to or affect respiration or breathing.

Smoking cessation—The act of quitting smoking or withdrawal from nicotine.

Stimulant—A drug or other substance that increases the rate of activity of a body system.

Tremor—A trembling, quivering, or shaking.

Withdrawal—Stopping of administration or use of a drug; the syndrome of sometimes painful physical and psychological symptoms that follow the discontinuance.

risk of a second tumor, especially if cancer in the lung, head, or neck has been successfully treated.

Description

Quitting smoking is one of the best things a person can do to increase their life expectancy. On average, male smokers who quit at 35 years old can be expected to live to be 76 years old instead of 69 years if they were still smoking. Women who quit would live to be 80 years old instead of 74 years.

Effects of smoking on the body

Nicotine acts as both a stimulant and a depressant on the body. Saliva and bronchial secretions increase along with bowel tone. Some inexperienced smokers may experience tremors or even convulsions with high doses of nicotine because of the stimulation of the central nervous system. The respiratory muscles are then depressed following stimulation.

Nicotine causes arousal as well as relaxation from stressful situations. Tobacco use increases the heart rate about 10–20 beats per minute; and because it constricts the blood vessels, it increases the blood pressure reading by 5–10 mm Hg.

Sweating, nausea, and diarrhea may also increase because of the effects of nicotine upon the central nervous system. Hormonal activities of the body are also affected. Nicotine elevates the blood glucose levels and increases insulin production; it can also lead to blood clots. Smoking does have some positive effects on the body by stimulating memory and alertness, and enhancing cognitive skills that require speed, reaction time, vigilance, and work performance. Smoking tends to alleviate boredom and reduce stress as well as reduce aggressive responses to stressful events because of its mood-altering ability. It also acts as an appetite suppressant, specifically decreasing the appetite for simple carbohydrates (sweets) and inhibiting the efficiency with which food is metabolized. The fear of weight gain prevents some people from quitting smoking. The addictive effects of tobacco have been well documented. It is considered mood- and behavior-altering, psychoactive, and prone to abuse. Tobacco's addictive potential is believed to be comparable to the addictive potentials of alcohol, cocaine, and morphine.

Health problems associated with smoking

In general, chronic use of nicotine may cause an acceleration of coronary artery disease, hypertension, reproductive disturbances, esophageal reflux, peptic ulcer disease, fetal illnesses and **death**, and delayed wound healing. The smoker is at greater risk of developing cancer (especially in the lung, mouth, larynx, esophagus, bladder, kidney, pancreas, and cervix); heart attacks and strokes; and chronic lung disease. Using tobacco during pregnancy increases the risk of miscarriage, intrauterine growth retardation (resulting in the birth of an infant small for gestational age), and the infant's risk for sudden infant death syndrome.

The specific health risks of tobacco use include: nicotine addiction, lung disease, lung cancer, emphysema, chronic bronchitis, coronary artery disease and angina, heart attack, atherosclerotic and peripheral vascular disease, aneurysms, hypertension, blood clots, strokes, oral/tooth/gum diseases including oral cancer, and cancer in the kidney, bladder, and pancreas. Nicotine is also associated with decreased senses of taste and smell. During pregnancy, nicotine may cause increased fetal death, premature labor, low birth weight infants, and sudden infant death syndrome.

Smoking is also increasingly harmful to a person's social acceptability. According to the National Institute on Drug Abuse (NIDA), students at the high school and college levels in the early twenty-first century are increasingly disapproving of smoking. In just one year, disapproval of smoking among high school seniors increased from 76.2% in 2004 to 79.8% in 2005. For young adults, smoking complicates finding housing, as many landlords will not rent to smokers and many potential roommates do not want to share their apartment with a smoker.

Nonsmokers who are regularly exposed to secondhand smoke also may experience specific health risks including:

- Increased risk of lung cancer.
- An increased frequency of respiratory infections in infants and children (e.g. bronchitis and pneumonia), asthma, and decreases in lung function as the lungs mature.
- Acute, sudden, and occasionally severe reactions including eye, nose, throat, and lower respiratory tract symptoms.

The specific health risks for smokeless tobacco users include many of the diseases of smokers, as well as a 50-fold greater risk for oral cancer with long-term or regular use.

In diabetics taking medication for high blood pressure, it has been reported that smoking may increase the risk of kidney disease and/or kidney failure.

Making a plan to quit

Long lead times for elective procedures like joint operations offer a good opportunity for doctors to encourage their patients to quit smoking, but only the smoker has the power to stop smoking. Before a smoker decides to quit, he should make sure he wants to quit smoking for himself, and not for other people. The following are some suggestions the smoker may want to consider:

- The first step is to set a quit date. Women should set their quit date to begin at the end of their period for best results.
- Make a written list of why you want to quit smoking.
- Consider using an aid to help you quit, which can be the patch, nicotine gum, Zyban, nicotine spray, soft laser therapy, nasal inhaler, or some other method. If you plan to use Zyban, set your quit date for one week after you begin to use it.
- Smoke only in certain places, preferably outdoors.
- Switch to a brand of cigarettes that you don't like.
- Buy a piggy bank or an attractive box or jar and put the money in it that you would ordinarily spend on cigarettes. At an average cost of $5 per pack, the money in your savings bank will quickly add up.
- Do not buy cigarettes by the carton.
- Cut coffee consumption in half. You will not need to give it up.
- Practice putting off lighting up when the urge strikes.
- Go for a walk every day or begin an exercise program.
- Stock up on non-fattening safe snacks to help with weight control after quitting.
- Enlist the support of family and friends.
- Clean and put away all ashtrays the day before quitting.

Smokers who are trying to quit should remind themselves that they are doing the smartest thing they have ever done. Because of the preparation for smoking cessation, the smoker won't be surprised by or fearful of quitting. The quitter will be willing to do what's necessary, even though it won't be easy. Remember, this will likely add years to the lifespan. The quitting smoker should be prepared to spend more time with nonsmoking friends, if other smokers don't support the attempt to quit.

Since hospitals are smoke-free environments, if a smoking patient is in the hospital for **elective surgery**, it may be a good opportunity to quit smoking. It might be best to set the quit date around the time of the surgery and let the attending doctor know. As the smoker takes the first step, professional hospital staff will be there to give the support and help needed.

Medical staff can start the patient on nicotine replacement therapy to help control the cravings and increase the chances of quitting permanently.

Methods of quitting

Cold turkey, or an abrupt cessation of nicotine, is one way to stop smoking. Cold turkey can provide cost savings because paraphernalia and smoking cessation aids are not required; however, not everyone can stop this way as tremendous willpower is needed.

Laser therapy is an entirely safe and pain free form of acupuncture that has been in use since the 1980s. Using a painless soft laser beam instead of needles the laser beam is applied to specific energy points on the body, stimulating production of endorphins. These natural body chemicals produce a calming, relaxing effect. It is the sudden drop in endorphin levels that leads to withdrawal symptoms and physical cravings when a person stops smoking. Laser treatment not only helps relieve these cravings, but helps with stress reduction and lung detoxification. Some studies indicate that laser therapy is the most effective method of smoking cessation, with an extraordinarily high success rate.

Acupuncture—small needles or springs are inserted into the skin—is another aid in smoking cessation. The needles or springs are sometimes left in the ears and touched lightly by the patient between visits.

Some smokers find hypnosis particularly useful, especially if there is any kind of mental conflict, such as phobias, panic attacks, or weight control. As a smoker struggles to stop smoking, the conscious mind, deciding to quit, battles the inner mind, which is governed by habit and body chemistry. Hypnosis, by talking directly to the inner mind, can help to resolve that inner battle.

Some people are helped to quit smoking by psychotherapy. As of 2007, cognitive behavioral therapy, or CBT, is considered the most effective form of psychotherapy for smoking cessation. A research team at Yale University reported in the fall of 2007 that CBT was more effective than brief behavioral interventions in helping adolescent smokers stay in a smoking cessation program as well as actually quitting smoking.

Aversion techniques attempt to make smoking seem unpleasant. This technique reminds the person of the distasteful aspects of smoking, such as the smell, dirty ashtrays, coughing, the high cost, and health issues. The most common technique prescribed by psychologists for "thought stopping"—stopping unwanted thoughts—is to wear a rubber band around the wrist. Every time there is an unwanted thought (a craving to smoke) the band is supposed to be pulled so that it hurts. The thought then becomes associated with pain and gradually neutralized.

Rapid smoking is a technique in which smoking times are strictly scheduled once a day for the first three days after quitting. Phrases are repeated such as "smoking irritates my throat" or "smoking burns my lips and tongue." This technique causes over-smoking in a way that makes the taste and sensations associated with smoking very unpleasant.

There are special mouthwashes available, which, when used before smoking, alter the taste, giving cigarettes a very unpleasant taste. The intention is to create a link in the smoker's mind between cigarettes and a bad taste in the mouth.

Smoking cessation aids wean a person off nicotine slowly, and the nicotine can be delivered where it does the least bodily harm. Unlike cigarettes, these aids do not introduce other harmful poisons to the body. They can be used for a short period of time; however, nicotine from any source (smoking, nicotine gum, or the nicotine patch) can make some health problems worse. These include heart or circulation problems, irregular heartbeat, chest pain, high blood pressure, overactive thyroid, stomach ulcers, or diabetes.

The four main brands of the patch are Nicotrol, Nicoderm, Prostep, and Habitrol. All four transmit low doses of nicotine to the body throughout the day. The patch comes in varying strengths ranging from 7 mg to 21 mg. The patch must be prescribed and used under a physician's care. Package instructions must be followed carefully. Other smoking cessation programs or materials should be used while using the patch.

Nicorette gum allows the nicotine to be absorbed through the membrane of the mouth between the cheek and gums. Past smoking habits determine the right strength to choose. The gum should be chewed slowly.

The nicotine nasal spray reduces cravings and withdrawal symptoms, allowing smokers to cut back slowly. The nasal spray acts quickly to stop the cravings, as it is rapidly absorbed through the nasal membranes. One of the drawbacks is a risk of addiction to the spray.

The nicotine inhaler uses a plastic mouthpiece with a nicotine plug, delivering nicotine to the mucous membranes of the mouth. It provides nicotine at about one-third the nicotine level of cigarettes.

Bupropion hydrochloride, sold under the trade name Zyban, is an oral medication that is making an impact in the fight to help smokers quit. It is a treatment for nicotine dependence. Another new medication, approved by the Food and Drug Administration (FDA) in 2006, is varenicline tartrate, sold under the trade name Chantix. Chantix is thought to work by affecting parts of the brain affected by nicotine in two ways: by providing some nicotine effects to ease withdrawal symptoms and by blocking the effects of nicotine from cigarettes if the patient resumes smoking. In November 2007, however, the FDA issued a warning regarding mood changes reported in persons taking Chantix. The drug is still considered safe, but anyone taking it in order to stop smoking should contact their doctor at once if they feel depressed or notice other sudden mood changes.

The nicotine lozenge is another smoking cessation aid recently added to the growing list of tools to combat nicotine withdrawal.

As of 2007, scientists are researching the possibility of developing medications that inhibit the function of CYP2A6, an enzyme that makes people more susceptible to nicotine addiction. Some people have a genetic variant that decreases the amount of CYP2A6 in the body, which is thought to protect these individuals against nicotine addiction. Thus medications that lower the amount of this enzyme might offer a new approach to smoking cessation.

Withdrawal symptoms

Generally, the longer one has smoked and the greater the number of cigarettes (and nicotine) consumed, the more likely it is that withdrawal symptoms will occur and the more severe they are likely to be. When a smoker switches from regular to low-nicotine cigarettes or significantly cuts back smoking, a milder form of nicotine withdrawal involving some or all of these symptoms can occur.

These are some of the withdrawal symptoms that most former smokers experience in the beginning of their new smoke-free life:

- dry mouth;
- mood swings;
- irritability;
- feelings of depression;
- gas in the digestive tract;
- tension;
- sleeplessness or sleeping too much;
- difficulty in concentration;
- intense cravings for a cigarette;
- increased appetite and weight gain; and
- headaches.

These side effects are all temporary conditions that will probably subside in a short time for most people. These symptoms can last from one to three weeks and are strongest during the first week after quitting. Drinking plenty of water during the first week can help detoxify the body and shorten the duration of the withdrawal symptoms. A positive attitude, drive, commitment, and a willingness to get help from health care professionals and support groups will help a smoker kick the habit.

Researchers from the University of California San Diego strongly suggest that any of the above cessation aids should be used in combination with other types of smoking cessation help, such as counseling and/or support programs. These products are not designed to help with the behavioral aspects of smoking, but only the cravings associated with them. Counseling and support groups can offer tips on coping with difficult situations that can trigger the urge to smoke.

Even a new heart can't break a bad habit

Why do some people who have heart transplants continue to smoke? In a three-year study at the University of Pittsburgh of 202 heart transplant recipients, 71% of the recipients were smokers before surgery. The overall rate of post-transplant smoking was 27%. All but one of the smokers resumed the smoking habit they had before the transplant. The biggest reason for resuming smoking was addiction to nicotine. Smoking is a complex behavior, involving social interactions, visual cues, and other factors. Those who smoked until less than six months before the transplant were much more likely to resume smoking early and to smoke more. One of the major causes of early relapse was because of depression and anxiety within two months after the transplant. Another strong predictor of relapse was having a caretaker who smoked. The knowledge of these risk factors could help develop strategies for identifying those in greatest need of early intervention. According to European studies, the five-year survival rate for post-transplant smokers is 37%, compared to 80% for nonsmoking recipients. Smokers can develop inoperable lung cancers within five years after a transplant, thus resulting in a shorter survival rate. There is an alarming incidence of head and neck cancers in transplant recipients who resume smoking.

Overall, there is a 90% relapse rate in the general population; however, the more times a smoker tries to quit, the greater the chance of success with each new try.

Resources

BOOKS

Abrams, David B., et al. *The Tobacco Dependence Treatment Handbook: A Guide to Best Practices*. New York: Guilford Press, 2003.

American Cancer Society. *Kicking Butts: Quit Smoking and Take Charge of Your Health.* Atlanta, GA: American Cancer Society, 2002.

Britton, John, ed. *ABC of Smoking Cessation.* Malden, MA: BMJ Books, 2004.

Dodds, Bill. *1440 Reasons to Quit Smoking: 1 For Every Minute of the Day.* Minnetonka, MN: Meadowbrook Press, 2000.

Mannoia, Richard J. *NBAC Program: Never Buy Another Cigarette: A Cigarette Smoking Cessation Program.* Paradise Publications, 2003.

National Institutes of Health. *Clearing the Air: Quit Smoking Today.* Bethesda, MD: National Institutes of Health, 2003.

Shipley, Robert H. *Quit Smart: Stop Smoking Guide With the Quitsmart System, It's Easier Than You Think!* Quitsmart, 2002.

PERIODICALS

Cavallo, D. A., J. L. Cooney, A. M. Duhig, et al. "Combining Cognitive Behavioral Therapy with Contingency Management for Smoking Cessation in Adolescent Smokers: A Preliminary Comparison of Two Different CBT Formats." *American Journal on Addictions* 16, no. 6 (November 2007): 468–474.

Lancaster, T., L. Stead, and K. Cahill. "An Update on Therapeutics for Tobacco Dependence." *Expert Opinion on Pharmacotherapy* 9, no. 1 (January 2008): 15–22.

Landman, Anne, Pamela M. Ling, and Stanton A. Glantz. "Tobacco Industry Youth Smoking Prevention Programs: Protecting the Industry and Hurting Tobacco Control." *American Journal of Public Health* 92, no. 6 (June 2002): 917–30.

Le Foll, B., and T. P. George. "Treatment of Tobacco Dependence: Integrating Recent Progress into Practice." *Canadian Medical Association Journal* 177, no. 11 (November 20, 2007): 1373–1380.

Mwenifumbo, J. C., and R. F. Tyndale. "Genetic Variability in CYP2A6 and the Pharmacokinetics of Nicotine." *Pharmacogenomics* 8, no. 10 (October 2007): 1385–1402.

Taylor, D. H., Jr., V. Hasselblad, S. J. Henley, M. J. Thun, and F. A. Sloan. "Research and Practice: Benefits of Smoking Cessation for Longevity." *American Journal of Public Health* 92, no. 6 (June 2002): 990–996.

OTHER

Illig, David. *Stop Smoking.* Audio CD. Seattle: WA: Successworld, 2001.

Mesmer. *Stop Smoking With America's Foremost Hypnotist.* Audio CD. Victoria, BC: Ace Mirage Entertainment, 2000.

"NIDA InfoFacts: Cigarettes and Other Tobacco Products." National Institute on Drug Abuse. July 2007. http://www.nida.nih.gov/infofacts/tobacco.html (April 7, 2008).

"Prevention and Cessation of Cigarette Smoking: Control of Tobacco Use," patient version. National Cancer Institute. 2008. http://www.cancer.gov/cancertopics/pdq/prevention/control-of-tobacco-use/Patient (April 7, 2008).

ORGANIZATIONS

Action on Smoking and Health, 2013 H Street, NW, Washington, DC, 20006, (202) 659-4310, http://ash.org.

American Cancer Society, 1875 Connecticut Avenue, NW, Suite 730, Washington, DC, 20009, (800) ACS-2345, http://www.cancer.org.

Centers for Disease Control and Prevention, Mail Stop K-50, 4770 Buford Highway, NE, Atlanta, GA, 30341, (800) 232-4636, http://www.cdc.gov/tobacco/osh/index.htm.

Crystal H. Kaczkowski, M.Sc.
Rebecca Frey, Ph.D.

Snoring surgery

Definition

Snoring is defined as noisy or rough breathing during sleep, caused by vibration of loose tissue in the upper airway. Surgical treatments for snoring include several different techniques for removing tissue from the back of the patient's throat, reshaping the nasal passages or jaw, or preventing the tongue from blocking the airway during sleep.

Purpose

The purpose of snoring surgery is to improve or eliminate the medical and social consequences of heavy snoring. Most insurance companies, however, regard surgical treatment of snoring as essentially a cosmetic procedure—which means that patients must cover its expenses themselves. The major exception is surgery to correct a deviated septum or other obstruction in the nose, on the grounds that nasal surgery generally improves the patient's breathing during the day as well as at night.

Snoring as a medical problem

The connection between heavy snoring, breathing disorders, and other health problems is a relatively recent discovery. Obstructive sleep apnea (OSA) is a breathing disorder that was first identified in 1965. OSA is marked by brief stoppages in breathing during sleep resulting from partial blockage of the airway. A person with OSA may stop breathing temporarily as often as 20–30 times per hour. He or she usually snores or makes choking and gasping sounds between these episodes. The person is not refreshed by nighttime sleep and may suffer from morning headaches as well as daytime sleepiness. He or she may be misdiagnosed

KEY TERMS

Continuous positive airway pressure (CPAP)—A ventilation device that blows a gentle stream of air into the nose during sleep to keep the airway open.

Deviated septum—An abnormal configuration of the cartilage that divides the two sides of the nose. It can cause breathing problems if left uncorrected.

Injection snoreplasty—A technique for reducing snoring by injecting a chemical that forms scar tissue near the base of the uvula, helping to anchor it and reduce its fluttering or vibrating during sleep.

Obstructive sleep apnea (OSA)—A potentially life-threatening condition characterized by episodes of breathing cessation during sleep alternating with snoring or disordered breathing. The low levels of oxygen in the blood of patients with OSA may eventually cause heart problems or stroke.

Palate—The roof of the mouth.

Polysomnography—A test administered in a sleep laboratory to analyze heart rate, blood circulation, muscle movement, brain waves, and breathing patterns during sleep.

Primary snoring—Simple snoring; snoring that is not interrupted by episodes of breathing cessation.

Somnoplasty—A technique that uses radiofrequency signals to heat a thin needle inserted into the tissues of the soft palate. The heat from the needle shrinks the tissues, thus enlarging the patient's airway. Somnoplasty is also known as radiofrequency volumetric tissue reduction (RFVTR).

Uvula—A triangular piece of tissue that hangs from the roof of the mouth above the back of the tongue. Primary snoring is often associated with fluttering or vibrating of the uvula during sleep.

Uvulopalatopharyngoplasty (UPPP)—An operation to remove the tonsils and other excess tissue at the back of the throat to prevent it from closing the airway during sleep.

as suffering from clinical depression when the real problem is physical tiredness. In addition, the high levels of carbon dioxide that build up in the blood when a person is not breathing normally may eventually lead to high blood pressure, irregular heartbeat, heart attacks, and stroke. In children, heavy snoring appears to be a major risk factor for attention-deficit/hyperactivity disorder.

Although people with OSA snore, not everyone who snores has OSA. It is thought that OSA affects about 4% of middle-aged males and 2% of middle-aged females. Most adults who snore have what is called primary snoring, which means that the loud sounds produced in the upper airway during sleep are *not* interrupted by episodes of breathing cessation. Other terms for primary snoring are simple snoring, benign snoring, rhythmical snoring, continuous snoring, and socially unacceptable snoring (SUS). Although primary snoring is not associated with severe disorders to the same extent as OSA, it has been shown to have some negative consequences for health, including such things as chronic daily headaches.

Snoring as a social problem

As the term SUS suggests, primary snoring can cause the same social problems for a person as does snoring associated with OSA. People who snore heavily often keep other family members, roommates, or even neighbors from getting a good night's sleep, which leads to considerable anger and resentment. Studies have found that the nonsnoring partner or roommate loses an average of an hour's sleep each night. According to Dr. Kingman Strohl, head of a sleep disorders program in a Veterans Administration hospital, even the average volume of snoring (60 decibels or dB) is as loud as normal speech. Some people, however, snore around 80–82 dB, the sound level of a loud yell; a few have been recorded as reaching 90 dB, the sound level of loud rock music. One study found that 80% of people married to heavy snorers end up sleeping in separate rooms. A group of Swedish researchers reported that heavy snoring has the same level of negative effects on quality of life among adult males as high blood pressure, chronic obstructive pulmonary disease, heart disease, and similar chronic medical conditions.

Risk factors for snoring

Some people are at higher risk of developing problem snoring than others. Risk factors in addition to sex and age include:

- Genetic factors. The size and shape of the uvula, soft palate, tonsils, and other parts of the airway are largely determined by heredity.
- Family history of heavy snoring.

- Obesity. Severe overweight increases a person's risk of developing OSA.
- Lack of exercise. Physical activity helps to keep the muscles of the throat firm and strong as well as the larger muscles of the body.
- Heavy consumption of alcohol and tobacco.
- A history of frequent upper respiratory infections or allergies.
- Trauma to the nose, face, or throat.

Demographics

Snoring is a commonplace problem in the general population in North America. About 19% to 37% of all Americans snore, and more than half of all middle-aged men snore. Men are more affected because of the architecture of their throat, and because of hormonal patterns and how those hormones affect fat distribution and the muscles of the upper airway. About 12% of children over the age of five are reported to snore frequently and loudly. Among adults, 45% snore occasionally, while 25% snore almost every night. The problem usually grows worse as people age; 50% of people over age 65 are habitual snorers.

Problem snoring is worse among males than among females in all age brackets. With regard to racial and ethnic differences, a sleep research study published in 2003 reported that frequent snoring is more common (in the United States) among African American women, Hispanic women, and Hispanic men than their Caucasian counterparts, even after adjusting for weight and body mass index (BMI). African American, Native American, and Asian American males have the same rates of snoring as Caucasian males. Further research is needed to determine whether these differences are related to variations in the rates and types of health problems in these respective groups.

According to international researchers, heavy snoring appears to be more common in persons of Asian origin than in persons of Middle Eastern, European, or African origin.

Description

With the exception of UPPP, all of the surgical treatments for snoring described in this section are outpatient or office-based procedures.

Uvulopalatopharyngoplasty (UPPP)

Uvulopalatopharyngoplasty, or UPPP, is the oldest and most invasive surgical treatment for snoring. It was first performed in 1982 by a Japanese surgeon named S. Fujita. UPPP requires **general anesthesia**, one to two nights of inpatient care in a hospital, and a minimum of two weeks of recovery afterward. In a uvulopalatopharyngoplasty, the surgeon resects (removes) the patient's tonsils, part of the soft palate, and the uvula. The procedure works by enlarging the airway and removing some of the soft tissue that vibrates when the patient snores. It is not effective in treating snoring caused by obstructions at the base of the tongue.

UPPP has several drawbacks in addition to its cost and lengthy recovery period. It can result in major complications, including severe bleeding due to removal of the tonsils as well as airway obstruction. In addition, the results may not be permanent; between 50% and 70% of patients who have been treated with UPPP report that short-term improvements in snoring do not last longer than a year.

Laser-assisted uvulopalatoplasty

Laser-assisted uvulopalatoplasty, or LAUP, is an outpatient surgical treatment for snoring in which a carbon dioxide laser is used to vaporize part of the uvula, a small triangular piece of tissue that hangs from the soft palate above the back of the tongue. The patient is seated upright in a comfortable chair in the doctor's office. The doctor first sprays a local anesthetic—usually lidocaine— over the back of the patient's throat, covering the patient's soft palate, tonsils, and uvula. The second step is the injection of more anesthetic into the muscle tissue in the uvula. After waiting for the anesthetic to take effect, the surgeon uses a carbon dioxide laser to make two vertical incisions in the soft palate on either side of the uvula. A third incision is used to remove the tip of the uvula. The surgeon also usually removes part of the soft palate itself. The total procedure takes about half an hour.

LAUP is typically performed as a series of three to five separate treatments. Additional treatment sessions, if needed, are spaced four to eight weeks apart.

LAUP was developed in the late 1980s by Dr. Yves-Victor Kamami, a French surgeon whose first article on the technique was published in 1990. Kamami claimed a high rate of success for LAUP in treating OSA as well as snoring. The procedure has become controversial because other surgeons found it less effective than the first reports indicated, and also because most patients suffer considerable pain for about two weeks after surgery. Although some surgeons report a success rate as high as 85% in treating snoring with LAUP, the effectiveness of the procedure is highly dependent on the surgeon's experience and ability.

Somnoplasty

Somnoplasty, or radiofrequency volumetric tissue reduction (RFVTR) is a newer technique in which the surgeon uses a thin needle connected to a source of radiofrequency signals to shrink the tissues in the soft palate, throat, or tongue. It was approved by the U.S. Food and Drug Administration (FDA) for the treatment of snoring in 1997. The needle is inserted beneath the surface layer of cells and heated to a temperature between 158°F and 176°F (70° and 80°C). The upper layer of cells is unaffected, but the heated tissue is destroyed and gradually reabsorbed by the body over the next four to six weeks. Somnoplasty stiffens the remaining layers of tissue as well as reducing the total volume of tissue. Some patients require a second treatment, but most find that their snoring is significantly improved after only one. The procedure takes about 30 minutes and is performed under **local anesthesia**.

Somnoplasty appears to have a higher success rate (about 85%) than LAUP and is considerably less painful. Most patients report two to three days of mild swelling after somnoplasty compared to two weeks of considerable discomfort for LAUP.

Tongue suspension procedure

The tongue suspension procedure, which is also known as the Repose™ system, is a minimally invasive surgical treatment for snoring that stabilizes the base of the tongue during sleep, preventing it from falling backward and obstructing the airway. The Repose system was approved by the FDA in 1998. It consists of a titanium screw inserted into the lower jaw on the floor of the mouth and a suture passed through the base of the tongue that is then attached to the screw. The attachment holds the tongue forward during sleep.

The Repose system is done as an outpatient procedure under total anesthesia. It takes about 15–20 minutes to complete. The advantages of the tongue suspension procedure include the fact that it is reversible, since no incision is made; and that it can be combined with UPPP, LAUP, or a **tonsillectomy**. Its disadvantages include its relatively long healing time (one to two weeks) and the fact that it appears to be more effective in treating OSA than primary snoring. One team of American and Israeli researchers who conducted a multicenter trial concluded that the tongue suspension procedure requires further evaluation.

Injection snoreplasty

Injection snoreplasty was developed by a team of Army physicians at Walter Reed Hospital and introduced to other ear, nose and throat specialists at a professional conference in 2000. In injection snoreplasty, the surgeon gives the patient a local anesthetic and then injects a hardening agent known as sodium tetradecyl sulfate underneath the skin of the roof of the mouth just in front of the uvula. The chemical, which is also used in sclerotherapy, creates a blister that hardens into scar tissue. The scar tissue pulls the uvula forward, reducing the vibration or flutter that causes snoring.

Preliminary research indicates that injection snoreplasty is safe, has a higher rate of success than LAUP (about 92%), and is also less painful. Most patients need only one treatment, and can manage the discomfort the next day with a mild **aspirin** substitute and throat spray. The primary drawback of injection snoreplasty is that it treats only tissues in the area of the uvula. Snoring caused by tissue vibrations elsewhere in the throat requires another form of treatment. Injection snoreplasty costs about $500 per treatment.

Diagnosis/Preparation

Diagnosis

The most important task in diagnosing a patient's snoring is to distinguish between primary snoring and obstructive sleep apnea. The reason for care in the diagnosis is that surgical treatment without the recommended tests for OSA can complicate later diagnosis of the disorder.

The sounds made when a person snores have a number of different physical causes. Snoring noises may result from one or more of the following:

- An unusually long soft palate and uvula. These structures narrow the airway between the nose and the throat. They act like noisy flutter valves when the person breathes in and out during sleep.
- Too much tissue in the throat. Large tonsils and adenoids can cause snoring, which is one reason why tonsillectomies are sometimes recommended to treat heavy snoring in children.
- Nasal congestion. When a person's nose is stuffy, their attempts to breathe create a partial vacuum in the throat that pulls the softer tissues of the throat together. This suction can also produce a snoring noise. Nasal congestion helps to explain why some people snore only when they have a cold or during pollen season.
- Anatomical deformations of the nose. People who have had their noses or cheekbones fractured or who have a deviated septum are more likely to snore, because their nasal passages develop a twisted or crooked shape and vibrate as air passes through them.

- Sleeping position. People are more likely to snore when they are lying on the back because the force of gravity draws the tongue and soft tissues in the throat backward and downward, blocking the airway.
- Obesity. Obesity adds to the weight of the tissues in the neck, which can cause partial blockage of the airway during sleep.
- Use of alcohol, sleeping medications, or tranquilizers. These substances relax the throat muscles, which may become soft or limp enough to partially close the airway.

Because snoring may be related to lifestyle factors, upper respiratory infections, seasonal allergies, and sleeping habits as well as the anatomy of the person's airway, a complete medical history is the first step in determining suitable treatments. In some cases the patient may have been referred by his or her dentist on the basis of findings during a dental procedure. A primary care doctor can take a history and perform a basic examination of the patient's nose and throat. In addition, the primary care doctor may give the patient one or more short questionnaires to evaluate the severity of daytime sleepiness and other problems related to snoring. The test most commonly used is the Epworth Sleepiness Scale (ESS), which was developed by an Australian physician, Dr. Murray Johns, in 1991. The ESS lists eight situations (reading, watching TV, etc.) and asks the patient to rate his or her chances of dozing off in each situation on a four-point scale (0–3, with 3 representing a high chance of falling asleep). A score of 6 or lower indicates that the person is getting enough sleep; a score higher than 9 is a danger sign. The ESS is often used to measure the effectiveness of various treatments for snoring as well as to evaluate patients prior to surgery.

The next stage in the differential diagnosis of snoring problems is a detailed examination of the patient's airway by an otolaryngologist, who is a physician who specializes in diagnosing and treating disorders involving the nose and throat. The American Sleep Apnea Association (ASAA) maintains that no one should consider surgery for snoring until their airway has been examined by a specialist. The otolaryngologist will be able to determine whether the size and shape of the patient's uvula, soft palate, tonsils and adenoids, nasal cartilage, and throat muscles are contributing factors, and to advise the patient on specific procedures. It may be necessary for the patient to undergo more than one type of treatment for snoring, as some surgical procedures correct only one or two structures in the nose or throat.

A complete airway examination consists of an external examination of the patient's face and neck; an endoscopic examination of the nasal passages and throat; the use of a laryngeal mirror or magnifying laryngoscope to study the lower portions of the throat; and various imaging studies. The otolaryngologist may use a nasopharyngoscope, which allows for evaluation of obstructions below the palate and the tongue, and may be performed with the patient either awake or asleep. The nasopharyngoscope is a flexible fiberoptic device that is introduced into the airway through the patient's nose. Other imaging studies that may be done include acoustic reflection, computed tomography (CT) scans, or **magnetic resonance imaging** (MRI).

In addition to the airway examination, patients considering surgical treatment for snoring must make an appointment for sleep testing in a specialized laboratory. The American Academy of Sleep Medicine recommends this step in order to exclude the possibility that the patient has obstructive sleep apnea. Sleep testing consists of an overnight stay in a special sleep laboratory. Before the patient goes to sleep, he or she will be connected to a polysomnograph, which is an instrument that monitors the patient's breathing, heart rate, temperature, muscle movements, airflow, body position, and other measurements that are needed to evaluate the cause(s) of sleep disorders. A technician records the data in a separate room. As of 2003, some companies are developing portable polysomnographs that allow patients to connect the device to a computer in their home and transmit the data to the sleep center over an Internet connection.

Preparation

Apart from the extensive diagnostic testing that is recommended, preparation for outpatient snoring surgery is usually limited to taking a mild sedative before the procedure. Preparation for UPPP requires a **physical examination**, EKG, blood tests, and a preoperation interview with the anesthesiologist to evaluate the patient's fitness for general anesthesia.

Aftercare

Aftercare following outpatient snoring surgery consists primarily of medication for throat discomfort, particularly when swallowing. The patient can resume normal work and other activities the same day as the procedure, and speaking is usually not affected.

Risks

In addition to the risk of an allergic reaction to the local anesthetic, snoring surgery is associated with the following risks:

- Severe pain following the procedure that lasts longer than two to three days. This complication occurs more frequently with LAUP than with somnoplasty or injection snoreplasty.
- Causation or worsening of obstructive sleep apnea. LAUP has been reported to cause OSA in patients who had only primary snoring before the operation.
- Nasal regurgitation. This complication refers to food shooting or leaking through the nose when the patient swallows.
- Dehydration. This complication has been reported with the tongue suspension procedure.
- Permanent change in the quality of the patient's voice.
- Recurrence of primary snoring.

Normal results

In general, surgical treatment for snoring appears to be most effective in patients whose primary problem is nasal obstruction. The results of snoring surgery depend to a large degree on a good "fit" between the anatomy of a specific patient's airway and the specific procedure performed, as well as on the individual surgeon's skills.

WHO PERFORMS THE PROCEDURE AND WHERE IS IT PERFORMED?

Snoring surgery is done by a head and neck surgeon, a plastic surgeon, or an otolaryngologist, who is a doctor with special training in treating disorders of the ear, nose, and throat. UPPP is performed under general anesthesia and requires an overnight hospital stay. LAUP, somnoplasty, the tongue suspension procedure, and injection snoreplasty are performed as outpatient surgery, usually in a doctor's office or other outpatient facility.

Prosthetic devices to alter the position of the jaw or restrain the tongue during sleep are prescribed and fitted by general dentists or orthodontists.

Polysomnography as a part of a diagnostic workup is done in a special sleep laboratory by experts who are trained in the use of the equipment and interpretation of the results. Advances in technology, however, may allow patients to be monitored at home with portable polysomnographs and a computer with an Internet connection.

Morbidity and mortality rates

Mortality rates for UPPP are related to complications of OSA rather than to the procedure itself. With regard to the outpatient procedures for snoring, mortality rates are very close to zero because these surgeries are performed under local anesthesia. Complication rates, however, are high with both UPPP and LAUP. According to one European study, as many as 42% of patients have complications following UPPP, with 14% reporting general dissatisfaction with the results of surgery. Specific complication rates for UPPP are 15% for recurrence of snoring; 13% for nasal regurgitation; 10% for excessive throat secretions; 9% for swallowing problems; and 7% for speech disturbances. Complications for LAUP have been estimated to be 30–40% for recurrence of snoring; 30% for causing or worsening of OSA; 5–10% for persistent nasal regurgitation; 1% for permanent change in vocal quality.

As of early 2003, no morbidity figures have been published for somnoplasty or injection snoreplasty.

Alternatives

Oral devices and appliances

Oral appliances are intended to reduce snoring by changing the shape of the oral cavity or preventing the tongue from blocking the airway. There are three basic types of mouthpieces: those that push the lower jaw forward; those that raise the soft palate; and those that restrain the tongue from falling backward during sleep. To work properly, oral appliances should be fitted by an experienced dentist or orthodontist and checked periodically for proper fit. Their major drawback is a low rate of patient compliance; one German study found that only 30% of patients fitted with these devices were still using them after four years. In addition, oral appliances cannot be used by patients with gum disease, **dental implants**, or teeth that are otherwise in poor condition.

Continuous positive airway pressure (CPAP) devices

CPAP devices are masks that fit over the nose during sleep and deliver air into the airway under enough pressure to keep the airway open. If used correctly, CPAP devices can be an effective alternative to surgery. Their main drawback is a relatively low rate of patient compliance; the mask must be used every night, and some people feel mildly claustrophobic when using it. In addition, patients are often asked to lose weight or stop smoking while using CPAP, which are lifestyle adjustments that some would rather not make.

QUESTIONS TO ASK THE DOCTOR

- How often have you performed surgery for primary snoring? Which procedures have you performed most frequently?
- What is your opinion of somnoplasty and injection snoreplasty?
- Am I likely to benefit from lifestyle changes or other less invasive alternatives?
- Should I talk to my dentist about an oral appliance to control snoring?

Lifestyle changes

Patients who snore only occasionally or who are light snorers may be helped by one or more of the following changes without undergoing surgery:

- Losing weight and getting adequate physical exercise.
- Avoiding tranquilizers, sleeping pills, antihistamines, or alcoholic beverages before bedtime.
- Quitting smoking.
- Sleeping on the side rather than the back. One do-it-yourself device that is sometimes recommended to keep the patient turned on his or her side is a tennis ball placed inside a sock and attached to the back of the pajamas or nightgown. This approach seems to work for some patients with simple snoring.
- Tilting the head of the bed upward about 4 in (10 cm).

Complementary and alternative (CAM) approaches

There are three forms of alternative treatment that have been shown to be helpful in reducing primary snoring in patients with histories of nasal congestion or swollen tissues in the throat. The first is acupuncture. Treatments for snoring usually focus on acupuncture points on the stomach, arms, and legs associated with the production of excess mucus. Insertion of the acupuncture needles at these points is thought to stimulate the body to release the excess moisture or phlegm.

Homeopathy and aromatherapy also appear to benefit some patients whose snoring is related to colds, allergies, or sore throats. Homeopathic remedies for snoring are available as nose drops and throat sprays as well as the traditional pill formulations. Aromatherapy formulas for snoring typically contain marjoram oil, which may be used alone or combined with lavender and other herbs that clear the nasal passages. Some people find aromatherapy preparations helpful alongside mainstream treatments because their fragrance is pleasant and relaxing.

Resources

BOOKS

Cummings, C. W., et al. *Otolaryngology: Head and Neck Surgery,* 4th ed. St. Louis: Mosby, 2004.

Goetz, Christopher G. *Textbook of Clinical Neurology,* 3rd ed. Philadelphia: Saunders, 2007.

PERIODICALS

Hoban T. F., and R. D. Chervin. "Sleep-Related Breathing Disorders of Childhood: Description and Clinical Picture Diagnosis, and Treatment Approaches." *Sleep Medicine Clinics* 2, no. 3 (September 2007): 445–462.

Norman, D., J. S. Loredo. "Obstructive sleep apnea in older adults." *Clinics of Geriatric Medicine* 24, no. 1 (February 2008): 151–165.

O'Brien, L. M., C. R. Holbrook, C. B. Mervis, et al. "Sleep and Neurobehavioral Characteristics of 5- to 7-Year-Old Children with Parentally Reported Symptoms of Attention-Deficit/Hyperactivity Disorder." *Pediatrics* 111, no. 3 (March 2003): 554–563.

O'Connor, G. T., B. K. Lind, E. T. Lee, et al. "Variation in Symptoms of Sleep-Disordered Breathing with Race and Ethnicity: The Sleep Heart Health Study." *Sleep* 26, no. 1 (February 1, 2003): 74–79.

Scher, A. I., R. B. Lipton, and W. F. Stewart. "Habitual Snoring as a Risk Factor for Chronic Daily Headache." *Neurology* 60, no. 8 (April 22, 2003): 1366–1368.

Velamuri K. "Upper Airway Resistance Syndrome." *Sleep Medicine Clinics* 1, no. 4 (December 2006): 475–482.

OTHER

"Considering Surgery for Snoring?" American Sleep Apnea Association. August 2000. http://www.sleepapnea.org/resources/pubs/snoring.html (May 10, 2003).

"What Is Sleep Apnea?" Diseases and Conditions Index. National Heart, Lung, and Blood Institute. February 2008. http://www.nhlbi.nih.gov/health/dci/Diseases/SleepApnea/SleepApnea_WhatIs.html (April 7, 2008).

ORGANIZATIONS

American Academy of Medical Acupuncture, 4929 Wilshire Boulevard, Suite 428, Los Angeles, CA, 90010, (323) 937-5514, http://www.medicalacupuncture.org.

American Academy of Otolaryngology—Head and Neck Surgery, One Prince Street, Alexandria, VA, 22314-3357, (703) 836-4444, http://www.entnet.org.

American Academy of Sleep Medicine, One Westbrook Corporate Center, Suite 920, Westchester, IL, 60154, (708) 492-0930, http://www.aasmnet.org.

American Dental Association, 211 East Chicago Avenue, Chicago, IL, 60611, (312) 440-2500, http://www.ada.org.

American Sleep Apnea Association, 1424 K Street NW, Suite 302, Washington, DC, 20005, (202) 293-3650, http://www.sleepapnea.org.

National Center on Sleep Disorders Research, Two Rockledge Centre, Suite 10038, 6701 Rockledge Drive, MSC 7920, Bethesda, MD, 20892-7920, (301) 435-0199, http://www.nhlbi.nih.gov/about/ncsdr/index.htm.

Rebecca Frey, Ph.D.

Sodium test *see* **Electrolyte tests**
Somnoplasty *see* **Snoring surgery**

Sphygmomanometer

Definition

A sphygmomanometer is a device for measuring blood pressure.

Purpose

The sphygmomanometer is designed to monitor blood pressure by measuring the force of the blood in the heart where the pressure is greatest. This occurs during the contraction of the ventricles, when blood is pumped from the heart to the rest of the body (systolic pressure). The minimal force is also measured. This occurs during the period when the heart is relaxed between beats and pressure is lowest (diastolic pressure).

A sphygmomanometer is used to establish a baseline at a healthcare encounter and on admission to a hospital. Checking blood pressure is also performed to monitor the effectiveness of medication and other methods to control hypertension, and as a diagnostic aid to detect various diseases and abnormalities.

Description

A sphygmomanometer consists of a hand bulb pump, a unit that displays the blood pressure reading, and an inflatable cuff that is usually wrapped around a person's upper arm. Care should be taken to ensure that the cuff size is appropriate for the person whose blood pressure is being taken. This improves the accuracy of the reading. Children and adults with smaller or larger than average-sized arms require special-sized cuffs appropriate for their needs. A **stethoscope** is also used in conjunction with the sphygmomanometer to hear the blood pressure sounds. Some devices have the stethoscope already built in.

A sphygmomanometer can be used or encountered in a variety of settings:

- home
- hospital
- primary care clinic or professional office
- ambulance
- dental office
- pharmacy and other retail establishment

There are three types of equipment in common use for monitoring blood pressure.

- A mercury-based unit has a manually inflatable cuff attached by tubing to the unit that is calibrated in millimeters of mercury. During blood pressure measurement, the unit must be kept upright on a flat surface and the gauge read at eye level. Breakage of the unit may cause dangerous mercury contamination and would require specialist removal for disposal. Due to the hazards of mercury, the use of mercury-based sphygmomanometers has declined sharply since 2000.
- An aneroid unit is mercury free and consists of a cuff that can be applied with one hand for self-testing; a stethoscope that is built in or attached; and a valve that inflates and deflates automatically with the data displayed on an easy-to-read gauge that will function in any position. The unit is sensitive and if dropped may require recalibration.
- An automatic unit is also mercury free and is typically battery operated. It has a cuff that can be applied with one hand for self-testing, and a valve that automatically inflates and deflates. Units with manual inflation are also available. The reading is displayed digitally and a stethoscope is not required. This is useful for persons who are hearing impaired, for emergency situations when staff is limited, and for automatic input into instruments for storage or graphical display. A wrist monitor is also available for home testing. Some more expensive models also remember and print out recordings. The automatic units tend to be more portable than bulkier mercury devices.

KEY TERMS

Aneroid monitor—A monitor that works without fluids, i.e. without mercury.

Blood pressure—The tension of the blood in the arteries, measured in millimeters of mercury (mm Hg) by a sphygmomanometer or by an electronic device.

Diastolic—Minimum arterial blood pressure during ventricular relaxation or rest.

Systolic—Maximum arterial blood pressure during ventricular contraction.

Operation

The flow, resistance, quality, and quantity of blood circulating through the heart and the condition of the arterial walls are all factors that influence blood pressure. If blood flow in the arteries is restricted, the reading will be higher.

Blood pressure should be routinely checked every one to two years. It can be checked at any time, but is best measured when a person has been resting for at least five minutes, so that exertion prior to the test will not unduly influence the outcome of the reading.

To record blood pressure, the person should be seated with one arm bent slightly, and the arm bare or with the sleeve loosely rolled up. With an aneroid or automatic unit, the cuff is placed level with the heart and wrapped around the upper arm, one inch above the elbow. Following the manufacturer's guidelines, the cuff is inflated and then deflated while an attendant records the reading.

If the blood pressure is monitored manually, a cuff is placed level with the heart and wrapped firmly but not tightly around the arm one inch (2–3 cm) above the elbow over the brachial artery. Wrinkles in the cuff should be smoothed out. Positioning a stethoscope over the brachial artery in front of the elbow with one hand and listening through the earpieces, the health professional inflates the cuff well above normal levels (to about 200 mm Hg), or until no sound is heard. Alternatively, the cuff should be inflated 10 mm Hg above the last sound heard. The valve in the pump is slowly opened. Air is allowed to escape no faster than 5 mm Hg per second to deflate the pressure in the cuff to the point where a clicking sound is heard over the brachial artery. The reading of the gauge at this point is recorded as the systolic pressure. The sounds continue as the pressure in the cuff is released and the flow of blood through the artery is no longer blocked. At this point, the noises are no longer heard. The reading of the gauge at this point is noted as the diastolic pressure. "Lub-dub" is the sound produced by the normal heart as it beats. Every time this sound is detected, it means that the heart is contracting once. The sounds are created when the heart valves click to close. When one hears "lub," the atrioventricular valves are closing. The "dub" sound is produced by the pulmonic and aortic valves.

With children, the clicking sound does not disappear but changes to a soft muffled sound. Because sounds continue to be heard as the cuff deflates to zero, the reading of the gauge at the point where the sounds change is recorded as the diastolic pressure.

Blood pressure readings are recorded with the systolic pressure first, then the diastolic pressure (e.g. 120/70).

Interpretation

Blood pressure readings must be interpreted in relation to a person's age, physical condition, medical history, and medications being used.

Maintenance

Devices should be checked and calibrated annually by a qualified technician to ensure accurate readings. This is especially important for automatic sphygmomanometers.

Normal results

One elevated reading does not mean that hypertension is present. Repeated measurements may be required if hypertension is suspected. The **blood pressure measurement** is recorded and compared with normal ranges for an individual's age and medical condition, and a decision is made on whether any further medical intervention is required.

Resources

BOOKS

Bickley, L. S., P. G. Szilagyi, and J. G. Stackhouse. *Bates' Guide to Physical Examination & History Taking*. 8th ed. Philadelphia: Lippincott Williams & Wilkins, 2002.

Chan, P. D., and P. J. Winkle. *History and Physical Examination in Medicine*. 10th ed. New York: Current Clinical Strategies, 2002.

Seidel, Henry M. *Mosby's Physical Examination Handbook*. 4th ed. St. Louis: Mosby-Year Book, 2003.

Swartz, Mark A., and William Schmitt. *Textbook of Physical Diagnosis: History and Examination*. 4th ed. Philadelphia: Saunders, 2001.

PERIODICALS

Doyle, L. W., B. Faber, C. Callanan, and R. Morley. "Blood Pressure in Late Adolescence and Very Low Birth Weight." *Pediatrics* 111, no. 2 (2003): 252–257.

Jones, D. W., L. J. Appel, S. G. Sheps, E. J. Roccella, and C. Lenfant. "Measuring Blood Pressure Accurately: New and Persistent Challenges." *Journal of the American Medical Association* 289, no. 8 (2003): 1027–1030.

O'Brien, E. "Demise of the Mercury Sphygmomanometer and the Dawning of a New Era in Blood Pressure Measurement." *Blood Pressure Monitoring* 8, no. 1 (2003): 19–21.

Pickering, T. G. "What Will Replace the Mercury Sphygmomanometer?" *Blood Pressure Monitoring* 8, no. 1 (2003): 23–25.

ORGANIZATIONS

American Academy of Family Physicians. 11400 Tomahawk Creek Parkway, Leawood, KS 66211-2672. (913) 906-6000. Email: fp@aafp.org. http://www.aafp.org.

American Academy of Pediatrics. 141 Northwest Point Boulevard, Elk Grove Village, IL 60007-1098. (847) 434-4000. Fax: (847) 434-8000. Email: kidsdoc@aap.org. http://www.aap.org/default.htm.

American College of Physicians. 190 N. Independence Mall West, Philadelphia, PA 19106-1572. (800) 523-1546, x 2600 or (215) 351-2600. http://www.acponline.org.

American Medical Association. 515 N. State Street, Chicago, IL 60610. (312) 464-5000. http://www.ama-assn.org.

OTHER

"High Blood Pressure." Medline Plus Health Information. [cited March 12, 2003]. http://www.nlm.nih.gov/medlineplus/highbloodpressure.html.

"Hypertension." The Franklin Institute Online. [cited March 12, 2003]. <http://sln.fi.edu/biosci/healthy/pressure.html>.

"Your Guide to Lowering High Blood Pressure." National Heart, Lung and Blood Institute (National Institutes of Health). [cited March 12, 2003]. http://www.nhlbi.nih.gov/hbp

L. Fleming Fallon, Jr., MD, DrPH

Sphygmomanometry *see* **Blood pressure measurement**

Spina bifida surgery *see* **Meningocele repair**

Spinal fluid analysis *see* **Cerebrospinal fluid (CSF) analysis**

Spinal fusion

Definition

Spinal fusion is a procedure that promotes the fusing, or growing together, of two or more vertebrae in the spine.

Purpose

Spinal fusion is performed to:

- Straighten a spine deformed by scoliosis, neuromuscular disease, cerebral palsy, or other disorder.
- Prevent further deformation.
- Support a spine weakened by infection or tumor.
- Reduce or prevent pain from pinched or injured nerves.
- Compensate for injured vertebrae or disks.

The goal of spinal fusion is to unite two or more vertebrae to prevent them from moving independently of each other. This may be done to improve posture, increase ability to ventilate the lungs, prevent pain, or treat spinal instability and reduce the risk of nerve damage.

Demographics

According to the American Academy of Orthopaedic Surgeons, approximately a quarter-million spinal fusions are performed each year, half on the upper and half on the lower spine.

Description

Spinal anatomy

The spine is a series of individual bones, called vertebrae, separated by cartilaginous disks. The spine is composed of seven cervical (neck) vertebrae, 12 thoracic (chest) vertebrae, five lumbar (lower back) vertebrae, and the fused vertebrae in the sacrum and coccyx that help to form the hip region.

While the shapes of individual vertebrae differ among these regions, each is essentially a short hollow tube containing the bundle of nerves known as the spinal cord. Individual nerves, such as those carrying messages to the arms or legs, enter and exit the spinal cord through gaps between vertebrae.

The spinal disks act as shock absorbers, cushioning the spine, and preventing individual bones from contacting each other. Disks also help to hold the vertebrae together.

The weight of the upper body is transferred through the spine to the hips and the legs. The spine is held upright through the work of the back muscles, which are attached to the vertebrae.

While the normal spine has no side-to-side curve, it does have a series of front-to-back curves, giving it a gentle "S" shape. The spine curves in at the lumbar region, back out at the thoracic region, and back in at the cervical region.

Surgery for scoliosis, neuromuscular disease, and cerebral palsy

Abnormal side-to-side curvature of the spine is termed scoliosis. An excessive lumbar curve is termed lordosis, and an excessive thoracic curve is kyphosis. "Idiopathic" scoliosis is the most common form of scoliosis; it has no known cause.

Scoliosis and other curves can be caused by neuromuscular disease, including Duchenne muscular dystrophy. Progressive and perhaps uneven weakening of the

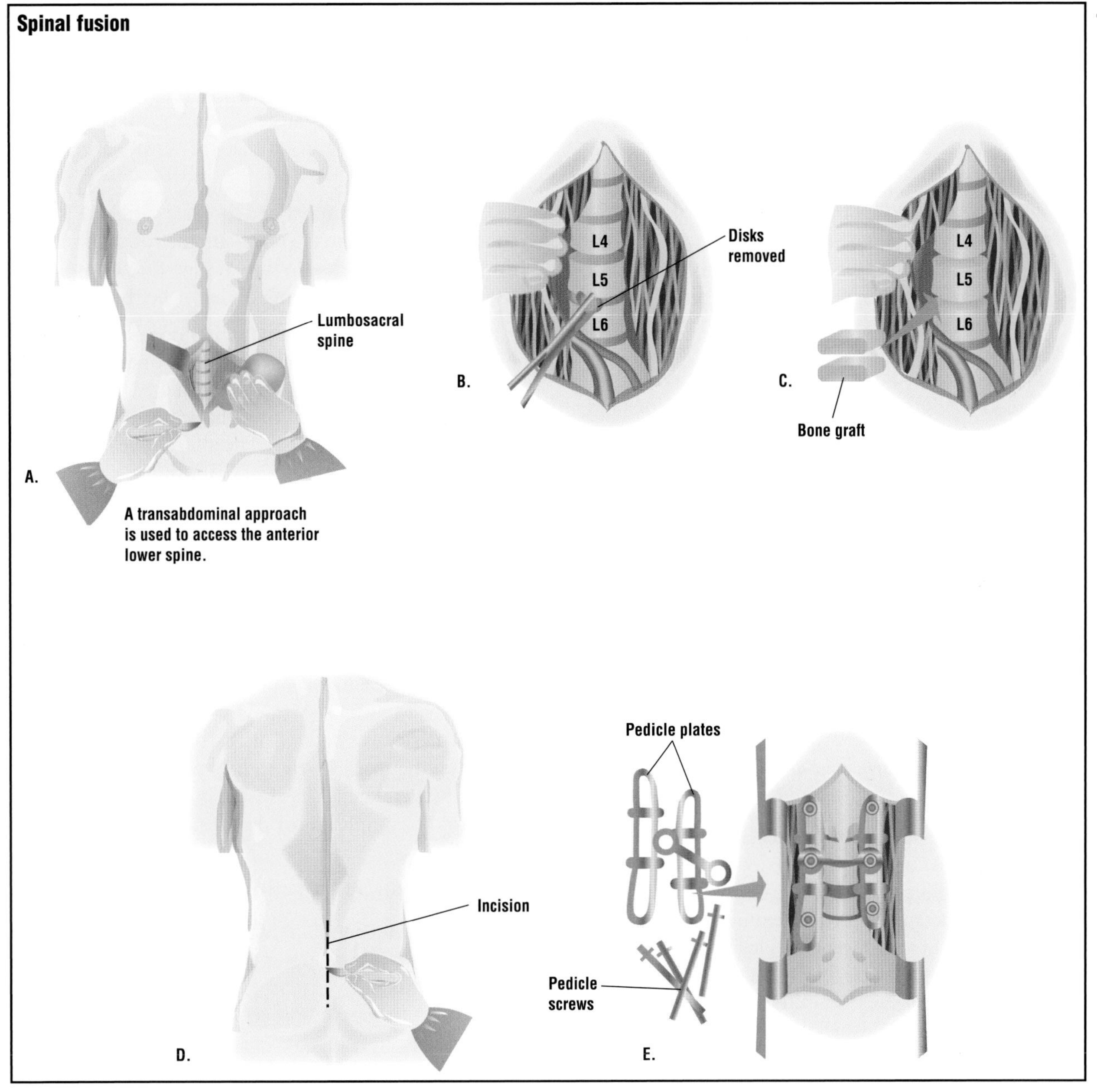

In this spinal fusion, the surgeon makes an incision in the lower abdomen to access the lumrosacral spine (A). The disks between the vertebrae are removed (B), and bone grafts are inserted into the spaces (C). Then another incision is made in the patient's back (D), and the vertebrae are exposed and fixed the pedicle plates and screws (E) *(Illustration by GGS Information Services. Cengage Learning, Gale.)*

spinal muscles leads to gradual inability to support the spine in an upright position. The weight of the upper body then begins to collapse the spine, inducing a curve. In addition to pain and disfigurement, severe scoliosis prevents adequate movement of air into and out of the lungs. Scoliosis also occurs in cerebral palsy, due to excess and imbalanced muscle activity pulling on the spine unevenly.

Idiopathic scoliosis, which occurs most often in adolescent girls, is usually managed with a brace that wraps the abdomen and chest, allowing the spine to develop straight. Spinal fusion is indicated in patients whose curves are more severe or are progressing rapidly. The indication for surgery in cerebral palsy is similar to that for idiopathic scoliosis.

KEY TERMS

Fusion—A union, joining together; e.g., bone fusion.

Herniated disk—A blister-like bulging or protrusion of the contents of the disk out through the fibers that normally hold them in place. Also called ruptured disk, slipped disk, or displaced disk.

Magnetic resonance imaging (MRI)—A test that provides pictures of organs and structures inside the body by using a magnetic field and pulses of radio wave energy to detect tumors, infection, and other types of tissue disease or damage, or conditions affecting blood flow. The area of the body being studied is positioned inside a strong magnetic field.

Vertebra—One of the bones that make up the back bone (spine).

Spinal fusion in Duchenne muscular dystrophy is usually indicated earlier than in otherwise healthy adolescents. This is because these patients lose ventilatory function rapidly through adolescence, making the surgery more dangerous as time passes. Surgery should occur before excess ventilatory function is lost.

Surgery for herniated disks, disk degeneration, and pain

As people age, their disks become less supple and more prone to damage. A herniated disk is one that has developed a bulge. The bulge can press against nerves located in the spinal cord or exiting from it, causing pain. Disks can also degenerate, losing mass and thickness, allowing vertebrae to contact each other. This can pinch nerves and cause pain. Disk-related pain is very common in the neck, which is subject to constant twisting forces, and the lower back, which experiences large compressive forces. In these cases, spinal fusion is employed to prevent the nerves from being damaged. The offending disk is removed at the same time. A fractured vertebra may also be treated with fusion to prevent it from causing future problems.

Sometimes, spinal fusion is used to treat back pain even when the anatomical source of the problem cannot be located. This is usually viewed as a last resort for intractable and disabling pain.

The spinal fusion operation

Spinal fusion is performed under **general anesthesia**. During the procedure, the target vertebrae are exposed. Protective tissue layers next to the bone are removed, and small chips of bone are placed next to the vertebrae. These bone chips can either be from the patient's hip or from a bone bank. The chips increase the rate of fusion. Using bone from the patient's hip (an autograft) is more successful than banked bone (an allograft), but it increases the stresses of surgery and loss of blood.

Fusion of the lumbar and thoracic vertebrae is done by approaching from the rear, with the patient lying face down. Cervical fusion is typically performed from the front, with the patient lying on his or her back.

Many spinal fusion patients also receive **spinal instrumentation**. During the fusion operation, a set of rods, wires, or screws will be attached to the spine. This instrumentation allows the spine to be held in place while the bones fuse. The alternative is an external brace applied after the operation.

An experimental treatment, called human recombinant bone morphogenetic protein-2, has shown promise for its ability to accelerate fusion rates without bone chips and instrumentation. This technique is only available through clinical trials at a few medical centers.

Spinal fusion surgery takes approximately four hours. The patient is intubated (tube placed in the trachea), and has an IV line and Foley (urinary) catheter in place. At the end of the operation, a drain is placed in the incision site to help withdraw fluids over the next several days. The fusion process is gradual and may not be completed for months after the operation.

Diagnosis/Preparation

A potential candidate for spinal fusion undergoes a long series of medical tests. In patients with scoliosis, x rays are taken over many months or years to track progress of the curve. Patients with disk herniation or degeneration may receive x rays, MRI studies, or other tests to determine the location and extent of injury.

Patients in good health may donate several units of their own blood in preparation for surgery. This may be done between six weeks and one week prior to the operation. The patient will probably be advised to take iron supplements to help replace lost iron in the donated blood. Sunburn or sores on the back should be avoided prior to surgery because they increase the risk of infection.

A variety of medical tests will be done shortly before surgery to ensure that the patient is in good health and prepared for the rigors of surgery. Blood and urine tests, x rays, and possibly photographs documenting the curvature will be done. An electroencephalogram (EEG) may be performed to test nerve function along the spine.

WHO PERFORMS THE PROCEDURE AND WHERE IS IT PERFORMED?

Spinal fusion is performed by an orthopedic surgeon or neurosurgeon in a hospital setting.

The patient will be admitted to the hospital the evening before surgery. No food is allowed after midnight in order to clear the gastrointestinal tract, which will be immobilized by anesthesia.

Aftercare

The patient will stay in the hospital for four to six days after the operation.

Post-operative pain is managed by intravenous pain medication. Many centers use **patient-controlled analgesia** (PCA) pumps, which allow patients to control the timing of pain medication.

For several days after the operation, the patient is unable to eat or drink because of the lasting effects of the anesthesia on the bowels. Fluids and nutrition are delivered via the IV line.

The nurse helps the patient sit up several times per day, and assists with other needs as well. Physical therapy begins several days after the operation.

Most activities are restricted for several weeks. Strenuous activities such as bike riding or running are usually resumed after six to eight months. The surgical incision should be protected from sunburn for approximately one year to promote healing of the scar.

Risks

Spinal fusion carries a risk of nerve damage. Rarely, delayed paralysis can occur, probably from loss of oxygen to the spine during surgery. Infection may occur. Bone from the bone bank carries a small risk of infection with transmissible diseases from the bone donor. Anesthesia also poses risks. Unsuccessful fusion (pseudoarthrosis) may occur, leaving the patient with the same problem after the operation.

Normal results

Spinal fusion for scoliosis is usually very successful in partially or completely correcting the deformity. Spinal fusion for pain is less uniformly successful because the cause of the pain cannot always be completely identified.

QUESTIONS TO ASK THE DOCTOR

How long will hospitalization be necessary?

Will patient-controlled analgesia (PCA) be used for pain?

How soon can the normal regime of school or work be resumed?

What outcome is expected?

Is there an alternative to surgery?

Morbidity and mortality rates

Unsuccessful fusion may occur in 5–25% of patients. Neurologic injury occurs in less than 1–5% of patients. Infection occurs in 1–8%. **Death** occurs in less than 1% of patients.

Alternatives

Bracing and "watchful waiting" is the alternative to scoliosis surgery. Disk surgery without fusion is possible for some patients. Strengthening exercises and physical therapy may help some back pain patients avoid back surgery.

Resources

BOOKS

Neuwirth, M.D., Michael. *The Scoliosis Sourcebook*. New York: McGraw-Hill, 2001.

PERIODICALS

Robinson, Richard. "Setting the Record Straight." *Quest Magazine* 4, no.1 (1997). http://www.mdausa.org/publications/Quest/q41scoliosis.html

ORGANIZATIONS

National Scoliosis Foundation. (800) NSF-MYBACK (673-6922). http://www.scoliosis.org.

Richard Robinson

Spinal instrumentation

Definition

Spinal instrumentation is a method of keeping the spine rigid after **spinal fusion** surgery by surgically attaching hooks, rods, and wire to the spine in a way that redistributes the stresses on the bones and keeps them in proper alignment while the bones of the spine fuse.

Purpose

Spinal instrumentation is used to treat instability and deformity of the spine. Instability occurs when the spine no longer maintains its normal shape during movement. Such instability results in nerve damage, spinal deformities, and disabling pain. Scoliosis is a side-to-side spinal curvature. Kyphosis is a front-to-back curvature of the upper spine, while lordosis is an excessive curve of the lower spine. More than one type of curve may be present.

Demographics

Spinal deformities may be caused by:

- birth defects
- fractures
- Marfan syndrome
- neurofibromatosis
- neuromuscular diseases
- severe injuries
- tumors
- idiopathic scoliosis (Idiopathic scoliosis is scoliosis of unknown origin. About 85% of cases occur in girls between the ages of 12 and 15 who are experiencing adolescent growth spurt.)

Description

Spinal instrumentation provides a stable, rigid column that encourages bones to fuse after spinal fusion surgery. Its purpose is to aid fusion. Without fusion, the metal will eventually fatigue and break, and so instrumentation is not itself a treatment for spine deformity.

Different types of spinal instrumentation are used to treat different spinal problems. Although the details of the insertion of rods, wires, screws, and hooks vary, the purpose of all spinal instrumentation is the same—to correct and stabilize the backbone while the bones of the spine fuse. The various instruments are all made of stainless steel, titanium, or titanium alloy.

The oldest form of spinal instrumentation is the Harrington rod. While it was simple in design, it required a long period of brace wearing after the operation, and did not allow segmental adjustment of correction. The Luque rod was developed to avoid the long postoperative bracing period. This system threads wires into the space within each vertebra. The risk of injury to the nerves and spinal cord is higher than with some other forms of instrumentation. Cotrel-Dubousset instrumentation uses hooks and rods in a cross-linked pattern to realign the spine and redistribute the biomechanical stress. The main advantage of Cotrel-Dubousset instrumentation is that because of the extensive cross-linking, the patient may not have to wear a cast or brace after surgery. The disadvantage is the complexity of the operation and the number of hooks and cross-links that may fail.

Several newer systems use screws that are embedded into the portion of the vertebra called the pedicle. Pedicle screws avoid the need for threading wires, but carry the risk of migrating out of the bone and contacting the spinal cord or the aorta (the major blood vessel exiting the heart). During the late 1990s, pedicle screws were the subject of several high-profile lawsuits. The controversies have since subsided, and pedicle screws remain an indispensible part of the spinal instrumentation. Many operations today are performed with a mix of techniques, such as Luque rods in the lower back and hooks and screws up higher. A physician chooses the proper type of instrumentation based on the type of disorder, the age and health of the patient, and the physician's experience.

The surgeon strips the tissue away from the area to be fused. The surface of the bone is peeled away. A piece of bone is removed from the hip and placed along side the area to be fused. The stripping of the bone helps the bone graft to fuse.

After the fusion site is prepared, the rods, hooks, screws, and wires are inserted. There is much variation in how this is done based on the spinal instrumentation chosen. Once the rods are in place, the incision is closed.

KEY TERMS

Lumbar vertebrae—The vertebrae of the lower back below the level of the ribs.

Marfan syndrome—A rare hereditary defect that affects the connective tissue.

Neurofibromatosis—A rare hereditary disease that involves the growth of lesions that may affect the spinal cord.

Osteoporosis—A bone disorder, usually seen in the elderly, in which the bones become increasingly less dense and more brittle.

Spinal fusion—An operation in which the bones of the spine are permanently joined together using a bone graft obtained usually from the hip.

Thoracic vertebrae—The vertebrae in the chest region to which the ribs attach.

WHO PERFORMS THE PROCEDURE AND WHERE IS IT PERFORMED?

Spinal instrumentation is performed by a neurosurgical and/or orthopedic surgical team with special experience in spinal operations. The surgery is done in a hospital under general anesthesia. It is done at the same time as spinal fusion.

QUESTIONS TO ASK THE DOCTOR

- What types of instrumentation will I be receiving?
- Why is this the best choice for my condition?
- How long will I be immobilized?
- Should I receive physical therapy to help me regain lost strength and mobility?

Diagnosis/Preparation

Spinal fusion with spinal instrumentation is major surgery. The patient will undergo many tests to determine the nature and exact location of the back problem. These tests are likely to include

- x rays
- magnetic resonance imaging (MRI)
- computed tomography scans (CT scans)
- myleograms

In addition, the patient will undergo a battery of blood and urine tests, and possibly an **electrocardiogram** to provide the surgeon and anesthesiologist with information that will allow the operation to be performed safely. In Harrington rod instrumentation, the patient may be placed in **traction** or an upper body cast to stretch contracted muscles before surgery.

Aftercare

After surgery, the patient will be confined to bed. A catheter is inserted so that the patient can urinate without getting up. **Vital signs** are monitored, and the patient's position is changed frequently so that **bedsores** do not develop.

Recovery from spinal instrumentation can be a long, arduous process. Movement is severely limited for a period of time. In certain types of instrumentation, the patient is put in a cast to allow the realigned bones to stay in position until healing takes place. This can be as long as six to eight months. Many patients will need to wear a brace after the cast is removed.

During the recovery period, the patient is taught respiratory exercises to help maintain respiratory function during the time of limited mobility. Physical therapists assist the patient in learning self-care and in performing strengthening and range-of-motion exercises. **Length of hospital stay** depends on the age and health of the patient, as well as the specific problem that was corrected. The patient can expect to remain under a physician's care for many months.

Risks

Spinal instrumentation carries a significant risk of nerve damage and paralysis. The skill of the surgeon can affect the outcome of the operation, so patients should look for a hospital and **surgical team** that has a lot of experience doing spinal procedures.

Since the hooks and rods of spinal instrumentation are anchored in the bones of the back, spinal instrumentation should not be performed on people with serious osteoporosis. To overcome this limitation, techniques are being explored that help anchor instrumentation in fragile bones.

After surgery there is a risk of infection or an inflammatory reaction due to the presence of the foreign material in the body. Serious infection of the membranes covering the spinal cord and brain can occur. In the long term, the instrumentation may move or break, causing nerve damage and requiring a second surgery. Some bone grafts do not heal well, lengthening the time the patient must spend in a cast or brace or necessitating additional surgery. Casting and wearing a brace may take an emotional toll, especially on young people. Patients who have had spinal instrumentation must avoid contact sports, and, for the rest of their lives, eliminate situations that will abnormally put stress on their spines.

Normal results

Many young people with scoliosis heal with significantly improved alignment of the spine. Results of spinal instrumentation done for other conditions vary widely.

Morbidity and mortality rates

Mortality rate for spinal fusion surgery is less than 1%. Neurologic injury may occur in 1–5% of cases. Delayed paralysis is possible but rare.

Alternatives

Not all patients require instrumentation with their spinal fusion. For some patients, a rigid external brace can provide the required rigidity to allow the bones to fuse.

Resources

BOOKS

"Cotrel-Dubousset Spinal Instrumentation." In *Everything You Need to Know About Medical Treatments.* Springhouse, PA: Springhouse Corp., 1996.

"Harrington Rod." In *Everything You Need to Know About Medical Treatments.* Springhouse, PA: Springhouse Corp., 1996.

ORGANIZATIONS

National Scoliosis Foundation. 5 Cabot Place, Stoughton, MA 020724. (800) 673-6922. http://www.scoliosis.org

OTHER

Orthogate [cited July 1, 2003]. <http://owl.orthogate.org/>.

Tish Davidson, A.M.
Richard Robinson

Spinal tap *see* **Cerebrospinal fluid (CSF) analysis**

Spirometry tests

Definition

Spirometry is the measurement of air flow into and out of the lungs.

Description

Spirometry requires that the nose is pinched off as the patient breathes through a mouthpiece attached to the spirometer. The patient is instructed on how to breathe during the procedure. Three breathing maneuvers are practiced before recording the procedure, and the highest of three trials is used for evaluation of breathing. This procedure measures air flow by electronic or mechanical displacement principles, and uses a microprocessor and recorder to calculate and plot air flow.

The test produces a recording of the patient's ventilation under conditions involving both normal and maximal effort. The recording, called a spirogram, shows the volume of air moved and the rate at which it travels into and out of the lungs. Spirometry measures several lung capacities. Accurate measurement is dependent upon the patient performing the appropriate maneuver properly. The most common measurements are:

- Vital capacity (VC). This is the amount of air (in liters) moved out of the lung during normal breathing. The patient is instructed to breathe in and out normally to attain full expiration. Vital capacity is usually about 80% of the total lung capacity. Because of the elastic nature of the lungs and surrounding thorax, a small volume of air will remain in the lungs after full exhalation. This volume is called the residual volume (RV).
- Forced vital capacity (FVC). After breathing out normally to full expiration, the patient is instructed to breathe in with a maximal effort and then exhale as forcefully and rapidly as possible. The FVC is the volume of air that is expelled into the spirometer following a maximum inhalation effort.
- Forced expiratory volume (FEV). At the start of the FVC maneuver, the spirometer measures the volume of air delivered through the mouthpiece at timed intervals of 0.5, 1.0, 2.0, and 3.0 seconds. The sum of these measurements normally constitutes about 97% of the FVC measurement. The most commonly used FEV measurement is FEV-1, which is the volume of air exhaled into the mouthpiece in one second. The FEV-1 should be at least 70% of the FVC.
- Forced expiratory flow 25–75% (FEF 25–75). This is a calculation of the average flow rate over the center portion of the forced expiratory volume recording. It is determined from the time in seconds at which 25% and 75% of the vital capacity is reached. The volume of air exhaled in liters per second between these two times is the FEF 25–75. This value reflects the status of the medium and small sized airways.
- Maximal voluntary ventilation (MVV). This maneuver involves the patient breathing as deeply and as rapidly as possible for 15 seconds. The average air flow (liters per second) indicates the strength and endurance of the respiratory muscles.

Normal values for FVC, FEV, FEF, and MVV are dependent on the patient's age, gender, and height.

Purpose

Spirometry is the most commonly performed pulmonary function test (PFT). The test can be performed at the bedside, in a physician's office, or in a pulmonary laboratory. It is often the first test performed when a problem with lung function is suspected. Spirometry may also be suggested by an abnormal x ray, arterial blood gas analysis, or other diagnostic pulmonary test result. The National Lung Health Education Program

KEY TERMS

Bronchodilator—A drug, usually self-administered by inhalation, that dilates the airways.

Forced expiratory volume (FEV)—The volume of air exhaled from the beginning of expiration to a set time (usually 0.5, 1, 2, and 3 seconds).

Forced vital capacity (FVC)—The volume of air that can be exhaled forceably after a maximal inspiration.

Hemoptysis—Spitting up of blood derived from the lungs or bronchial tubes as a result of pulmonary or bronchial hemorrhage.

Thrombosis—Formation or presence of a thrombus; clotting within a blood vessel that may cause infarction of tissues supplied by the vessel.

Thrombotic—Relating to, caused by, or characterized by thrombosis.

Vital capacity (VC)—The volume of air that can be exhaled following a full inspiration.

recommends that regular spirometry tests be performed on persons over 45 years old who have a history of smoking. Spirometry tests are also recommended for persons with a family history of lung disease, chronic respiratory ailments, and advanced age.

Spirometry measures ventilation, the movement of air into and out of the lungs. The spirogram will identify two different types of abnormal ventilation patterns, obstructive and restrictive.

Common causes of an obstructive pattern are cystic fibrosis, asthma, bronchiectasis, bronchitis, and emphysema. These conditions may be collectively referred to by using the acronym CABBE. Chronic bronchitis, emphysema, and asthma result in dyspnea (difficulty breathing) and ventilation deficiency, a condition known as chronic obstructive pulmonary disease (COPD). COPD is the fourth leading cause of **death** among Americans.

Common causes of a restrictive pattern are pneumonia, heart disease, pregnancy, lung fibrosis, pneumothorax (collapsed lung), and pleural effusion (compression caused by chest fluid).

Obstructive and restrictive patterns can be identified on spirographs using both a "y" and "x" axis. Volume (liters) is plotted on the y-axis versus time (seconds) on the x-axis. A restrictive pattern is characterized by a normal shape showing reduced volumes for all parameters. The reduction in volumes indicates the severity of the disease. An obstructive pattern produces a spirogram with an abnormal shape. Inspiration volume is reduced. The volume of air expelled is normal but the air flow rate is slower, causing an elongated tail to the FVC.

A flow-volume loop spirogram is another way of displaying spirometry measurements. This requires the FVC maneuver followed by a forced inspiratory volume (FIV). Flow rate in liters per second is plotted on the y-axis and volume (liters) is plotted on the x-axis. The expiration phase is shown on top and the inspiration phase on the bottom. The flow-volume loop spirogram is helpful in diagnosing upper airway obstruction, and can differentiate some types of restrictive patterns.

Some conditions produce specific signs on the spirogram. Irregular inspirations with rapid frequency are caused by hyperventilation associated with stress. Diffuse fibrosis of the lung causes rapid breathing of reduced volume, which produces a repetitive pattern known as the penmanship sign. Serial reduction in the FVC peaks indicates air trapped inside the lung. A notch and reduced volume in the early segments of the FVC is consistent with airway collapse. A rise at the end of expiration is associated with airway resistance.

Spirometry is used to assess lung function over time, and often to evaluate the efficacy of bronchodilator inhalers such as albuterol. It is important for the patient to refrain from using a bronchodilator prior to the evaluation. Spirometry is performed before and after inhaling the bronchodilator. In general, a 12% or greater improvement in both FVC and FEV-1, or an increase in FVC by 0.2 liters, is considered a significant improvement for an adult patient.

Precautions

The patient should inform the physician of any medications he or she is taking, or of any medical conditions that are present; these factors may affect the validity of the test. The patient's smoking habits and history should be thoroughly documented. The patient must be able to understand and respond to instructions for the breathing maneuvers. Therefore, the test may not be appropriate for very young, unresponsive, or physically impaired persons.

Spirometry is contraindicated in patients whose condition will be aggravated by forced breathing, including:

- hemoptysis (spitting up blood from the lungs or bronchial tubes)
- pneumothorax (free air or gas in the pleural cavity)
- recent heart attack
- unstable angina
- aneurysm (cranial, thoracic, or abdominal)

- thrombotic condition (such as clotting within a blood vessel)
- recent thoracic or abdominal surgery
- nausea or vomiting

The test should be terminated if the patient shows signs of significant head, chest, or abdominal pain while the procedure is in progress.

Spirometry is dependent upon the patient's full compliance with breathing instructions, especially his or her willingness to extend a maximal effort at forced breathing. Therefore, the patient's emotional state must be considered.

Preparation

The patient's age, gender, and race are recorded, and height and weight are measured before the procedure begins. The patient should not have eaten heavily within three hours of the test. He or she should be instructed to wear clothing that fits loosely over the chest and abdominal area. The respiratory therapist or other testing personnel should explain and demonstrate the breathing maneuvers to the patient. The patient should practice breathing into the mouthpiece until he or she is able to duplicate the maneuvers successfully on two consecutive attempts.

Aftercare

In most cases, special care is not required following spirometry. Occasionally, a patient may become lightheaded or dizzy. Such patients should be asked to rest or lie down, and should not be discharged until after the symptoms subside. In rare cases, the patient may experience pneumothorax, intracranial hypertension, chest pain, or uncontrolled coughing. In such cases, additional care directed by a physician may be required.

Normal results

The results of spirometry tests are compared to predicted values based on the patient's age, gender, and height. For example, a young adult in good health is expected to have the following FEV values:

- FEV-0.5—50-60% of FVC
- FEV-1—75-85% of FVC
- FEV-2—95% of FVC
- FEV-3—97% of FVC

In general, a normal result is 80–100% of the predicted value. Abnormal values are:

- mild lung dysfunction—60–79%
- moderate lung dysfunction—40–59%
- severe lung dysfunction—below 40%

QUESTIONS TO ASK THE DOCTOR

What preparation is needed before the test?

What results are expected?

When will the results be available?

What are the risks of the test in this particular case?

Resources

BOOKS

Braunwald, Eugene et al., editors. *Harrison's Principles of Internal Medicine*. Philadelphia: McGraw-Hill, 2001.

PERIODICALS

Blonshine, S. and J.B. Fink. "Spirometry: Asthma and COPD Guidelines Creating Opportunities for RTs." *AARC Times* (January 2000): 43-7.

ORGANIZATIONS

National Lung Health Education Program (NLHEP). 1850 High Street, Denver, CO 80218. http://www.nlhep.org.

OTHER

Gary, T., et al. "Office Spirometry for Lung Health Assessment in Adults: A Consensus Statement for the National Lung Health Education Program." (March 2000): 1146-61.

National Institutes of Health. [cited April 4, 2003] http://www.nlm.nih.gov/medlineplus/encyclopedia.html.

"Spirometry—AARC Clinical Practice Guide." American Association for Respiratory Care. 1130 Ables Lane, Dallas, TX 75229. [cited April 4, 2003] http://www.muhealth.org/~shrp/rtwww/rcweb/aarc/spirocpg.html.

Robert Harr
Paul Johnson
Mark A. Best

Spleen removal *see* **Splenectomy**

Splenectomy

Definition

A splenectomy is the total or partial surgical removal of the spleen, an organ that is part of the lymphatic system.

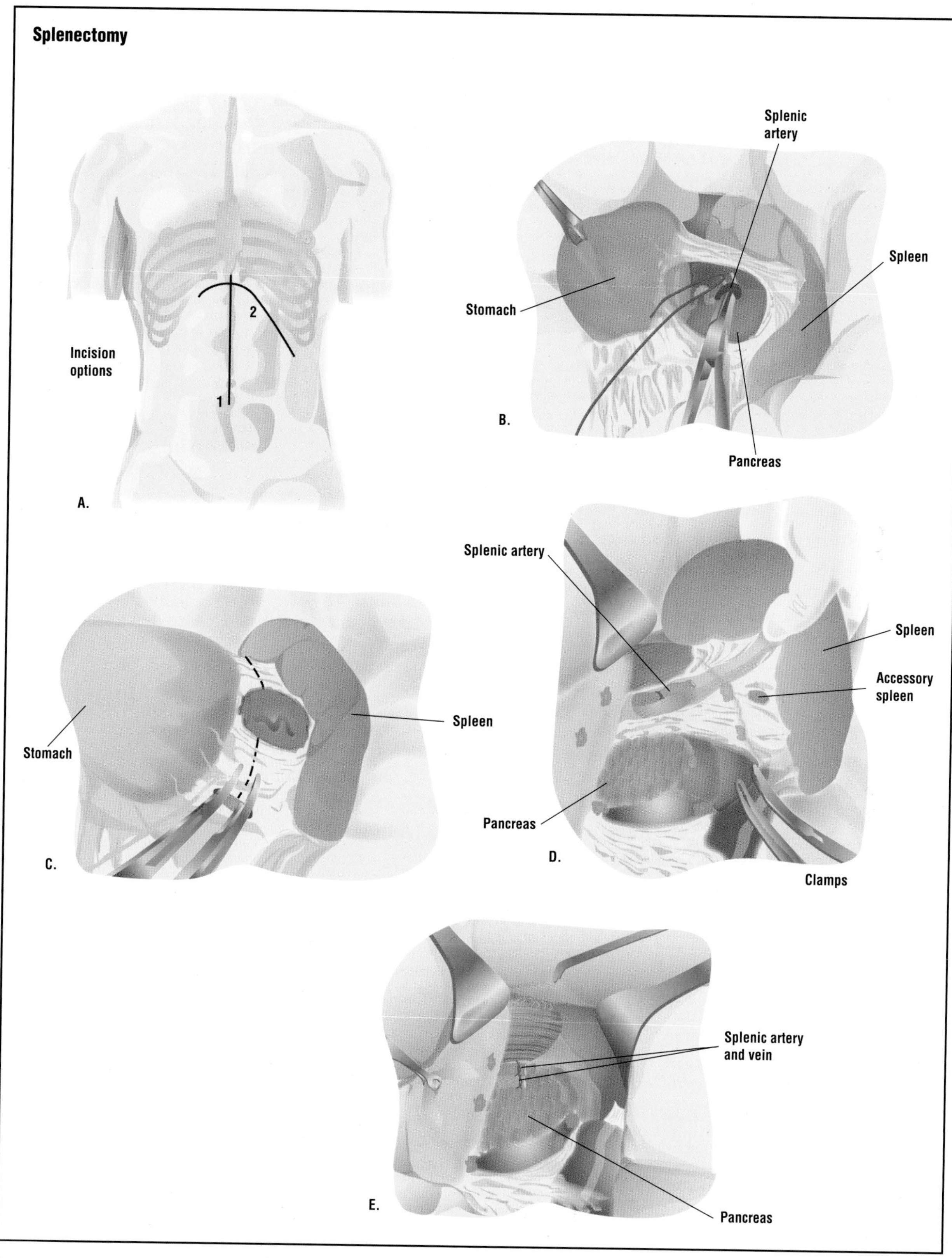

There are two options for accessing the spleen for a splenectomy (A, 1 and 2). After the abdomen is entered, the spleen is located, and the artery leading to it is tied off (B). The ligament connecting the stomach and spleen is cut (C), as is the ligament connecting the spleen and colon (D). This frees the spleen for removal (E). *(Illustration by GGS Information Services. Cengage Learning, Gale.)*

Purpose

The human spleen is a dark purple, bean-shaped organ located in the upper left side of the abdomen just behind the bottom of the rib cage. In adults, the spleen is about 4.8 X 2.8 X 1.6 in (12 X 7 X 4 cm) in size, and weighs about 4–5 oz (113–141 g). The spleen plays a role in the immune system of the body. It also filters foreign substances from the blood and removes worn-out blood cells. The spleen regulates blood flow to the liver and sometimes stores blood cells—a function known as sequestration. In healthy adults, about 30% of blood platelets are sequestered in the spleen.

Splenectomies are performed for a variety of different reasons and with different degrees of urgency. Most splenectomies are done after a patient has been diagnosed with hypersplenism. Hypersplenism is not a specific disease but a syndrome (group or cluster of symptoms) that may be associated with different disorders. Hypersplenism is characterized by enlargement of the spleen (splenomegaly), defects in the blood cells, and an abnormally high turnover of blood cells. It is almost always associated with such specific disorders as cirrhosis of the liver or certain cancers. The decision to perform a splenectomy depends on the severity and prognosis of the disease that is causing the hypersplenism.

Splenectomy always required

There are two diseases for which a splenectomy is the only treatment—primary cancers of the spleen and a blood disorder called hereditary spherocytosis (HS). In HS, the absence of a specific protein in the red blood cell membrane leads to the formation of relatively fragile cells that are easily damaged when they pass through the spleen. The cell destruction does not occur elsewhere in the body and ends when the spleen is removed. HS can appear at any age, even in newborns, although doctors prefer to put off removing the spleen until the child is five to six years old.

Splenectomy usually required

There are some disorders for which a splenectomy is usually recommended. They include:

- Immune (idiopathic) thrombocytopenic purpura (ITP). ITP is a disease in which platelets are destroyed by antibodies in the body's immune system. A splenectomy is the definitive treatment for this disease and is effective in about 70% of cases of chronic ITP.
- Trauma. The spleen can be ruptured by blunt as well as penetrating injuries to the chest or abdomen. Car accidents are the most common cause of blunt traumatic injury to the spleen.
- Abscesses. Abscesses of the spleen are relatively uncommon but have a high mortality rate.
- Rupture of the splenic artery. This artery sometimes ruptures as a complication of pregnancy.
- Hereditary elliptocytosis. This is a relatively rare disorder. It is similar to HS in that it is characterized by red blood cells with defective membranes that are destroyed by the spleen.

Splenectomy sometimes required

Other disorders may or may not necessitate a splenectomy. These include:

- Hodgkin's disease, a serious form of cancer that causes the lymph nodes to enlarge. A splenectomy is often performed in order to find out how far the disease has progressed.
- Autoimmune hemolytic disorders. These disorders may appear in patients of any age but are most common in adults over 50. The red blood cells are destroyed by antibodies produced by the patient's own body (autoantibodies).
- Myelofibrosis. Myelofibrosis is a disorder in which bone marrow is replaced by fibrous tissue. It produces severe and painful splenomegaly. A splenectomy does not cure myelofibrosis but may be performed to relieve pain caused by the swelling of the spleen.
- Thalassemia. Thalassemia is a hereditary form of anemia that is most common in people of Mediterranean origin. A splenectomy is sometimes performed if the patient's spleen has become painfully enlarged.

Demographics

In the United States, splenomegaly affects as many as 30% of full-term newborns and about 10% of healthy children. Approximately 3% of healthy first-year college students also have spleens that are large enough to be felt when a doctor palpates the abdomen. Some specific causes of splenomegaly are more common in certain racial or ethnic groups. For example, splenomegaly is a common complication of sickle cell disease in patients of African or Mediterranean ancestry. In other parts of the world, splenomegaly is frequently caused by malaria, schistosomiasis, and other infections in areas where these diseases are endemic.

Hereditary spherocytosis (HS) is a disorder is most common in people of northern European descent but has been found in all races. A family history of HS increases the risk of developing this disorder.

Immune thrombocytopenic purpura (ITP) is much more common in children, with male and female children being equally afflicted. Female predominance

KEY TERMS

Computed tomography (CT) scan—An imaging technique that creates a series of pictures of areas inside the body, taken from different angles. The pictures are created by a computer linked to an x-ray machine.

Embolization—A treatment in which foam, silicone, or other substance is injected into a blood vessel in order to close it off.

Endemic—Present in a specific population or geographical area at all times. Some diseases that may affect the spleen are endemic to certain parts of Africa or Asia.

Hereditary spherocytosis—A hereditary disorder that leads to a chronic form of anemia (too few red blood cells) due to an abnormality in the red blood cell membrane.

Idiopathic thrombocytopenia purpura (ITP)—A rare autoimmune disorder characterised by an acute shortage of platelets with resultant bruising and spontaneous bleeding.

Laparoscopy—A procedure in which a laparoscope (a thin, lighted tube) is inserted through an incision in the abdominal wall to evaluate the presence or spread of disease. Tissue samples may be removed for biopsy.

Lymphatic system—The tissues and organs that produce and store cells that fight infection, together with the network of vessels that carry lymph. The organs and tissues in the lymphatic system include the bone marrow, spleen, thymus gland, and lymph nodes.

Palpate—To examine by means of touch.

Platelet—A disk-shaped structure found in blood that binds to fibrinogen at the site of a wound to begin the clotting process.

Sequestration—A process in which the spleen withdraws blood cells from the circulation and stores them.

Spleen—An organ that produces lymphocytes, filters the blood, stores blood cells and destroys those that are aging. It is located on the left side of the abdomen near the stomach.

Splenomegaly—Enlargement of the spleen.

begins at puberty and continues in adult patients. Overall, 70% of patients with ITP are female; 72% of women diagnosed with ITP are over 40 years old.

Description

Complete splenectomy

REMOVAL OF ENLARGED SPLEEN. A splenectomy is performed under **general anesthesia**. The most common technique is used to remove greatly enlarged spleens. After the surgeon makes a cut (incision) in the abdomen, the artery to the spleen is tied to prevent blood loss and reduce the size of the spleen. Tying the splenic artery also keeps the spleen from further sequestration of blood cells. The surgeon detaches the ligaments holding the spleen in place and removes the organ. In many cases, tissue samples will be sent to a laboratory for analysis.

REMOVAL OF RUPTURED SPLEEN. When the spleen has been ruptured by trauma, the surgeon approaches the organ from its underside and ties the splenic artery before removing the ruptured organ.

Partial splenectomy

In some cases, the surgeon removes only part of the spleen. This procedure is considered by some to be a useful compromise that reduces pain caused by an enlarged spleen while leaving the patient less vulnerable to infection.

Laparoscopic splenectomy

Laparoscopic splenectomy, or removal of the spleen through several small incisions, has been performed more frequently in recent years. Laparoscopic surgery, which is sometimes called keyhole surgery, is done with smaller **surgical instruments** inserted through very short incisions, with the assistance of a tiny camera and video monitor. Laparoscopic procedures reduce the **length of hospital stay**, the level of postoperative pain, and the risk of infection. They also leave smaller scars.

As of 2003, however, a laparoscopic procedure is contraindicated if the patient's spleen is greatly enlarged. Most surgeons will not remove a spleen longer than 20 cm (as measured by a CT scan) by this method.

Diagnosis/Preparation

The most important part of a medical assessment in disorders of the spleen is the measurement of splenomegaly. The normal spleen cannot be felt when the doctor palpates the patient's abdomen. A spleen that is large enough to be felt indicates splenomegaly. In some cases, the doctor will hear a dull sound when he or she thumps (percusses) the patient's abdomen near the ribs on the left side. Imaging studies that can be used to confirm splenomegaly include **ultrasound** tests, technetium-99m sulfur colloid imaging, and **CT scans**. The rate of platelet or red blood cell destruction by the spleen can also be measured by tagging blood cells with radioactive chromium or platelets with radioactive indium.

Preoperative preparation for a splenectomy procedure usually includes:

- Correction of abnormalities of blood clotting and the number of red blood cells.
- Treatment of any infections.
- Control of immune reactions. Patients are usually given protective vaccinations about a month before surgery. The most common vaccines used are Pneumovax or Pnu-Imune 23 (against pneumococcal infections) and Menomune-A/C/Y/W-135 (against meningococcal infections).

Aftercare

Immediately following surgery, patients are given instructions for **incision care** and medications intended to prevent infection. Blood transfusions may be indicated for some patients to replace defective blood cells. The most important part of aftercare, however, is long-term caution regarding vulnerability to infection. Patients are asked to see their doctor at once if they have a fever or any other sign of infection, and to avoid travel to areas where exposure to malaria or similar diseases is likely. Children with splenectomies may be kept on antibiotic therapy until they are 16 years old. All patients can be given a booster dose of pneumococcal vaccine five to 10 years after undergoing a splenectomy.

Risks

The main risk of a splenectomy procedure is overwhelming bacterial infection, or postsplenectomy sepsis. This condition results from the body's decreased ability to clear bacteria from the blood, and lowered levels of a protein in blood plasma that helps to fight viruses (immunoglobulin M). The risk of **dying** from infection after undergoing a splenectomy is highest in children, especially in the first two years after surgery. The risk of postsplenectomy sepsis can be reduced by vaccinations before the operation. Some doctors also recommend a two-year course of penicillin following splenectomy, or long-term treatment with ampicillin.

WHO PERFORMS THE PROCEDURE AND WHERE IS IT PERFORMED?

A splenectomy is performed by a surgeon trained in gastroenterology, the branch of medicine that deals with the diseases of the digestive tract. An anesthesiologist is responsible for administering anesthesia and the operation is performed in a hospital setting.

Other risks associated with the procedure include inflammation of the pancreas and collapse of the lungs. In some cases, a splenectomy does not address the underlying causes of splenomegaly or other conditions. Excessive bleeding after the operation is an additional possible complication, particularly for patients with ITP. Infection of the incision immediately following surgery may also occur.

Normal results

Results depend on the reason for the operation. In blood disorders, the splenectomy will remove the cause of the blood cell destruction. Normal results for patients with an enlarged spleen are relief of pain and the complications of splenomegaly. It is not always possible, however, to predict which patients will respond well or to what degree.

Recovery from the operation itself is fairly rapid. Hospitalization is usually less than a week (one to two days for laparoscopic splenectomy), and complete healing usually occurs within four to six weeks. Patients are encouraged to return to such normal activities as showering, driving, climbing stairs, light lifting and work as soon as they feel comfortable. Some patients may return to work in a few days while others prefer to rest at home a little longer.

Morbidity and mortality rates

The outcome of the procedure varies with the underlying disease or the extent of other injuries. Rates of complete recovery from the surgery itself are excellent, in the absence of other severe injuries or medical problems.

Splenectomy for HS patients is usually delayed in children until the age of five to prevent unnecessary infections; reported outcomes are very good.

Studies of patients with ITP show that 80%–90% of children achieve spontaneous and complete remission

QUESTIONS TO ASK THE DOCTOR

- What happens on the day of surgery?
- What type of anesthesia will be used?
- How long will it take to recover from the surgery?
- When can I expect to return to work and resume normal activities?
- What are the risks associated with a splenectomy?
- How many splenectomies do you perform in a year?
- Will I have a large scar?

in two to eight weeks. A small percentage develop chronic or persistent ITP, but 61% show complete remission by 15 years. No deaths in patients older than 15 have been attributed to ITP.

Alternatives

As of 2003 there are no medical alternatives to removing the spleen.

Splenic embolization is a surgical alternative to splenectomy that is used in some patients who are poor candidates for surgery. Embolization involves plugging or blocking the splenic artery with synthetic substances to shrink the size of the spleen. The substances that are injected during this procedure include polyvinyl alcohol foam, polystyrene, and silicone.

Resources

BOOKS

Hiatt, J. R., Phillips, E. H., and L. Morgenstern, eds. *Surgical Diseases of the Spleen*. New York: Springer Verlag, 1997.

Wilkins, B. S., and D. H. Wright. *Illustrated Pathology of the Spleen*. Cambridge, UK: Cambridge University Press, 2000.

PERIODICALS

Al-Salem A. H., and Z. Nasserulla. "Splenectomy for Children with Thalassemia." *Internal Surgery* 87 (October-December 2002): 269-273.

Duperier, T., J. Felsherm, and F. Brody. "Laparoscopic Splenectomy for Evans Syndrome." *Surgical Laparoscopy, Endoscopy & Percutaneous Techniques* 13 (February 2003): 45-47.

Schwartz, J., M. D. Leber, S. Gillis, et al. "Long-Term Follow-Up After Splenectomy Performed for Immune Thrombocytopenic Purpura (ITP)." *American Journal of Hematology* 72 (February 2003): 94-98.

Svarch, E., I. Nordet, J. Valdes, et al. "Partial Splenectomy in Children with Sickle Cell Disease." *Haematologica* 88 (February 2003): 281-287.

ORGANIZATIONS

American College of Gastroenterology. 4900 B South 31st St., Arlington, VA 22206. (703) 820-7400. www.acg.gi.org

American Gastroenterological Association (AGA). 4930 Del Ray Avenue, Bethesda, MD 20814. (301) 654-2055. www.gastro.org

National Cancer Institute (NCI). NCI Public Inquiries Office, Suite 3036A, 6116 Executive Boulevard, MSC8322 Bethesda, MD 20892-8322. (800) 422-6237. www.cancer.gov

OTHER

The Body Homepage. *Spleen Cancer*. www.thebody.com/Forums/AIDS/Cancer/Archive/othertypes/Q141422.html.

Your surgery.com. *Splenectomy*. www.yoursurgery.com/ProcedureDetails.cfm?BR=1&Proc=46.

Teresa Norris, RN

Monique Laberge, Ph. D.

Stapedectomy

Definition

Stapedectomy is a surgical procedure in which the innermost bone (stapes) of the three bones (the stapes, the incus, and the malleus) of the middle ear is removed, and replaced with a small plastic tube surrounding a short length of stainless-steel wire (a prosthesis). The operation was first performed in the United States in 1956.

Purpose

A stapedectomy is performed to improve the movement of sound to the inner ear. It is done to treat progressive hearing loss caused by otosclerosis, a condition in which spongy bone hardens around the base of the stapes. This condition fixes the stapes to the opening of the inner ear, so that the stapes no longer vibrates properly. Otosclerosis can also affect the malleus, the incus, and the bone that surrounds the inner ear. As a result, the transmission of sound to the inner ear is disrupted. Untreated otosclerosis eventually results in total deafness, usually in both ears.

Demographics

Otosclerosis affects about 10% of the United States population. It is an autosomal dominant disorder with variable penetrance. These terms mean that a child having one parent with otosclerosis has a 50% chance of inheriting the gene for the disorder, but that not everyone who has the gene will develop otosclerosis. In addition, some researchers think that the onset of the disorder is triggered when a person who has the gene for otosclerosis is infected with the measles virus. This hypothesis is supported by the finding that the incidence of otosclerosis has been steadily declining in countries with widespread measles vaccination.

Otosclerosis develops most frequently in people between the ages of 10 and 30. In most cases, both ears are affected; however, about 10–15% of patients diagnosed with otosclerosis have loss of hearing in only one ear. The disorder affects women more frequently than men by a ratio of two to one. Pregnancy is a risk factor for onset or worsening of otosclerosis.

With regard to race, Caucasian and Asian Americans are more likely to develop otosclerosis than African Americans.

Description

A stapedectomy does not require any incisions on the outside of the body, as the entire procedure is performed through the ear canal. With the patient under local or **general anesthesia**, the surgeon opens the ear canal and folds the eardrum forward. Using an operating microscope, the surgeon is able to see the structures in detail, and evaluates the bones of hearing (ossicles) to confirm the diagnosis of otosclerosis.

Next, the surgeon separates the stapes from the incus; freed from the stapes, the incus and malleus bones can now move when pressed. A laser or small drill may be used to cut through the tendon and arch of the stapes bone, which is then removed from the middle ear.

The surgeon then opens the window that joins the middle ear to the inner ear and acts as the platform for the stapes bone. The surgeon directs the laser's beam at the window to make a tiny opening, and gently clips the prosthesis to the incus bone. A piece of tissue is taken from a small incision behind the ear lobe and used to help seal the hole in the window and around the prosthesis. The eardrum is then gently replaced and repaired, and held there by absorbable packing ointment or a gelatin sponge. The procedure usually takes about an hour and a half.

Good candidates for the surgery are those who have a fixed stapes from otosclerosis and a conductive hearing loss of at least 20 dB. Patients with a severe hearing loss might still benefit from a stapedectomy, if only to improve their hearing to the point where a hearing aid can be of help. The procedure can improve hearing in more than 90% of cases.

KEY TERMS

Audiologist—A health care professional who performs diagnostic testing of impaired hearing.

Cochlea—The hearing part of the inner ear. This snail-shaped structure contains fluid and thousands of microscopic hair cells tuned to various frequencies, in addition to the organ of Corti (the receptor for hearing).

Conductive hearing loss—A type of medically treatable hearing loss in which the inner ear is usually normal, but there are specific problems in the middle or outer ears that prevent sound from getting to the inner ear in a normal way.

Footplate—A flat oval plate of bone that fits into the oval window on the wall of the inner ear; the base of the stapes.

Incus—The middle of the three bones of the middle ear. It is also known as the "anvil."

Malleus—One of the three bones of the middle ear. It is also known as the "hammer."

Ossicles—The three small bones of the middle ear: the malleus (hammer), the incus (anvil) and the stapes (stirrup). These bones help carry sound from the eardrum to the inner ear.

Otology—The branch of medicine that deals with the diagnosis and treatment of ear disorders.

Otosclerosis—Formation of spongy bone around the footplate of the stapes, resulting in conductive hearing loss.

Stapedotomy—A procedure in which a small hole is cut in the footplate of the stapes.

Tinnitus—A sensation of noise in the ears, usually a buzzing, ringing, clicking, or roaring sound.

Vertigo—A feeling of dizziness together with a sensation of movement and a feeling of rotating in space.

Diagnosis/Preparation

Diagnosis

Diagnosis of otosclerosis is based on a combination of the patient's family history, the patient's symptoms, and the results of hearing tests. Some patients notice only a gradual loss of hearing, but others experience dizziness, tinnitus (a sensation of buzzing, ringing, or hissing in the ears), or balance problems. The hearing tests should be administered by an ear specialist (audiologist or otologist) rather than the patient's family doctor. The examiner will need to determine whether the patient's hearing loss is conductive (caused by a lesion or disorder in the ear canal or middle ear) or sensorineural (caused by a disorder of the inner ear or the eighth cranial nerve).

Two tests that are commonly used to distinguish conductive hearing loss from sensorineural are Rinne's test and Weber's test. In Rinne's test, the examiner holds the stem of a vibrating tuning fork first against the mastoid bone and then outside the ear canal. A person with normal hearing will hear the sound as louder when it is held near the outer ear; a person with conductive hearing loss will hear the tone as louder when the fork is touching the bone.

In Weber's test, the vibrating tuning fork is held on the midline of the forehead and the patient is asked to indicate the ear in which the sound seems louder. A person with conductive hearing loss on one side will hear the sound louder in the affected ear.

A computed tomography (CT) scan or x-ray study of the head may also be done to determine whether the patient's hearing loss is conductive or sensorineural.

Preparation

Patients are asked to notify the surgeon if they develop a cold or sore throat within a week of the scheduled surgery. The procedure should be postponed in order to minimize the risk of infection being carried from the upper respiratory tract to the ear.

Some surgeons prefer to use general anesthesia when performing a stapedectomy, although an increasing number are using **local anesthesia**. A sedative injection is given to the patient before surgery.

Aftercare

The patient is asked to have a friend or relative drive them home after the procedure. **Antibiotics** are given up to five days after surgery to prevent infection; packing and sutures are removed about a week after surgery.

It is important that the patient not put pressure on the ear for a few days after surgery. Blowing one's nose, lifting heavy objects, swimming underwater, descending rapidly in high-rise elevators, or taking an airplane flight should be avoided.

Right after surgery, the ear is usually quite sensitive, so the patient should avoid loud noises until the ear retrains itself to hear sounds properly.

WHO PERFORMS THE PROCEDURE AND WHERE IS IT PERFORMED?

Stapedectomies are usually done by otologists or otolaryngologists, who are surgeons with advanced training in treating ear disorders. A stapedectomy is usually performed as an outpatient procedure in an ambulatory surgery facility or same-day surgery clinic.

It is extremely important that the patient avoid getting the ear wet until it has completely healed. Water in the ear could cause an infection; most seriously, water could enter the middle ear and cause an infection within the inner ear, which could then lead to a complete hearing loss. When taking a shower, and washing the hair, the patient should plug the ear with a cotton ball or lamb's wool ball, soaked in Vaseline. The surgeon should give specific instructions about when and how this can be done.

Usually, the patient may return to work and normal activities about a week after leaving the hospital, although if the patient's job involves heavy lifting, three weeks of home rest is recommend. Three days after surgery, the patient may fly in pressurized aircraft.

Risks

The most serious risk is an increased hearing loss, which occurs in about 1% of patients. Because of this risk, a stapedectomy is usually performed on only one ear at a time.

Less common complications include:

- temporary change in taste (due to nerve damage) or lack of taste
- perforated eardrum
- vertigo that may persist and require surgery
- damage to the chain of three small bones attached to the eardrum
- partial facial nerve paralysis
- ringing in the ears

Severe dizziness or vertigo may be a signal that there has been an incomplete seal between the fluids of the middle and inner ear. If this is the case, the patient needs immediate bed rest, an examination by the ear surgeon, and (rarely) an operation to reopen the eardrum to check the prosthesis.

QUESTIONS TO ASK THE DOCTOR

- What is your opinion of medication treatments for otosclerosis?
- Am I a candidate for a stapedotomy without prosthesis?
- What are the chances of my hearing getting worse if I postpone surgery?
- How many stapedectomies have you performed?
- What are the possible complications I could expect following a stapedectomy?

Normal results

Most patients are slightly dizzy for the first day or two after surgery, and may have a slight headache. Hearing improves once the swelling subsides, the slight bleeding behind the ear drum dries up, and the packing is absorbed or removed, usually within two weeks. Hearing continues to get better over the next three months.

About 90% of patients will have markedly improved hearing following the procedure, while 8% experience only minor improvement. About half the patients who had tinnitus before surgery will experience significant relief within six weeks after the procedure.

Morbidity and mortality rates

Stapedectomy is a very safe procedure with a relatively low rate of complications. With regard to hearing, about 2% of patients may have additional hearing loss in the operated ear following a stapedectomy; fewer than 1% lose hearing completely in the operated ear. About 9% of patients experience disturbances in their sense of taste. Infection, damage to the eardrum, and facial nerve palsy are rare complications that occur in fewer than 0.1% of patients.

Alternatives

Alternatives to a stapedectomy include:

- Watchful waiting. Some patients with only a mild degree of hearing loss may prefer to postpone surgery.
- Medications. Although there is no drug that can cure otosclerosis, some compounds containing fluoride or calcium are reported to be effective in preventing further hearing loss by slowing down abnormal bone growth. The medication most commonly recommended for the purpose is a combination of sodium fluoride and calcium carbonate sold under the trade name Florical. The medication is taken twice a day over a two-year period, after which the patient's hearing is reevaluated. Florical should not be used during pregnancy, however.
- Hearing aids.
- Stapedotomy. A stapedotomy is a surgical procedure similar to a stapedectomy except that the surgeon uses the laser to cut a hole in the stapes in order to insert the prosthesis rather than removing the stapes. In addition, some ear surgeons use the laser to free the stapes bone without inserting a prosthesis. This variation, however, works best in patients with only mild otosclerosis.

Resources

BOOKS

"Approach to the Patient with Ear Problems." In *The Merck Manual of Diagnosis and Therapy*, edited by Mark H. Beers, M.D., and Robert Berkow, M.D. Whitehouse Station, NJ: Merck Research Laboratories, 2001.

"Congenital Anomalies." In *The Merck Manual of Diagnosis and Therapy*, edited by Mark H. Beers, M.D., and Robert Berkow, M.D. Whitehouse Station, NJ: Merck Research Laboratories, 2001.

"Otosclerosis." In *The Merck Manual of Diagnosis and Therapy*, edited by Mark H. Beers, M.D., and Robert Berkow, M.D. Whitehouse Station, NJ: Merck Research Laboratories, 2001.

PERIODICALS

Brown, D. J., T. B. Kim, E. M. Petty, et al. "Characterization of a Stapes Ankylosis Family with an NOG Mutation." *Otology and Neurotology* 24 (March 2003): 210–215.

House, H. P., M. R. Hansen, A. A. Al Dakhail, and J. W. House. "Stapedectomy Versus Stapedotomy: Comparison of Results with Long-Term Follow-Up." *Laryngoscope* 112 (November 2002): 2046–2050.

Nadol, J. B., Jr. "Histopathology of Residual and Recurrent Conductive Hearing Loss After Stapedectomy." *Otology and Neurotology* 22 (March 2001): 162–169.

Shea, J. J. Jr., and X Ge. "Delayed Facial Palsy After Stapedectomy." *Otology and Neurotology* 22 (July 2001): 465–470.

Shohet, Jack A., M.D., and Frank Sutton, Jr., M.D. "Middle Ear, Otosclerosis." *eMedicine*, July 17, 2001 [cited May 3, 2003]. http://www.emedicine.com/ent/topic218.htm.

Vincent, R., J. Oates, and N. M. Sperling. "Stapedotomy for Tympanosclerotic Stapes Fixation: Is It Safe and Efficient? A Review of 68 Cases." *Otology and Neurotology* 23 (November 2002): 866–872.

ORGANIZATIONS

American Academy of Audiology. 11730 Plaza America Drive, Suite 300, Reston, VA 20190. (703) 790-8466. http://www.audiology.org.

American Academy of Otolaryngology-Head and Neck Surgery, Inc. One Prince St., Alexandria VA 22314-3357. (703) 836-4444. http://www.entnet.org

Better Hearing Institute. 515 King Street, Suite 420, Alexandria, VA 22314. (703) 684-3391.

National Institute on Deafness and Other Communication Disorders (NIDCD), National Institutes of Health. 31 Center Drive, MSC 2320. Bethesda, MD 20892-2320. http://www.nidcd.nih.gov.

OTHER

National Institute on Deafness and Other Communication Disorders (NIDCD). *Otosclerosis.* August 1999 [May 2, 2003]. NIH Publication No. 99-4234. http://www.nidcd.nih.gov/health/hearing/otosclerosis/otosclerosis.htm.

Carol A. Turkington
Rebecca J. Frey, Ph.D.

Staples *see* **Stitches and staples**

Stem cell transplant *see* **Bone marrow transplantation**

Stents, biliary *see* **Biliary stenting**

Stents, coronary *see* **Coronary stenting**

Stents, ureteral *see* **Ureteral stenting**

Stereotactic radiosurgery

Definition

Stereotactic radiosurgery is the use of a precise beam of radiation to destroy tissue in the brain.

Purpose

This procedure is used to treat brain tumors, arteriovenous malformations in the brain, and in some cases, benign eye tumors or other disorders within the brain.

Demographics

Stereotactic radiosurgery is used to treat a variety of disorders with widely differing demographic profiles.

Description

"Radiosurgery" refers to the use of a high-energy beam of radiation. "Stereotactic" refers to the three-dimensional targeting system used to deliver the beam to the precise location desired. Stereotactic radiosurgery is primarily confined to the head and neck, because the patient must be kept completely still during the delivery of the radiation in order to prevent damage to surrounding tissue. The motion of the patient's head and neck are restricted by a stereotactic frame that holds them in place. It is difficult to immobilize other body regions in this way.

The high energy of the radiation beam disrupts the DNA of the targeted cells, killing them. Multiple weak beams are focused on the target area, delivering maximum energy to it while keeping surrounding tissue safe. Since the radiation passes through the skull to its target, there is no need to cut open the skull to perform the surgery. The beam can be focused on any structure in the brain, allowing access to tumors or malformed blood vessels that cannot be reached by open-skull surgery.

Two major forms of stereotactic radiosurgery are in use as of 2003. The Gamma Knife® is a stationary machine that is most useful for small tumors, blood vessels, or similar targets. Because it does not move, it can deliver a small, highly localized and precise beam of radiation. Gamma knife treatment is done all at once in a single hospital stay. The second type of radiosurgery uses a movable linear accelerator-based machine that is preferred for larger tumors. This treatment is delivered in several small doses given over

KEY TERMS

Angiography—A technique for the diagnostic imaging of blood vessels that involves the injection of contrast material.

Fractionated radiosurgery—Radiosurgery in which the radiation is delivered in several smaller doses over a period of time rather than the full amount in a single treatment.

Metastatic—Referring to the spread of cancer from one organ in the body to another not directly connected to it.

Radiosurgery—Surgery that uses ionizing radiation to destroy tissue rather than a surgical incision.

Simulation scan—The process of making a mask for the patient and other images in order to plan the radiation treatment.

Stereotactic—Characterized by precise positioning in space. When applied to radiosurgery, stereotactic refers to a system of three-dimensional coordinates for locating the target site.

WHO PERFORMS THE PROCEDURE AND WHERE IS IT PERFORMED?

Stereotactic radiosurgery is performed by a radiosurgeon, who is a neurosurgeon with advanced training in the use of a gamma knife or linear accelerator-based machine. The radiosurgeon's dose plan is checked by a physicist before the treatment is administered to the patient. Stereotactic radiosurgery is done in a hospital that has the necessary specialized equipment.

several weeks. Radiosurgery that is performed with divided doses is known as fractionated radiosurgery. The total dose of radiation is higher with a linear accelerator-based machine than with gamma knife treatment.

Disorders treated by stereotactic radiosurgery include:

- benign brain tumors, including acoustic neuromas and meningiomas
- malignant brain tumors, including gliomas and astrocytomas
- metastatic brain tumors
- trigeminal neuralgia
- Parkinson's disease
- essential tremor
- arteriovenous malformations
- pituitary tumors

Diagnosis/Preparation

A patient requiring radiosurgery has already been diagnosed with a specific disorder that affects the brain. As preparation for radiosurgery, he or she will undergo neuroimaging studies to determine the precise location of the target area in the brain. These studies may include **CT scans**, MRI scans, and others. Imaging of the blood vessels (**angiography**) or the brain's ventricles (ventriculography) may be done as well. These require the injection of either a harmless radioactive substance or a contrast dye.

Prior to the procedure, the patient will be fitted with a stereotactic frame or rigid mask to immobilize the head. This part of the treatment may be uncomfortable. The patient may receive a simulation scan to establish the precise relationship of the mask or frame to the head to help plan the treatment.

QUESTIONS TO ASK THE DOCTOR

- What are the alternatives, if any, to radiosurgery for my specific condition?
- How many radiosurgical procedures have you performed?
- What is your success rate?
- What side effects have your patients reported?

The patient may be given a sedative and an anti-nausea agent prior to the simulation scan or treatment.

Aftercare

Stereotactic radiosurgery does not produce some of the side effects commonly associated with radiation treatment, such as reddening of the skin or hair loss. Most patients can return to their usual daily activities following treatment without any special precautions.

Risks

The risks of stereotactic radiosurgery include mild headache, tiredness, nausea and vomiting, and recurrence of the tumor. Questions have been raised as to whether radiosurgery can cause secondary tumors, but as of 2003, there is little detailed information about this potential risk.

Normal results

Stereotactic radiosurgery does not cause pain; and because the skull is not opened, there is no long hospital stay or risk of infection. Recovery is very rapid; most patients go home the same day they are treated, although follow-up imaging and retreatment may be necessary in some cases. This form of surgery appears to be quite successful in extending the length of survival in cancer patients; one study found that gamma knife radiosurgery controlled tumor growth in 96% of patients with kidney cancer that had spread to the brain, and added an average of 15 months to the patients' survival.

Morbidity and mortality rates

Stereotactic radiosurgery has a low reported rate of serious complications with minimal mortality. One German study reported a 4.8% rate of temporary morbidity in patients under treatment for brain tumors, with no permanent morbidity and no mortality. An American group of researchers found that less than

2% of patients who had eye tumors treated with radiosurgery suffered damage to the optic nerve from the dose of radiation.

Mild side effects following gamma knife radiosurgery are not uncommon, however. One group of British researchers found that 47 out of a group of 65 patients treated with gamma knife surgery had mild or moderate side effects within two weeks of treatment. Of these patients, more than half suffered headaches and a fifth reported unusual tiredness or nausea and vomiting.

Alternatives

With certain types of brain tumors, whole-brain radiation treatment (WBRT) is an option; however, it has a number of severe side effects. Surgical removal of the tumor is another option, but it carries a higher risk of tumor recurrence. For other tumors, gamma knife radiosurgery is the only treatment available as of 2003.

Resources

BOOKS

"Acoustic Neuroma." Section 7, Chapter 85 in *The Merck Manual of Diagnosis and Therapy*, edited by Mark H. Beers, MD, and Robert Berkow, MD. Whitehouse Station, NJ: Merck Research Laboratories, 1999.

"Radiation Injury of the Nervous System." Section 14, Chapter 177 in *The Merck Manual of Diagnosis and Therapy*, edited by Mark H. Beers, MD, and Robert Berkow, MD. Whitehouse Station, NJ: Merck Research Laboratories, 1999.

PERIODICALS

Chua, D. T., J. S. Sham, P. W. Kwong, et al. "Linear Accelerator-Based Stereotactic Radiosurgery for Limited, Locally Persistent, and Recurrent Nasopharyngeal Carcinoma; Efficacy and Complications." *International Journal of Radiation Oncology, Biology, Physics* 56 (May 1, 2003): 177-183.

Ganz, J. C. "Gamma Knife Radiosurgery and Its Possible Relationship to Malignancy: A Review." *Journal of Neurosurgery* 97 (December 2002) (5 Suppl): 644-652.

Muacevic, A., and F. W. Kreth. "Significance of Stereotactic Biopsy for the Management of WHO Grade II Supratentorial Glioma." [in German] *Der Nervenarzt* 74 (April 2003): 350-354.

O'Neill, B. P., N. J. Iturria, M. J. Link, et al. "A Comparison of Surgical Resection and Stereotactic Radiosurgery in the Treatment of Solitary Brain Metastases." *International Journal of Radiation Oncology, Biology, Physics* 55 (April 1, 2003): 1169-1176.

St. George, E. J., J. Kudhail, J. Perks, and P. N. Plowman. "Acute Symptoms After Gamma Knife Radiosurgery." *Journal of Neurosurgery* 97 (December 2002) (5 Suppl): 631-634.

Sheehan, J. P., M. H. Sun, D. Kondziolka, et al. "Radiosurgery in Patients with Renal Cell Carcinoma Metastasis to the Brain: Long-Term Outcomes and Prognostic Factors Influencing Survival and Local Tumor Control." *Journal of Neurosurgery* 98 (February 2003): 342-349.

Stafford, S. L., B. E. Pollock, J. A. Leavitt, et al. "A Study on the Radiation Tolerance of the Optic Nerve and Chiasm After Stereotactic Radiosurgery." *International Journal of Radiation Oncology, Biology, Physics* 55 (April 1, 2003): 1177-1181.

ORGANIZATIONS

International Radiosurgery Support Association (IRSA). 3005 Hoffman Street, Harrisburg, PA 17110. (717) 260-9808. www.irsa.org.

Johns Hopkins Radiosurgery. Weinberg 1469, 600 North Wolfe Street, Baltimore, MD 21287. (410) 614-2886. www.hopkinsmedicine.org/radiosurgery/treatmentoptions/stereotacticradiosurgery.cfm.

Richard Robinson

Sterilization, female *see* **Tubal ligation**

Sterilization, male *see* **Vasectomy**

Stethoscope

Definition

The stethoscope is an instrument used for auscultation, or listening to sounds produced by the body. It is used primarily to listen to the lungs, heart, and intestinal tract. It is also used to listen to blood flow in peripheral vessels and the heart sounds of developing fetuses in pregnant women.

Purpose

A stethoscope is used to detect and study heart, lung, stomach, and other sounds in adult humans, human fetuses, and animals. Using a stethoscope, the listener can hear normal and abnormal respiratory, cardiac, pleural, arterial, venous, uterine, fetal and intestinal sounds.

Demographics

All health care providers and students learn to use a stethoscope.

Description

Stethoscopes vary in their design and material. Most are made of Y-shaped rubber tubing. This shape allows sounds to enter the device at one end, travel up the tubes and through to the ear pieces. Many stethoscopes have a two-sided sound-detecting device or head that listeners can reverse, depending on whether they need to hear high or low frequencies. Some newer models have only one pressure-sensitive head. The various types of instruments include: binaural stethoscopes, designed for use with both ears; single stethoscopes, designed for use with one ear; differential stethoscopes, which allow listeners to compare sounds at two different body sites; and electronic stethoscopes, which electronically amplify tones. Some stethoscopes are designed specifically for hearing sounds in the esophagus or fetal heartbeats.

Diagnosis/Preparation

Training

Stethoscope users must learn to assess what they hear. When listening to the heart, one must listen to the left side of the chest, where the heart is located. Specifically, the heart lies between the fourth and sixth ribs, almost directly below the breast. The stethoscope must be moved around. A health care provider should listen for different sounds coming from different locations. The bell (one side of the head) of the instrument is generally used for listening to low-pitched sounds. The diaphragm (the other side of the head) of the instrument is used to listen to different areas of the heart. The sounds from each area will be different. "Lub-dub" is the sound produced by the normal heart as it beats. Every time this sound is detected, it means that the heart is contracting once. The noises are created when the heart valves click to close. When one hears "lub," the atrioventricular valves are closing. The "dub" sound is produced by the pulmonic and aortic valves. Other heart sounds, such as a quiet "whoosh," are produced by "murmurs." These sounds are produced when there are irregularities in the path of blood flow through the heart. The sounds reflect turbulence in normal blood flow. If a valve remains closed rather than opening completely, turbulence is created and a murmur is produced. Murmurs are not uncommon; many people have them and are unaffected. They are frequently too faint to be heard and remain undetected.

The lungs and airways require different listening skills from those used to detect heart sounds. The stethoscope must be placed over the chest, and the person being examined must breathe in and out deeply and slowly. Using the bell, the listener should note different sounds in various areas of the chest. Then, the diaphragm should be used in the same way. There will be no wheezes or crackles in normal lung sounds.

KEY TERMS

Atrioventricular—Referring to the valves regulating blood flow from the upper chambers of the heart (atria) to the lower chambers (ventricles). There are two such valves, one connecting the right atrium and ventricle and one connecting the left atrium and ventricle.

Auscultation—The act of listening to sounds produced by the body.

Bell—The cup-shaped portion of the head of a stethoscope, useful for detecting low-pitched sounds.

Borborygmi—Sounds created by the passage of food, gas or fecal material in the stomach or intestines.

Diaphragm—The flat-shaped portion of the head of a stethoscope, useful for detecting high-pitched sounds.

Murmur—The sound made as blood moves through the heart when there is turbulence in the flow of blood through a blood vessel, or if a valve does not completely close.

Crackles or wheezes are abnormal lung sounds. When the lung rubs against the chest wall, it creates friction and a rubbing sound. When there is fluid in the lungs, crackles are heard. A high-pitched whistling sound called a wheeze is often heard when the airways are constricted.

When the stethoscope is placed over the upper left portion of the abdomen, gurgling sounds produced by the stomach and small intestines can usually be heard just below the ribs. The large intestines, in the lower part of the abdomen, can also be heard. The noises they make are called borborygmi and are entirely normal. Borborygmi are produced by the movement of food, gas or fecal material.

Operation

Some stethoscopes must be placed directly on the skin, while others can work effectively through clothing. For the stethoscopes with a two-part sound detecting device in the bell, listeners press the rim against the skin, using the bowl-shaped side, to hear low-pitched sounds. The other flat side, called the diaphragm, detects high-pitched sounds.

A stethoscope is used in conjunction with a device to measure blood pressure (**sphygmomanometer**). The stethoscope detects sounds of blood passing though an artery.

WHO PERFORMS THE PROCEDURE AND WHERE IS IT PERFORMED?

Any member of a health care team participating in a physical examination uses a stethoscope. It is used to detect and transmit sounds created within the body.

QUESTIONS TO ASK THE DOCTOR

Are the sounds being heard normal or abnormal?

Have the sounds changed since the last examination?

Has a murmur, if present, changed in pitch or loudness?

Examination with a stethoscope is noninvasive but very useful. It can assist members of the health care team in localizing problems related to the patient's complaints.

Maintenance

Stethoscopes should be cleaned after each use in order to avoid the spread of infection. This precaution is especially important when they are placed directly onto bare skin.

Aftercare

A stethoscope is a sensitive instrument. It should be handled with some care to avoid damage. It requires periodic cleaning.

Risks

There are no risks to persons being examined with a stethoscope. Users of a stethoscope may be exposed to loud noise if the bell is accidentally dropped or struck against a hard surface while the earpieces are in the user's ears.

Normal results

Stethoscopes produce important diagnostic information when used by a person with training and experience.

Morbidity and mortality rates

Normal use of a stethoscope is not associated with injury to either an examiner or a person being examined.

Alternatives

A tube formed by a roll of paper will function in the same manner as a stethoscope. This improvised instrument was the first form of the modern stethoscope invented by René Laënnec (1781-1826), a French physician. An inverted glass will also function as a stethoscope by placing the open portion on the surface to be listened to and the ear of the examiner on the bottom of the glass. Due to their shape, wine glasses with stems are more effective than flat-bottomed tumblers.

Resources

BOOKS

Bickley, L. S., P. G. Szilagyi, and J. G. Stackhouse, eds. *Bates' Guide to Physical Examination & History Taking*, 8th ed. Philadelphia, PA: Lippincott Williams & Wilkins, 2002.

Blaufox, MD. *An Ear to the Chest: An Illustrated History of the Evolution of the Stethoscope*. Boca Raton, FL: CRC Press-Parthenon Publishers, 2001.

Duffin, J. *To See with a Better Eye*. Princeton, NJ: Princeton University Press, 1998.

Duke, M. *Tales My Stethoscope Told Me*. Santa Barbara, CA: Fithian Press, 1998.

PERIODICALS

Conti, C. R. "The Ultrasonic Stethoscope: The New Instrument in Cardiology?" *Clinical Cardiology* 25 (December 2002): 547-548.

Guinto, C. H., E. J. Bottone, J. T. Raffalli, et al. "Evaluation of Dedicated Stethoscopes as a Potential Source of Nosocomial Pathogens." *American Journal of Infection Control* 30 (December 2002): 499-502.

Hanna, I. R., and M. E. Silverman. "A History of Cardiac Auscultation and Some of its Contributors." *American Journal of Cardiology* 90 (August 1, 2002): 259-267.

Savage, G. J. "On the Stethoscope." *Delaware Medical Journal* 74 (October 2002): 415-416.

ORGANIZATIONS

American Academy of Family Physicians. 11400 Tomahawk Creek Parkway, Leawood, KS 66211-2672. (913) 906-6000. E-mail: fp@aafp.org. www.aafp.org.

American Academy of Pediatrics. 141 Northwest Point Boulevard, Elk Grove Village, IL 60007-1098. (847) 434-4000. Fax: (847) 434-8000. E-mail: kidsdoc@aap.org. www.aap.org.

American College of Physicians. 190 N. Independence Mall West, Philadelphia, PA 19106-1572. (800) 523-1546, x2600 or (215) 351-2600. www.acponline.org.

American College of Surgeons. 633 North St. Clair Street, Chicago, IL 60611-3231. (312) 202-5000. Fax: (312) 202-5001. E-mail: postmaster@facs.org. www.facs.org.

OTHER

British Broadcasting Company. www.bbc.co.uk/radio4/science/guessingtubes.shtml. (March 1, 2003)

Institution of Electrical Engineers. www.iee.org/News/PressRel/z18oct2002.cfm. (March 1, 2003)

McGill University Virtual Stethoscope. www.music.mcgill.ca/auscultation/auscultation.html. (March 1, 2003)

University of Minnesota Academic Health Center. www.ahc.umn.edu/rar/MNAALAS/Steth.html. (March 1, 2003)

L. Fleming Fallon, Jr., MD, DrPH

Stomach resection *see* **Gastrectomy**

Stomach stapling *see* **Vertical banded gastroplasty**

Stomach tube insertion *see* **Gastrostomy**

Strabismus repair *see* **Eye muscle surgery**

Stress test

Definition

A stress test is primarily used to identify coronary artery disease. It requires patients to **exercise** on a treadmill or exercise bicycle while their heart rate, blood pressure, **electrocardiogram** (ECG), and symptoms are monitored.

Purpose

The body requires more oxygen during exercise than when it is at rest. To deliver more oxygen during exercise, the heart has to pump more oxygen-rich blood. Because of the increased stress on the heart, exercise can reveal coronary problems that are not apparent when the body is at rest. This is why the stress test, though not perfect, remains the best initial, noninvasive, practical coronary test.

The stress test is particularly useful for detecting ischemia (inadequate supply of blood to the heart muscle) caused by blocked coronary arteries. Less commonly, it is used to determine safe levels of exercise in people with existing coronary artery disease.

Description

A technician affixes electrodes to the patient's chest, using adhesive patches with a special gel that conducts electrical impulses. Typically, electrodes are placed under each collarbone and each bottom rib, and six electrodes are placed across the chest in a rough outline of the heart. Wires from the electrodes are connected to an ECG, which records the electrical activity picked up by the electrodes.

The technician runs resting ECG tests while the patient is lying down, then standing up, and then breathing heavily for half a minute. These baseline tests can later be compared with the ECG tests performed while the patient is exercising. The patient's blood pressure is taken and the blood pressure cuff is left in place so that blood pressure can be measured periodically throughout the test.

The patient begins riding a stationary bicycle or walking on a treadmill. Gradually the intensity of the exercise is increased. For example, if the patient is walking on a treadmill, then the speed of the treadmill increases and the treadmill is tilted upward to simulate an incline. If the patient is on an exercise bicycle, then the resistance or "drag" is gradually increased. The patient continues exercising at increasing intensity until reaching the target heart rate (generally set at a minimum of 85% of the maximal predicted heart rate based on the patient's age) or experiences severe fatigue, dizziness, or chest pain. During the test, the patient's heart rate, ECG, and blood pressure are monitored.

Sometimes other tests, such as **echocardiography** or thallium scanning, are used in conjunction with the exercise stress test. For instance, studies suggest that

KEY TERMS

Angina—Chest pain from a poor blood supply to the heart muscle due to stenosis (narrowing) of the coronary arteries.

Cardiac arrhythmia—An irregular heart rate (frequency of heartbeats) or rhythm (the pattern of heartbeats).

Defibrillator—A device that delivers an electric shock to the heart muscle through the chest wall in order to restore a normal heart rate.

False negative—Test results showing no problem when one exists.

False positive—Test results showing a problem when one does not exist.

Hypertrophy—The overgrowth of muscle.

Ischemia—Dimished supply of oxygen-rich blood to an organ or area of the body.

women have a high rate of false negatives (results showing no problem when one exists) and false positives (results showing a problem when one does not exist) with the stress test. They may benefit from another test, such as exercise echocardiography. People who are unable to exercise may be injected with drugs, such as adenosine, which mimic the effects of exercise on the heart, and then given a thallium scan. The thallium scan or echocardiogram are particularly useful when the patient's resting ECG is abnormal. In such cases, interpretation of exercise-induced ECG abnormalities is difficult.

Preparation

Patients are usually instructed not to eat or smoke for several hours before the test. They should be advised to inform the physician about any medications they are taking, and to wear comfortable sneakers and exercise clothing.

Aftercare

After the test, the patient should rest until blood pressure and heart rate return to normal. If all goes well, and there are no signs of distress, the patient may return to his or her normal daily activities.

Risks

There is a very slight risk of myocardial infarction (a heart attack) from the exercise, as well as cardiac arrhythmia (irregular heart beats), angina, or cardiac arrest (about one in 100,000). The exercise stress test carries a very slight risk (one in 100,000) of causing a heart attack. For this reason, exercise stress tests should be attended by health care professionals with immediate access to defibrillators and other emergency equipment.

Patients are cautioned to stop the test should they develop any of the following symptoms:

- unsteady gait;
- confusion;
- skin that is grayish or cold and clammy;
- dizziness or fainting;
- a drop in blood pressure;
- angina (chest pain); and
- cardiac arrhythmias (irregular heartbeat).

Normal results

A normal result of an exercise stress test shows normal electrocardiogram tracings and heart rate, blood pressure within the normal range, and no angina, unusual dizziness, or shortness of breath.

A number of abnormalities may appear on an exercise stress test. Examples of exercise-induced ECG abnormalities are ST segment depression or heart rhythm disturbances. These ECG abnormalities may indicate deprivation of blood to the heart muscle (ischemia) caused by narrowed or blocked coronary arteries. Stress test abnormalities generally require further diagnostic evaluation and therapy.

Patient education

Patients must be well prepared for a stress test. They should not only know the purpose of the test, but also signs and symptoms that indicate the test should be stopped. Physicians, nurses, and ECG technicians can ensure patient safety by encouraging them to immediately communicate discomfort at any time during the stress test.

Resources

BOOKS

Grainger R. G., D. J. Allison, and A. K. Dixon. *Grainger & Allison's Diagnostic Radiology: A Textbook of Medical Imaging,* 4th ed. Philadelphia: Churchill Livingstone, 2001.

Mettler, F. A. *Essentials of Radiology,* 2nd ed. Philadelphia: Saunders, 2005.

Zipes, D. P., P. Libby, R. Bonow, and E. Braunwald. *Braunwald's Heart Disease: A Textbook of Cardiovascular Medicine,* 8th ed. Philadelphia: Saunders, 2007.

ORGANIZATIONS

American Heart Association, National Center 7272 Greenville Avenue, Dallas, TX, 75231, (800) 242-8721, http://www.americanheart.org.

National Heart, Lung, and Blood Institute, Information CenterP.O. Box 30105, Bethesda, MD, 20824-0105, (301) 592-8573, http://www.nhlbi.nih.gov.

Barbara Wexler
Lee A. Shratter, M.D.

Sulfonamides

Definition

Sulfonamides are a group of anti-infective drugs that prevent the growth of bacteria in the body by interfering with their metabolism. Bacteria are one-celled disease-causing microorganisms that commonly multiply by cell division.

Purpose

Sulfonamides are used to treat many kinds of infections caused by bacteria and certain other microorganisms. Physicians may prescribe these drugs to treat urinary tract infections, ear infections, frequent or long-lasting bronchitis, bacterial meningitis, certain eye infections, *Pneumocystis carinii* pneumonia (PCP), traveler's diarrhea, and a number of other infections. These drugs will, however, *not* work for colds, flu, and other infections caused by viruses.

Description

Sulfonamides, which are also called sulfa medicines, are available only with a physician's prescription. They are sold in tablet and liquid forms. Some commonly used sulfonamides are sulfisoxazole (Gantrisin) and the combination drug sulfamethoxazole and trimethoprim (Bactrim, Cotrim, Septra).

Although the sulfonamides have been largely replaced by **antibiotics** for treatment of infections, some bacteria have developed resistance to antibiotics but can still be treated with sulfonamides because the bacteria have not been exposed to these drugs in the past.

Silver sulfadiazine, an ointment containing a sulfonamide, is valuable for the treatment of infections associated with severe burns. The combination drug trimethoprim/sulfamethoxazole (TMP-SMZ) remains in use for many infections, including those associated with HIV infection (AIDS). TMP-SMZ is particularly useful for prevention and treatment of *Pneumocystis carinii* pneumonia, which has been the most dangerous of the infections associated with HIV infection.

Recommended dosage

The recommended dosage depends on the type of sulfonamide, the strength of the medication, and the medical problem for which it is being taken. Patients should check the correct dosage with the physician who prescribed the drug or the pharmacist who filled the prescription.

Patients should always take sulfonamides exactly as directed. To make sure the infection clears up completely, the full course of the medicine must be taken. Patients should not stop taking the drug just because their symptoms begin to improve, because the symptoms may return if the drug is stopped too soon.

Sulfonamides work best when they are at constant levels in the blood. To help keep blood levels constant, patients should take the medicine in doses spaced evenly through the day and night without missing any doses. For best results, sulfa medicines should be taken with a full glass of water, and the patient should drink several more glasses of water every day. This precaution is necessary because sulfa drugs do not dissolve in tissue fluids as easily as some other anti-infective medications. Drinking plenty of water will help prevent some of the medicine's side effects.

KEY TERMS

Anemia—A deficiency of hemoglobin in the blood. Hemoglobin is the compound in blood that carries oxygen from the lungs throughout the body.

Anticoagulant—A type of medication given to prevent blood from clotting. Anticoagulants are also known as blood thinners.

Bronchitis—Inflammation of the air passages of the lungs.

Diuretic—A type of medication given to increase urinary output.

HIV infection—An infectious disease that impairs the immune system. It is also known as acquired immune deficiency syndrome or AIDS.

Inflammation—A condition in which pain, redness, swelling, and warmth develop in a tissue or organ in response to injury or illness.

Meningitis—Inflammation of tissues that surround the brain and spinal cord.

***Pneumocystis carinii* pneumonia (PCP)**—A lung infection that affects people with weakened immune systems, such as patients with AIDS or people taking medicines that weaken the immune system.

Porphyria—A disorder in which porphyrins build up in the blood and urine.

Porphyrin—A dark red pigment, sensitive to light, that is found in chlorophyll as well as in a substance in hemoglobin known as heme.

Stevens-Johnson syndrome—A severe inflammatory reaction that is sometimes triggered by sulfa medications. It is characterized by blisters and eroded areas in the mouth, nose, eyes, and anus; it may also involve the lungs, heart, and digestive tract. Stevens-Johnson syndrome is also known as erythema multiforme.

Urinary tract—The passage through which urine flows from the kidneys out of the body.

Precautions

Symptoms should begin to improve within a few days of beginning to take a sulfa drug. If they do not, or if they get worse, the patient should consult the physician who prescribed the medicine.

Although major side effects are rare, some people have had severe and life-threatening reactions to sulfonamides. These include sudden and severe liver damage; serious blood problems; breakdown of the outer layer of the skin; and a condition called Stevens-Johnson syndrome (erythema multiforme), in which people get blisters around the mouth, eyes, or anus. The patient may be unable to eat and may develop ulcerated areas in the eyes or be unable to open the eyes. It is important to consult a dermatologist and an ophthalmologist as quickly as possible if a patient develops Stevens-Johnson syndrome, to prevent lasting damage to the patient's eyesight. In addition, the syndrome is sometimes fatal.

A physician should be called immediately if any of these signs of a dangerous reaction occur:

- skin rash or reddish or purplish spots on the skin;
- such other skin problems as blistering or peeling;
- fever;
- sore throat;
- cough;
- shortness of breath;
- joint pain;
- pale skin; or
- yellow skin or eyes.

Sulfa drugs may also cause dizziness. Anyone who takes sulfonamides should not drive, use machines or do anything else that might be dangerous until they have found out how these drugs affect them.

Sulfonamides may cause blood problems that can interfere with healing and lead to additional infections. Patients should try to avoid minor injuries while taking these medicines, and be especially careful not to injure the mouth when brushing or flossing the teeth or using a toothpick. They should not have dental work done until their blood is back to normal.

Sulfa medications may increase the skin's sensitivity to sunlight. Even brief exposure to sun can cause a severe sunburn or a rash. During treatment with these drugs, patients should avoid exposure to direct sunlight, especially high sun between 10 A.M. and 3 P.M.; wear a hat and tightly woven clothing that covers the arms and legs; use a sunscreen with a skin protection factor (SPF) of at least 15; protect the lips with a lip balm containing sun block; and avoid the use of tanning beds, tanning booths, or sunlamps.

Babies under two months should not be given sulfonamides unless their physician has specifically ordered these drugs.

Older people may be especially sensitive to the effects of sulfonamides, increasing the chance of such unwanted side effects as severe skin problems and blood disorders. Patients who are taking water pills (**diuretics**) at the same time as sulfonamides may also be more likely to have these problems.

Special conditions

People with certain medical conditions or who are taking other medicines may have problems if they take sulfonamides. Before taking these drugs, the patient must inform the doctor about any of these conditions:

ALLERGIES. Anyone who has had unusual reactions to sulfonamides, diuretics, diabetes medicines, or glaucoma medications in the past should let his or her physician know before taking sulfonamides. The physician should also be told about any allergies to foods, dyes, preservatives, or other substances.

PREGNANCY. Some sulfonamides have been found to cause birth defects in studies of laboratory animals. The drugs' effects on human fetuses have not been studied. Pregnant women are advised not to use sulfa drugs around the time of labor and delivery, because they can cause side effects in the baby. Women who are pregnant or who may become pregnant should check with their physicians about the safety of using sulfonamides during pregnancy.

LACTATION. Sulfonamides pass into breast milk and may cause liver problems, anemia, and other problems in nursing babies whose mothers take the medicine. Because of those problems, women should not breast-feed their babies when they are under treatment with sulfa drugs. Women who are breast-feeding but require treatment with sulfonamides should check with their physicians to find out how long they should stop breast-feeding.

OTHER MEDICAL CONDITIONS. People with any of the following medical problems should make sure their physicians are aware of their conditions before they take sulfonamides:

- anemia or other blood problems;
- kidney disease;
- liver disease;
- asthma or severe allergies;
- alcohol abuse;
- poor nutrition;
- abnormal intestinal absorption;

- porphyria;
- folic acid deficiency; and
- deficiency of an enzyme known as glucose-6-phosphate dehydrogenase (G6PD).

Side effects

The most common side effects are mild diarrhea, nausea, vomiting, dizziness, headache, loss of appetite, and tiredness. These problems usually go away as the body adjusts to the drug and do not require medical treatment.

More serious side effects are not common, but may occur. If any of the following side effects occur, the patient should check with a physician immediately:

- itching or skin rash;
- reddish or purplish spots on the skin;
- such other skin problems as redness, blistering, or peeling;
- severe, watery or bloody diarrhea;
- muscle or joint aches;
- fever;
- sore throat;
- cough;
- shortness of breath;
- unusual tiredness or weakness;
- unusual bleeding or bruising;
- pale skin;
- yellow eyes or skin; or
- swallowing problems.

Other rare side effects may occur. Anyone who has unusual symptoms while taking sulfonamides should get in touch with his or her physician.

Interactions

Sulfonamides may interact with a large number of other medicines. When an interaction occurs, the effects of one or both of the drugs may change or the risk of side effects may be greater. Anyone who takes sulfonamides should give the physician a list of all other medicines that he or she is taking. Among the drugs that may interact with sulfonamides are:

- acetaminophen (Tylenol);
- medicines to treat an overactive thyroid gland;
- male hormones (androgens);
- female hormones (estrogens);
- other medicines used to treat infections;
- birth control pills;
- such medicines for diabetes as glyburide (Micronase);
- warfarin (Coumadin) and other anticoagulants;
- disulfiram (Antabuse), a drug used to treat alcohol abuse;
- amantadine (Symmetrel), used to treat influenza and also Parkinson's disease;
- hydrochlorothiazide (HCTZ, HydroDIURIL) and other diuretics;
- the anticancer drug methotrexate (Rheumatrex); and
- valproic acid (Depakote, Depakene) and other antiseizure medications.

The list above does not include every drug that may interact with sulfonamides. Patients should be careful to check with a physician or pharmacist before combining sulfonamides with any other prescription or nonprescription (over-the-counter) medicine. This precaution includes herbal preparations. Some herbs, such as bearberry, parsley, dandelion leaf, and sarsaparilla, have a diuretic effect and should not be used while taking sulfa drugs. Basil, which is commonly used in cooking to flavor salad **dressings**, stews, and tomato recipes, is reported to affect the absorption of sulfonamides.

Resources

BOOKS

Cohen J., and W. G. Powderly. *Infectious Diseases,* 2nd ed. St. Louis: Mosby, 2003.

Gershon A. A., P. J. Hotez, and S. L. Katz. *Krugman's Infectious Diseases of Children,* 11th ed. St. Louis: Mosby, 2003.

Long S. S., L. K. Pickering, and C. G. Prober. *Principles and Practice of Pediatric Infectious Diseases,* 3rd ed. London: Churchill Livingstone, 2008.

Mandell G. L., J. E. Bennett, and R. Dolin. *Principles and Practice of Infectious Diseases,* 6th ed. London: Churchill Livingstone, 2004.

ORGANIZATIONS

American Society of Health-System Pharmacists, 7272 Wisconsin Avenue, Bethesda, MD, 20814, (301) 657-3000, http://www.ashp.org.

United States Food and Drug Administration, 5600 Fishers Lane, Rockville, MD, 20857-0001, (888) INFO-FDA, http://www.fda.gov.

Nancy Ross-Flanigan
Sam Uretsky, Pharm.D.

Surgical debridement *see* **Debridement**

Surgical instruments

Definition

Surgical instruments are tools or devices that perform functions such as cutting, dissecting, grasping, holding, retracting, or suturing. Most surgical instruments are made from stainless steel. Other metals, such as titanium, chromium, vanadium, and molybdenum, are also used.

Purpose

Surgical instruments facilitate a variety of procedures and operations. Specialized surgical packs contain the most common instruments needed for particular surgeries.

In the United States, surgical instruments are used in all hospitals, outpatient facilities, and most professional offices. Instrument users include surgeons, dentists, physicians, and many other health-care providers. Millions of new and replacement instruments are sold each year. Many modern surgical instruments have electronic or computerized components.

Description

Basic categories of surgical instruments include specialized implements for the following functions:

- cutting, grinding, and dissecting;
- clamping;
- grasping and holding;
- probing;
- dilating or enlarging;
- retracting; and
- suctioning.

Scissors are an example of cutting instruments. Dissecting instruments are used to cut or separate tissue. Dissectors may be sharp or blunt. One example of a sharp dissector is a scalpel. Examples of blunt dissectors include the back of a knife handle, curettes, and elevators. Clamps, tenacula, and forceps are grasping and holding instruments. Probing instruments are used to enter natural openings, such as the common bile duct, or fistulas. Dilating instruments expand the size of an opening, such as the urethra or cervical os. Retractors assist in the visualization of the operative field while preventing trauma to other tissues. Suction devices remove blood and other fluids from a surgical or dental operative field.

Sharps and related items should be counted four times: prior to the start of the procedure, before closure of a cavity within a cavity, before wound closure begins, and at skin closure or the end of the procedure. In addition, a count should be taken any time surgical personnel are replaced before, during, or after a procedure. Instruments, sharps, and sponges should be counted during all procedures in which there is a possibility of leaving an item inside a patient.

The misuse of surgical instruments frequently causes alignment problems. Instruments should always be inspected before, during, and after surgical or dental procedures. Inspection is an ongoing process that must be carried out by all members of a **surgical team**.

Scissors must be sharp and smooth, and must cut easily. Their edges must be inspected for chips, nicks, or dents.

After a procedure, staff members responsible for cleaning and disinfecting the instruments should also inspect them. The instruments should be inspected again after cleaning and during packaging. Any instrument that is not in good working order should be sent for repair. Depending on use, surgical instruments can last for up to 10 years given proper care.

KEY TERMS

Autoclave—A heavy vessel that uses pressurized steam for disinfecting and sterilizing surgical instruments.

Curette—A scoop-shaped surgical instrument for removing tissue from body cavities.

Dilation—The process of enlarging, usually applied to relatively circular openings.

Forceps—An instrument designed to grasp or hold. Forceps usually have a locking mechanism so that they continue to hold tissue when put down by an operator.

Instruments—Tools or devices that perform such functions as cutting, dissecting, grasping, holding, retracting, or suturing.

Sharps—Surgical implements with thin cutting edges or a fine point. Sharps include suture needles, scalpel blades, hypodermic needles, and safety pins.

Sponges—Pieces of absorbent material, usually cotton gauze, used to absorb fluids, protect tissue, or apply pressure and traction.

Tenaculum (plural, tenacula)—A small, sharp-pointed hook set in a handle, used to seize or pick up pieces of tissue during surgical operations.

Preparation

Instruction in the use and care of surgical instruments may range from the medical training required by physicians and dentists to on-the-job training for orderlies and aides.

Surgical instruments are prepared for use according to strict institutional and professional protocols. Instruments are maintained and sterilized prior to use.

Surgical instruments must be kept clean during a procedure. This is accomplished by carefully wiping them with a moist sponge and rinsing them frequently in sterile water. Periodic cleaning during the procedure prevents blood and other tissues from hardening and becoming trapped on the surface of an instrument.

Instruments must be promptly rinsed and thoroughly cleaned and sterilized after a procedure. Ultrasonic cleaning and automatic washing often follow the manual cleaning of instruments. Instruments may also be placed in an autoclave after manual cleaning. The manufacturer's instructions must be followed for each type of machine. Staff members responsible for cleaning instruments should wear protective gloves, waterproof aprons, and face shields to protect themselves and maintain instrument sterility.

Aftercare

Observation of the patient after surgical or dental procedures provides the best indication that correct instrument handling and **aseptic technique** was followed during surgery. After an operation or dental procedure, individuals should show no evidence of the following:

- retained instruments or sponges; or
- infection at the site of the incision or operation.

Risks

Risks associated with surgical instruments include improper use or technique by an operator, leaving an instrument inside a person after an operation, and transmitting infection or disease due to improper cleaning and sterilization techniques. Improperly cleaned or sterilized instruments may contribute to postoperative infections or mortality. Improper use of surgical instruments may contribute to postoperative complications.

Resources

BOOKS

Brunicardi, F. C., D. K. Anderson, D. L. Dunn, J. G. Hunter, and R. E. Pollock. *Schwartz's Manual of Surgery,* 8th ed. New York: McGraw Hill, 2006.

Ellis, H., R. Caine, and C. Watson. *General Surgery: Lecture Notes,* 11th ed. New York: Wiley, 2006.

Lawrence, P. F. *Essentials of General Surgery,* 4th ed. Philadelphia: Lippincott Williams & Wilkins, 2005.

Townsend, C.M., R. D. Beauchamp, B. M. Evers, and K. Mattox. *Sabiston Textbook of Surgery,* 17th ed. Philadelphia: Saunders, 2004.

PERIODICALS

Downey, C. "Counting as caring." *Canadian Operating Room Nursing Journal* 25, no. 3 (September 2007): 6–13.

Egorova, N. N., A. Moskowitz, A. Gelijns, A. Weinberg, et al. "Managing the Prevention of Retained Surgical Instruments: What Is the Value of Counting?" *Annals of Surgery* 247, no. 1 (January 2008): 13–18.

Sabrosky, P. "Spiraling instrument costs present many challenges." *Materials Management in Health Care* 16, no. 7 (July 2007): 66–74.

Sroga, J., S. D. Patel, and T. Falcone. "Robotics in reproductive medicine." *Frontiers in Bioscience* 13 (January 2008): 1308–1317.

OTHER

"Orange County's 1st robotics-assisted surgery performed at UCI Medical Center." University of California-Irvine Healthcare. May 3, 2002. http://www.ucihealth.com/News/Releases/DaVinci2.htm (January 3, 2008).

"Surgical Instruments from Ancient Rome." University of Virginia Health System. October 30, 2007. http://www.healthsystem.virginia.edu/internet/library/wdc-lib/historical/artifacts/roman_surgical/ (January 3, 2008).

"Surgical Technologists." *Occupational Outlook Handbook*. United States Bureau of Labor, Bureau of Labor Statistics. December 18, 2007. http://www.bls.gov/oco/ocos106.htm (January 3, 2008).

ORGANIZATIONS

American Board of Surgery, 1617 John F. Kennedy Boulevard, Suite 860, Philadelphia, PA, 19103, (215) 568-4000, (215) 563-5718, http://www.absurgery.org.

American College of Surgeons, 633 North Saint Claire Street, Chicago, IL, 60611, (312) 202-5000, http://www.facs.org/.

Association of Perioperative Registered Nurses, 2170 South Parker Road, Suite 300, Denver, CO, 80231, (800) 755-2676, (303) 750-3212, http://www.aorn.org.

Association of Surgical Technologists, 6 West Dry Creek Circle, Suite 200, Littleton, CO, 80120-8031, (303) 694-9130, (303) 694-9169, http://www.ast.org.

L. Fleming Fallon, Jr., M.D., Dr.P.H.

Surgical mesh

Definition

Surgical mesh is a sterile woven piece of netting that is used in surgical procedures to help repair sites of surgical incision, tissue herniation, or to provide support to internal parts of the body.

Demographics

Surgical mesh is used in many different types of surgical procedures. Hernia repair is one of the most frequently performed general surgeries world wide, and usually involves the use of surgical mesh. Mesh is also used to assist in surgical correction of urinary incontinence, uterine suspension, vertebral reconstruction, tissue reconstruction, vaginal prolapse, and provides support for devices implanted to support the heart.

Description

Surgical mesh can be used in many different surgical procedures to provide wound closure or support for internal body parts. Also known as a patch or screen, surgical mesh is implanted in the body for repair or reinforcement. Surgical mesh may be absorbable or non-absorbable. Some types of repair procedures using surgical mesh may also be called a "Lichtenstein Repair," because of a surgeon named Irving Lichtenstein whose influence in the medical field increased the widespread use of surgical mesh. A Lichtenstein Repair is specifically a flat piece of surgical mesh used as a patch placed on top of a tissue defect.

Surgical mesh is usually a sterile, woven material made of a type of synthetic plastic. Surgical mesh can be made of various different types of synthetic material, such as Gore-Tex, polyprolene, or knitted polyester. Mesh is very sturdy and strong, yet extremely thin. It is soft and flexible to allow it to easily conform to the movement of the body. Surgical mesh is available in various measurements and can be cut to size for each surgical application. Depending on the type of repair that is needed, a patch of mesh is placed under, over, or within a defect in the body and sewn in place by a few sutures. The mesh acts as a type of scaffold for the body tissue that grows around and into the mesh. Mesh is also used like a sling to support internal body parts and hold them in place.

Once inserted, mesh is eventually incorporated into the surrounding tissue as if it is part of the body. For this reason, mesh is considered a tension-free type of repair, as opposed to sutures. Sutures hold flesh together through the tension they create by pulling tissues together to close a wound. Because sutures create tension in the tissue they repair, too much movement early on in the recovery period after surgery can re-open the repair site and cause internal bleeding. Mesh is different in that it does not rely on tension to hold tissue together. Rather the mesh itself fills the wound and allows tissue to grow into and around it. Patients in which surgical mesh has been used may resume activity much sooner after the surgical procedure than is usually seen with tension repair techniques such as sutures. Surgical mesh may be used in the form of a patch that goes under or over a weakness in body tissues, or a plug that goes inside a hole in the tissue. The patient cannot feel the internal mesh, and is able to move freely.

Mesh Used for Tissue Support

Surgical mesh may be used to help physically support body tissues that are weak or damaged in some way. One example of a procedure that may benefit from mesh in this way is uterine suspension. Uterine suspension is necessary when the uterus is tipped out of its normal position and causes medical complications. Uterine suspension is performed to put the uterus back into its normal position. Surgical mesh may be used as a sling to support the uterus and hold it in place. A second example of mesh used for tissue support is as a sling for the urethra in some types of urinary incontinence where the urethra has fallen out of its normal position. In surgery done for urinary incontinence, a sling is put in place to lift the urethra back into its normal position and create a type of pressure that helps prevent the incontinence. A mesh sling may be used and attached to the abdominal wall, where the body tissue will grow around and into it to provide strength and support.

Mesh Used for Hernia Repair

Hernia repair is the most common use for surgical mesh. A hernia is a protrusion of body tissues through a defect in a muscle or other containing body parts. Mesh may be used to repair the defect that allowed the herniation of body tissue. Hernias used to be commonly repaired using sutures and other types of tension-based tissue closure techniques. However, sutures do not allow for free movement as soon after the surgery. Sutures also create a higher post-operative intra-abdominal pressure and consequent breathing problems than mesh. Sutures are associated with a higher rate of hernia recurrence than mesh. Mesh hernia repair also causes less pain after surgery than suture repair. Mesh hernia repair clearly has many advantages over hernia repair using sutures.

Almost all hernia repairs are performed today using tension-free surgical mesh. Polyprolene is one of the most commonly used synthetic meshes in hernia repair, with each type of mesh material having advantages and disadvantages for hernia repair. Some hernia repair techniques using mesh include the Lichtenstien Repair where mesh is placed over the defect in the tissue, the Kugel Method where mesh is placed behind the defect, and the Prolene Hernia System where two

KEY TERMS

Adhesions—Scar tissue.

Intra-abdominal Pressure—The pressure present in the abdominal cavity that affects the pressure on the diaphragm and the ability to breathe easily.

Prolapse—A condition where the organs fall out of their normal location in the body.

Sutures—Stiches that are used in surgical procedures to bring two pieces of flesh together or close a wound.

Urinary Incontinence—Disorder where urination is uncontrolled and involuntary.

Uterine Suspension—Procedure that places a sling under the uterus and holds it in place.

Vertebral Reconstruction—Procedure for reconstruction and support of the vertebrae of the skeletal system.

layers of mesh are placed around the defect, one behind and one over the defect. Another method of mesh-based hernia repair is the Plug and Patch Method, where mesh is placed like a plug into the tissue defect and then covered over the top with another mesh patch. Hernia repairs using mesh may be done as same day surgery using only **local anesthesia**. Because surgical mesh is a type of tension-free repair, patients can resume normal physical activity much sooner after the operation.

Risks Associated with Surgical Mesh

While the use of surgical mesh has many advantages over other techniques, it is also associated with risk of some medical complications. One of the greatest risks of the use of surgical mesh is mesh infection. Mesh infections tend to be resistant to **wound care** techniques and **antibiotics**, and are generally removed upon discovery. Removal of infected mesh necessitates a new surgical procedure and the replacement of the mesh with a new repair. Surgical mesh may also cause tissue inflammation, which can be painful. Mesh may also cause adhesions, or scar tissue. Adhesions sometimes cause medical problems in the surrounding area. For example, adhesions in the abdominal cavity may cause obstruction of the bowels, and adhesions in the pelvic region may contribute to infertility in females. All types of hernia repair are associated with the risk of hernia recurrence, the protrusion of tissue through the repaired defect from failure of the mesh or suture repair. Mesh repairs have a lower risk of hernia recurrence than sutures.

Resources

BOOKS

Kumar, Vinay, Nelson Fausto, and Abul Abbas. *Robbins & Cotran: Pathologic Basis of Disease,* Seventh Edition. Saunders, Elsevier, 2005.

PERIODICALS

Burger, J. W. A., R. W. Luijendijk, W. Hop, J. A. Halm, E. G. Verdaasdonk, J. Jeekel. "Long-term Follow-up of a Randomized Controlled Trial of Suture Versus Mesh Repair of Incisional Hernia." *Ann Surg* 240(4):578-585, 2004.

Frey, D. M., A. Wildisen, C. T. Hamel, M. Zuber, D. Oertli, J. Metzger. "Randomized Clinical Trial of Lichtenstein's Operation Versus Mesh Plug for Inguinal Hernia Repair." *Br J Surg*. 2007;94:36-41.

OTHER

"Health Adhesions, General and After Surgery." eMedicine. October 16, 2005. http://www.emedicinehealth.com/adhesions_general_and_after_surgery/article_em.htm [Accessed April 15, 2008].

Maria Basile, PhD

Surgical oncology

Definition

Surgical oncology is a specialized area of oncology that engages surgeons in the cure and management of cancer.

Purpose

Cancer has become a medical specialty warranting its own surgical area because of advances in the biology, pathophysiology, diagnostics, and staging of malignant tumors. Surgeons have traditionally treated cancer patients with resection and radical surgeries of tumors, and left the management of the cancer and the patient to other specialists. Advances in the early diagnosis of cancer, the staging of tumors, microscopic analyses of cells, and increased understanding of cancer biology have broadened the range of nonsurgical cancer treatments. These treatments include systematic chemotherapy, hormonal therapy, and radiotherapy as alternatives or adjunctive therapy for patients with cancer.

Not all cancer tumors are manageable by surgery, nor does the removal of some tumors or metastases

KEY TERMS

Biopsy—The surgical excision of tissue to diagnose the size, type, and extent of a cancerous growth.

Cancer surgery—Surgery in which the goal is to excise a tumor and its surrounding tissue found to be malignant.

Resection—Cutting out tissue to eliminate a cancerous tumor; usually refers to a section of the organ, (e.g., colon, intestine, lung, stomach) that must be cut to remove the tumor and its surrounding tissue.

Tumor staging—The method used by oncologists to determine the risk from a cancerous tumor. A number—ranging from 1A–4B— is assigned to predict the level of invasion by a tumor, and offer a prognosis for morbidity and mortality.

necessarily lead to a cure or longer life. The oncological surgeon looks for the relationship between tumor excision and the risk presented by the primary tumor. He or she is knowledgeable about patient management with more conservative procedures than the traditional excision or resection.

Demographics

According to the American Cancer Society and the National Cancer Institute, about 559,650 people were projected to die of cancer in the year 2007. 66% of those diagnosed with cancer within the year 2007 are expected to survive for at least five years after diagnosis. The most common newly diagnosed cancers for males in the United States during 2007, with total of over 766,860 cases for all races, were:

- prostate—29%;
- lung—15%;
- colon and rectum—10%;
- bladder—7%; and
- non-Hodgkin's lymphoma—4%.

The most common newly diagnosed cancers for females in the United States during 2007, with total of over 678,060 cases for all races, were:

- breast—26%;
- lung—15%;
- colon and rectum—11%;
- uterine corpus—6%; and
- non-Hodgkin's lymphoma—4%.

Description

Surgical oncology is guided by principles that govern the routine procedures related to the cancer patient's cure, palliative care, and quality of life. Surgical oncology performs its most efficacious work by local tumor excision, regional lymph node removal, the handling of cancer recurrence (local or widespread), and in rare cases, with surgical resection of metastases from the primary tumor. Each of these areas plays a different role in cancer management.

Excision

Local excision has been the hallmark of surgical oncology. Excision refers to the removal of the cancer and its effects. Resection of a tumor in the colon can end the effects of obstruction, for instance, or removal of a breast carcinoma can stop the cancer. Resection of a primary tumor also stops the tumor from spreading throughout the body. The cancer's spread into other body systems, however, usually occurs before a local removal, giving resection little bearing upon cells that have already escaped the primary tumor. Advances in oncology through pathophysiology, staging, and biopsy offer a new diagnostic role to the surgeon using excision. These advances provide simple diagnostic information about size, grade, and extent of the tumor, as well as more sophisticated evaluations of the cancer's biochemical and hormonal features.

Regional lymph node removal

Lymph node involvement provides surgical oncologists with major diagnostic information. The sentinel node biopsy is superior to any biological test in terms of prediction of cancer mortality rates. Nodal biopsy offers very precise information about the extent and type of invasive effects of the primary tumor. The removal of nodes, however, may present pain and other morbid conditions for the patient.

Local and regional recurrence

Radical procedures in surgical oncology for local and regional occurrences of a primary tumor provide crucial information on the spread of cancer and prognostic outcomes; however, they do not contribute substantially to the outcome of the cancer. According to most surgical oncology literature, the ability to remove a local recurrence must be balanced by the patient's goals related to aesthetic and pain control concerns. Historically, more radical procedures have not improved the chances for survival.

Surgery for distant metastases

In general, a cancer tumor that spreads further from its primary site is less likely to be controlled by surgery. According to research, except for a few instances where metastasis is confined, surgical removal of a distant metastasis is not warranted. Since the rapidity of discovering a distant metastasis has little bearing upon cancer survival, the usefulness of surgery is not time dependent. In the case of liver metastasis, for example, a cure is related to the pathophysiology of the original cancer and level of cancer antigen in the liver rather than the size or time of discovery. While surgery of metastatic cancer may not increase life, there may be indications for it such as pain relief, obstruction removal, control of bleeding, and resolution of infection.

Diagnosis/Preparation

Surgery removes cancer cells and surrounding tissues. It is often combined with radiation therapy and chemotherapy. It is important for the patient to meet with the surgical oncologist to talk about the procedure and begin preparations for surgery. Oncological surgery may be performed to biopsy a suspicious site for malignant cells or tumor. It is also used for **tumor removal** from organs such as the tongue, throat, lung, stomach, intestines, colon, bladder, ovary, and prostate. Tumors of limbs, ligaments, and tendons may also be treated with surgery. In many cases, the biopsy and surgery to remove the cancer cells or tissues are done at the same time.

The impact of a surgical procedure depends upon the diagnosis and the area of the body that is to be treated by surgery. Many cancer surgeries involve major organs and require open abdominal surgery, which is the most extensive type of surgical procedure. This surgery requires medical tests and work-ups to judge the health of the patient prior to surgery, and to make decisions about adjunctive procedures like radiation or chemotherapy. Preparation for cancer surgery requires psychological readiness for a hospital stay, postoperative pain, sometimes slow recovery, and anticipation of complications from tumor excision or resection. It also may require consultation with stomal therapists if a section of the urinary tract or bowel is to be removed and replaced with an outside reservoir or conduit called an ostomy.

Aftercare

After surgery, the type and duration of side effects and the elements of recovery depend on where in the body the surgery was performed and the patient's general health. Some surgeries may alter basic functions in the urinary or gastrointestinal systems. Recovering full use of function takes time and patience. Surgeries that remove conduits such as the colon, intestines, or urinary tract require appliances for urine and fecal waste and the help of a stomal therapist. Breast or prostate surgeries yield concerns about cosmetic appearance and intimate activities. For most cancer surgeries, basic functions like tasting, eating, drinking, breathing, moving, urinating, defecating, or neurological ability may be changed in the short-term. Resources to attend to deficits in daily activities need to be set up before surgery.

WHO PERFORMS THE PROCEDURE AND WHERE IS IT PERFORMED?

A surgeon who specializes in cancer surgery or oncology performs oncology surgery in a general hospital or cancer research center.

Risks

The type of risks that cancer surgery presents depends almost entirely upon the part of the body being biopsied or excised. Risks of surgery can be great when major organs are involved, such as the gastrointestinal system or the brain. These risks are usually discussed explicitly when surgerical decisions are made.

Normal results

Most cancers are staged; that is, they are described by their likelihood of being contained, spreading at the original site, or recurring or invading other bodily systems. The prognosis after surgery depends upon the stage of the disease, and the pathology results on the type of cancer cell involved. General results of cancer surgery depend in large part on norms of success based upon the study of groups of patients with the same diagnosis. The results are often stated in percentages of the chance of cancer recurrence or its spread after surgery. After five disease-free years, patients are usually considered cured. This is because the recurrence rates decline drastically after five years. The benchmark is based upon the percentage of people known to reach the fifth year after surgery with no recurrence or spread of the primary tumor.

Morbidity and mortality rates

Morbidity and mortality of oncological surgery are high if there is organ involvement or extensive

QUESTIONS TO ASK THE DOCTOR

Who is recommended for a second opinion?

What are the alternatives to surgery for this cancer?

What is the likelihood that this surgery will entirely eliminate the cancer?

Is this a surgical procedure that is often performed in this hospital or surgical center?

excision of major parts of the body. Because there is an ongoing disease process and many patients may be very ill at the time of surgery, the complications of surgery may be quite complex. Each procedure is understood by the surgeon for its likely complications or risks, and these are discussed during the initial surgical consultations.

There are comprehensive surgical procedures for many cancers, and complications may be extensive due to the use of general anesthetic and the opening of body cavities. Open surgery has general risks associated with it that are not related to the type of procedure. These risks include possibility of blood clots and cardiac events.

There is an extensive body of literature about the complication and morbidity rates of surgery performed by high-volume treatment centers. Data show that in general, large volumes of surgery affect the quality outcomes of surgery, with smaller hospitals having lower rates of procedural success and higher operative and postoperative complications than larger facilities. It is not known whether the surgeon's experience or the advantages of institutional resources in operative or **postoperative care** contributes to these statistics.

Alternatives

Alternatives to cancer surgery exist for almost every cancer treated in the United States. Research into alternatives has been very successful for some—but not all—cancers. There are many alternatives to surgery, and chemotherapy and radiation after surgery. Most organizations dealing with cancer patients suggest alternative treatments. Physicians and surgeons expect to be asked about alternatives to surgery, and are usually quite knowledgeable about their use as cancer treatments or as adjuncts to surgery.

Resources

BOOKS

Abeloff, M. D., J. Armitage, J. Niederhuber, M. Kastan, and W. G. McKenna. *Clinical Oncology,* 3rd ed. Philadelphia: Elsevier, 2004.

Cummings, C. W., et al.*Otolaryngology: Head and Neck Surgery,* 4th ed. St. Louis: Mosby, 2004.

Katz V. L., G. Lentz, R. A. Lobo, and D. Gershenson. *Comprehensive Gynecology,* 5th ed. St. Louis: Mosby, 2007.

Khatri, V. P., and J. A. Asensio. *Operative Surgery Manual,* 1st ed. Philadelphia: Saunders, 2002.

Townsend, C.M., R. D. Beauchamp, B. M. Evers, and K. Mattox. *Sabiston Textbook of Surgery,* 17th ed. Philadelphia: Saunders, 2004.

Wein, A. J., L. R. Kavoussi, A. C. Novick, A. W. Partin, and C. A. Peters. *Campbell-Walsh Urology,* 9th ed. Philadelphia: Saunders, 2006.

OTHER

Cancer Trends Progress Report—2007 Update. National Cancer Institute. December 2007. http://progressreport.cancer.gov/ (April 7, 2008).

ORGANIZATIONS

American Cancer Society, 1875 Connecticut Avenue, NW, Suite 730, Washington, DC, 20009, (800) ACS-2345, http://www.cancer.org.

National Breast Cancer Coalition, 1101 17th Street, NW, Suite 1300, Washington, DC, 20036, (800) 622-2838, (202) 265-6854, http://www.stopbreastcancer.org/.

Office of Cancer Complementary and Alternative Medicine, National Cancer Institute, 6116 Executive Boulevard, Suite 609, MSC 8339, Bethesda, MD, 20892, (800) 422-6237, http://www.cancer.gov/cam/.

Nancy McKenzie, Ph.D.
Rosalyn Carson-DeWitt, M.D.

Surgical risk

Definition

Surgical risk is the set of potential adverse medical circumstances that may arise from having surgery, or the dangers and harm that may occur. Risk is determined by surgical risk factors, which are any set of circumstances that increase the risk of surgical complications. Surgical complications are any negative medical results that deviate from the normal expected outcomes of surgery, or the expected recovery scenario.

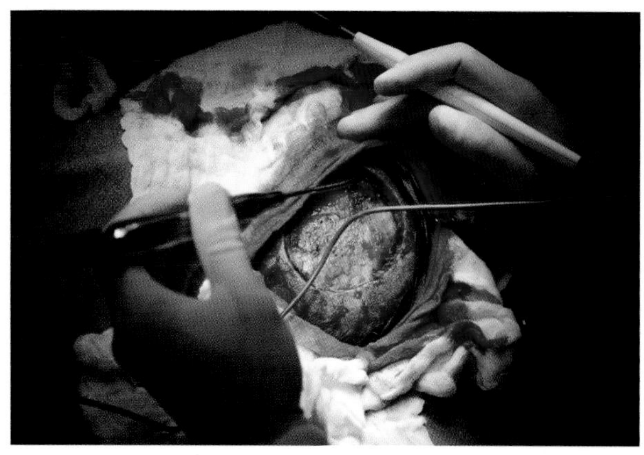

Surgeon using electrocautery to stop bleeding. *(PHOTOTAKE Inc. / Alamy)*

Demographics

Specific subsets of the population are at higher risk for serious complications after surgery. People who are more vulnerable to surgical complications and therefore have a higher risk include the elderly, the obese, people who are in very poor physical condition from disease, lack of **exercise**, or malnourishment, people who have a compromised immune system such as AIDS patients, people with certain heart conditions, and smokers.

Benefits and Risk

By nature, surgery is a risky business. However, those risks have been greatly minimized by modern technology and the high standard of physician **surgical training**. Surgeons usually undergo the rigors of nearly a decade of intensive training and education before they perform surgeries on their own. Experience is key to becoming a qualified surgeon, and so is included even in the early training stages of a surgeon's career. A qualified surgeon is a highly trained and skilled professional who can serve certain patients to improve or even save their lives. It can be overwhelming to read the long list of potential complications that may arise from having surgery. However, it is important to note that most of these complications are anticipated and measures are taken to avoid harm to the patient. Surgery saves many lives each year, and should be viewed in light of considering the potential benefits as well as the potential risks.

Description

The degree of surgical risk varies between different surgical procedures, as well as with the individual medical aspects associated with each patient. The risk a patient takes when having a surgical procedure is a combination of the risks associated with the procedure itself as well as risks associated with specific patient-based factors regarding surgery. Patient-based risk factors are an important part of surgical risk, and help determine the likelihood of a surgical complication occurring. The decision to perform any surgical procedure is based on whether or not potential benefits outweigh the sum of the potential risks.

Procedure-Based Risk

Any patient undergoing surgery is at risk for medical complications that arise from the procedure itself. The specific factors that may potentially cause these complications are called procedure-based risk factors. The surgical procedures associated with the highest level of risk include cardiac surgery, lung surgery, prostate removal, and some major orthopedic surgeries such as **hip replacement**.

Patient-Based Risk

Many patient-based factors increase the risk of having complications during or after a surgical procedure. Patient-based factors that generally increase risk include advanced age, obesity, poor physical condition, smoking, a compromised immune system, recent heart attack or unstable heart conditions, and malnourishment. Some specific types of surgical procedures may have their own specific types of patient-based risk factors. Specific complications are also associated with certain patient-based risk factors. For example, obesity increases the risk for wound and pulmonary complications after surgery. **Smoking cessation** for six weeks before surgery decreases the incidence of pulmonary complications.

Risk of Excessive Bleeding

Excessive bleeding is risk factor of undergoing surgery. During any surgical procedure, there may be accidental damage to a major blood vessel. If that damage is not effectively repaired, it may result in excessive blood loss. If procedural damage is done to smaller blood vessels as an expected part of the surgery but is not properly controlled, there may be excessive blood loss. Even without surgical damage to blood vessels, if a patient undergoes too much physical activity soon after having a surgical procedure, they may accidentally open some of the internal or external surgical sites and cause bleeding. Excessive bleeding may result in the patient becoming anemic. Anemia, and the resulting fatigue associated with anemia, is a risk of surgical procedures. If a very large amount of blood is lost, it can lead to complications much more serious than anemia. A very large loss of blood risks the patient going into a state of shock.

Disorders of blood clotting predispose a surgical patient to bleeding complications. If the patient's blood has a defective ability to clot, the body cannot properly close small wounds in a normal manner. Instead, even small cuts that are part of the surgical procedure can result in excessive or prolonged bleeding that may be life threatening. If surgery is a necessity in this type of patient, physicians can appropriately manage these conditions prior to the procedure to minimize the risk for bleeding complications.

Risk of Seroma Formation

A seroma is an internal collection of bodily fluids at a surgical site. Seromas may result from improper wound closure or as a complication of the specific procedure. For example, breast surgery is associated with a high risk of seroma formation, even when performed properly. The presence of a seroma may delay wound healing and also increases the risk of developing an infection. Seromas are more likely to form in obese individuals, or individuals whose body forms an excessive volume of fluids that need to be drained from the surgical site during the recovery period.

Risk of Infection

Hospitals may contain types of bacteria that the average person in the United States is not normally exposed to, or mutated strains of common bacteria. Having surgery and staying in the hospital may increase the risk of being exposed to these types of bacteria. Additionally, the emergence of antibiotic resistant strains of bacteria complicates the risk of infection after surgery. Infections with mutated strains of bacteria that are resistant to available **antibiotics** are especially difficult to prevent, treat, or control.

Risk of infection is associated with any type of surgical procedure. To minimize the chance of a patient contracting a bacterial infection, some surgical procedures involve prophylactic application of antibiotics. Surgical procedures that may involve **antibiotic prophylaxis** include bowel surgery, procedures that include insertion of prosthetic material, surgeries on patients with impaired immune systems, **neurosurgery**, cardiac surgery, and ophthalmic surgery. In addition to antibiotics, proper surgical technique in an appropriately clean **operating room** setting also minimizes risk of infection. Surgeons "scrub in" to surgery, meaning that they follow specific protocols of hand washing and dressing in surgical gowns that minimize risk of infection. The surgical site on the patient's body also needs to be effectively disinfected before the procedure can be performed. However, even with proper protective measures taken, there is risk of contracting a bacterial infection at surgical sites after having a procedure.

Bacterial infections after surgery may also occur in the urinary tract when a urinary catheter is used, in the respiratory tract if the patient needs to be on a respirator after the procedure, or may be systemic infections that lead to sepsis. Patients with compromised immune systems are at especially high risk of contracting bacterial infections that healthier individuals are usually able to resist. Other patient-based risk factors for post-surgery infection include a preexisting infection before surgery, low levels of certain non-immune blood components, advanced age, obesity, smoking, diagnosis of diabetes, certain cardiovascular diseases, a physiological state of shock, excessive physical trauma, and requiring a blood **transfusion**. The organism most often associated with infection of surgical sites in the hospital is *Staphylococcus aureus*, which may be resistant to many current antibiotics such as methicillin.

Risk of Neurological Damage

Surgical procedures may involve risk of neurological damage, or damage to the nervous system. Depending on the type of surgery, nerve damage may be a result of direct injury to the brain, spinal cord, or peripheral nerves. Nerve damage from a surgical procedure may also occur secondary to the administration of spinal, epidural, or regional anesthesia, or from a temporary reduction of oxygen flow to a specific part of the body. Depending on the part of the nervous system that sustains damage, the results may be mild to severe, temporary or permanent. For example, head and neck surgery is associated with risk of injury to numerous delicate nerves, some of which may result in a permanent state of Bell's palsy if damage occurs.

Risk of Postoperative Delirium

Although most patients experience a temporary state of confusion when they come out of anesthesia, having a surgical procedure may carry the risk of postoperative delirium. Delirium is a severe state of mental confusion, disorientation, agitation, and general incoherence. Delirium may also include hallucinations. Postoperative delirium is a temporary state of delirium that may be caused by multiple factors relating to the surgical procedure. A postoperative temporary state of delirium may occur if the patient experiences a lack of oxygen, hypotension, or sepsis as a result of the surgical procedure. Patient-based risk factors for postoperative delirium include advanced age, pre-existing dementia, chronic drug or alcohol abuse, certain metabolic disorders, side effects of certain medications such as merperidine, and sleep deprivation. Because individuals of advanced age are at higher risk for postoperative delirium, the mental status of elderly patients is frequently assessed in postoperative recovery. If delirium occurs, the patient's oxygen levels are checked, and all non-essential drugs are temporarily discontinued. With proper treatment, post-operative delirium usually goes away within 72 hours.

Risk of Anesthesia Complications

A patient undergoing **general anesthesia** for a surgical procedure runs the risk of a temporary, minor disturbance in mental function after the procedure. Patients may experience slight confusion, disorientation, and decreased general mental acuity after having anesthesia for a surgical procedure. This mental state may take up to a week to fully dissipate, and may affect the patient's ability to work or operate an automobile. Patient-based factors that increase the likelihood of anesthesia complications include advanced age, obesity, and kidney or liver insufficiencies resulting in poor metabolism of the anesthetic agent.

Risk of Cardiac Complications

Cardiac complications are another surgical risk factor. Certain types of anesthesia such as halothane may cause a cardiac arrhythmia during the induction of anesthesia. Additionally there are other factors that may contribute to cardiac complications after surgery. Certain drugs, excessive pain, certain acid-base imbalances, and problems with oxygen delivery during surgery may lead to arrhythmias. Post-operative hypertension may also occur as a result of poor **pain management** after a surgical procedure. Patient-based risk factors for post-operative hypertension include advanced age, congestive heart failure, and angina.

There is a slight risk of heart attack associated with non-cardiac surgeries, and a greater risk associated with cardiac or vascular surgeries. Risk factors for heart attack associated with surgery are pre-existing congestive heart failure, angina, atherosclerosis, pre-existing anemia, hypotension or anemia as a result of blood loss during surgery, defective oxygen delivery during surgery, and advanced patient age.

Risk of Other Organ-Based Complications

Any surgical procedure performed on or around an organ system has some risk of damage to that system. The following are examples of organ-based surgical risk factors. Pancreatitis (inflammation of the pancreas) is a rare complication as a result of surgery. However, within the cases of pancreatitis that do exist, approximately 10% are related to injury during surgical procedures. When a surgical procedure is performed in the physical vicinity of the pancreas, approximately 1-3% of patients may develop pancreatitis. If the surgical procedure involves maneuvering the actual biliary tract, the incidence of pancreatitis rises. Patient surgical risk factors that predispose to pancreatitis include previous history of pancreatitis, parathyroid surgery which alters blood levels of calcium very quickly and in a short period of time, cardiopulmonary bypass, and renal transplantation.

Surgeries involving the contents of the abdomen have risk for temporarily disrupting the normal movement of the intestines, a condition known as postoperative intestinal ileus. If the intestines are handled too much or are damaged, or certain types of postoperative pain medications are overused, the normal propulsive movements of the bowels may cease completely. While this condition is temporary and treatable, the patient cannot eat or drink until normal intestinal movement is restored. Postoperative ileus may cause abdominal distention, pain, constipation, and vomiting; require a prolonged hospital stay; or contribute to a regional bacterial infection.

Risk of Vascular Complications

Several vascular complications may result from a surgical procedure. If a procedure involves the placement of a central line, air may be introduced into the body cavity outside of the lung, and then collapse the lung. If a catheter is left open air may enter the blood stream, travel to, and affect the proper functioning of the heart.

Deep Venous Thrombosis (DVT) is a condition where a blood clot (thrombus) forms in a blood vessel. DVT occurs in approximately 40% of postoperative patients. Clots usually form in the lower extremities. To prevent DVT, support hose and compression devices are used during surgical procedures. DVT is dangerous because if a clot becomes an embolus (clot that detaches from the vessel wall and travels through the bloodstream) and goes into the pulmonary system (pulmonary embolus) it can be life threatening. It is one of the most common causes of sudden **death** in hospitalized patients and is a risk factor if a surgical procedure requires a long period of bed rest during recovery.

Pulmonary emboli may be caused by multiple types of clots in addition to DVT, and are a type of surgical risk. For example pulmonary emboli may also be caused fat droplets entering the bloodstream during joint replacement surgery. Patient-based risk factors for a pulmonary embolus during surgery include advanced age, heart disease, obesity, and varicose veins.

Risk Associated with Blood Transfusions

Patients undergoing some surgical procedures carry the risk of needing a blood transfusion. Blood transfusions may cause a dangerous immune system reaction against the blood type or other blood components of the transfusion. These reactions can make the patient very sick or may even become anaphylactic and life threatening. To prevent the likelihood of an immune reaction, blood is carefully matched to the patient in a way that minimizes risk. Although the blood used for blood transfusions is screened for known viruses, transmission of an unknown virus is a possibility.

Risk of Pulmonary Complications

Pulmonary complications are a main cause of postoperative illness. Pulmonary complications may be caused by patient-based risk factors or surgical procedure-based risk factors. Many pulmonary complications after surgery involve part of the respiratory system partially collapsing, usually within 48 hours of a surgical procedure. Other potential respiratory/pulmonary complications involve lung infections, difficulty breathing, or aspirating (breathing in) regurgitated gastric secretions while under general anesthesia. While under anesthesia the parts of the body that normally protect the respiratory system from taking in food or fluids (the epiglottis and esophageal sphincter) are relaxed. Therefore safeguards have to be set in place for protection. Endotracheal tubes are tubes placed in the throat to minimize the risk of breathing regurgitated stomach contents down into the respiratory tract. If food or fluids from the stomach enter the respiratory tract, it may result in pulmonary complications associated with high mortality rates. In order to avoid these complications patients are asked to fast from food before surgical procedures requiring general anesthesia, are positioned carefully for surgery, and carefully fitted with an endotracheal tube.

Patient-based risk factors associated with different types of pulmonary complications include advanced age, obesity, pre-existing chronic lung disease, and smoking history. Surgical procedure-based risk factors include procedures requiring a long duration of anesthesia, prolonged **mechanical ventilation**, thoracic or upper abdomen surgery, abdominal distention, inadequate pain control that results in the patient not coughing effectively after the procedure, oversedation due to administration of too much anesthesia, excessive postsurgical pain killer use, or an endotracheal tube that is not positioned correctly.

QUESTIONS TO ASK YOUR DOCTOR

- Why do I need a surgical procedure?
- What are alternative options to surgery?
- What are the potential benefits of this procedure?
- What are the potential risks of this procedure?
- What outcomes are anticipated if I do not have the surgical procedure?
- Who would perform the procedure?
- How many times has my surgeon performed this procedure before?
- Are there any patient-based risk factors that could be altered to minimize risk?
- Will any of my medications, over-the-counter medicines, and nutritional or herbal supplements affect my recovery from this procedure?
- How long should recovery be expected to take?
- Will I have to stay in the hospital after the procedure?

Tool-Based Risk

The tools used during surgery pose a risk for damage to organs, nerves, or blood vessels. Scalpels, cauterizers, needles, and clamps may be mishandled and accidentally cut, burn, pierce, or cause blunt trauma to the body. Even minimal access surgeries such as a **laparoscopy** involve tool-based surgical risk. Tool-based risks of laparoscopies include the use of **trocars**, a tool used to make the first incision or entry into the abdominal cavity. If a classic trocars is used in the first "blind jab" into the abdomen, before a camera can be inserted, the physician may push too hard on the trocars and damage blood vessels or internal organs. Any surgical tool poses a risk for damage, and is only as safe as the skill of the surgeon wielding it.

Hospital Screening Tests to Minimize Surgical Risk

Hospitals may perform laboratory tests before admitting a patient for surgery in order to catch patient-based risk factors that predispose for surgical complications and treat them. Pre-surgery tests such as **urinalysis**, chest x-rays, or complete blood counts may identify potential risk factors that could lead to complications. Commonly performed pre-surgery tests include:

KEY TERMS

Acquired Immunodeficiency Syndrome (AIDS)—A disease syndrome in which the patient's immune cells are destroyed by HIV virus, leaving the patient open to opportunistic infections that a healthy immune system could keep at bay.

Anaphylactic—A serious allergic reaction to a foreign protein or other material.

Anemia—A physiological state in which the number of red blood cells or amount of hemoglobin in the blood is abnormally low, leading to a decrease in the capacity of the blood to carry oxygen to the tissues.

Angina—Disease involving decreased oxygen flow to the heart and often constricting chest pain.

Aspiration—The act of inspiring or sucking foreign fluid or vomit into the airways.

Atherosclerosis—Disease involving irregularly deposited fat within the arteries that results in medical complications.

Bell Palsy—One-sided paralysis of the face that may be due to damage to the facial nerve.

Cardiac Arrhythmia—An irregular heartbeat.

Cardiac Pulmonary Bypass—A procedure where heart blood is diverted into an inserted pump in order to maintain appropriate blood flow.

Catheter—A flexible tube inserted into the body to allow passage of fluids in or out.

Central Line—A catheter passed through a vein into large blood vessels of the chest or the heart; used in various medical procedures.

Deep Venous Thrombosis (DVT)—Blood clot that usually forms in the lower extremities after prolonged inactivity.

Delirium—An altered state of consciousness that includes confusion, disorientation, incoherence, agitation, and defective perception (such as hallucinations).

Electrocardiogram (ECG)—A medical tool used to monitor the electrical impulses released by the beating heart. The results are drawn out in graphical fashion to visualize the function of the heart.

Embolus—A plug of blood cell components, bacteria, or foreign body that travels through the bloodstream, lodges, and occludes a blood vessel.

Endotracheal Tube—Tube inserted in the throat during general anesthesia to prevent aspiration of gastric contents into the respiratory tract.

Epidural Anesthesia—Regional anesthesia produced by injecting the anesthetic agent into an area near the spinal cord.

- Chest x-rays for patients with shortness of breath, chest pain, or a cough
- Electrocardiogram (ECG) for patients with chest pain or abnormal heart signs
- Urinalysis for patients with urinary problems, side pain, kidney disease, or diabetes
- White blood cell count for patients with a suspected infection, or on medications known to affect white blood cell counts
- Platelet count for patients with excessive blood loss, alcoholism, or on medications known to affect platelet count
- Glucose levels for patients with excessive sweating, tremors, diabetes, cystic fibrosis, an altered mental status, or alcoholism
- Potassium levels for patients with congestive heart failure, kidney failure, muscle weakness, diabetes, or on medications known to affect potassium levels
- Sodium levels for patients with pulmonary disease, central nervous system disease, congestive heart failure, or some types of liver disease

Resources

BOOKS

The Merck Manual of Diagnosis and Therapy Eighteenth Edition. 2006.

General Surgery Board Review Series. Lippincott Williams & Wilkins. 2000.

The Merck Manual Home Edition 2004.

PERIODICALS

Cheadle, W. G. "Risk Factors for Surgical Site Infection." *Surgical Infections* 7, no. 1 (2006).

Weinstein, Robert A. "Nosocomial Infection Update." *Emerging Infectious Diseases, Special Issue* 4, no. 3 (July-September 1998; updated April 3, 2008). http://www.cdc.gov/ncidod/eid/vol4no3/weinstein.htm [accessed April 3, 2008].

ORGANIZATIONS

American Association for the Surgery of Trauma, 633 N Saint Clair St, Suite 2400, Chicago, Illinois, 60611, (312)202-5252, (800)789-4006, (312)202-5013, http://www.aast.org/index.aspx.

American Academy of Orthopaedic Surgery, 6300 North River Road, Rosemont, Illinois, 60018-4262, (847)823-7186, (847)823-8125, http://www.aaos.org.

Epiglottis—A leaf-shaped piece of cartilage lying at the root of the tongue that protects the respiratory tract from aspiration during the swallowing reflex.

Esophageal Sphincter—Muscle at the opening to the stomach that keeps the stomach contents from traveling into the esophagus.

Glucose—A form of sugar used by the body for energy.

Hypotension—Low blood pressure.

Hypovolemia—An abnormally low amount of blood in the body.

Intestinal Ileus—Mechanical or dynamic obstruction of the bowel causing pain, abdominal distention, vomiting, and often fever.

Laparoscopy—Minimally invasive surgical procedure in which small incisions are made in the abdominal or pelvic cavity and surgical tools are used with a miniature camera for guidance.

Merperidine—A type of narcotic pain killer that may be used after surgical procedures.

Methicillin-resistant *Staphylococcus aureus* (MRSA)—A strain of Staph. bacteria that is resistant to methicillin and hence poses a greater health threat because it is difficult to control or kill.

Pancreatitis—Inflammation of the pancreas.

Parathyroid Gland—An endocrine gland that modulates calcium in the body.

Platelet—A blood component responsible for normal clotting mechanisms that seal small wounds.

Prophylaxis—The prevention of disease or infection, or of a process that can lead to disease or infection.

Sepsis—A dangerous physiological state of extensive, systemic bacterial infection.

Seroma—A seroma is an internal collection of fluid at a surgical site.

Spinal Anesthesia—Regional anesthesia produced by injecting the anesthetic agent into an area directly around the spinal cord.

Thrombus—A blood clot attached to a blood vessel wall.

Trocars—A surgical tool shaped as a hollow cylinder that is sometimes used to make an initial incision into a body cavity and through which other surgical tools are then passed.

White Blood Cell—A component of the blood involved in the immune response.

American Academy for Thoracic Surgery, 900 Cummings Center, Suite 221-U, Beverly, Massachusetts, 01915, (978)927-8330, (978)524-8890, http://www.aats.org.

Maria Basile, PhD

Surgical team

Definition

The surgical team is a unit providing the continuum of care beginning with **preoperative care**, and extending through perioperative (during the surgery) procedures, and postoperative recovery. Each specialist on the team, whether surgeon, anesthesiologist or nurse, has advanced training for his or her role before, during, and after surgery.

Purpose

Surgery, whether elective, required, or emergency, is done for a variety of conditions that include:

- cosmetic procedures
- diagnostic and exploratory procedures
- treatment of acute, chronic, and infectious diseases of tissue or organs
- transplantation of organs
- resposition and enhancement of bone, ligaments, tendons, or organ conduits
- replacement or implantation of artificial or electronic devices

The crucial elements of surgery—surgical and operative procedures, pain control, patient safety, and blood and wound control—require individual expertise and high levels of concentration and coordination. Through a team effort, the patient is treated and monitored as he or she undergoes significant acts of bodily invasion and pain control that make up the surgical experience, whether they be the most benign and superficial operations, or the most intense.

Demographics

According to the Centers for Disease Control (CDC) and Prevention and the National Center for Health Statistics, 45 million inpatient surgical procedures were performed in the United States in 2005, followed closely by 31.5 million outpatient surgeries. Leading surgeries included:

- digestive system surgeries: 12 million
- musculoskeletal system surgeries: 7.4 million
- cardiovascular system surgeries: 6.8 million
- eye surgeries: 5.4 million

Description

The components of the surgical team depend on the type of surgery, the precise procedures, and the location and the type of anesthesia utilized. The team may include surgeons, anesthesiologists, and nursing and technical staff who are trained in **general surgery** or in a particular surgical specialty. Intense surgeries require larger teams and more comprehensive recovery care. Even though minimally invasive procedures (e.g., **laparoscopy** or endoscopy) are conducted with small instruments and a video camera probe, they require specialized expertise and high technology knowledge. These procedures utilize smaller teams, create less extensive wounds, and yield quicker healing, but often require more operating time and may result in operative injuries.

Types of surgery

Many surgeries are categorized as general surgery, and are associated primarily with accidents, emergencies, and trauma care. Hospitals have general surgeons that staff their emergency rooms or trauma centers. As surgical technology and knowledge have advanced, other surgical specialties have developed for each function and organ of the body. They involve special surgical techniques and anesthesiology requirements, and sometimes require subspecialists with in-depth knowledge of organ function, operative techniques, complex anesthesiology procedures, and specialized nursing care.

The basic surgical specialties include:

- General surgery. General surgeons manage a broad spectrum of surgical conditions that involve almost any part of the body. They confirm the diagnoses provided by primary care or emergency physicians and radiologists, and perform procedures necessary to correct or alleviate the problem.
- Cardiothoracic surgery. A major surgical specialty with very high demands, The cardiothoracic surgical team oversees the preoperative, operative, and critical care of patients with pathologic conditions within the chest, including the heart and its valves, cancers of the lung, esophagus, and chest wall, and chest vessels.
- Neurosurgery. Neurosurgical teams specialize in surgery of the nervous system, including the brain, spine, and peripheral nervous system, and their supporting structures.
- Oral and maxillofacial surgery. Head and neck surgical teams provide treatment for problems of the ears, sinuses, mouth, pharynx, jaw, and other structures of the head and neck.
- Reconstructive and plastic surgery. Reconstructive surgery is performed on abnormal structures of the body due to injury, birth defects, infection, tumors, or disease. Cosmetic surgery is performed to improve a patient's appearance.
- Transplantation. Transplant surgical teams specialize in specific organ transplant techniques, such as heart and heart-lung transplants, liver transplants, and kidney/pancreas transplants. These highly intricate surgeries require very advanced training and technological support.
- Urology and renal transplantation. Also known as gastrointestinal surgery, the team specializes in problems of the digestive tract (stomach, bowels, liver,

KEY TERMS

Anesthesiologist—A physician with advanced training in anesthesia (and sometimes other medical specialties) who administers or oversees the administration of anesthesia to the patient and monitors care after surgery.

Anesthetist—A nurse trained in anesthesiology who, working as an assistant to an anesthesiologist, administers the anesthesia in surgery and monitors the patient after surgery.

Minimally invasive surgery—Surgical techniques, especially the use of small instruments and tiny video cameras, that allow surgery to take place without a full operative wound.

Operative nurse—A nurse specially trained to assist the surgeon and work in all areas of the surgical event to care for the patient.

and gallbladder) with intensive use of or coordination with transplant team members.

- Vascular surgery. Vascular surgery offers diagnosis and treatment of arterial and venous disorders such as aneurysms, lower extremity revascularization, and other problems.
- Pediatric surgery. Pediatric surgical teams are specially trained to treat a broad range of conditions affecting infants and children. They work closely with specially trained anesthesiologists, and are experts in childhood diseases of the head, neck, chest, and abdomen, with training in birth defects and injuries. Many pediatric surgeons work to increase the use of minimally invasive techniques with children.

Surgical techniques

Open surgeries requiring invasive procedures within the abdominal cavity, brain, or extensive limb areas require a hospital stay overnight or up to two weeks. Hospitalization allows the clinical staff to monitor patient recovery (and provide medical attention in the case of a complication), while allowing patients to regain organ functions.

Surgery has been revolutionized by new technology. Ambulatory or outpatient surgeries account for an increasing percentage of surgeries in the United States. Imagery with miniature videoscopes that pass into the patient via tiny incisions is an example of how minimally invasive procedures are replacing open surgeries. Minimally invasive surgeries reduce recovery time and increase the speed of healing. Outpatient or ambulatory surgery environments often allow patients to recover and go home the same day. In specialty surgery centers, such as those designed for ophthalmology, surgery is performed as part of a physician's office practice. These centers contain their own operating rooms and recovery areas.

Minimally invasive procedures that involve the use of a videoscope as an exploratory as well as viewing instrument, include the following:

- Arthroscopy allows viewing of the interior of joints, especially the knee joint.
- Cystoscopy is used to examine the urethra and bladder.
- Endoscopy uses an endoscope in gastrointestinal surgeries of the esophagus, stomach, and colon.
- Laparoscopy uses an illuminated tube with a video camera inserted in small incisions in the abdomen.
- Sigmoidoscopy is used for examining the rectum and sigmoid colon.

Types of anesthesia

Surgical procedures and the surgical setting may be associated with different types of anesthesia:

- General anesthesia renders the patient unconscious during surgery. The anesthesia is either inhaled or given intravenously. A breathing tube may be inserted into the windpipe (trachea) to facilitate breathing. The patient is carefully monitored and wakes up in the recovery room.
- Regional anesthesia numbs the surgical section of the body. This is usually accomplished via injection through the spinal canal (spinal anesthesia) or through a catheter to the lower part of the back (epidural). Regional anesthetics numb the area of the nerves that provide feeling to the designated part of the body.
- Local anesthesia medicates only the direct operative site, and is administered through injection. The patient remains conscious during the operation.

Surgical team

The basic surgical team consists of experts in operative procedure, **pain management**, and overall or specific patient care. Team members include the surgeon, anesthesiologist, and **operating room** nurse. In teaching hospitals attached to medical schools, the team may be added to by those in training, such as interns, residents, and nursing students.

SURGEON. The surgeon performs the operation, and leads the surgical team. Surgeons have medical degrees, specialized **surgical training** of up to seven years, and, in most cases, have passed national board certification exams. Board certification means that the surgeon has passed written and oral examinations of academic competence. The American Board of Surgery, a professional organization that strives to improve the quality of care for patients, is the certifying board for surgeons. As a peer review organization, the College has advanced standards to certify surgical competence by allowing examined surgeons to become a fellow of the organization. Fellows of the American College of Surgeons (FACS) are the elite members of the profession. An FACS designation after a physician's name and degree denotes attainment of the profession's highest training and expertise. Surgeons' credentials may be explored through the Official American Board of Medical Specialties, available at libraries or online.

ANESTHESIOLOGIST. Anesthesiologists are physicians with at least four years of advanced training in anesthesia. They may attain further specialization in surgical procedures, such as **neurosurgery** or **pediatric surgery**. They are directly or indirectly involved in all three stages of surgery, preoperative, operative, and postoperative, due to their focus on pain management and patient safety.

CERTIFIED REGISTERED NURSE ANESTHETIST (CRNA). The certified nurse anesthetist supports the anesthesiologists and, in an increasing number of hospitals, takes full control of the anesthesia for the operation. Registered nurses must graduate from an approved nursing program and pass a licensing examination. They may be licensed in more than one state. While states determine the training and certification requirements of nurses, the work setting determines their daily responsibilities. Certified registered nurse anesthetists must have advanced education and clinical practice experience in anesthesiology.

OPERATING NURSE. The general nursing staff is a critical feature of the surgical team. The nursing staff performs comprehensive care, assistance, and pain management during each surgical phase. He or she is usually the team member providing the most continuity between the stages of care. The operating nurse is the general assistant to the surgeon during the actual operation phase, and usually has advanced training.

Preparation

The surgical team admits the patient to the hospital or surgery center. Many surgeons and anesthesiologists have privileges at more than one hospital and may admit the patient to a center of the patient's choosing. Surgical preparation is the preoperative phase of surgery, and involves special team activities that include monitoring **vital signs**, and administering medications and tests needed immediately before the procedure. In preparation for surgery, the patient meets with the surgeon, anesthesiologist, and surgical nurse. Each team member discusses his or her role in the surgery, and obtains from the patient pertinent information.

Aftercare

After the surgical procedure has been performed, the patient is brought to a **recovery room** where post-anesthesia staff take over from the surgical team under the guidance of the surgeon and anesthesiologist. The staff carefully monitors the patient by checking vital signs, the surgical wound and its **dressings**, IV medications, swallowing ability, level of consciousness, and any tubes or drains. Clinical staff also manages the patient's pain and body positioning.

Risks

Because of its risks, surgery should be the option chosen when the benefit includes the removal of life-threatening conditions or improvement in quality of daily life. Radical surgeries for some types of cancer may offer less than a 20% chance of cure, and the operation may pose the same percentage of mortality risk. A failed operation may shorten time with loved ones and friends, or a successful operation may lead to major positive changes in daily life.

Surgery often brings quicker relief from many conditions than other medical treatment. The risks of surgery depend upon a number of factors, including the experience of the surgical team. In a *New England Journal of Medicine* article, researchers found that mortality decreased as patient volume in a surgical setting increased. The study's messages were that patients should choose surgical centers where a large number of the type of surgery they need is performed, and that physicians working in low-volume hospitals should find ways to increase volume and reduce their morbidity and mortality rates.

Mortality rates are lower and the care more extensive in teaching hospitals with a house staff made up of interns and residents in training.

Healthcare facilities keep records of the procedures they perform. By contacting the Joint Commission on Accreditation of Healthcare Organizations (JCAHO), a center's success with surgical care, mortality and morbidity rates, and surgical complications can be determined.

The Institute of Medicine estimates that today's anesthesia care is nearly 50 times safer than it was 20 years ago, with one anesthesia-related **death** per 200,000–300,000 cases. Despite this record of progress, many questions remain about anesthetic safety. Certified registered nurse anesthetists administer over 65% of anesthesia in the United States, and are often the primary anesthetists for rural communities and delivery rooms.

Independent of surgical team expertise and experience, patient status, and the level of technological advancement in surgical procedures, cardiac events, blood clots, and infection pose surgical risks. These risks accompany all surgeries and, while great progress has been achieved, they remain factors that are part of any surgical invasion and any use of anesthesia.

Alternatives

Alternatives to surgery should be investigated with the referring physician or primary care physician. Many medical conditions benefit from changes in lifestyle, such as losing weight, increasing **exercise**, and undergoing physical rehabilitation. This is especially true for chronic conditions of the gastrointestinal tract, cardiovascular system, urologic system, and bone and joint issues. Research and other resources offer alternatives to surgery including pharmaceutical and medical remedies.

Patients should obtain a **second opinion** before undergoing most major surgeries. It is very important that patients understand that a second opinion offers them the ability to obtain a confirming or differing diagnosis as well as new treatment options. A study of New York City employees and retirees who sought second opinions found that 30% of the second opinions differed from the first. Many health plans have mandatory second opinion clauses. Second opinions should involve physicians in other facilities or even other cities. A change in surgeon will mean a change in the surgical team.

Resources

BOOKS

Khatri, V. P., and J. A. Asensio. *Operative Surgery Manual*, 1st ed. Philadelphia: Saunders, 2003.

Miller, R. D. *Miller's Anesthesia*, 6th ed. Philadelphia: Elsevier, 2005.

Townsend, C. M., et al. *Sabiston Textbook of Surgery*, 17th ed. Philadelphia: Saunders, 2004.

PERIODICALS

Birkmeyer, J.D., E.V. Finlayson, and C.M. Birkmeyer. "Volume Standards for High-risk Surgical Procedures: Potential Benefits of the Leapfrog Initiative." *Surgery* (130) (September 2001): 415–22.

Finlayson, E.V., and J.D. Birkmeyer. "Operative Mortality with Elective Surgery in Older Adults." *Effective Clinical Practice* 4 (July 2001): 172–7.

ORGANIZATIONS

American Board of Medical Specialties. 1007 Church Street, Suite 404, Evanston, IL 60201. (847) 491-9091. http://www.abms.org/ (accessed April 8, 2008).

American Board of Surgery. 1617 John F. Kennedy Boulevard, Suite 860, Philadelphia, PA 19103. (215) 568-4000. Fax: (215) 563-5718.

American College of Surgeons. 633 North St. Clair Street, Chicago, IL 60611-32311. (312) 202-5000. Fax: (312) 02-5001. http://www.facs.org/ (accessed April 8, 2008).

American Society of Anesthesiologists. 520 N. Northwest Highway Park Ridge, IL 60068-2573. (847) 825-5586. Fax: (847) 825-1692. http://www.asahq.org (accessed April 8, 2008).

OTHER

Joint Commission on Accreditation of HealthCare Organizations. One Renaissance Blvd., Oakbrook Terrace, IL 60181. (630) 792-5000. http://www.jcaho.org/ (accessed April 8, 2008).

Nancy McKenzie, PhD

Surgical training

Definition

Surgical training encompasses the acquisition of knowledge and skills required for a physician to operate on people in a safe and therapeutically successful manner.

Purpose

The purpose of surgical training is to prepare a physician to specialize in surgery.

An individual's first formal exposure to surgery occurs during the third year of medical school. Every medical student spends 12 weeks in a surgical clerkship. During this period, students are exposed to patients with conditions that can be addressed using surgery. Medical students accompany surgeons. Initially, they observe. Gradually, they are allowed to assist with simple activities such as changing **bandages** or wound **dressings** or holding instruments. Under constant direct supervision, they may be allowed to close wounds by placing sutures. During this period, students read about surgery and are taught and quizzed by the surgeons that they are accompanying.

The next phase surgical training occurs after a physician has graduated from medical school. This phase is called residency training and lasts for five years. The first year of residency training is often referred to as an internship year. During this time, surgical residents receive intensive training in the medical management of patients. Their surgical duties include additional observation of surgical procedures. As their skills improve and knowledge base grows, they are allowed to perform simple surgical procedures such as establishing a surgical field, making initial incisions, placing drains in wounds and closing wounds when surgical procedures have been completed.

During the second through fifth years, surgical residents continue to read, acquire additional skills and manage patients. Throughout the five years of surgical training, residents are constantly observed and evaluated. In the fifth year, each trainee serves as a Chief Resident. In this capacity, residents learn about leadership. They are responsible for assigning cases (patients) to other surgical residents, instructing other surgical residents and teaching medical students.

After completing the five years of resident training, trainees must pass an examination. The testing involves a written component that covers medical and surgical knowledge and an oral component that covers surgical skills and patient management. When they

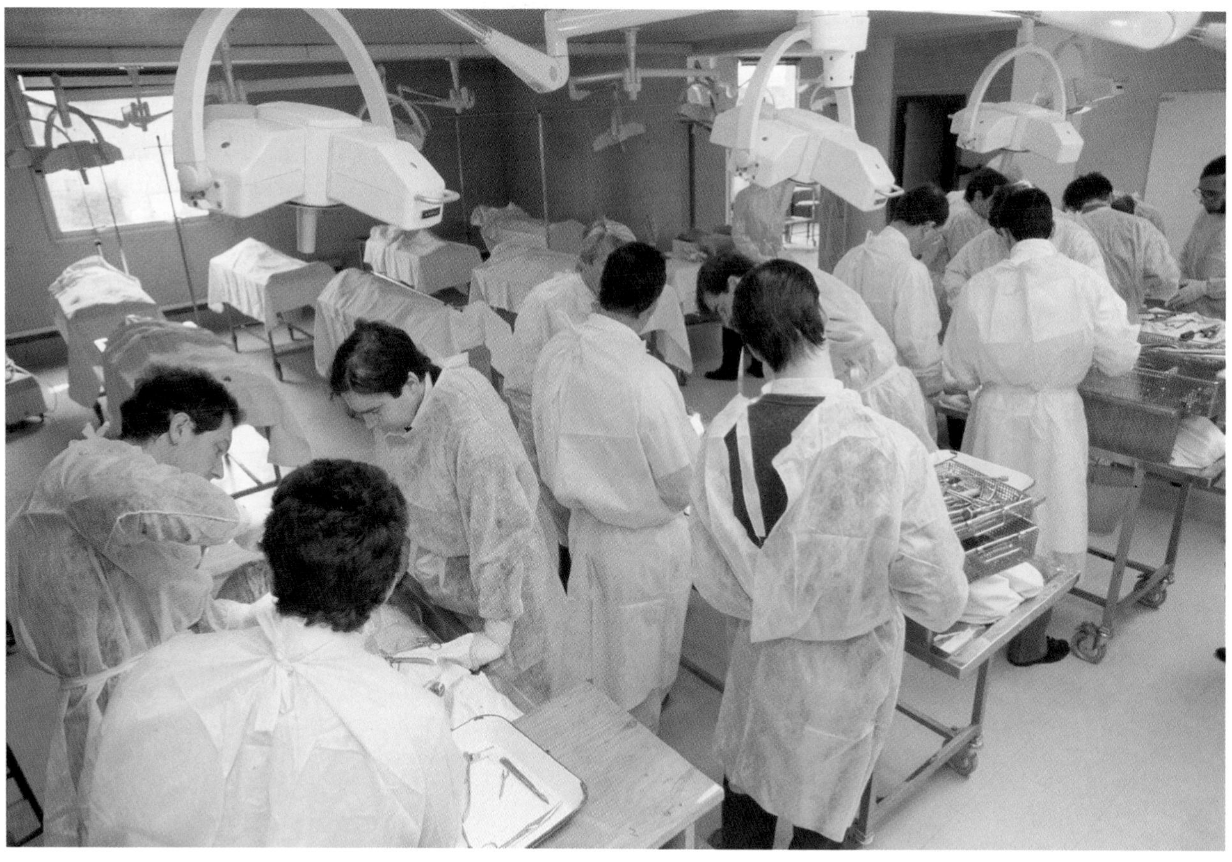

Surgeons at medical school. *(BSIP / Phototake. Reproduced by permission.)*

pass this examination, they receive Fellowship status in the American College of Surgeons. With this, they are entitled to call themselves surgeons and use the letters FACS after their names. At this point, surgeons are also board certified.

Some surgeons begin regular work in a surgical practice or as employees in a hospital or other similar organization. Some surgeons opt for obtaining additional specialized training and enter fellowships. (This is not to be confused with their Fellowship status in the American College of Surgeons.) Fellowship training is focused on a particular aspect of surgery. Fellowship training lasts from one to two years. At the completion of fellowship training, surgeons take another round of examinations. When they successfully complete the written and oral components, they receive an additional board certification as specialists.

Examples of surgical fellowship training include cardiac surgery (specialize on the heart), **thoracic surgery** (specialize on the lungs), **plastic surgery** (specialize on reconstructive and **cosmetic surgery**), **orthopedic surgery** (specialize on bones and joints), trauma surgery (specialize on hands or other body parts), gynecological surgery (specialize on the female reproductive system), ophthalmic surgery (specialize on the eye), and **transplant surgery** (specialize on the kidneys, pancreas, liver and lungs), and **neurosurgery** (specialize on the brain and nervous system).

Demographics

As of 2008, there were 61,516 Fellows in the American College of Surgeons.

More males than females enter surgical training. This is a long-standing pattern. As a result, the great majority of surgeons in the United States are males.

Description

An individual's first formal exposure to surgery occurs during the third year of medical school. Every medical student spends 12 weeks in a a surgical clerkship. During this period, students are exposed to patients with conditions that can be addressed using surgery. Medical students accompany surgeons. Initially, they observe. Gradually, they are allowed to assist with simple activities such as changing bandages or wound dressings or holding instruments. Under constant direct supervision, they may be allowed to close wounds by placing sutures. During this period, students read about surgery and are taught and quizzed by the surgeons that they are accompanying.

The next phase surgical training occurs after a physician has graduated from medical school. This phase is called residency training and lasts for five years. The first year of residency training is often referred to as an internship year. During this time, surgical residents receive intensive training in the medical management of patients. Their surgical duties include additional observation of surgical procedures. As their skills improve and knowledge base grows, they are allowed to perform simple surgical procedures such as establishing a surgical field, making initial incisions, placing drains in wounds and closing wounds when surgical procedures have been completed.

During the second through fifth years, surgical residents continue to read, acquire additional skills and manage patients. Throughout the five years of surgical training, residents are constantly observed and evaluated. In the fifth year, each trainee serves as a Chief Resident. In this capacity, residents learn about leadership. They are responsible for assigning cases (patients) to other surgical residents, instructing other surgical residents and teaching medical students.

After completing the five years of resident training, trainees must pass an examination. The testing involves a written component that covers medical and surgical knowledge and an oral component that covers surgical skills and patient management. When they pass this examination, they receive Fellowship status in the American College of Surgeons. With this, they are entitled to call themselves surgeons and use the letters FACS after their names. At this point, surgeons are also board certified.

Some surgeons begin regular work in a surgical practice or as employees in a hospital or other similar organization. Some surgeons opt for obtaining additional specialized training and enter fellowships. (This is not to be confused with their Fellowship status in the American College of Surgeons.) Fellowship training is focused on a particular aspect of surgery. Fellowship training lasts from one to two years. At the completion of fellowship training, surgeons take another round of examinations. When they successfully complete the written and oral components, they receive an additional board certification as specialists.

Examples of surgical fellowship training include cardiac surgery (specialize on the heart), thoracic surgery (specialize on the lungs), plastic surgery (specialize on reconstructive and cosmetic surgery), orthopedic surgery (specialize on bones and joints), trauma surgery (specialize on hands or other body parts), gynecological surgery (specialize on the female reproductive system), ophthalmic surgery (specialize on the eye), and transplant surgery (specialize on the kidneys, pancreas, liver and lungs), and neurosurgery (specialize on the brain and nervous system).

QUESTIONS TO ASK YOUR SURGEON

- Are you board certified?
- When did you complete your surgical training?
- What is your complication rate?
- How many times have you completed the surgical procedure that you are recommending for me?

Diagnosis/Preparation

Prior to entering medical school, individuals interested in becoming surgeons usually complete four years of undergraduate training in a college or university. During their premedical education, future physicians complete a core curriculum that includes a minimum of one year of biology, one year of physics, one year of mathematics (including a semester of calculus), and two years of chemistry (including a year of inorganic chemistry and a year of organic chemistry). So-called premeds often complete a bachelor degree in biology or chemistry although this is not now required. Medical schools seek persons that can think in a logical manner. Thus, persons with degrees in any undergraduate major are welcomed as long as they have completed the ten courses of a core currriculul already described.

Candidates must take and submit scores from the Medical College Admission Test (MCAT).

Risks

Risks associated with surgical training include disappointment for candidates that are unsuccessful in gaining admission to medical school. Risks associated with surgical training from medical school through fellowship training include fatigue and occupational injuries. Occupational injuries associated with surgery include accidental needle sticks, accidental cuts from scalpels or other instruments and exposure to pathogens acquired from patients. Risks associated with surgical training include fatigue, occupational injuries and malpractice suits.

KEY TERMS

Fellowship training—Additional specialty training that follows completion of residency training; fellowships are one to two years in length.

Internship—The first year of residency training

Residency training—A five-year period of additional training that follows completion of medical school.

Surgeon—A physician that has completed surgical residency training, passed all examinations and is a Fellow of the American College of Surgeons.

Normal results

The normal result of surgical training is successfully mastering the knowledge presented in medical school and residency, learning the techniques of surgery, and becoming a productive surgeon.

Morbidity and mortality rates

Morbidity for surgeons includes occupational injuries on the job. They experience the same risks of life as do all individuals. In 2008, mortality from on-the-job related events includes exposure to AIDS through an accidental needle-stick or cut by a contaminated instrument.

Alternatives

To become a surgeon, there are no alternatives to receiving surgical training.

Resources

BOOKS

Brunicardi, F. C., D. K. Anderson, T. R. Billiar, D. L. Dunn, J. G. Hunter, and R. E. Pollock. *Schwartz's Manual of Surgery*. 8th ed. New York: McGraw Hill, 2006.

Ellis, H., R. Caine, and C. Watson. *General Surgery: Lecture Notes*. 11th ed. New York: Wiley, 2006.

Lawrence, P. F. *Essentials of General Surgery*. 4th ed. Philadelphia: Lippincott Williams & Wilkins, 2005.

Townsend, C.M., R. D. Beauchamp, B. M. Evers, and K. Mattox. *Sabiston Textbook of Surgery*. 17th ed. Philadelphia: Saunders, 2004.

Toy, E. C., T. H. Liu, and A. R. Campbell. *Case Files: Surgery*. New York: McGraw Hill, 2006.

PERIODICALS

Allen, T. K., A. S. Habib, G. L. Dear, W. White, D. A. Lubarsky, and T. J. Gan. "How much are patients willing to pay to avoid postoperative muscle pain associated with succinylcholine?" *Journal of Clinical Anesthesia* 19, no. 8 (2007): 601–608.

Halpern, L. R., and S. Feldman. "Perioperative risk assessment in the surgical care of geriatric patients." *Oral and Maxillofacial Surgery Clinics of North America* 18, no. 1 (2006): 19–34.

Siddiqui, T., A. MacDonald, P. S. Chong, and J. T. Jenkins. "Early versus delayed laparoscopic cholecystectomy for acute cholecystitis: a meta-analysis of randomized clinical trials." *American Journal of Surgery* 195, no. 1 (2008): 40–47.

Vergis, A., L. Gillman, S. Minor, M. Taylor, and J. Park. "Structured assessment format for evaluating operative reports in general surgery." *American Journal of Surgery* 195, no. 1 (2008): 24–29.

ORGANIZATIONS

American Board of Surgery. 1617 John F. Kennedy Boulevard, Suite 860, Philadelphia, PA 19103. (215) 568-4000; Fax: (215) 563-5718. http://www.absurgery.org.

American College of Surgeons. 633 North St. Clair Street, Chicago, IL 60611-32311. (312) 202-5000; Fax: (312) 202-5001. Web site: http://www.facs.org. E-mail: <postmaster@facs.org>.

American Medical Association. 515 N. State Street, Chicago, IL 60610. (312) 464-5000. http://www.ama-assn.org.

American Society for Aesthetic Plastic Surgery. 11081 Winners Circle, Los Alamitos, CA 90720. (800) 364-2147 or (562) 799-2356. http://www.surgery.org.

American Society for Dermatologic Surgery. 5550 Meadowbrook Dr., Suite 120, Rolling Meadows, IL 60008. (847) 956-0900. http://www.asds.net.

American Society of Plastic Surgeons. 444 E. Algonquin Rd., Arlington Heights, IL 60005. (847) 228-9900. http://www.plasticsurgery.org.

OTHER

Archives of Surgery (American Medical Association) [cited December 23, 2007]. http://archsurg.ama-assn.org/.

MedScape General Surgery [cited December 23, 2007]. http://www.medscape.com/generalsurgery.

National Medical Society [cited December 23, 2007]. http://www.medical-library.org/j_surg.htm.

Wake Forest University School of Medicine [cited December 23, 2007]. http://www.bgsm.edu/surg-sci/atlas/atlas.html.

L. Fleming Fallon, Jr, MD, DrPH

Surgical triage

Definition

Triage (from the French verb trier "to sort") is the assessment of medical condition performed by health care providers to screen for the most critically ill patients out of a group of people. Surgical triage focuses on establishing priority with respect to which surgeries are most critical in a time-sensitive manner. Triage is a necessary process when health care resources are limited and not every patient can be treated at once.

Purpose

Triage is performed to prioritize medical treatment so that the most endangered patients are treated first, while the number of lives saved is maximized. Triage is especially important in emergency situations where the amount of resources are limited and so have to be distributed in a selective manner. For example, a patient with a chest wound requiring immediate surgery to maintain life will take priority over a patient who needs surgery for a benign tumor.

Demographic

Surgical triage is performed on any patient presenting with a condition that may be amenable to surgical repair. Surgical triage is performed, when medically necessary, regardless of age, gender, or race.

Description

Triage is a system of screening, evaluating, and classifying the sick or wounded. It may be done during war, disaster situations, or in the emergency room of a hospital. Regardless of where it is performed, triage for any medical treatment is dependent on available medical resources. Medical resources include medications, **operating room** space, hospital space, **bandages** or other materials, as well as a physician's time. Medical resources are all limiting factors to the medical treatment available for patients. Surgical triage takes both the acuity (severity) of the patient's medical condition, as well as available medical resources into account.

Emergency Surgical Triage

There are multiple grading systems or standards for triaging patients in an emergency setting. In emergency situations, each patient is evaluated (including obtaining a brief history when possible) and given a rapid physical exam specifically geared toward **vital signs** and areas of critical injury or illness. The components of the initial triage history include a specific set of information that is important: allergies to specific medications; current medications need to be established in case new medications are indicated; when the patient last ate is pertinent due to the risk of vomiting and breathing in the vomit during **general anesthesia** and the surgical procedure. Establishing an airway and taking basic life support measures is a priority. Other priority items include stopping any arterial bleeding before the patient goes into shock. **Emergency surgery** procedures apply the general principles of emergency triage in addition to information about the specific medical condition involved in order to determine which surgeries need to be performed first.

Emergency surgical procedures may be necessary due to trauma (with the patient being critically injured) or a critical phase of a disease state (such as immediately life-threatening heart failure that is caused by a condition amenable to surgical repair). It is essential that triage be performed rapidly and accurately, because in emergency situations a single minute could make the difference between survival and **death**. The rationale of surgical triage is to first treat patients that are in the most critical need of care in order to preserve life. Topics that factor into the order in which patients are triaged includes vital signs, clinical history, mechanism of injury or pre-hospital course of disease, age, co-morbid conditions, and whether they have open airways through which to breathe. A patient may be given priority if their vital signs are unstable, they have a clinical history of cardiac or pulmonary disease, have serious injuries, closed airways, are very young or very old, have lost consciousness, or are showing signs of neurological injuries.

An initial assessment of the patient involves running a primary survey, during which the airway, breathing, circulation/hemorrhage, and mental disability are evaluated. The purpose of the primary survey is for the initial management of life-threatening conditions. If the airway is obstructed, the patient may immediately go into an emergency surgery procedure to remove the obstruction. Next the patient's ability to breathe independently is evaluated. If the patient cannot breathe due to a surgically amenable condition such as internal bleeding into the chest cavity they may be triaged into emergency surgery. If the patient has obstructed circulation, such as in cardiac tamponade where the heart sac is filled with blood and the heart cannot pump properly, emergency surgery would be required. Mental disability in the context of a primary survey refers to the current mental status of the patient. If the patient has serious neurological disability due to a head or spinal cord injury, **neurosurgery** may be necessary.

If the patient has not been triaged in the primary survey as having an immediately life-threatening condition, a secondary survey is performed. The secondary survey is a more thorough **physical examination** covering the entire body of the patient. Blood tests may be run to check the basic functioning of the patient's bodily systems. At this point, triage is performed and the patients are prioritized for surgery.

Trauma patients being triaged for surgery may need diagnostic tests such as a Computed Tomography (CT) scan to help diagnose what is wrong with them and initiate appropriate surgery. However, if a patient has initially been brought to a smaller hospital without an appropriate surgeon present, this aspect of surgical triage may be temporarily put aside. Diagnostic tools such as **CT scans** take time and may delay the transfer of the patient to an appropriate trauma facility.

Non-emergency Surgical Triage

Triage also takes place in non-emergency department situations when scheduling operations in the hospital. While non-emergent procedures are generally scheduled on a first-come first-serve basis, if a patient is identified who medically requires a procedure in a time-sensitive manner, it may take precedence over a previously scheduled surgery. For example, if a current patient is identified during a routine examination with an aggressive tumor that requires surgery, a non-emergent procedure may be rescheduled to make room for the tumor patient. Hence, initial triage decisions may take place outside of the emergency department of the hospital.

Who Performs the Triage Procedure

An initial triage officer is a health care professional who performs triage on a patient arriving at the hospital. In the emergency department, the initial triage officer is often a triage nurse, who identifies the critically ill and sends them for further evaluation by a physician. Sometimes the triage officer is a resident, a full medical doctor who is in training for their specialty. For surgical triage, it is often a surgical resident that first determines whether a new patient requires surgery immediately.

Once a patient has undergone a surgical procedure, the triage process continues in the Surgical **Intensive Care Unit** (SICU). The SICU is a special hospital unit dedicated to patients undergoing surgery until they are deemed well enough to be transferred to other parts of the hospital or discharged. The surgical specialties of each hospital support the SICU, and may include the specialties of trauma surgery, neurosurgery, cardiothoracic surgery, **transplant surgery**, **orthopedic surgery**, ear nose and **throat surgery**, **plastic surgery**, **vascular surgery**, **general surgery**, and obstetrics and gynecological surgery. While the SICU is run by numerous types of health care providers, some systems utilize a Surgical Intensivist to triage which patients need to stay in the SICU and which may leave. A Surgical Intensivist is an MD who is both a general surgeon and has special training in intensive care practices.

In addition to the triage needs of each individual patient, the Surgical Intensivist must also manage a balance between the supply and demand of factors such as operating room time, post-anesthesia care unit availability, and bed space. It is a challenge for the Surgical Intensivist to properly assess which patients require SICU admission and which ones can be either denied admission or discharged safely for home. Patients who are inappropriately judged ready for discharge have been associated with a higher level or mortality, so triage on this level has a critical impact on healthcare. The Surgical Intensivist's triage decisions may be supported by the surgeons on the patient's primary surgical care team.

Triage Systems

Triage systems of classification may have from two to five categories into which to place patients. Many hospitals in the U.S. use three level systems with the categories of Emergency, Urgent, and Non-Urgent. However, studies have shown that five level systems are the most effective. Five level systems include the categories of Resuscitation (when breathing or pulse is not detected), Emergent, Urgent, Non-urgent, and Referred (minimal medical resources are required). One well-known five level triage system that is employed by emergency departments of the United States is the Emergency Severity Index (ESI). The ESI categorizes patients presenting to the emergency department by both health threat acuity and the resources available. The ESI scale ranges from one to five, with a lower number indicating greater severity. A triage nurse is usually the one who initiates the ESI when a patient presents to the emergency department. The acuity of a patient's medical condition is determined by the stability of the patient's vital signs and the potential for threat to life, limbs, or organs. If the patient meets high acuity level criteria (level 1 or 2), they need immediate treatment possibly including surgery. If the patient does not meet high acuity level criteria, the triage nurse then proceeds to evaluate the expected resources needed for treatment to help determine a triage level (level 3, 4, or 5). The ESI is a method for emergency departments to triage patients in a validated manner. It is one of the only triage systems that specifically categorizes based on resources available. A general triage system such as the ESI is only one factor in the process of surgical triage. Patients with high acuity levels and conditions amenable to surgery are then given over to more specific surgical triage done by the appropriate surgical specialty.

Surgical Triage after Trauma

Triage decisions are based on many factors, and may include a patient's trauma score. These scores are an approximate way to aid assessment of how critical a patient's medical condition is after physical trauma. There are many different trauma-scoring systems that may assist in the process of triage. The Revised Trauma Score (RTS) is one commonly used system to aid triage decisions. The RTS is based on physiological parameters, including vital signs. Blood pressure, respiratory rate, and level of consciousness all contribute to the RTS. Each parameter is worth a certain number of points, with higher points being better. An RTS score lower than 11 requires admission of the patient to a trauma center. Other types of trauma scoring systems may be geared toward different types of injuries: The Injury Severity Score (ISS), Penetrating Abdominal Trauma Index (PATI), Systemic Inflammatory Response Syndrome (SIRS), and ICD-based Injury Severity Score (ICISS) are all examples. The Abbreviated Injury Score (AIS) is often used to assist in triage for trauma surgery. The AIS is an anatomically based system of grading injuries from one to six, with one being minor injury and six being lethal injury. For trauma conditions that are amenable to surgery, an appropriate trauma-scoring system may greatly influence who is brought to the trauma center and surgical triage decisions.

Triage Coding in Disasters

Triage officers in mass casualty situations may utilize the Simple Triage and Rapid Treatment (START) system. The START system is a very simple four category triage system that groups medical conditions as severe, urgent, minor, and beyond medical assistance. In advanced systems, patients triaged in emergency or mass casualty situations are often given a color-coded tag to help identify their status to other health care workers. Triage tag systems vary from country to country. In general, there are five categories each assigned to a color: immediate care required with possible positive outcome anticipated, urgent care required but may be briefly delayed, care required but may be extensively delayed, and immediate care required but the patient is realistically beyond saving.

Red is the color tag used for the group of patients requiring immediate care without which they would not survive. The red triage tag indicates that the patient is in an immediate medical crisis, and may be realistically saved given the medical facilities available. Red-tagged triage patients are given top priority over other colored tags. In surgical triage a red-tagged patient would generally be one who requires immediate surgery to save their life. If the medical facilities are substantial enough, some types of crippling injuries that are not life threatening may be given a red triage tag. For example, amputations may be triaged as red because surgical reattachment of severed or partially severed limbs must take place within minutes of the injury, in order to be salvaged.

Yellow is the color tag used for patients who require medical care urgently but who are not in immediate danger of losing their life. Yellow triage groups may be able to wait hours for medical treatment, but not days. Yellow is the group known as delayed priority. In surgical triage, yellow-tagged patients may require surgery within a specific time frame in order to maintain life. While yellow-tagged patients may be stable for the moment, triage is a dynamic process and medical conditions may deteriorate rapidly. A patient in the yellow triage category needs to be monitored while awaiting treatment and re-triaged if necessary.

Green is the color tag used for patients for whom medical care is a minor priority, and who may wait a number of days before treatment without risking life. An example of a green triage condition is a broken bone without compound fracture, which needs to be treated but will not endanger a patient's life. The green category is sometimes referred to as the "walking wounded". White is the color tag used for patients who have such minor injuries that a doctor's care is not required. These patients are dismissed and would not be placed in a surgical triage situation.

Black is the triage color category that causes the most difficult ethical dilemma. The black triage tag is given to patients who are in immediate danger of losing their lives from injury or disease, but for whom medical treatment is unlikely to be successful. This category of triage is often given lowest priority when medical resources are scarce. The purpose of triage is to maintain the health of the greatest number of people. Resources devoted to black-tagged patients are often considered resources taken away from patients who may have benefited from them. For surgical triage, black-tagged patients are patients for whom surgery is unlikely to salvage. Potential examples of black-tagged surgical triage would be patients with extremely extensive burns or crush injuries.

Ethical Considerations of Triage

Triage systems have been developed to ensure the greatest number of people requiring medical care

KEY TERMS

Cardiac Disease—Any disease involving the heart.

Cardiac Tamponade—A condition in which the sac around the heart is filled with blood and keeps the heart from functioning properly.

Cardiothoracic Surgery—Surgery involving the chest body cavity known as the thoracic cavity.

Co-morbid Conditions—Diseases or disorders that exist simultaneously in one patient.

Computed Tomography (CT scan)—A computer uses x-rays across many different directions on a given cross section of the body, and combines all the cross sections to create one image. CT scans can be used to visualize bodily organs including the brain, blood vessels, bones, and the spinal cord. Contrast dye is sometimes administered to the patient to help visualize structures.

Hemorrhage—Excessive blood loss through blood vessel walls.

Mental Disability—The inability to mentally function due to injury, illness, or toxicity.

Neurological—Pertaining to the nervous system: peripheral nervous system, brain, and spinal cord.

Neurosurgery—Surgery involving the nervous system: peripheral nervous system, brain, and spinal cord.

Obstetrics and Gynecological Surgery—Surgery involving the reproductive organs or pregnancy.

Orthopedic Surgery—Surgery involving the musculoskeletal system, which includes muscles, tendons, joints, and bones.

Physiological—Pertaining to the normal vital life functions of a living organism.

Pulmonary Disease—Any disease involving the lungs.

Trauma Surgery—Surgery performed as a result of injury.

Vascular Surgery—Surgery involving blood vessels.

Vital Signs—The physiological aspects of body function basic to life. They are temperature, pulse, breathing rate, and blood pressure.

survive disease or injury. Unfortunately, medical resources are often limited, and not enough to give each and every patient ideal medical care. For black-tagged triage patients who are unlikely to survive despite medical care, this dilemma is especially poignant. Physicians are generally trained to see any patient under their care as one to whom the physician demonstrates fidelity by acting in the best interests of the patient over the interests of others. However in emergency triage situations it is necessary for triage officers to assign priority based on established guidelines. Any care given to black-tagged triage patients is considered care taken away from other patients who might have survived or suffered less severe disability if the resources had been used on them. In essence, physicians may greatly desire to treat any patient that requires help. However, in emergency situations they may need to put certain patients aside so as to use the available medical resources to save the lives of others. Since a physician's time is considered a limited medical resource, especially in emergency or mass casualty situations, a patient may even be coded as black-tagged for triage if the amount of time necessary to save them is very long. With limited time to save as many as possible, a twenty-four hour procedure for one person may mean losing five others that could have been treated in the same time period. Triage is essentially designed to do the greatest good for the greatest number of patients in any given situation. However, accomplishing this goal often puts physicians in difficult ethical situations and an emotionally painful decision-making process.

Resources

PERIODICALS

Dries, David J., Perry, John F. "Initial Evaluation of the Trauma Patient." Emedicine (February 8, 2007). http://www.emedicine.com/med/topic3221.htm [accessed April 7, 2008].

Funderburke, P. "Exploring Best Practice for Triage." *Journal of Emergency Nursing* 34 (2008): 180-82.

Good, L. "Ethical Decision Making in Disaster Triage." *Journal of Emergency Nursing* 34 (2008): 112-15.

Iserson, K.V., Moskop, J.C. "Triage in Medicine, Part I: Concept, History, and Types." *Annals of Emergency Medicine* 49, no. 3 (2007): 275-81.

Iserson, K.V., Moskop, J.C. "Triage in Medicine, Part II: Underlying Values and Principles." *Annals of Emergency Medicine* 49, no. 3 (2007): 282-87.

Pohlman, Timothy H. "Trauma Scoring Systems." Emedicine (July 16, 2007). http://www.emedicine.com/med/TOPIC3214.HTM [accessed April 7, 2008].

Stawicki, P.S., Pryor, J.P., Hyams, E.S., Gupta, R., Gracias, V.H., Schwab, C.W. "The Surgeon and the Intensivist: Reaching Consensus in Intensive Care Triage." *Journal of Surgical Education* 64, no. 5 (2007): 289-93.

OTHER

Gilboy, N., Tanabe, P., Travers, D.A., Rosenau, A.M., Eitel, D.R. "Emergency Severity Index, Version 4: Implementation Handbook." AHRQ Publication No.

05-0046-2, May 2005. Agency for Healthcare Research and Quality, Rockville, MD. http://www.ahrq.gov/research/esi/esi1.htm [Accessed April 7, 2008].

Maria Basile, PhD

Sweat test *see* **Electrolyte tests**

Sympathectomy

Definition

Sympathectomy is a surgical procedure that destroys nerves in the sympathetic nervous system. The procedure is performed to increase blood flow and decrease long-term pain in certain diseases that cause narrowed blood vessels. It can also be used to decrease excessive sweating. This surgical procedure cuts or destroys the sympathetic ganglia, which are collections of nerve cell bodies in clusters along the thoracic or lumbar spinal cord.

Purpose

The autonomic nervous system controls involuntary body functions such as breathing, sweating, and blood pressure. It is subdivided into two components, the sympathetic and the parasympathetic nervous systems.

The sympathetic nervous system speeds the heart rate, narrows (constricts) blood vessels, and raises blood pressure. Blood pressure is controlled by means of nerve cells that run through sheaths around the arteries. The sympathetic nervous system can be described as the "fight or flight" system because it allows humans to respond to danger by fighting off an attacker or running away. When danger threatens, the sympathetic nervous system increases heart and respiratory rates and blood flow to muscles, and decreases blood flow to other areas such as skin, digestive tract, and limb veins. The net effect is an increase in blood pressure.

Sympathectomy is performed to relieve intermittent constricting of blood vessels (ischemia) when the fingers, toes, ears, or nose are exposed to cold (Raynaud's phenomenon). In Raynaud's phenomenon, the affected extremities turn white, then blue, and red as the blood supply is cut off. The color changes are accompanied by numbness, tingling, burning, and pain. Normal color and feeling are restored when heat is applied. The condition sometimes occurs without direct cause but is more often caused by an underlying medical condition, such as rheumatoid arthritis. Sympathectomy is usually less effective when Raynaud's syndrome is caused by an underlying medical condition. Narrowed blood vessels in the legs that cause painful cramping (claudication) are also treated with sympathectomy.

KEY TERMS

Causalgia—A severe burning sensation sometimes accompanied by redness and inflammation of the skin. Causalgia is caused by injury to a nerve outside the spinal cord.

Claudication—Cramping or pain in a leg caused by poor blood circulation, frequently caused by hardening of the arteries (atherosclerosis). Intermittent claudication occurs only at certain times, usually after exercise, and is relieved by rest.

Fiberoptics—In medicine, fiberoptics uses glass or plastic fibers to transmit light through a specially designed tube inserted into organs or body cavities where it transmits a magnified image of the internal body structures.

Hyperhidrosis—Excessive sweating. Hyperhidrosis can be caused by heat, overactive thyroid glands, strong emotion, menopause, or infection.

Parasympathetic nervous system—The division of the autonomic (involuntary) nervous system that slows heart rate, increases digestive and glandular activity, and relaxes the sphincter muscles that close off body organs.

Percutaneous—Performed through the skin. It is derived from two Latin words, *per* (through) and *cutis* (skin).

Pneumothorax—A collection of air or gas in the chest cavity that causes a lung to collapse. Pneumothorax may be caused by an open chest wound that admits air.

Sympathectomy may be helpful in treating reflex sympathetic dystrophy (RSD), a condition that sometimes develops after injury. In RSD, the affected limb is painful (causalgia) and swollen. The color, temperature, and texture of the skin changes. These symptoms are related to prolonged and excessive sympathetic nervous system activity.

Sympathectomy is also effective in treating excessive sweating (hyperhidrosis) of the palms, armpits, or face.

Demographics

Experts estimate that 10,000–20,000 sympathectomy procedures are performed each year in the United States.

Description

Sympathectomy for hyperhidrosis is accomplished by making a small incision under the armpit and introducing air into the chest cavity. The surgeon inserts a fiberoptic tube (endoscope) that projects an image of the operation on a video screen. The ganglia are cut with fine scissors attached to the endoscope. Laser beams may also be used to destroy the ganglia.

If only one arm or leg is affected, it may be treated with a percutaneous radiofrequency technique. In this technique, the surgeon locates the ganglia by a combination of x-ray and electrical stimulation. The ganglia are destroyed by applying radio waves through electrodes on the skin.

Diagnosis/Preparation

A reversible block of the affected nerve cell (ganglion) determines if sympathectomy is needed. This procedure interrupts nerve impulses by injecting the ganglion with a steroid and anesthetic. If the block has a positive effect on pain and blood flow in the affected area, the sympathectomy will probably be helpful. The surgical procedure should be performed only if conservative treatment has not been effective. Conservative treatment includes avoiding exposure to stress and cold, and the use of physical therapy and medications.

Sympathectomy is most likely to be effective in relieving reflex sympathetic dystrophy if it is performed soon after the injury occurs. The increased benefit of early surgery must be balanced against the time needed to promote spontaneous recovery and responses to more conservative treatments.

Patients should discuss expected results and possible risks with their surgeons. They should inform their surgeons of all medications they are taking, and provide a complete medical history. Candidates for surgery should have good general health. To improve general health, a surgical candidate may be asked to lose weight, give up smoking or alcohol, and get the proper amount of sleep and **exercise**. Immediately before the surgery, patients will not be permitted to eat or drink, and the surgical site will be cleaned and scrubbed.

Aftercare

The surgeon informs the patient about specific aftercare needed for the technique used. Doppler ultrasonography, a test using sound waves to measure blood flow, can help to determine whether sympathectomy has had a positive result.

The operative site must be kept clean until the incision closes.

WHO PERFORMS THE PROCEDURE AND WHERE IS IT PERFORMED?

A sympathectomy is usually performed by a general surgeon, neurosurgeon, or surgeon with specialty training in head and neck surgery.

Sympathectomy was traditionally performed on an inpatient under general anesthesia. An incision was made on the mid-back, exposing the ganglia to be cut. Recent techniques are less invasive. As a result, the procedure may be performed under local anesthesia in an outpatient surgical facility.

Risks

Side effects of sympathectomy may include decreased blood pressure while standing, which may cause fainting. After sympathectomy in men, semen is sometimes ejaculated into the bladder, possibly impairing fertility. After a sympathectomy is performed by inserting an endoscope in the chest cavity, some persons may experience chest pain with deep breathing. This problem usually disappears within two weeks. They may also experience pneumothorax (air in the chest cavity).

Normal results

Studies show that sympathectomy relieves hyperhidrosis in more than 90% of cases and causalgia in up to 75% of cases. The less invasive procedures cause very little scarring. Most persons stay in the hospital for less than one day and return to work within a week.

Morbidity and mortality rates

In 30% of cases, surgery for hyperhidrosis may cause increased sweating on the chest. In 2% of cases, the surgery may cause increased sweating in other areas, including increased facial sweating while eating. Less frequent complications include Horner's syndrome, a condition of the nervous system that causes the pupil of the eye to close, the eyelid to droop, and sweating to decrease on one side of the face. Other rare complications are nasal blockage and pain to the nerves supplying the skin between the ribs. Mortality is extremely rare, and usually attributable to low blood pressure.

Alternatives

Nonsurgical treatments include physical therapy, medications, and avoidance of stress and cold.

QUESTIONS TO ASK THE DOCTOR

How will a sympathectomy affect daily activities after recovery?

Is the surgeon board certified?

What alternative procedures are available?

How many sympathectomy procedures has the surgeon performed?

What is the surgeon's complication rate?

These measures reduce or remove the likelihood of triggering a problem mediated by the sympathetic nervous system.

Resources

BOOKS

Bland, K.I., W.G. Cioffi, and M.G. Sarr. *Practice of General Surgery*.Philadelphia: Saunders, 2001.

Grace, P.A., A. Cuschieri A, D. Rowley, N. Borley, and A. Darzi. *Clinical Surgery,* 2nd ed. Londin, 2003.

Schwartz, S.I., J.E. Fischer, F.C. Spencer, G.T. Shires, and J.M. Daly. *Principles of Surgery,* 7th ed. New York: McGraw Hill, 1998.

Townsend, C., K.L. Mattox, R.D. Beauchamp, B.M. Evers, and D.C. Sabiston. *Sabiston's Review of Surgery,* 3rd ed. Philadelphia: Saunders, 2001.

PERIODICALS

Atkinson, J.L., and R.D. Fealey. "Sympathotomy Instead of Sympathectomy for Palmar Hyperhidrosis: Minimizing Postoperative Compensatory Hyperhidrosis." *Mayo Clinic Proceedings* 78, no. 2 (2003): 167-72.

Gossot, D., D. Galetta, A. Pascal, D. Debrosse, R. Caliandro, P. Girard, J.B. Stern, and D. Grunenwald. "Long-Term Results of Endoscopic Thoracic Sympathectomy for Upper Limb Hyperhidrosis." *Annals of Thoracic Surgery* 75, no. 4 (2003): 1075-9.

Matthews, B.D., H.T. Bui, K.L.Harold, K.W.Kercher, M.A. Cowan, C.A. Van der Veer, and B.T. Heniford. "Thoracoscopic Sympathectomy for Palmaris Hyperhidrosis." *Southern Medical Journal* 96, no. 3 (2003): 254-8.

Singh, B., J. Moodley, A.S. Shaik, and J.V. Robbs. "Sympathectomy for Complex Regional Pain Syndrome." *Journal of Vascular Surgery* 37, no.3 (2003): 508-11.

Urschel, H.C., and A. Patel. "Thoracic Outlet Syndromes." *Current Treatment Options in Cardiovascular Medicine* 5, no. 2 (2003): 163-8.

ORGANIZATIONS

American Academy of Neurology. 1080 Montreal Avenue, St. Paul, Minnesota 55116. (651) 695-1940. Fax: (651) 695-2791. E-mail: info@aan.org. http://www.aan.com/

American Board of Surgery. 1617 John F. Kennedy Boulevard, Suite 860, Philadelphia, PA 19103. (215) 568-4000. Fax: 215-563-5718. http://www.absurgery.org/.

American College of Surgeons. 633 North St. Clair Street, Chicago, IL 60611-32311. (312) 02-5000. Fax: (312) 202-5001. E-mail: postmaster@facs.org. http://www.facs.org/.

OTHER

Columbia University College of Physicians and Surgeons. [cited May 15, 2003] http://www.columbiasurgery.org/divisions/cardiothoracic/dd_hydrosis_ endoscopic.html.

"Excessive Sweating." [cited May 15, 2003] http://www.excessive-sweating.net/sympathectomy_history.html.

New York Presbyterian Hospital. [cited May 15, 2003] http://www.masc.cc/sympathectomy.htm.

University of Maryland School of Medicine. [cited May 15, 2003] http://www.umm.edu/thoracic/thoracic5a.html.

University of Southern California School of Medicine. [cited May 15, 2003] <http://uscneurosurgery.com/glossary/s/sympathectomy.htm>.

L. Fleming Fallon, Jr., M.D., Dr.PH.

Syndactyly surgery *see* **Webbed finger or toe repair**

Syringe and needle

Definition

Syringes and needles are sterile devices used to inject solutions into or withdraw secretions from the body. A syringe is a calibrated glass or plastic cylinder with a plunger at one and an opening that attaches to a needle. The needle is a hollow metal tube with a pointed tip.

Purpose

A syringe and needle assembly is used to administer drugs when a small amount of fluid is to be injected; when a person cannot take the drug by mouth; or when the drug would be destroyed by digestive secretions. A syringe and needle may also be used to withdraw various types of body fluids, most commonly tissue fluid from swollen joints or blood from veins.

Description

The modern hypodermic needle was invented in 1853 by Alexander Wood, a Scottish physician, and independently in the same year by Charles Pravaz, a French surgeon. As of 2003, there are many different types and sizes of syringes used for a variety of purposes. Syringe sizes may vary from 0.25 mL to 450 mL, and can be made from glass or assorted plastics. Latex-free syringes eliminate the exposure of health care professionals and patients to allergens to which they may be sensitive. The most common type of syringe is the piston syringe. Pen, cartridge, and dispensing syringes are also extensively used.

One common type of syringe consists of a hollow barrel with a piston at one end and a nozzle at the other end that connects to a needle. Other syringes have a needle already attached. These devices are often used for subcutaneous injections of insulin and are single-use (i.e., disposable). Syringes have markings etched or printed on their sides, showing the graduations (i.e., in milliliters) for accurate dispensing of drugs or removal of body fluids. Cartridge syringes are intended for multiple uses, and are often sold in kits containing a pre-filled drug cartridge with a needle inserted into the piston syringe. Syringes may also have anti-needlestick features, as well as positive stops that prevent accidental pullouts.

There are three types of nozzles:

- Luer-lock, which locks the needle onto the nozzle of the syringe.
- Slip tip, which secures the needle by compressing the slightly tapered hub onto the syringe nozzle.
- Eccentric, which secures with a connection that is almost flush with the side of the syringe.

A hypodermic needle is a hollow metal tube, usually made of stainless steel and sharpened at one end. It has a female connection at one end that fits into the male connection of a syringe or intravascular administration set. The size of the diameter of the needle ranges from the largest gauge (13) to the smallest (27). The length of the needle ranges from 3.5 inches (8 cm) for the 13-gauge to 0.25 inch (0.6 cm) for the 27-gauge. The needle consists of a hub with a female connection at one end that attaches to the syringe. The bevel, which is a slanted opening on one side of the needle tip, is located at the other end.

Needles are almost always disposable. Reusable needle assemblies are available for home use.

Operation

Syringes and needles are used for injecting or withdrawing fluids from a person. The most common procedure for removing fluids is venipuncture or drawing blood from a vein. In this procedure, the syringe and a needle of the proper size are used with a vacutainer. A vacutainer is a tube with a rubber top from which air has been removed. Fluids enter the container without pressure applied by the person withdrawing the blood. A vacutainer is used to collect blood as it is drawn. The syringe and needle can be left in place while the health care provider changes the vacutainer, allowing for multiple samples to be drawn during a single procedure.

Fluids can be injected by intradermal injection, subcutaneous injection, intramuscular injection, or Z-track injection. For all types of injections, the size of syringe should be chosen based on the amount of fluid being delivered; the gauge and length of needle should be chosen based on the size of the patient and type of medication. A needle with a larger gauge may be chosen for drawing up the medication into the syringe, and a smaller-gauge needle used to replace the larger one for administering the injection. Proper procedures for infection control should be strictly followed for all injections.

Maintenance

Syringes and needles are normally sterile products and should be stored in appropriate containers. Care should be taken prior to using them. The care provider should ensure that the needles have not been blunted and that the packaging is not torn, as poor handling or

KEY TERMS

Aseptic—Free from infection or diseased material; sterile.

Bevel—The slanted opening on one side of the tip of a needle.

Hypodermic—Applied or administered beneath the skin. The modern hypodermic needle was invented to deliver medications below the skin surface.

Piston—The plunger that slides up and down inside the barrel of a syringe.

Sharps—A general term for needles, lancets, scalpel blades, and other medical devices with points or sharp edges requiring special disposal precautions.

Sterile—Free from living microorganisms.

Subcutaneous—Beneath the skin.

Vacutainer—A tube with a rubber top from which air has been removed.

Z-track injection—A special technique for injecting a drug into muscle tissue so that the drug does not leak (track) into the layers of tissue just beneath the skin.

storage exposes the contents to air and allows contamination by microorganisms.

Safety

All health care personnel must be offered vaccines against such bloodborne infections as hepatitis B and C.

Used syringes and needles should be discarded quickly in appropriate containers. If a needlestick injury occurs, it must be reported immediately and proper treatment administered to the injured person.

Training

Health care instructors should ensure that staff members are skilled in up-to-date methods of **aseptic technique** as well as the correct handling and use of syringes and needles. All persons administering injections should be aware of current methods of infection prevention.

Teaching the correct use of syringes and needles, as well as their disposal, is important to protect medical staff and people receiving injections from needlestick injuries and contamination from bloodborne infections. As of 2003, some of the more serious infections are human immunodeficiency virus (HIV), hepatitis B (HBV), and hepatitis C (HCV).

Needles are defined as "sharps" for purposes of public health regulation, and must be broken or otherwise "rendered unrecognizable" before being placed in a puncture-proof container labeled with the universal biohazard symbol. This precaution is intended to prevent drug addicts from reusing the needles as well as to protect the hospital environment from contamination by medical waste.

Resources

BOOKS

Basford, Lynn, and Oliver Slevin. *Theory and Practice of Nursing: An Integrated Approach*, 2nd ed. London, UK: Stanley Thornes, 2003.

Ferri, Fred F.*Practical Guide to the Care of the Medical Patient*, 5th ed. St. Louis, MO: Mosby, 2001.

Nettina, Sandra M. *The Lippincott Manual of Nursing Practice*, 7th ed. Philadelphia, PA: Lippincott Williams & Wilkins, 2001.

Perry, Anne G., and Patricia A. Potter. *Clinical Nursing Skills & Techniques*, 5th ed. St. Louis, MO: Mosby, 2001.

PERIODICALS

Clarke, S. P., D. M. Sloane, and L. H. Aiken. "Needlestick Injuries to Nurses, in Context." *Leonard Davis Institute of Health Economics Issue Brief* 8 (September 2002): 1-4.

Metules, T. "What If You're Stuck by a Needle?" *Registered Nurse* 65 (November 2002): 34-37.

Perry, J., and J. Jagger. "Safer Needles: Not Optional." *Nursing* 32 (October 2002): 20-22.

Ratzlaff, J. I. "Needle Safety Technology." *Spinal Cord Injury Nursing* 19 (Spring 2002): 17-20.

ORGANIZATIONS

American Academy of Family Physicians. 11400 Tomahawk Creek Parkway, Leawood, KS 66211-2672. (913) 906-6000. E-mail: fp@aafp.org. www.aafp.org.

American Academy of Pediatrics. 141 Northwest Point Boulevard, Elk Grove Village, IL 60007-1098. (847) 434-4000. Fax: (847) 434-8000. E-mail: kidsdoc@aap.org. www.aap.org.

American College of Physicians. 190 N. Independence Mall West, Philadelphia, PA 19106-1572. (800) 523-1546, x2600 or (215) 351-2600. www.acponline.org.

American College of Surgeons. 633 North St. Clair Street, Chicago, IL 60611-3231. (312) 202-5000. Fax: (312) 202-5001. E-mail: postmaster@facs.org. www.facs.org.

American Medical Association. 515 N. State Street, Chicago, IL 60610. (312) 464-5000. www.ama-assn.org.

American Nurses Association. 600 Maryland Avenue, SW, Suite 100 West, Washington, DC 20024. (202) 651-7000 or (800) 274-4262. www.nursingworld.org.

OTHER

American College of Allergy, Asthma, and Immunology. [cited March 13, 2003]. www.allergy.mcg.edu/advice/latex.html.

American Nurses Association. [cited March 13, 2003]. www.nursingworld.org/readroom/fsneedle.htm.

National Institute of Occupational Safety and Health (NIOSH). [cited March 13, 2003]. www.cdc.gov/niosh/2000-135.html.

Occupational Safety and Health Administration (OSHA). [cited March 13, 2003]. www.osha-slc.gov/SLTC/needlestick.

L. Fleming Fallon, Jr., MD, DrPH

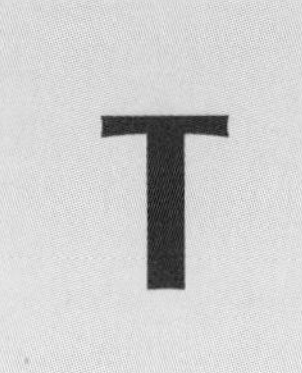

T-PA *see* **Thrombolytic therapy**

Talking to the doctor

Definition

Talking to the doctor is a fundamental requirement for an accurate exchange of information between patient and healthcare provider. It includes communicating private or potentially sensitive information, and requires a climate of trust. Without trust and accurate information, treatment and healing are difficult at best and impossible at worst.

Purpose

The purpose of talking to a doctor is to exchange information and obtain a cure or relief from pain and suffering. This outcome can only occur in an atmosphere of openness and mutual confidence.

Description

Talking is a basic human mode of communication. Talking to a doctor should be easy, but for many people, this is not the case. Barriers to straightforward communication include inhibition (shyness), fear, and guilt. These barriers may be present whether the patient is an adult who can speak for him- or herself or a child or elderly person whose history and symptoms must be described by another family member.

Inhibition

People often hold physicians in high regard. The stated reason for this feeling is a difference in educational level. Doctors have more educational credentials than most people in the general population. This differential tends to make patients self-conscious and hesitant to offer information.

Inhibition is further fueled by the sense of hurry and urgency that many health professionals project. Patients feel uncomfortable when they sense that they are being rushed by their doctor. As a result, they are reluctant to speak freely.

Fear

Apart from vaccinations or routine physical checkups, people in the United States do not ordinarily visit a doctor when they are well. The norm is to make an appointment when something hurts or does not function or feel right. It is natural for people to feel anxious in these circumstances—they are afraid of receiving bad news.

Guilt

Many patients' health complaints are often the direct consequences of their own behavior. Obesity often results from a combination of overeating and inadequate **exercise**. The leading cause of lung cancer is smoking tobacco. Casual sex can lead to unwanted pregnancies and sexually transmitted diseases. Having to accept responsibility for choices that lead to undesirable consequences is painful. Having to tell a person who is an authority figure as well as a trusted confidant often arouses guilt feelings.

Establishing trust

Trust requires time to develop, but it is also a two-way interaction. People seeking the advice of a doctor may reveal only a portion of their symptoms at first. While it is the doctor's task to elicit relevant information, the patient who is answering the questions must be open.

Doctors often assume that patients do not give completely honest answers. Women typically understate their body weight, while men overstate their strength. Smokers rarely admit to the true number of cigarettes that they smoke per day. Drinkers underestimate the amount of alcohol that they consume.

Preparation

Important elements of any doctor-patient conversation are honesty and openness. Some people may have to make a conscious decision to be open with their doctors. To avoid wasting time and feeling pressured, people should decide to be completely frank before they enter a doctor's office. In addition, inaccurate or incomplete information may lead the doctor to make an incorrect diagnosis or treatment decision.

Bringing records from visits to other healthcare providers is very useful to a doctor. People who have known their doctors for long periods of time are a steadily shrinking minority. Providing a new doctor with copies of one's medical history saves time and usually improves diagnostic accuracy. For example, old photographs are especially invaluable when evaluating skin problems.

Results

The passage of time, repeated positive interactions, and good outcomes from the information provided by the patient help to establish mutual trust. Trust then enhances the therapeutic interaction. The result may well be better health for the patient.

Preventive care should be part of the interaction between doctor and patient. A frank exchange of information is one form of prevention. If a conversation with one's doctor accomplishes nothing else, it will reduce inhibition, fear and guilt.

Resources

BOOKS

Bickley, L. S., and P. G. Szilagyi. *Bates' Guide to Physical Examination and History Taking*, 9th ed. Philadelphia: Lippincott Williams and Wilkins, 2007.

Jarvis, C. *Physical Examination and Health Assessment*, 5th ed. Philadelphia: Saunders, 2007.

Seidel, H. M., J. Ball, J. Dains, and W. Bennedict. *Mosby's Physical Examination Handbook*, 6th ed. St. Louis: Mosby, 2006.

Swartz, M. H. *Textbook of Physical Diagnosis: History and Examination*, 5th ed. Philadelphia: Saunders, 2005.

PERIODICALS

Arar, N. H., C. P. Wang, and J. A. Pugh. "Self-Care Communication during Medical Encounters: Implications for Future Electronic Medical Records." *Perspectives in Health Information Management* 24, no. 3 (2006): 3–12.

Buzaglo, J. S., J. L. Millard, C. G. Ridgeway, E. A. Ross, S. P. Antaramian, S. M. Miller, and N. J. Meropol. "An internet method to assess cancer patient information needs and enhance doctor-patient communication: a pilot study." *Journal of Cancer Education* 22, no. 4 (2007): 233–240.

Hassan, I., R. McCabe, and S. Priebe. "Professional-patient communication in the treatment of mental illness: a review." *Communication and Medicine* 4, no. 2 (2007): 141–152.

Mills, P., J. Neily, and E. Dunn. "Teamwork and Communication in Surgical Teams: Implications for Patient Safety." *Journal of the American College of Surgery* 206, no. 1 (2008): 107–112.

ORGANIZATIONS

American Academy of Family Physicians. 11400 Tomahawk Creek Parkway, Leawood, KS 66211-2672. (913) 906-6000. E-mail: fp@aafp.org. http://www.aafp.org (accessed April 8, 2008).

American Academy of Pediatrics. 141 Northwest Point Boulevard, Elk Grove Village, IL 60007-1098. (847) 434-4000. Fax: (847) 434-8000. E-mail: kidsdoc@aap.org. http://www.aap.org (accessed April 8, 2008).

American College of Physicians. 190 N. Independence Mall West, Philadelphia, PA 19106-1572. (800) 523-1546, x2600 or (215) 351-2600. http://www.acponline.org (accessed April 8, 2008).

American College of Surgeons. 633 North St. Clair Street, Chicago, IL 60611-3231. (312) 202-5000. Fax: (312) 202-5001. E-mail: postmaster@facs.org. http://www.facs.org (accessed April 8, 2008).

American Hospital Association. One North Franklin, Chicago, IL 60606-3421. (312) 422-3000. http://www.aha.org/ (accessed April 8, 2008).

American Medical Association. 515 N. State Street, Chicago, IL 60610. (312) 464-5000. http://www.ama-assn.org (accessed April 8, 2008).

OTHER

Agency for Healthcare Research and Quality. Information about Talking to the Doctor. 2008 [cited January 3, 2008]. http://www.ahrq.gov/CONSUMER/quicktips/doctalk.htm (accessed April 8, 2008).

Cable News Network (CNN). *Is Technology Changing the Doctor/Patient Relationship?* 2008 [cited January 3, 2008]. http://www.cnn.com/HEALTH/9906/30/internet.house.calls/ (accessed April 8, 2008).

National Library of Medicine. *Talking with Your Doctor* 2008 [cited January 3, 2008]. http://www.nlm.nih.gov/medlineplus/talkingwithyourdoctor.html (accessed April 8, 2008).

L. Fleming Fallon, Jr., MD, DrPH

Tarsorrhaphy

Definition

Tarsorrhaphy is a rare procedure in which the eyelids are partially sewn together to narrow the opening.

KEY TERMS

Cornea—The clear part of the front of the eye through which vision occurs.

Enophthalmos—A condition in which the eye falls back into the socket and inhibits proper eyelid function.

Exophthalmos—A condition in which the eyes bulge out of their sockets and inhibit proper eyelid function.

Palpebral fissure—Eyelid opening.

Sjögren's syndrome—A connective tissue disease that hinders the production of tears and other body fluids.

Purpose

The eye needs the lid for protection. It also needs tears and periodic blinking to cleanse it and keep it moist. There are many conditions that impair these functions and threaten the eye, specifically the cornea, with drying. Sewing the eyelids partially together helps protect the eye until the underlying condition can be corrected.

A partial list of the conditions that can require tarsorrhaphy includes:

- Paralysis or weakness of the eyelids so that they cannot close or blink adequately. Bell's palsy is a nerve condition that weakens the muscles of the face, including the eyelids. It is usually temporary. Myasthenia gravis also weakens facial muscles, but it is usually treatable. A stroke can also weaken eyelids so that they do not close.
- Exophthalmos (eyes bulging out of their sockets) occurs with Graves' disease of the thyroid, and with tumors behind the eyes. If the eyes bulge out too far, the lids cannot close over them.
- Enophthalmos is a condition in which the eye falls back into the socket, making the eyelid ineffective.
- Several eye and corneal diseases cause swelling of the cornea, and require temporary added protection until the condition resolves.
- Sjögren's syndrome reduces tear flow to the point where it can endanger the cornea.
- Dendritic ulcers of the cornea caused by viruses may need to be covered with the eyelid while they heal.

Demographics

People of all ages can suffer from paralysis or corneal diseases that may benefit from tarsorrhaphy.

WHO PERFORMS THE PROCEDURE AND WHERE IS IT PERFORMED?

Ophthalmologists perform the procedure on an outpatient basis in a hospital, or sometimes in their offices.

For that reason, physicians can perform tarsorrhaphy on patients of any age. However, it is viewed as a last alternative for many patients, and is not indicated until after other treatments (e.g., patching and eye ointments) have been attempted.

Description

Stitches are carefully placed at the corners of the eyelid opening (palpebral fissure) to narrow it. This provides the eye with improved lubrication and less air exposure. Eyeball motion can help bathe the cornea in tears when it rolls up under the lid. The outpatient procedure is done under local anesthetic.

Diagnosis/Preparation

The use of eye drops and contact lenses to moisten and protect the eyes must be considered before tarsorrhaphy is performed. Tarsorrhaphy is a minor procedure done under **local anesthesia**. Special preparation is not necessary.

Aftercare

Patients should avoid rubbing the eye and refrain from wearing make-up until given permission from the physician. Driving should be restricted until approval from the ophthalmologist.

Pathways in the home should be cleared of obstacles, and patients should be aware of peripheral vision loss. They will need to compensate by turning their head fully when looking at an object.

An analgesic may be used to ease pain, but severe pain is not normal, and the physician must be alerted. Sutures will be removed in two weeks.

Eye drops or ointment may still be needed to preserve the cornea or treat accompanying disease.

Risks

Tarsorrhaphy carries few risks. Complications may include minor eyelid swelling and superficial infection.

QUESTIONS TO ASK THE DOCTOR

How long will the eyes be closed with sutures?

Will it be painful?

Will the condition be remedied after the procedure?

Normal results

The procedure succeeds in protecting the eye and returning moisture to dry eyes.

Morbidity and mortality rates

This is a safe procedure. Only superficial infections have been reported.

Alternatives

Eye drops and contact lenses are widely used to treat conditions that once warranted tarsorrhaphy. The procedure is now considered a last option for treatment.

Resources

BOOKS

Cassel, M.D., H. Gary, Michael D. Billig, O.D., and Harry G. Randall, M.D. *The Eye Book: A Complete Guide to Eye Disorders and Health*. Baltimore, MD: Johns Hopkins University Press, 1998.

Daly, Stephen, ed. *Everything You Need to Know About Medical Treatments*. Springhouse, PA: Springhouse Corp., 1996.

Sardegna, Jill Otis, et al. *The Encyclopedia of Blindness and Vision Impairment*, 2nd ed. New York: Facts on File Inc., 2002.

J. Ricker Polsdorfer, M.D.
Mary Bekker

Telesurgery

Definition

Telesurgery, also called remote surgery, is performed by a surgeon at a site removed from the patient. Surgical tasks are directly performed by a robotic system controlled by the surgeon at the remote site. The word telesurgery is derived from the Greek words *tele*, meaning "far off," and *cheirourgia*, meaning "working by hand."

Description

In the early 2000s, several projects investigating the possibility and practicality of telesurgery were successful in performing complete surgical procedures on human patients from remote locations.

Preceding technologies

Telesurgery became a possibility with the advent of laparoscopic surgery in the late 1980s. **Laparoscopy** (also called minimally invasive surgery) is a surgical procedure in which a laparoscope (a thin, lighted tube) and other instruments are inserted into the abdomen through small incisions. The internal operating field may then be visualized on a video monitor connected to the scope. In certain cases, the technique may be used in place of more invasive surgical procedures that require more extensive incisions and longer recovery times.

Computer-assisted surgery premiered in the mid-1990s; it was the next step toward the goal of remote surgery. The ZEUS Surgical System, developed in 1995 by Computer Motion, Inc., was approved by the Federal Drug Administration (FDA) in 2002 for use in general and laparoscopic surgeries with the patient and surgeon in the same room. ZEUS comprises three table-mounted robotic arms—one holding the AESOP endoscope positioner, which provides a view of the internal operating field, the others holding **surgical instruments**. The robotic arms are controlled by the surgeon, who sits at a console several meters away. Visualization of the operating field is controlled by voice activation, while the robotic arms are controlled by movements of the surgeon's hands and wrists.

Computer-assisted surgery, which is generally called telerobotic surgery as of 2007, has a number of advantages over traditional laparoscopic surgery. The computer interface provides a method for filtering out the normal hand tremors of the surgeon. Two- and three-dimensional visualization of the operating field is possible. The surgeon can perform a maneuver on the console, review it to be sure of its safety and efficacy, then instruct the remote device to perform the task. The surgeon is also seated in an ergonomic position with arms supported by arm rests for the duration of the operation. One limitation on telerobotic surgery as of the early 2000s is the cost of the robots; the Da Vinci surgical robot, a new model with four arms, costs $2.2 million.

Operation Lindbergh

While the concept of telesurgery seems like a logical technological progression, there is a major constraint that could lead to disastrous results during surgery, namely time delay. In the case of computer-assisted surgery, the computer console and remote surgical device are directly connected by several feet (meters) of cable; there is therefore virtually no delay in the transmission of data from the console to the surgical device back to the console. The surgeon views his or her movements on the computer interface as they are happening. If the surgical system were removed to a more distant site, however, it would introduce a time delay. Visualization of the operating field could be milliseconds or even seconds behind the real-time manipulations of the surgeon. Studies showed that a delay of more than 150–200 milliseconds would be dangerous; satellite transmission, for example, would introduce a delay of more than 600 milliseconds.

In order to make telesurgery a reality, expert surgeons would need to work with the telecommunication industry to develop secure, reliable, high-speed transmission of data over large distances with imperceptible delays. In January 2000, such a project, labeled Operation Lindbergh, began under the direction of Dr. Jacques Marescaux, director of the European Institute of Telesurgery; Moji Ghodoussi, project manager at Computer Motions, Inc.; and communication experts from France Télécom. Testing began on a prototype remote system (a modified version of the ZEUS Surgical System called ZEUS TS) in September 2000, with data being relayed between Paris and Strasbourg, France—a distance of approximately 625 mi (1,000 km). Once an acceptable length of time delay was established, trials began in July 2001 between New York City and Strasbourg.

On September 7, 2001, Operation Lindbergh culminated in the first complete remote surgery on a human patient (a 68-year-old female), performed over a distance of 4,300 mi (7,000 km). The patient and surgical system were located in an **operating room** in Strasbourg, while the surgeon and remote console were situated in a high-rise building in downtown New York. A team of surgeons remained at the patient's side to step in if need arose. The procedure performed was a laparoscopic **cholecystectomy** (gall bladder removal), considered the standard of care in minimally invasive surgery. The established time delay during the surgery was 135 ms—remarkable considering that the data traveled a distance of more than 8,600 mi (14,000 km) from the surgeon's console to the surgical system and back to the console. The patient left the hospital within 48 hours—a typical stay following laparoscopic cholecystectomy—and had an uneventful recovery.

Limitations that still need to be overcome in order to make telesurgery more widely available include the establishment of international compatibility of equipment and training to overcome linguistic difficulties. Another concern is the need for a backup human surgeon at the remote location in case the robot malfunctions or there is an interruption in telecommunications.

Applications

Operation Lindbergh has paved the way for wide-ranging applications of telesurgery technology. On February 28, 2003, the first hospital-to-hospital telerobotic-assisted surgery took place in Ontario, Canada, over a distance of 250 mi (400 km). Two surgeons worked together to perform a Nissen fundoplication (surgery to treat chronic acid reflux), with one situated at the patient's side and the other controlling a robotic surgical system from a remote hospital site. Such a scenario may eventually allow surgeons in rural areas to receive expert assistance during minimally invasive procedures. Since the first telesurgery in Canada, Dr. Mehran Anvari, the founder of the Centre for Minimal Access Surgery (CMAS) in Ontario, has performed a number of remote surgeries between St. Joseph's Hospital in Hamilton, Ontario, and a community hospital in North Bay, about 250 miles from Hamilton. Dr. Anvari uses a virtual private network (VPN) over a non-dedicated fiber-optic connection that shares bandwidth with regular telecommunications data.

Other applications of telesurgery include:

- Training new surgeons. CMAS has developed a program in advanced minimal access surgery for Canadian surgeons, which combines lectures, laboratory sessions, and live surgery. As of 2007, about 160 surgeons have completed the program.
- Assisting and training surgeons in developing countries.
- Treating injured soldiers on or near the battlefield.
- The expanded use of telerobotic surgery. Telerobotic surgery offers the advantages of allowing surgery to be performed during an epidemic (such as the SARS outbreak of 2002–2003) without having to bring patients from remote and uninfected communities into cities affected by the epidemic.
- Performing surgical procedures in space or underwater. CMAS joined forces in 2006 with the National Aeronautics and Space Administration (NASA), the U.S. Army Telemedicine and Advanced Technology Research Center (TATRC), and the National Space

Biomedical Research Institute (NSBRI) to work on NASA's Extreme Environment Mission Operation 9, or NEEMO 9. Dr. Anvari at CMAS tested remote surgery with a next-generation surgical robot and a patient simulator in the Aquarius Undersea Habitat, an underwater laboratory operated by the National Undersea Research Center at the University of North Carolina at Wilmington (UNCW) for the National Oceanic and Atmospheric Administration (NOAA). The laboratory is located on the ocean floor off Key Largo in the Florida Keys, 70 feet beneath the surface. The mission lasted 18 days. A two-second time delay was built into the telecommunications system to simulate the time delay that would be present in a manned lunar exploration mission.

- Collaborating and mentoring during surgery by surgeons around the globe. Telementoring has been used in Canada since 2004 with financial assistance from a government partnership program. Telementoring involves an experienced surgeon in an advanced treatment facility in a major city using a two-way telecommunications link to guide the remote surgeon during an operation.

Resources

BOOKS

Telesurgery, 1st ed. New York: Springer, 2007.

PERIODICALS

Birch, D. W., C. Sample, and R. Gupta. "The Impact of a Comprehensive Course in Advanced Minimal Access Surgery on Surgeon Practice." *Canadian Journal of Surgery* 50 (February 2007): 9–12.

Gondziola, Jason. "Telerobotic Surgery: Harnessing the Many-Armed Beast." *National Review of Medicine* 1 (September 23, 2004). Available online at http://www.nationalreviewofmedicine.com/issue/2004/09_23/feature05_17.html [cited January 7, 2008, accessed April 8, 2008].

Marescaux, J., et al. "Transatlantic Robotic Assisted Remote Telesurgery." *Nature* 413, no. 6854 (September 27, 2001): 379–80.

ORGANIZATIONS

Centre for Minimal Access Surgery (CMAS). 50 Charlton Avenue E., Hamilton, Ontario L8N 4A6 Canada. (905) 522-1155 x 5144. http://www.cmas.ca/ (accessed April 8, 2008).

Computer Motion, Inc. 130-B Cremona Dr., Goleta, CA 93117. (805) 968-9600.

European Institute of TeleSurgery (EITS). Hôpitaux Universitaires 1, place de l'Hôpital 67091 Strasbourg Cedex, France. +33 (0)3 88 11 90 00. http://www.eits.fr/homepage.php (accessed April 8, 2008).

OTHER

Canada Health Infrastructure Partnership Program (CHIPP). *Project: Centre for Minimal Access Surgery*, 2005. http://www.hc-sc.gc.ca/hcs-sss/pubs/chipp-ppics/2004-surg-support-network/synopsis/index_e.html [cited January 7, 2008, accessed April 8, 2008].

Ghodoussi, Moji. http://isandtcolloq.gsfc.nasa.gov/spring2002/speakers/ghodoussi.html (accessed April 8, 2008).

Intuitive Surgery, Mountain View, CA. *Da Vinci Telerobotic Surgical System*. http://www.teleroboticsurgeons.com/davinci.htm [cited January 7, 2008, accessed April 8, 2008].

Kay, Sharon. "Remote Surgery." *Light Speed Special Report*. http://www.pbs.org/wnet/innovation/episode7_essay1.html [cited January 7, 2008, accessed April 8, 2008].

Malik, Tariq. "NASA's NEEMO 9: Remote Surgery and Mock Moonwalks on the Sea Floor." *SPACE.com*, April 19, 2006 [cited January 7, 2008]. http://www.space.com/businesstechnology/060419_neemo9_techwed.html (accessed April 8, 2008).

NEEMO 9/Centre for Minimal Access Surgery. http://www.cmas.ca/neemo9/NEEMO9-CentreforMinimalAccessSurgery.htm [cited January 7, 2008, accessed April 8, 2008].

Stephanie Dionne Sherk
Rebecca Frey, PhD

Temperature measurement

Definition

Temperature measurement is the quantification of a person's **body temperature**, which is an important indicator of a person's physiological state. Temperature measurement is done to assess whether body temperature is within a narrow, safe range. An abnormally high temperature is a fever, a sign that the body is mounting an immune response.

Description of Body Temperature

Normal body temperature varies from person to person. Gender, age, recent physical activity, having a meal, and the menstrual cycle all affect body temperature within the normal range. Body temperature measurement also varies based on which part of the body it is taken from. The average normal body temperature is 98.6°F (37°C) when taken orally. However, body temperature may vary slightly more than one degree higher or lower and still be in the normal range. Normal body temperature can range from 97 to 100°F (36.1 to 37.8°C). A temperature higher than normal is considered a fever (hyperthermia). A temperature lower than 96°F is considered a state of hypothermia. Temperature varies with the age of a person. Younger people tend to have higher body temperatures. Temperature also varies by the time of day it is taken. Body temperature is usually lowest in the morning and highest in the evening. Temperature can also be elevated by **exercise**, stress or strong emotions, eating food, heavy clothing, certain medications, or high room temperature. All of these factors need to be taken into account when temperature is measured because they affect the interpretation of temperature-measurement results.

Locations for Body Temperature Measurement

Oral

Temperature is often measured orally by placing a **thermometer** in the heat pocket under the tongue in the back of the mouth. The mouth is closed and the patient breathes through their nose for several minutes until the temperature is measured. Oral temperatures that are 1 to 1.5°F above a patient's normal body temperature are considered a fever.

Rectal

The most accurate method of assessing body temperature is rectally using a glass or electronic digital thermometer. A lubricated electronic probe is inserted about 1 to 1.5 inches into the anal canal. Normal rectal temperature is usually 0.5 to 1.0°F higher than oral temperature. A rectal body temperature above 100.5°F is considered a fever in adults. In infants and children, a normal rectal temperature may approach 101°F. Rectal temperature measurement is a convenient alternative for patients who are unable to hold an oral thermometer in a closed mouth due to illness or being unconscious. It is also used for infants or very young children who cannot safely hold a thermometer in their mouth.

Armpit

Another temperature measurement method sometimes employed by pediatricians is placing a thermometer in the armpit. While less invasive than rectal temperature measurement, this location is the least accurate and takes the longest time to measure. Normal temperature in the armpit tends to be 0.5 to 1.0°F lower than oral temperature.

Ear

Thermometers made for the ear can be used to assess the body's core temperature, which approximates the temperature of the internal organs. Ear thermometers may measure the temperature of the eardrum or the ear canal. Normal ear temperature tends to be about 1.4°F higher than oral temperature.

Why Temperature is Measured in the Hospital

Temperature measurement is done to monitor a person's body temperature. Body temperature, heart rate, breathing rate, and blood pressure are all considered **vital signs**. If body temperature is abnormal, it is an important indicator of the physiological state of the body. A fever is the body mounting an immune defense against a foreign invader to help fight infection or disease. A fever can be a critical sign that the body is fighting a battle, such as a post-surgical bacterial infection or cancer. It can also be used to assess whether a treatment is working, such as in antibiotic treatment of infections. The extent of a fever does not necessarily correlate with the severity of the illness. However, temperature measurement is still an important tool used in the hospital to monitor a patient's health.

Measuring and monitoring body temperature can be done at specific time points in the process of diagnosing and treating illness. Physicians sometimes use repeated temperature measurements to follow patterns in body temperature such as how frequently a fever occurs and how long it lasts. These measurements may provide diagnostic insights into body processes during illness. Temperature measurement is especially important for the management of a critically ill patient, where trends in body temperature are significant. Careful temperature measurement is also essential in the health management of elderly people. Because the elderly may have difficulty mounting a high fever as an immune response against infection, a low-grade fever is often the only early sign that something is wrong. Elderly people are also more prone to hypothermia than younger individuals.

How Temperature is Measured

Mercury Thermometers

Traditionally temperature was measured orally with a graded glass thermometer containing mercury. The level to which the mercury would rise on the graded scale was an indication of temperature. According to the Environmental Protection Agency (EPA), mercury is a toxic substance that is poisonous to both humans and the environment. The dangers associated with mercury if the thermometer breaks in a patient's body and the cost of disposing of mercury led to the development of modern mercury-free thermometers that do not pose such health risks.

Electronic Digital Thermometers

Digital thermometers with an electronic probe are far more accurate at measuring body temperature than the old mercury thermometers. They are usually a lightweight plastic and shaped like a broad pencil, with the electronic temperature probe at the tip. A digital temperature display window at the other end measures temperature down to a tenth of a decimal point. Electronic thermometers are designed for use in the mouth, rectum, or armpit. Rectal thermometers may have a colored probe to help distinguish them from silver-tipped oral thermometers. They are accurate and easy to use in the hospital. In addition to antiseptic, disposable protective guards are often used to cover the probe to help prevent the spread of infection between patients.

Infrared Ear Thermometers

Digital ear thermometers use infrared energy to measure body temperature instead of an electronic probe. They are made in different shapes. One design has a small cone-shaped end that is placed within the ear. An infrared beam is then aimed at the eardrum. Ear thermometers only take seconds to measure body temperature, whereas other types of thermometers require minutes for accurate temperature measurement.

Disposable Thermometers

Hospitals often use disposable thermometers to decrease risk of transmitting infection from patient to patient. Disposable thermometers are thin pieces of plastic with a colored grid of dots representing temperature on one end. The color change displayed in the grid is how temperature measurement is visualized. Disposable thermometers are accurate and safe since they contain no glass or mercury. One thermometer can be reused on the same patient until it is no longer needed. Disposable thermometers are designed for use in the mouth, armpit, or rectum. A disposable thermometer in patch form has been designed for use on infants whose temperature needs to be monitored for long periods of time.

When Temperature is Measured

In the hospital routine temperature measurement takes place twice a day. The first measurement is usually done in the morning between 7 and 10 am. The second measurement takes place in the afternoon around 2 pm. If a patient is suspected to have an illness causing fever or is critically ill, temperature measurement may be performed up to four times an hour to closely monitor the situation. Interpretation of temperature measurement is influenced by when the measurement is taken. In the early morning, normal adult body temperature may be as low as 96.4°F (35.8°C). In the evening normal temperature may be as high as 99.1°F (37.3°C).

What Abnormal Results of Temperature Measurement Mean

An abnormally high body temperature means that the patient has a fever. Fever is not an illness itself but rather a defense mechanism of the body to fight disease or infection. Higher body temperatures are less hospitable for most bacteria and viruses, and also allow the body's immune system to mobilize against disease more readily. However, if the body temperature is raised too high for a prolonged period of time, then fever may pose a threat to the body. In infants and children, a very high fever may occur even in response to minor infections.

Abnormally High Body Temperature Potential Causes

- Infection by Bacteria, Viruses, or Parasites
- Medications
- Response to Surgical Procedures without having an Infection
- Drugs used during Surgery
- Metabolic Disorders such as Hyperthyroidism
- Heat Stroke
- Extreme Dehydration
- Cancer
- Inflammatory Conditions and Autoimmune Disorders
- Physical Trauma
- Certain Blood Disorders

Abnormally Low Body Temperature Potential Causes

- Hypothermia from Cold Exposure
- Medications
- Metabolic Disorders such as Hypothyroidism
- Excessive Alcohol Intake
- Starvation

KEY TERMS

Autoimmune Disorders—Disorder in which the immune system mounts a response against some aspect of its own body.

Hypothermia—State of abnormally low body temperature that can be fatal if left untreated.

Hyperthyroidism—Disease of the thyroid gland involving overproduction of thyroid hormones. Hyperthyroidism affects body temperature.

Hypothyroidism—Disease of the thyroid gland involving underproduction of thyroid hormones. Hypothyroidism affects body temperature.

Immune Response—Any response of the immune system against something identified by the immune system as being foreign.

Infrared—A type of energy wave given off as heat.

Physiological State—The status of the normal vital life functions of a living organism.

Vital Signs—The physiological aspects of body function basic to life. They are temperature, pulse, breathing rate, and blood pressure.

Resources

BOOKS

Bates Guide to Physical Examination and History Taking, Eighth Edition. Lippincott Williams & Wilkins 2003.

Cecil Essentials of Medicine, Sixth Edition. Saunders 2004.

Harrison's Principles of Internal Medicine, Sixteenth Edition. McGraw-Hill 2005.

Merck Manual of Diagnosis and Therapy, Eighteenth Edition 2006.

Oxford Textbook of Geriatric Medicine, Second Edition. Oxford University Press 2000.

Maria Basile, PhD

Tendon repair

Definition

Tendon repair refers to the surgical repair of damaged or torn tendons, which are cord-like structures made of strong fibrous connective tissue that connect muscles to bones. The shoulder, elbow, knee, and ankle are the joints most commonly affected by tendon injuries.

Purpose

The goal of tendon repair is to restore the normal function of joints or their surrounding tissues following a tendon laceration.

Demographics

Tendon injuries are widespread in the general adult population. They are more common among people whose occupations or recreational athletic activities require repetitive motion of the shoulder, knee, elbow, or ankle joints. Injuries to the tendons in the shoulder often occur among baseball players, window washers, violinists, dancers, carpenters, and some assembly line workers. Rowers are at increased risk for injuries to the forearm tendons. The repetitive stresses of classical ballet, running, and jogging may damage the Achilles tendon at the back of the heel. So-called tennis elbow, which occurs in many construction workers, highway crews, maintenance workers, and baggage handlers as well as professional golfers and tennis players, is thought to affect 5% of American adults over the age of 30.

Women in all age brackets are at greater risk than men for injuries to the tendons in the elbow and knee joints. It is thought that injuries in these areas are related to the slightly greater looseness of women's joints compared to those in men.

Description

Local, regional or **general anesthesia** is administered to the patient depending on the extent and location of tendon damage. With a general anesthetic, the patient is asleep during surgery. With a regional anesthetic, a specific region of nerves is anesthetized; with a local anesthetic, the patient remains alert during the surgery, and only the incision location is anesthetized.

After the overlying skin has been cleansed with an antiseptic solution and covered with a sterile drape, the surgeon makes an incision over the injured tendon. When the tendon has been located and identified, the surgeon sutures the damaged or torn ends of the tendon together. If the tendon has been severely injured, a tendon graft may be required. This is a procedure in which a piece of tendon is taken from the foot or other part of the body and used to repair the damaged tendon. If required, tendons are reattached to the surrounding connective tissue. The surgeon inspects the area for injuries to nerves and blood vessels, and closes the incision.

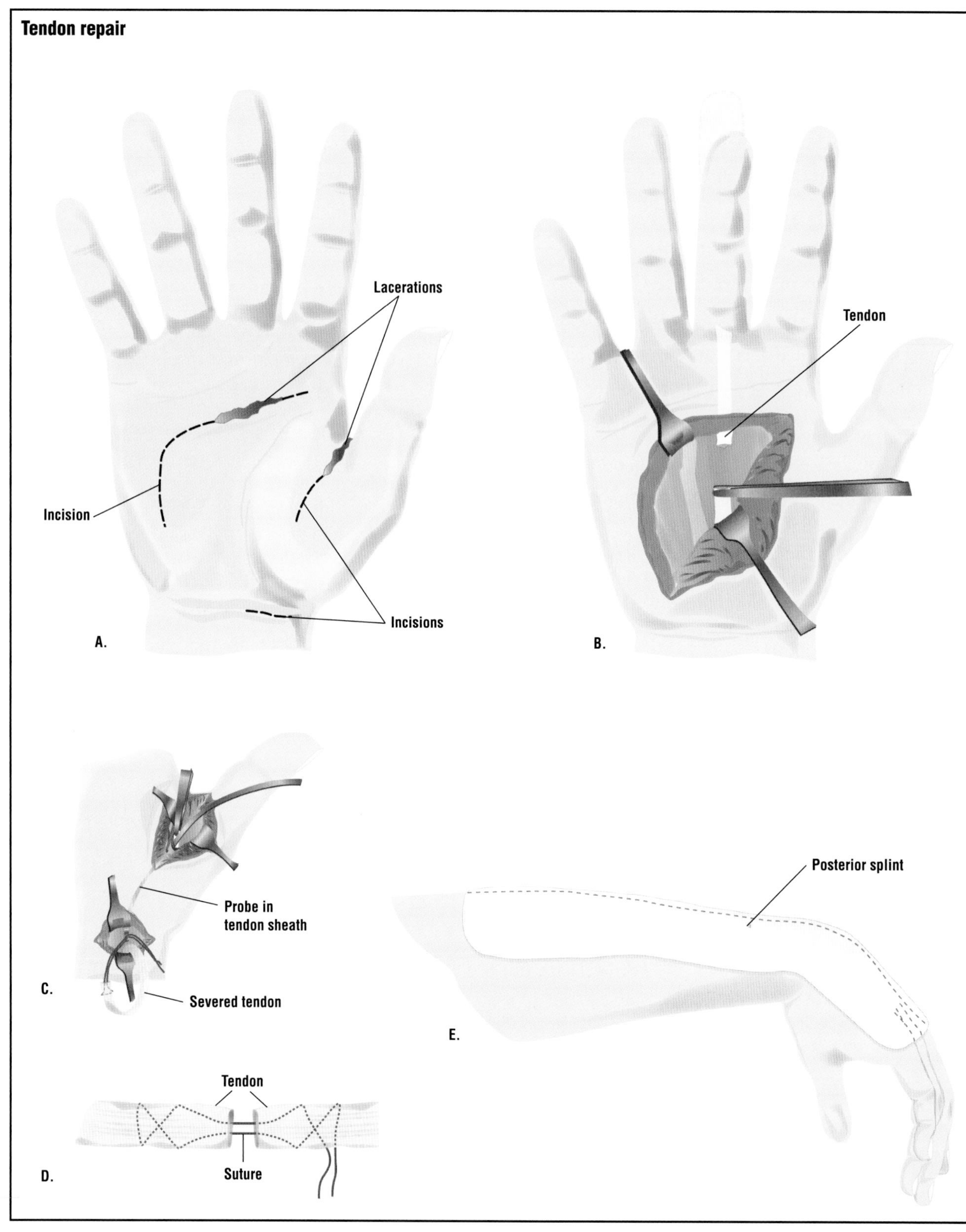

To repair a torn tendon, incisions are made to expose the area for repair (A). Some tendon can be reattached through one incision (B), while others require two to access the severed point and the remaining tendon (C). A special splint that minimizes stretching the tendons may be worn after surgery (E). *(Illustration by GGS Information Services. Cengage Learning, Gale.)*

KEY TERMS

Anesthesia—Loss of normal sensation or feeling induced by anesthetic drugs.

Collagen—Any of a group of about 14 proteins found outside cells. Collagens are a major component of connective tissue, providing its characteristic strength and flexibility.

Contracture—A condition of high resistance to the passive stretching of a muscle, resulting from the formation of fibrous tissue in a joint or from a disorder of the muscle tissue itself.

Fibroblast—A type of cell found in connective tissue involved in collagen production as well as tendon formation and healing.

Laceration—A physical injury that results in a jagged tearing or mangling of the skin.

Meniscus (plural, menisci)—One of two crescent-shaped pieces of cartilage attached to the upper surface of the tibia. The menisci act as shock absorbers within the knee joint.

Prolotherapy—A technique for stimulating collagen growth in injured tissues by the injection of glycerin or dextrose.

Tendon—A fibrous cord of strong connective tissue that connects muscle to bone.

Diagnosis/Preparation

Diagnosis of a tendon injury is usually made when the patient consults a doctor about pain in the injured area. The doctor will usually order radiographs and other imaging studies of the affected joint as well as taking a history and performing an external **physical examination** in the office. In some cases, fluid will be aspirated (withdrawn through a needle) from the joint to check for signs of infection, bleeding, or arthritis.

In the hours prior to surgery, the patient is asked not to eat or drink anything, even water. A few days before the operation, patients are also instructed to stop taking such over-the-counter (OTC) pain medications as **aspirin** or ibuprofen. If the patient has a splint or cast, it is removed before surgery.

To prepare for surgery, the patient typically reports to a preoperative nursing unit. Next, the patient is taken to a preoperative holding area, where an anesthesiologist administers an intravenous sedative. The patient is then taken to the **operating room**.

Aftercare

Healing may take as long as six weeks, during which the injured part may be immobilized in a splint or cast. Patients are asked not to use the injured tendon until the physician gives permission. The physician will decide how long to rest the tendon. It should not be used for lifting heavy objects or walking. Patients are also asked to avoid driving until the physician gives the go-ahead. To reduce swelling and pain, they should keep the injured limb lifted above the level of the heart as much as possible for the first few days after surgery.

Splints or **bandages** should be left in place until the next checkup. Patients are advised to keep bandages clean and dry. If patients have a cast, they are asked not to get it wet. Fiberglass casts that get wet may be dried with a hair dryer. Patients are also instructed not to push or lean on the cast to avoid breaking it. If patients have a splint that is held in place with an Ace bandage, they are instructed to ensure that the bandage is not too tight. They are also asked to ensure that splints remain in exactly the same place. Medications prescribed by the doctor should be taken exactly as directed. Patients who have been given **antibiotics** should take the complete course even if they feel well; this precaution is needed to minimize the risk of drug resistance developing in the disease organism. If patients are taking medicine that makes them feel drowsy, they are advised against driving or using heavy equipment.

Aftercare may also include physical therapy for the affected joint. There are a variety of exercises, wraps, splints, braces, bandages, ice packs, massages, and other treatments that physical therapists may recommend or use in helping a patient recover from tendon surgery.

Risks

Tendon repair surgery includes the risks associated with any procedure requiring anesthesia, such as reactions to medications and breathing difficulties. Risks associated with any surgery are also present, such as bleeding and infection. Additional risks specific to tendon repair include formation of scar tissue that may prevent smooth movements (adequate tendon gliding), nerve damage, and partial loss of function in the involved joint.

Normal results

Tendon injuries represent a difficult and frustrating problem. Conservative treatment has little if any

WHO PERFORMS THE PROCEDURE AND WHERE IS IT PERFORMED?

Tendon repairs are usually performed in an outpatient setting. Hospital stays, if any, are short—no longer than a day. Tendon repairs are performed by orthopedic surgeons. Orthopedics is the medical specialty that focuses on the diagnosis, care and treatment of patients with disorders of the bones, joints, muscles, ligaments, tendons, nerves and skin.

QUESTIONS TO ASK THE DOCTOR

- What happens on the day of surgery?
- What type of anesthesia will be used?
- How long will it take to recover from the surgery?
- Can I expect normal flexibility in the affected area?
- What are the risks associated with tendon repair surgery?
- How many tendon repair procedures do you perform in a year?
- Will there be a scar?

chance of restoring optimal range of motion in the injured area. Even after surgical repair, a full range of motion is usually not achieved. Permanent loss of motion, joint contractures, and weakness and stiffness may be unavoidable. Scar tissue tends to form between the moving surfaces within joints, resulting in adhesions that hamper motion. The surgical repair may also split apart or loosen. Revision surgery may be required to remove scar tissue, insert tendon grafts, or perform other reconstructive procedures. Thus, successful tendon repair depends on many factors. Recovery of the full range of motion is less likely if there is a nerve injury or a broken bone next to the tendon injury; if a long period of time has elapsed between the injury and surgery; if the patient's tissues tend to form thick scars; and if the damage was caused by a crush injury. The location of the injury is also an important factor in determining how well a patient will recover after surgery.

Morbidity and mortality rates

Mortality rates for tendon repairs are very low, partly because some of these procedures can be performed with local or regional anesthesia, and partly because most patients with tendon injuries are young or middle-aged adults in good general health. Morbidity varies according to the specific tendon involved; ruptures of the Achilles tendon or shoulder tendons are more difficult to repair than injuries to smaller tendons elsewhere in the body. In addition, some postoperative complications result from patient noncompliance; in one study, two out of 50 patients in the study sample had new injuries within three weeks after surgery because they did not follow the surgeon's recommendations. In general, tendon repairs performed in the United States are reported as having an infection rate of about 1.9%, with other complications ranging between 5.8% and 9.5%.

Alternatives

There are no alternatives to surgery for tendon repair as of 2008; however, research is providing encouraging findings. Although there is no presently approved drug that targets this notoriously slow and often incomplete healing process, a cellular substance recently discovered at the Lawrence Berkeley National Laboratory may lead to a new drug that would improve the speed and durability of healing for injuries to tendons and ligaments. The substance, called Cell Density Signal-1, or CDS-1, by its discoverer, cell biologist Richard Schwarz, acts as part of a chemical switch that turns on procollagen production. Procollagen is a protein manufactured in large amounts by embryonic tendon cells. It is transformed outside the cell into collagen, the basic component of such connective tissues as tendons, ligaments or bones. Amgen Inc. is planning to use genetic engineering to bring CDS-1 into mass production.

Prolotherapy represents a less invasive alternative to surgery. It is a form of treatment that stimulates the repair of injured or damaged structures. It involves the injection of dextrose or natural glycerin at the exact site of an injury to stimulate the immune system to repair the area. Thus, prolotherapy causes an inflammatory reaction at the exact site of injuries to such structures as ligaments, tendons, menisci, muscles, growth plates, joint capsules, and cartilage to stimulate these structures to heal. Specifically, prolotherapy causes fibroblasts to multiply rapidly. Fibroblasts are the cells that actually make up ligaments and tendons. The rapid production of new fibroblasts means that strong, fresh collagen tissue is formed, which is what is needed to repair injuries to ligaments or tendons.

Resources

BOOKS

Browner, B. D., et al. *Skeletal Trauma: Basic Science, Management, and Reconstruction*, 3rd ed. Philadelphia: Elsevier, 2003.

Canale, S. T., ed. *Campbell's Operative Orthopaedics*, 10th ed. St. Louis: Mosby, 2003.

DeLee, J. C., and D. Drez. *DeLee and Drez's Orthopaedic Sports Medicine*, 2nd ed. Philadelphia: Saunders, 2005.

PERIODICALS

Beredjiklian, P. K. "Biologic Aspects of Flexor Tendon Laceration and Repair." *Journal of Bone and Joint Surgery, American Volume* 85 (March 2003): 539–550.

Forslund, C. "BMP Treatment for Improving Tendon Repair. Studies on Rat and Rabbit Achilles Tendons." *Acta Orthopedica Scandinavica Supplement* 74 (February 2003): 1–30.

Harrell, R. M., Tong, J., Weinhold, P. S., and L. E. Dahners. "Comparison of the Mechanical Properties of Different Tension Band Materials and Suture Techniques." *Journal of Orthopedic Trauma* 17 (February 2003): 119–122.

Joseph, T. A., Defranco, M. J., and G. G. Weiker. "Delayed Repair of a Pectoralis Major Tendon Rupture with Allograft: A Case Report." *Journal of Shoulder and Elbow Surgery* 12 (January–February 2003): 101–104.

ORGANIZATIONS

Academic Orthopaedic Society (AOS). 6300 N. River Rd., Suite 505, Rosemont, IL 60018. (847) 318-7330. http://www.a-o-s.org/ (accessed April 10, 2008).

American Academy of Orthopaedic Surgeons (AAOS). 6300 North River Road, Rosemont, Illinois 60018-4262. (847) 823-7186; (800) 346-AAOS. http://www.aaos.org (accessed April 10, 2008).

American Physical Therapy Association (APTA). 1111 North Fairfax Street, Alexandria, VA 22314. (703)684-APTA or (800) 999-2782. http://www.apta.org (accessed April 10, 2008).

OTHER

MedlinePlus. "Tendon Repair." http://www.nlm.nih.gov/medlineplus/ency/article/002970.htm (accessed Apirl 10, 2008).

Tendon Homepage. http://www.eatonhand.com/ten/ten000.htm (accessed April 10, 2008).

Monique Laberge, Ph D

Tenotomy

Definition

Tenotomy is the cutting of a tendon. This and related procedures are also called tendon release, tendon lengthening, and heel-cord release (for tenotomy of the Achilles tendon).

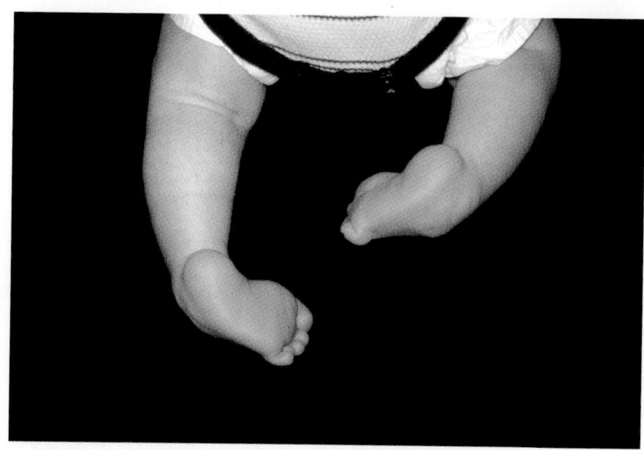

A baby with club foot: a candidate for tenotomy surgery. *(Medical-on-Line / Alamy)*

Purpose

Tenotomy is performed in order to lengthen a muscle that has developed improperly, or become shortened and is resistant to stretch.

Clubfoot is a common developmental deformity in which the foot is turned inward, with shortening of one or more of the muscles controlling the foot and possibly some bone deformity as well.

A muscle can become shortened and resistant to stretch when it remains in a shortened position for many months. When this occurs, the tendon that attaches muscle to bone can shorten, and the muscle itself can develop fibrous tissue within it, preventing it from stretching to its full range of motion. This combination of changes is called contracture.

Contracture commonly occurs in upper motor neuron syndrome, following spinal cord injury, traumatic brain injury, stroke, multiple sclerosis, or cerebral palsy. Damage to the nerves controlling muscles lead to an imbalance of opposing muscle forces across a joint, which may allow one muscle to pull harder than another. For instance, excess pull from the biceps, unless opposed by the triceps, can bend the elbow joint. If the shortened bicep remains in this position, it will develop contracture, becoming resistant to stretching. Tenotomy is performed to lengthen the tendon, allowing the muscle to return to its normal length and allowing the joint to straighten.

When one muscle pulls much more strongly than its opposing muscle, it may cause the joint to become partially dislocated, which is called subluxation. Tenotomy is also performed to prevent or correct subluxation, especially of the hip joint in cerebral palsy.

Chronic pain or bone deformity may prevent a person from moving a joint through its full range of motion, leading to contracture.

Contracture also occurs in a variety of neuromuscular diseases, including muscular dystrophies and polio. Degeneration of one muscle can allow the opposing muscle to pull too hard across the joint, shortening the muscle.

Demographics

Tenotomy is performed in infants with clubfoot, and in older patients who develop contractures or subluxations from neuromuscular disease, the upper motor neuron syndrome, or other disorders.

Description

During a tenotomy, the tendon is cut entirely or part-way through, allowing the muscle to be stretched. Tenotomy may be performed through the skin (percutaneous tenotomy) or by surgically exposing the tendon (open tenotomy). The details of the operation differ for each tendon.

During a percutaneous lengthening of the Achilles tendon, a thin blade is inserted through the skin to partially sever the tendon in two or more places. This procedure is called a Z-plasty, and is very rapid, requiring only a few minutes. It may be performed under **local anesthesia**.

More severe contracture may be treated with an open procedure. In this case, the tendon may be cut lengthwise, and the two pieces joined lengthwise to form a single longer tendon. This procedure takes approximately half an hour. This type of tenotomy is usually performed under **general anesthesia**.

If multiple joints are to be treated (for example, ankle, knee, and hip), these are often performed at the same time.

Diagnosis/Preparation

Patients requiring tenotomy are those with contracture or developmental deformity leading to muscle shortening that has not responded sufficiently to treatment with casts, splints, stretching exercises, or medication. Tests performed before surgery include determining the range of motion of the joint involved, and possibly x rays to determine if there is a bone deformity impeding movement or subluxation.

Patients undergoing general anesthesia will probably be instructed not to eat anything for up to 12 hours before the procedure.

WHO PERFORMS THE PROCEDURE AND WHERE IS IT PERFORMED?

Tenotomy is performed by an orthopedic surgeon in a hospital.

Aftercare

After tenotomy, the patient may receive pain medication. This may range from over-the-counter (OTC) **aspirin** to intravenous morphine, depending on the severity of the pain. Ice packs may also be applied. The patient will usually spend the night in the hospital, especially children with swallowing or seizure disorders, who need to be monitored closely after anesthesia.

Casts are applied to the limb receiving the surgery. Before the cast is applied, the contracted muscle is stretched to its normal or near-normal extension. The cast then holds it in that position while the tendon regrows at its extended length. Braces or splints may also be applied.

After the casts come off (typically two to three weeks), intensive physical therapy is prescribed to strengthen the muscle and keep it stretched out.

Risks

Tenotomy carries a small risk of excess bleeding and infection. Tenotomy performed under general anesthesia carries additional risks associated with the anesthesia itself.

Normal results

Tenotomy allows the muscle to stretch out, proving more complete range of motion to the affected joint. This promotes better posture and movement and may improve the ability to walk, stand, reach, or perform other activities, depending on the location of the procedure. Pain may be reduced as well. Clubfoot is usually completely fixed by proper treatment. Contracture and subluxation may be only partially remedied, depending on the degree of muscle shortening and fibrotic changes within the muscle before the procedure.

Morbidity and mortality rates

Properly performed, tenotomy does not carry the risk of mortality. It may cause temporary pain and bleeding, but these are usually easily managed.

QUESTIONS TO ASK THE DOCTOR

- How will any pain be managed?
- How long will the cast(s) stay on?
- What will the physical therapy program be like afterward?

Alternatives

Tenotomy is usually recommended only after other treatments have failed, or when the rate and severity of contracture or subluxation progression indicates no other, more conservative treatment is likely to be effective. Aggressive stretching programs can sometimes prevent or delay development of contracture.

Resources

BOOKS

Browner, B. D., et al. *Skeletal Trauma: Basic Science, Management, and Reconstruction*, 3rd ed. Philadelphia: Elsevier, 2003.

Canale, S. T., ed. *Campbell's Operative Orthopaedics*, 10th ed. St. Louis: Mosby, 2003.

DeLee, J. C., and D. Drez. *DeLee and Drez's Orthopaedic Sports Medicine*, 2nd ed. Philadelphia: Saunders, 2005.

ORGANIZATIONS

Muscular Dystrophy Association. 3300 E. Sunrise Dr. Tucson, AZ 85718. (800) 572-1717. http://www.mdausa.org (accessed April 10, 2008).

Richard Robinson

Testicular cancer surgery *see* **Orchiectomy**

Testicular torsion repair *see* **Orchiopexy**

Tetracyclines

Definition

Tetracyclines are broad-spectrum **antibiotics** that kill bacteria, which are one-celled disease-causing microorganisms that commonly multiply by cell division. Tetracyclines are also used to treat infections caused by such subcategories of bacteria as rickettsiae and spirochetes. The older tetracyclines became less useful in the early 2000s because many bacteria have developed resistance to this group of drugs; however, a new subgroup of tetracyclines known as glycylcyclines was introduced in June 2005 to treat infections that are resistant to other antibiotics, including the older tetracyclines. The name tetracycline comes from the four (*tetra* in Greek) hydrocarbon rings found in the chemical structure of these antibiotics.

Tetracyclines are classified as antibiotics, which are chemical substances produced by a microorganism that are able to kill other microorganisms without being toxic to the person, animal, or plant being treated. They were first discovered in the 1940s when a scientist at Lederle Laboratories isolated chlortetracycline from a bacterium in the soil known as *Streptomyces aureofaciens*; the drug was given the trade name Aureomycin. Oxytetracycline (Terramycin) was then derived from the bacterium *Streptomyces rimosus*. After the chemical structure of oxytetracycline was worked out, researchers were able to make synthetic tetracyclines in the laboratory. In the early 2000s, some tetracyclines are derived directly from a bacterium known as *Streptomyces coelicolor*, while others are made in the laboratory from chlortetracycline or oxytetracycline. One of these semi-synthetic drugs, minocycline, was used to develop tigecycline (Tygacil), the first glycylcycline to receive regulatory approval for use in the United States. Tigecycline was the first new tetracycline to be approved since the early 1980s.

Purpose

Tetracyclines are called broad-spectrum antibiotics, because they can be used to treat a wide variety of infections. Physicians may prescribe these drugs to treat eye infections, pneumonia, gonorrhea, syphilis, chlamydia, bubonic plague, anthrax, brucellosis, malaria, Rocky Mountain spotted fever, urinary tract infections, travelers' diarrhea, Lyme disease, and other infections caused by bacteria. These drugs are also used to treat acne and rosacea (a chronic inflammatory skin condition marked by flushing and redness). Tigecycline is used to treat skin and soft-tissue infections, as well as infections inside the abdomen. The tetracyclines will not work, however, for colds, flu, and other infections caused by viruses.

Description

Tetracyclines are available only with a physician's prescription. They are sold in capsule, tablet, liquid, and injectable forms. Some commonly used medicines in this group are tetracycline (Achromycin V, Sumycin), demeclocycline (Declomycin), minocycline (Minocin), oxytetracycline (Terramycin), and doxycycline (Doryx, Vibramycin, Vivox). Tigecycline (Tygacil) is not available in oral form, but must be given as a slow intravenous infusion over a period of 30–60 minutes.

Tetracyclines have been used for treatment of gum infections in dental surgery. In **orthopedic surgery**, they have been used as markers to identify living bone. The patient is given a tetracycline antibiotic for several weeks prior to surgery. Some of the tetracycline is absorbed into the bone during this period. Since tetracyclines glow under ultraviolet light, this absorption helps the surgeon distinguish the living bone from the dead tissue that must be removed.

Tetracycline may also be mixed with bone cement for prevention of infection in bone surgery. In nasal surgery, tetracycline ointments are used to help prevent postsurgical infections.

Recommended dosage

The recommended dosage depends on the specific tetracycline, its strength, and the disease agent and severity of infection for which it is being taken. Patients should check with the physician who prescribed the drug or the pharmacist who filled the prescription for the correct dosage.

To make sure an infection clears up completely, patients should take the full course of antibiotic medication. It is important to not stop taking the drug just because symptoms begin to improve.

Tetracyclines are most effective at constant levels in the blood. To keep blood levels constant, the medicine should be taken in doses spaced evenly throughout the day and night. It is important to not miss any doses.

These medicines work best when taken on an empty stomach with a full glass of water. The water will help prevent irritation of the stomach and esophagus (the tube-like structure that runs from the throat to the stomach). If the medicine still causes stomach upset, the patient may take it with food. Tetracyclines should never be taken with milk or milk products, however, as these foods may prevent the drugs from working properly. Patients should not drink or eat milk or dairy products within one to two hours of taking tetracyclines (except doxycycline and minocycline).

Precautions

There are specific warnings that apply to tetracycline preparations taken by mouth to treat infections; they do not apply to topical ointments or tetracyclines mixed with bone cement. Also, these warnings apply primarily to tetracycline itself. Some members of the tetracycline family, particularly doxycycline and

KEY TERMS

Antibiotic—A chemical substance produced by a microorganism that is able to kill other microorganisms without being toxic to the host. Antibiotics are used to treat diseases in humans, other animals, and plants.

Bacterium (plural, bacteria)—A one-celled microorganism that typically multiplies by cell division and whose nucleus is contained within a cell wall. Most diseases treated with tetracyclines are caused by bacteria.

Brucellosis—An infectious disease transmitted to humans from farm animals, most commonly goats, sheep, cattle, and dogs. It is marked by high fever, pains in the muscles and joints, heavy sweating, headaches, and depression.

Glycylcyclines—The name of a new subgroup of tetracyclines derived from minocycline, a semisynthetic tetracycline. As of 2007, the only drug in this class approved for use is tigecycline.

Gonorrhea—A sexually transmitted disease (STD) that causes infection in the genital organs and may cause disease in other parts of the body.

Microorganism—An organism that is too small to be seen with the naked eye.

Orthopedics—The medical specialty concerned with treatment of diseases of bone.

Rickettsia (plural, rickettsiae)—A microorganism belonging to a subtype of gram-negative bacteria that multiply only within the cells of a living host. Rickettsiae are usually transmitted to humans and other animals through the bites of ticks, fleas, and lice. They are named for Howard Ricketts (1871–1910), an American doctor.

Rocky Mountain spotted fever—An infectious disease that is caused by a rickettsia and spread by ticks. Its symptoms include high fever, muscle pain, and spots on the skin.

Rosacea—A chronic inflammatory skin condition primarily affecting the skin of the nose, forehead, and cheeks, marked by flushing and reddening of the affected areas.

Salicylates—A group of drugs that includes aspirin and related compounds. Salicylates are used to relieve pain and reduce inflammation or fever.

Spirochete—A spiral-shaped bacterium. Spirochetes cause such diseases as syphilis and Lyme disease.

minocycline, have different adverse effects and precautions. Patients should consult their physician or pharmacist about these specific drugs.

Taking outdated tetracyclines can cause serious side effects, particularly damage to the kidneys. Patients should not take these medicines when:

- the color, appearance, or taste have changed
- the drug has been stored in a warm or damp area
- the expiration date on the label has passed

Outdated tetracyclines should be thrown out. Patients should check with their physician or pharmacist if they have any doubts about the effectiveness of their drugs.

Patients should not take antacids, calcium supplements, such salicylates as Magan or Trilisate, magnesium-containing **laxatives**, or sodium bicarbonate (baking soda) within one to two hours of taking tetracyclines. Patients should also not take any medicines that contain iron (including multivitamin and mineral supplements) within two to three hours of taking tetracyclines.

Some people feel dizzy when taking these drugs. Tetracyclines may also cause blurred vision or interfere with color vision. Because of these possible side effects, anyone who takes these drugs should not drive, use machines, or do anything else that might be dangerous until they have found out how the drugs affect them.

Birth control pills may not work properly while tetracyclines are being taken. To prevent pregnancy, women should use alternative methods of birth control while taking tetracyclines.

Tetracyclines may increase the skin's sensitivity to sunlight. Even brief exposure to sun can cause severe sunburn or a rash. During treatment with these drugs, patients should avoid exposure to direct sunlight, especially high sun between 10 A.M. and 3 P.M.; wear a hat and tightly woven clothing that covers the arms and legs; use a sunscreen with a skin protection factor (SPF) of at least 15; protect the lips with a lip balm containing sun block; and avoid the use of tanning beds, tanning booths, or sunlamps. Sensitivity to sunlight and sunlamps may continue for two weeks to several months after stopping the medicine, so patients must continue to be careful about sun exposure.

Tetracyclines may permanently discolor the teeth of people who took the medicine in childhood. The drugs may also slow down the growth of children's bones. Tetracyclines should not be given to infants or children under eight years of age unless directed by the child's physician.

Special conditions

People with certain medical conditions or who are taking other medicines may have problems if they take tetracyclines. Before taking these drugs, the patient must inform the doctor about any of these conditions.

FOOD OR MEDICATION ALLERGIES. Anyone who has had unusual reactions to tetracyclines in the past should inform his or her physician before taking the drugs again. The physician should also be told about any allergies to foods, dyes, preservatives, or other substances.

PREGNANCY AND LACTATION. Pregnant women should not take tetracyclines during the last four months of pregnancy. These drugs can prevent the baby's bones and teeth from developing properly and may cause the baby's adult teeth to be permanently discolored. Tetracyclines can also cause liver problems in pregnant women.

Women who are breastfeeding should also not take tetracyclines. The drugs pass into breast milk and can affect the nursing baby's teeth and bones. They may also make the baby more sensitive to sunlight and may increase its risk of contracting fungal infections.

OTHER CONDITIONS. Before using tetracyclines, people with any of these medical problems should make sure their physicians have been informed:

- diabetes
- liver disease
- kidney disease

Side effects

The most common side effects of tetracyclines are stomach cramps or a burning sensation in the stomach, mild diarrhea, nausea, or vomiting. These problems usually go away as the body adjusts to the drug and do not require medical treatment. Less common side effects, such as a sore mouth or tongue and itching of the rectal or genital areas, may occur. These reactions do not need medical attention, however, unless they do not go away or are bothersome.

Other rare side effects have been reported, including inflammation of the pancreas, impairment of the kidneys, skin peeling, headache, intracranial hypertension, and ulceration of the esophagus. Anyone who has unusual symptoms during or after treatment with tetracyclines should consult his or her physician.

Interactions

Tetracyclines may interact with other medicines. When an interaction occurs, the effects of one or both of the drugs may change or the risk of side effects may be greater. Anyone who takes tetracyclines should give the doctor a list of all other medications that they take on a regular basis, including over-the-counter (OTC) drugs, herbal preparations, traditional Chinese medicines, or other alternative medicines. Standard medications that may interact with tetracyclines include:

- antacids
- calcium supplements
- medicines that contain iron (including multivitamin and mineral supplements)
- laxatives containing magnesium
- digoxin
- cholesterol-lowering drugs, including cholestyramine (Questran) and colestipol (Colestid)
- salicylates
- penicillin compounds
- birth control pills

Herbal preparations containing St. John's wort have been reported to increase sensitivity to sunlight in patients taking tetracyclines. People who have been using St. John's wort to relieve mild depression should discontinue it while they are taking tetracyclines.

Resources

BOOKS

Deglin, Judith Hopfer, and April Hazard Vallerand. *Davis's Drug Guide for Nurses*, 10th ed. Philadelphia: F. A. Davis, 2007.

Neal, Michael J. *Medical Pharmacology at a Glance*, 5th ed. Malden, MA: Blackwell Publishing, 2005.

Pelletier, Kenneth R., MD. *The Best Alternative Medicine*, Part I, Chapter 6, "Western Herbal Medicine." New York: Simon & Schuster, 2002.

PERIODICALS

Gottehrer, N. R. "Managing Risk Factors in Successful Nonsurgical Treatment of Periodontal Disease." *Dentistry Today* 22 (January 2003): 64–69.

Kasbekar, N. "Tigecycline: A New Glycylcycline Antimicrobial Agent." *American Journal of Health-System Pharmacy* 63 (July 1, 2006): 1235–1243.

Moore, D. E. "Drug-Induced Cutaneous Photosensitivity: Incidence, Mechanism, Prevention and Management." *Drug Safety* 25 (2002): 345–372.

Rose, W. E., and M. J. Rybak. "Tigecycline: First of a New Class of Antimicrobial Agents." *Pharmacotherapy* 26 (August 2006): 1099–1110.

Wormser, G. P., R. Ramanathan, J. Nowakowski, et al. "Duration of Antibiotic Therapy for Early Lyme Disease. A Randomized, Double-Blind, Placebo-Controlled Trial." *Annals of Internal Medicine* 138 (May 6, 2003): 697–704.

ORGANIZATIONS

American Society of Health-System Pharmacists (ASHP). 7272 Wisconsin Avenue, Bethesda, MD 20814. (301) 657-3000. http://www.ashp.org (accessed April 10, 2008).

United States Food and Drug Administration (FDA). 5600 Fishers Lane, Rockville, MD 20857-0001. (888) INFO-FDA. http://www.fda.gov (accessed April 10, 2008).

U.S. Pharmacopoeia (USP). 12601 Twinbrook Parkway, Rockville, MD 20852–1790. (800) 227–8772. http://www.usp.org/ (accessed April 10, 2008).

Nancy Ross-Flanigan
Sam Uretsky, PharmD
Rebecca Frey, PhD

Tetralogy of Fallot *see* **Heart surgery for congenital defects**

Therapeutic abortion *see* **Abortion, induced**

Thermometer

Definition

A thermometer is a device used to measure temperature.

Purpose

A thermometer is used in health care to measure and monitor **body temperature**. In an office, hospital or other health care facility, it allows a caregiver to record a baseline temperature when a patient is admitted. Repeated measurements of temperature are useful to detect deviations from normal levels. Repeated measurements are also useful in monitoring the effectiveness of current medications or other treatments.

The patient's temperature is recorded to check for pyrexia or monitor the degree of hypothermia present in the body.

Demographics

All health care professionals use thermometers. All health care facilities have thermometers. Most homes also have thermometers.

Description

A thermometer can use any of several methods to register temperature. These include mercury; liquid-in-glass; electronic with digital display; infrared or tympanic; and disposable dot matrix. A thermometer

KEY TERMS

Axillary—Pertaining to the armpit.

Hypothermia—Body temperature below 96°F (35.5°C).

Oral—Pertaining to the mouth.

Pyrexia—A temperature of 101°F (38.3°C) or higher in an infant younger than three months or above 102°F (38.9°C) for older children and adults.

Rectal—Pertaining to the rectum.

Sublingual—Under the tongue.

can be used in a clinical or emergency setting or at home. Thermometers can record body temperatures in the mouth (oral), armpit (axillary), eardrum (tympanic membrane), or anus (rectal).

A mercury thermometer consists of a narrow glass stem approximately 5 in (12.7 cm) in length with markings along one or both sides indicating the temperature scale in degrees Fahrenheit, Centigrade or both. Liquid mercury is held in a reservoir bulb at one end and rises through a capillary tube when the glass chamber is placed in contact with the body. Mercury thermometers are not used in modern clinical settings.

Electronic thermometers can record a wide range of temperatures between 94°F and 105°F (35°C and 42°C) and can record oral, axillary, or rectal temperatures. They have temperature sensors inside round-tipped probes that can be covered with disposable guards to prevent the spread of infection. The sensor is connected to a container housing the central processing unit. The information gathered by the sensor is then shown on a display screen. Some electronic models have such other features as memory recall of the last recording or a large display screen for easy reading. To use an electronic thermometer, the caregiver places the probe under the patient's arm or tongue, or in the patient's rectum. The probe is left in place for a period of time that depends on the model used. The device will beep when the peak temperature is reached. The time required to obtain a reading varies from three to 30 seconds.

A tympanic thermometer has a round-tipped probe containing a sensor that can be covered with a disposable guard to protect against the spread of ear infections. It is placed in the ear canal for 1 sec while an infrared sensor records the body heat radiated by the eardrum. The reading then appears on the unit's screen.

Digital and tympanic thermometers should be used in accordance with the manufacturer's guidelines.

Disposable thermometers are plastic strips with dots on the surface that have been impregnated with temperature-sensitive chemicals. The strips are sticky on one side to adhere to the skin under the armpit and prevent slippage. The dots change color at different temperatures as the chemicals in them respond to body heat. The temperature is readable after two to three minutes, depending on the instrument's guidelines. These products vary in length of use; they may be disposable, reusable, or used continuously for up to 48 hours. Disposable thermometers are useful for children, as they can record temperatures while children are asleep.

Diagnosis/Preparation

Training

Caregivers should be given training appropriate for the type of device used in their specific clinical setting.

Operation

The patient should sit or lie in a comfortable position to ensure that temperature readings are taken in similar locations each time and to minimize the effects of stress or excitement on the reading.

The manufacturer's guidelines should be followed when taking a patient's temperature with a digital, tympanic, or disposable thermometer. Dot-matrix thermometers are placed next to the skin and usually held in place by an adhesive strip. With the tympanic thermometer, caregivers should ensure that the probe is properly inserted into the ear to allow an optimal reading. The reading will be less accurate if the sensor cannot accurately touch the tympanic membrane or if the ear canal is clogged by wax or debris.

A mercury thermometer can be used to monitor a temperature in three body locations:

- Axillary.
- Oral or sublingual. This placement is never used with infants.
- Rectal. This method is used with infants. The tip of a rectal mercury thermometer is usually colored blue to distinguish it from the silver tip of an oral/axillary thermometer.

Before recording a temperature using a mercury thermometer, the caregiver shakes the mercury down by holding the thermometer firmly at the clear end and flicking it quickly a few times with a downward wrist motion toward the silver end. The mercury should be shaken down below 96°F (35.5°C) before the patient's temperature is taken.

In axillary placement, the silver tip of the thermometer is placed under the patient's right armpit, with the patient's arm pressing the instrument against the chest. The thermometer should stay in place for six to seven minutes. The caregiver can record the patient's other **vital signs** during this waiting period. After the waiting period has elapsed, the caregiver removes the thermometer and holds it at eye level to read it. The mercury will have risen to a level indicating the patient's temperature.

The procedure for taking a patient's temperature by mouth with a mercury thermometer is similar to the axillary method except that the silver tip of the thermometer is placed beneath the tongue for four to five minutes before being read. In both cases, the thermometer is wiped clean and stored in an appropriate container to prevent breakage.

To record the patient's rectal temperature with a mercury thermometer, a rectal thermometer is shaken down as described earlier. A small amount of water-based lubricant is placed on the colored tip of the thermometer to make it easier to insert. Infants must be positioned lying on their stomachs and held securely by the caregiver. The tip of the thermometer is inserted into the rectum no more than 0.5 in (1.3 cm) and held there for two to three minutes. The thermometer is removed, read as before, and cleansed with an antibacterial wipe. It is then stored in an appropriate container to prevent breakage. This precaution is important as mercury is poisonous when swallowed.

Liquid-in-glass thermometers contain alternatives to mercury (such as colored alcohol), but are used and stored in the same manner as mercury thermometers.

Maintenance

Many digital and infrared thermometers are self-calibrating and need relatively little care. To ensure accuracy, mercury thermometers should be shaken down prior to every use and left in place for at least three minutes. They require careful storage to prevent breakage and thorough cleaning after each use to prevent cross-infection.

As of early 2003, there is a nationwide initiative to ban the sale of thermometers and blood pressure monitors containing mercury. Health activists are concerned about mercury from broken or unwanted instruments contaminating the environment. A mercury thermometer contains 0.7g (0.025 oz) of mercury; 1 g of the substance is enough to contaminate a 20-acre lake. Several states have banned the use of products containing mercury. Most retail stores have stopped selling mercury thermometers. In October 1999, the Environmental Protection Agency (EPA) advised using alternative products to avoid the need for increased regulations in years to come and to protect human health and wildlife by reducing unnecessary exposure to mercury. According to a 2001 study by the Mayo Clinic, mercury-free devices can monitor information without compromising accuracy.

WHO PERFORMS THE PROCEDURE AND WHERE IS IT PERFORMED?

Most health professionals are trained in the proper operation of thermometers used in clinical settings. Most families have and use thermometers in the home.

Aftercare

A thermometer should be cleaned, disinfected and placed in an appropriate container for storage.

Risks

Breakage of a glass thermometer creates a risk of cuts from broken glass and possible mercury poisoning. Improper operation of a tympanic thermometer can cause injury to the middle ear. As digital devices have replaced glass thermometers, however, the number of injuries has declined.

An additional risk is that old or broken thermometers may give inaccurate results.

Normal results

A normal body temperature is defined as approximately 98.6°F (37°C). Body temperature is not constant throughout a 24-hour period. Some variation (0.3°F) is normal. Individuals also vary in their basal temperatures (0.3°F). A fever is defined as a temperature of 101°F (38.3°C) or higher in an infant younger than three months or above 102°F (38.9°C) for older children and adults. Hypothermia is recognized as a temperature below 96°F (35.5°C).

Morbidity and mortality rates

Injuries caused by properly inserted and normally functioning thermometers are extremely rare.

QUESTIONS TO ASK THE DOCTOR

What is the patient's temperature?

In the opinion of the professional, is the recorded temperature abnormal?

Based on the recorded temperature, what actions would the professional recommend?

Alternatives

There are no convenient alternatives to using a thermometer to measure body temperature.

Resources

BOOKS

Bickley, L. S., P. G. Szilagyi, and J. G. Stackhouse, eds. *Bates' Guide to Physical Examination & History Taking*, 8th ed. Philadelphia, PA: Lippincott Williams & Wilkins, 2002.

Chan, P. D., and P. J. Winkle. *History and Physical Examination in Medicine*, 10th ed. New York, NY: Current Clinical Strategies, 2002.

Seidel, Henry M. *Mosby's Physical Examination Handbook*, 4th ed. St. Louis, MO: Mosby-Year Book, 2003.

Swartz, Mark A., and William Schmitt. *Textbook of Physical Diagnosis: History and Examination*, 4th ed. Philadelphia, PA: Saunders, 2001.

PERIODICALS

Dowding, D., S. Freeman, S. Nimmo, et al. "An Investigation Into the Accuracy of Different Types of Thermometers." *Professional Nurse* 18 (November 2002): 166-168.

Drake-Lee, A., I. Mantella, and A. Bridle. "Infrared Ear Thermometers Versus Rectal Thermometers." *Lancet* 360 (December 7, 2002): 1883-1886.

Moran, D. S., and L. Mendal. "Core Temperature Measurement: Methods and Current Insights." *Sports Medicine* 32 (2002): 879-885.

Pompei, F. "Insufficiency in Thermometer Data." *Anesthesia and Analgesia* 96 (March 2003): 908-909.

ORGANIZATIONS

American Academy of Family Physicians. 11400 Tomahawk Creek Parkway, Leawood, KS 66211-2672. (913) 906-6000. www.aafp.org. E-mail: fp@aafp.org

American Academy of Pediatrics. 141 Northwest Point Boulevard, Elk Grove Village, IL 60007-1098. (847) 434-4000; FAX: (847) 434-8000. www.aap.org. E-mail: kidsdoc@aap.org

American College of Physicians. 190 N. Independence Mall West, Philadelphia, PA 19106-1572. (800) 523-1546, x2600 or (215) 351-2600. www.acponline.org.

American Medical Association. 515 N. State Street, Chicago, IL 60610. (312) 464-5000. www.ama-assn.org.

American Nurses Association. 600 Maryland Avenue, SW, Suite 100 West, Washington, DC 20024. (202) 651-7000 or (800) 274-4262. www.nursingworld.org.

OTHER

About.com. [cited March 1, 2003]. www.inventors.about.com/library/inventors/blthermometer.htm.

AskLynnRN. [cited March 1, 2003]. www.asklynnrn.com/html/healthmon_bbt_thermometer.htm.

How Stuff Works. [cited March 1, 2003]. www.howstuffworks.com/therm.htm.

Rice University. [cited March 1, 2003]. www.es.rice.edu/ES/humsoc/Galileo/Things/thermometer.html.

L. Fleming Fallon, Jr., MD, DrPH

Thoracic surgery

Definition

Thoracic surgery is any surgery performed in the chest (thorax).

Purpose

The purpose of thoracic surgery is to treat diseased or injured organs in the thorax, including the esophagus (muscular tube that passes food to the stomach), trachea (windpipe that branches to form the right bronchus and the left bronchus), pleura (membranes that cover and protect the lung), mediastinum (area separating the left and right lungs), chest wall, diaphragm, heart, and lungs.

General thoracic surgery is a field that specializes in diseases of the lungs and esophagus. The field also encompasses accidents and injuries to the chest, esophageal disorders (esophageal cancer or esophagitis), lung cancer, **lung transplantation**, and surgery for emphysema.

Description

The most common diseases requiring thoracic surgery include lung cancer, chest trauma, esophageal cancer, emphysema, and lung transplantation.

Lung cancer

Lung cancer is one of the most significant public health problems in the world. Approximately 213,380 new cases of lung and bronchial cancer occurred in 2007. It is the leading cause of cancer deaths among

KEY TERMS

Diaphragm—A membrane in the thorax that moves to assist the breathing cycle.

Dyspnea—Difficulty breathing.

Hemothorax—Blood in the pleural cavity.

Mediastinum—The portion of the thorax that consists of the heart, thoracic parts of the great vessels, and thoracic parts of the trachea, esophagus, thymus, and lymph nodes.

both men and women, killing more than 160,390 people annually. The overall five-year survival rate for all types of lung cancer is about 15.5%, as compared to 64.8% for colon cancer, 89% for breast cancer, and 99.9% for prostate cancer.

Lung cancer develops primarily by exposure to toxic chemicals. Cigarette smoking is the most important risk factor responsible for the disease. Other environmental factors that may predispose a person to lung cancer include industrial substances such as arsenic, nickel, chromium, asbestos, radon, organic chemicals, air pollution, and radiation.

Most cases of lung cancer develop in the right lung because it contains the majority (55%) of lung tissue. Additionally, lung cancer occurs more frequently in the upper lobes of the lung than in the lower lobes. The tumor receives blood from the bronchial artery (a major artery in the pulmonary system).

Adenocarcinoma of the lung is the most frequent type of lung cancer, accounting for 45% of all cases. This type of cancer can spread (metastasize) earlier than another type of lung cancer called squamous cell carcinoma (which occurs in approximately 30% of lung cancer patients). Approximately 66% of squamous cell carcinoma cases are centrally located. They expand against the bronchus, causing compression. Small-cell carcinoma accounts for 20% of all lung cancers; and the majority (80%) are centrally located. Small-cell carcinoma is a highly aggressive lung cancer, with early metastasis to distant sites such as the brain and bone marrow (the central portion of certain bones, which produce formed elements that are part of blood).

Most lung tumors are not treated with thoracic surgery since patients seek medical care later in the disease process. Chemotherapy increases the rate of survival in patients with limited (not advanced) disease. Surgery may be useful for staging or diagnosis. Pulmonary resection (removal of the tumor and neighboring lymph nodes) can be curative if the tumor is less than or equal to 1.8 in (3 cm), and presents as a solitary nodule. Lung tumors spread to other areas through neighboring lymphatic channels. Even if thoracic surgery is performed, postoperative chemotherapy may also be indicated to provide comprehensive treatment (i.e., to kill any tumor cells that may have spread via the lymphatic system).

Genetic engineering has provided insights related to the growth of tumors. A genetic mutation called a k-ras mutation frequently occurs, and is implicated in 90% of genetic mutations for adenocarcinoma of the lung. Mutations in the cancer cells make them resistant to chemotherapy, necessitating the use of multiple chemotherapeutic agents.

Chest trauma

Chest trauma is a medical/surgical emergency. Initially, the chest should be examined after an airway is maintained. The mortality (**death**) rate for trauma patients with respiratory distress is approximately 50%. This figure rises to 75% if symptoms include both respiratory distress and shock. Patients with respiratory distress require **endotracheal intubation** (passing a plastic tube from the mouth to the windpipe) and mechanically assisted ventilator support. Invasive thoracic procedures are necessary in emergency situations.

Trauma requiring urgent thoracic surgery may include any of the following problems: a large clotted hemothorax, massive air leak, esophageal injury, valvular cardiac (heart) injury, proven damage to blood vessels in the heart, or chest wall defect.

Esophageal cancer

The number of new cases of esophageal cancer is slowly rising, with about 14,500 people diagnosed annually. While the cause of esophageal cancer is not precisely known, the greatly increased rate of esophageal cancer seems to be tied to the epidemic of obesity in the United States. Obesity results in acid reflux into the esophagus, chronic esophageal irritation, and progression to abnormal cell types that result in esophageal cancer, specifically of adenocarinoma of the esophagus. Smoking and alcohol seem to also result in chronic esophageal irritation, leading to an association with squamous cell carcinoma of the esophagus.

Difficulty swallowing (dysphagia) is the cardinal symptom of esophageal cancer. Radiography, endoscopy, computerized axial tomography (CT scan), and ultrasonography are part of a comprehensive diagnostic evaluation. The standard operation for patients with resectable esophageal carcinoma includes removal of the tumor from the esophagus, a portion of the stomach, and the lymph nodes (within the cancerous region).

Emphysema

Lung volume reduction surgery (LVRS) is the term used to describe surgery for patients with emphysema. LVRS is intended to help persons whose disabling dyspnea (difficulty breathing) is related to emphysema and does not respond to medical management. Breathlessness is a result of the structural and functional pulmonary and thoracic abnormalities associated with emphysema. Surgery will assist the patient, but the primary pathogenic process that caused the emphysema is permanent because lung tissues lose the capability of elastic recoil during normal breathing (inspiration and expiration).

Patients are usually transferred out of the **intensive care unit** (ICU) within one day of surgery. Physical therapy and rehabilitation (coughing and breathing exercises) begin soon after surgery, and the patient is discharged when deemed clinically stable.

Lung transplantation

There are various types of lung transplantations: unilateral (one lung, the most common type); bilateral (both lungs); heart-lung; and living donor lobe transplantation.

The survival rate for persons receiving a single lung transplant is more than 82% at one year, almost 60% at three years, and more than 43% at five years. Double-lung transplants have similar success rates: 82% at one year, 64% at three years, and 48% at five years. A successful outcome is highly dependent on the patient's general medical condition. Those who have symptomatic osteoporosis (severe disease of the musculoskeletal system) or are users of **corticosteroids** may not have favorable outcomes.

The death rate occurs due to infections (pulmonary infections) or chronic rejection (bronchiolitis obliterans) if the donor lung was not a perfect genetic match. Patients are given postoperative **antibiotics** to prevent bacterial infections during the early period following surgery.

Bacterial pneumonia is usually severe. A bacterial genus known as *Pseudomonas* accounts for 75% of post-transplant pneumonia cases. Patients can also acquire viral and fungal infections, and an infection caused by a cell parasite known as *Pneumocystis carinii.* Infections are treated with specific medications intended to destroy the invading microorganism. Viral infections require treatment of symptoms.

Acute (quick onset) rejection is common within the first weeks after lung transplantation. Acute rejection is treated with steroids (bolus given intravenously), and is effective in 80% of cases. Chronic rejection is the most common problem, and typically begins with symptoms of fatigue and a vague feeling of illness. Treatment is difficult, and the results are unrewarding. There are several immunosuppressive protocols currently utilized for cases of chronic rejection. The goal of immunosuppressive therapy is to prevent the host's immune reaction from destroying the genetically foreign organ.

Diagnosis/Preparation

The surgeon may use two common incisional approaches: sternotomy (incision through and down the breastbone) or via the side of the chest (**thoracotomy**).

An operative procedure known as video-assisted thoracoscopic surgery (VATS) is minimally invasive. During VATS, a lung is collapsed and the thoracoscope and **surgical instruments** are inserted into the thorax through any of three or four small incisions in the chest wall.

Another approach involves the use of a mediastinoscope or bronchoscope to visualize the internal anatomical structures during thoracic surgery or diagnostic procedures.

Preoperative evaluation for most patients (except emergency cases) must include cardiac tests, blood chemistry analysis, and **physical examination**. Like most operative procedures, the patient should not eat or drink food 10–12 hours prior to surgery. Patients who undergo thoracic surgery with the video-assisted approach tend to have shorter inpatient hospital stays.

Aftercare

Patients typically experience severe pain after surgery, and are given appropriate pain medications. In uncomplicated cases, chest and urine (Foley catheter) tubes are usually removed within 24–48 hours. A highly trained and comprehensive team of respiratory therapists and nurses is vital for **postoperative care** that results in improved lung function via deep breathing and coughing exercises.

Risks

Precautions for thoracic surgery include coagulation blood disorders (disorders that prevent normal blood clotting) and previous thoracic surgery. Risks include hemorrhage, myocardial infarction (heart attack), stroke, nerve injury, embolism (blood clot or

WHO PERFORMS THE PROCEDURE AND WHERE IS IT PERFORMED?

Thoracic surgery is performed in a hospital by a specialist in general surgery who has received advanced training in thoracic surgery.

air bubble that obstructs an artery), and infection. Total lung collapse can occur from fluid or air accumulation, as a result of chest tubes that are routinely placed after surgery for drainage.

Resources

BOOKS

Abeloff, M. D., et al. *Clinical Oncology*, 3rd ed. Philadelphia: Elsevier, 2004.

Khatri, V. P., and J. A. Asensio. *Operative Surgery Manual*, 1st ed. Philadelphia: Saunders, 2003.

Libby, P., et al. *Braunwald's Heart Disease*, 8th ed. Philadelphia: Saunders, 2007.

Marx, John A., et al. *Rosen's Emergency Medicine*, 6th ed. St. Louis, MO: Mosby, Inc., 2006.

Mason, R. J., et al. *Murray & Nadel's Textbook of Respiratory Medicine*, 4th ed. Philadelphia: Saunders, 2007.

Townsend, C. M., et al. *Sabiston Textbook of Surgery*, 17th ed. Philadelphia: Saunders, 2004.

PERIODICALS

Krupnick, A. S. "Operative Thoracic Surgery," 5th ed. *Journal of the American College of Surgery* 204, no. 5 (May 2007).

Ng, T. "Evolution to video-assisted thoracic surgery lobectomy after training: Initial results of the first 30 patients." *Journal of the American College of Surgery* 203, no. 4 (October 2006).

ORGANIZATIONS

American Association for Thoracic Surgery. 900 Cummings Center, Suite 221-U, Beverly, MA 01915. (978) 927-8330. Fax: (978) 524-8890. E-mail: aats@prri.com.

Laith Farid Gulli, MD, MS
Abraham F. Ettaher, MD
Nicole Mallory, MS, PA-C

Thoracotomy

Definition

Thoracotomy is the process of making of an incision (cut) into the chest wall.

Purpose

A physician gains access to the chest cavity (called the thorax) by cutting through the chest wall. Reasons for the entry are varied. Thoracotomy allows for study of the condition of the lungs; removal of a lung or part of a lung; removal of a rib; and examination, treatment, or removal of any organs in the chest cavity. Thoracotomy also provides access to the heart, esophagus, diaphragm, and the portion of the aorta that passes through the chest cavity.

Lung cancer is the most common cancer requiring a thoracotomy. Tumors and metastatic growths can be removed through the incision (a procedure called resection). A biopsy, or tissue sample, can also be taken through the incision, and examined under a microscope for evidence of abnormal cells.

A resuscitative or emergency thoracotomy may be performed to resuscitate a patient who is near **death** as a result of a chest injury. An emergency thoracotomy provides access to the chest cavity to control injury-related bleeding from the heart, cardiac compressions to restore a normal heart rhythm, or to relieve pressure on the heart caused by cardiac tamponade (accumulation of fluid in the space between the heart's muscle and outer lining).

Demographics

Thoracotomy may be performed to diagnose or treat a variety of conditions; therefore, no data exist as to the overall incidence of the procedure. Lung cancer, a common reason for thoracotomy, is diagnosed in approximately over 196,000 people each year and affects more men than women (108,355 diagnoses in men compared to 87,897 in women).

Description

The thoracotomy incision may be made on the side, under the arm (axillary thoracotomy); on the front, through the breastbone (median sternotomy); slanting from the back to the side (posterolateral thoracotomy); or under the breast (anterolateral thoracotomy). The exact location of the cut depends on the reason for the surgery. In some cases, the physician is able to make the incision between ribs (called an intercostal approach) to minimize cuts through bone, nerves, and muscle. The incision may range from just under 5–10 in (12.7–25 cm).

During the surgery, a tube is passed through the trachea. It usually has a branch to each lung. One lung is deflated for examination and surgery, while the

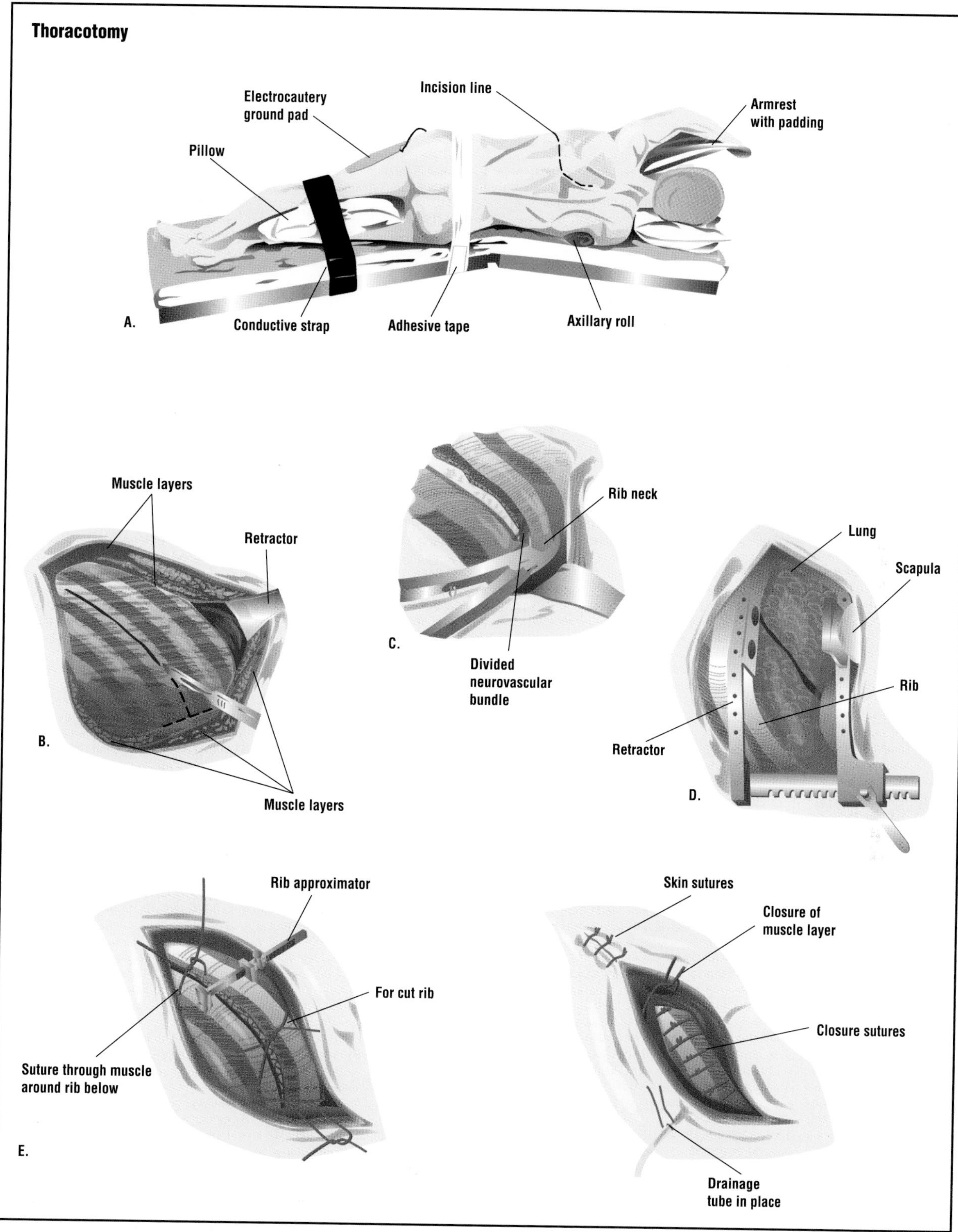

For a thoracotomy, the patient lies on his or her side with one arm raised (A). An incision is cut into the skin of the ribcage (B). Muscle layers are cut, and a rib may be removed to gain access to the cavity. (C). Retractors hold the ribs apart, exposing the lung (D). After any repairs are made, the cut rib is replaced and held in place with special materials (E). Layers of muscle and skin are stitched. *(Illustration by GGS Information Services. Cengage Learning, Gale.)*

KEY TERMS

Aorta—The major artery carrying blood away from the heart.

Catheter—A tube inserted into a body cavity to drain fluid. An example would be a urinary catheter used to drain urine from the urethra.

Diaphragm—The large flat muscle that runs horizontally across the bottom of the chest cavity.

Esophagus—The muscular tube that connects the mouth and the stomach.

Trachea—The tube made of cartilage that carries air from the nose and mouth to the lungs.

Urethra—The tube that carries urine from the bladder to the outside of the body.

other one is inflated with the assistance of a mechanical device (a ventilator).

A number of different procedures may be commenced at this point. A lobectomy removes an entire lobe or section of a lung (the right lung has three lobes and the left lung has two). It may be done to remove cancer that is contained by a lobe. A **segmentectomy**, or wedge resection, removes a wedge-shaped piece of lung smaller than a lobe. Alternatively, the entire lung may be removed during a **pneumonectomy**.

In the case of an emergency thoracotomy, the procedure performed depends on the type and extent of injury. The heart may be exposed so that direct cardiac compressions can be performed; the physician may use one hand or both hands to manually pump blood through the heart. Internal paddles of a defibrillating machine may be applied directly to the heart to restore normal cardiac rhythms. Injuries to the heart causing excessive bleeding (hemorrhaging) may be closed with **staples** or **stitches**.

Once the procedure that required the incision is completed, the chest wall is closed. The layers of skin, muscle, and other tissues are closed with stitches or staples. If the breastbone was cut (as in the case of a median sternotomy), it is stitched back together with wire.

Diagnosis/Preparation

Patients are told not to eat after midnight the night before surgery. They must tell their physicians about all known allergies so that the safest anesthetics can be selected. Older patients must be evaluated for heart ailments before surgery because of the additional strain on the heart.

WHO PERFORMS THE PROCEDURE AND WHERE IS IT PERFORMED?

Thoracotomy may be performed by a thoracic surgeon, a medical doctor who has completed surgical training in the areas of general surgery and surgery of the chest area, or an emergency room physician (in the case of emergency thoracotomy). The procedure is generally performed in a hospital operating room, although emergency thoracotomies may be performed in an emergency department or trauma center.

Aftercare

Opening the chest cavity means cutting through skin, muscle, nerves, and sometimes bone. It is a major procedure that often involves a hospital stay of five to seven days. The skin around the drainage tube to the thoracic cavity must be kept clean, and the tube must be kept unblocked.

The pressure differences that are set up in the thoracic cavity by the movement of the diaphragm (the large muscle at the base of the thorax) make it possible for the lungs to expand and contract. If the pressure in the chest cavity changes abruptly, the lungs can collapse. Any fluid that collects in the cavity puts a patient at risk for infection and reduced lung function, or even collapse (called a pneumothorax). Thus, any entry to the chest usually requires that a chest tube remain in place for several days after the incision is closed.

The first two days after surgery may be spent in the **intensive care unit** (ICU) of the hospital. A variety of tubes, catheters, and monitors may be required after surgery.

Risks

The rich supply of blood vessels to the lungs makes hemorrhage a risk; a blood **transfusion** may become necessary during surgery. **General anesthesia** carries risks such as nausea, vomiting, headache, blood pressure issues, or allergic reaction. After a thoracotomy, there may be drainage from the incision. There is also the risk of infection; the patient must learn how to keep the incision clean and dry as it heals.

After the chest tube is removed, the patient is vulnerable to pneumothorax. Physicians strive to reduce the risk of collapse by timing the removal of the tube. Doing so at the end of inspiration (breathing

QUESTIONS TO ASK THE DOCTOR

Why is thoracotomy being recommended?

What diagnostic tests will be performed to determine if thoracotomy is necessary?

What type of incision will be used and where will it be located?

What type of procedure will be performed?

How long is the recovery time and what is expected during this period?

If a biopsy is the only reason for the procedure, is a thoracoscopy or a guided needle biopsy an option (instead of thoracotomy)?

in) or the end of expiration (breathing out) poses less risk. Deep breathing exercises and coughing should be emphasized as an important way that patients can improve healing and prevent pneumonia.

Normal results

The results following thoracotomy depend on the reasons why it was performed. If a biopsy was taken during the surgery, a normal result would indicate that no cancerous cells are present in the tissue sample. The procedure may indicate that further treatment is necessary; for example, if cancer was detected, chemotherapy, radiation therapy, or more surgery may be recommended.

Morbidity and mortality

One study following lung cancer patients undergoing thoracotomy found that 10–15% of patients experienced heartbeat irregularities, readmittance to the ICU, or partial or full lung collapse; 5–10% experienced pneumonia or extended use of the ventilator (greater than 48 hours); and up to 5% experienced wound infection, accumulation of pus in the chest cavity, or blood clots in the lung. The mortality rate in the study was 5.8%, with patients **dying** as a result of the cancer itself or of postoperative complications.

Alternatives

Video-assisted **thoracic surgery** (VATS) is a less invasive alternative to thoracotomy. Also called thoracoscopy, VATS involves the insertion of a thoracoscope (a thin, lighted tube) into a small incision through the chest wall. The surgeon can visualize the structures inside the chest cavity on a video screen. Instruments such as a stapler or grasper may be inserted through other small incisions. Although initially used as a diagnostic tool (to visualize the lungs or to remove a sample of lung tissue for further examination), VATS is being increasingly used to remove some lung tumors, and is usually appropriate for those under 2.4 in (6 cm). In some practices, as many as 8% of all lobectomies are now performed using VATS technique.

An alternative to emergency thoracotomy is a tube thoracostomy, a tube placed through chest wall to drain excess fluid. Over 80% of patients with a penetrating chest wound can be successfully managed with a thoracostomy.

Resources

BOOKS

Khatri, V. P., and J. A. Asensio. *Operative Surgery Manual*, 1st ed. Philadelphia: Saunders, 2003.

Mason, R. J., et al. *Murray & Nadel's Textbook of Respiratory Medicine*, 4th ed. Philadelphia: Saunders, 2007.

Townsend, C. M., et al. *Sabiston Textbook of Surgery*, 17th ed. Philadelphia: Saunders, 2004.

PERIODICALS

Blewett, C. J., et al. "Open Lung Biopsy as an Outpatient Procedure." *Annals of Thoracic Surgery* (April 2001): 1113–1115.

Handy, John R., et al. "What Happens to Patients Undergoing Lung Cancer Surgery? Outcomes and Quality of Life Before and After Surgery." *Chest* 122, no.1 (August 14, 2002): 21–30.

Swanson, Scott J. and Hasan F. Batirel. "Video-Assisted Thoracic Surgery (VATS) Resection for Lung Cancer." *Surgical Clinics of North America* 82, no.3 (June 1, 2002): 541–9.

ORGANIZATIONS

American Cancer Society. 1599 Clifton Rd. NE, Atlanta, GA 30329-4251. (800) 227-2345. http://www.cancer.org (accessed April 10, 2008).

Society of Thoracic Surgeons. 663 N. Saint Clair St., Suite 2320, Chicago, IL 60611-3658. (312) 202-5800. http://www.sts.org (accessed April 10, 2008).

OTHER

"Detailed Guide: Lung Cancer." *American Cancer Society* [cited April 28, 2003]. http://www.cancer.org/docroot/CRI/CRI_2_3x.asp?dt=15 (accessed April 10, 2008).

Diane M. Calabrese
Stephanie Dionne Sherk

Thrombocyte count *see* **Complete blood count**

Thrombolytic therapy

Definition

Thrombolytic therapy is the use of drugs that dissolve blood clots. The name "thrombolytic" comes from two Greek words that mean "clot" and "loosening."

Purpose

When a blood clot forms in a blood vessel, it may cut off or severely reduce blood flow to parts of the body that are served by that blood vessel. This event can cause serious damage to those parts of the body. If the clot forms in an artery that supplies blood to the heart, for example, it can cause a heart attack. A clot that cuts off blood to the brain can cause a stroke. Thrombolytic therapy is used to dissolve blood clots that could cause serious, and possibly life-threatening, damage if they are not removed. Research suggests that when used to treat stroke, thrombolytic therapy can prevent or reverse paralysis and other problems that otherwise might result.

In heart attacks, thrombolytic therapy is an alternative to stenting, a procedure in which a spring-like device is inserted into a blocked blood vessel. In general, stenting is the preferred treatment, since it both removes the clot and opens the blood vessel, which may have internal cholesterol deposits. Thrombolytic therapy only removes the clot, but it can be administered in hospitals with fewer resources than are required for insertion of a stent.

Thrombolytic therapy is also used to dissolve blood clots that form in catheters or tubes put into people's bodies for medical treatments, such as dialysis or chemotherapy.

Description

Thrombolytic therapy uses drugs called thrombolytic agents, such as alteplase (Activase), anistreplase (Eminase), streptokinase (Streptase, Kabikinase), urokinase (Abbokinase), and tissue plasminogen activator (TPA) to dissolve clots. These drugs are given as injections, and given only under a physician's supervision.

Recommended dosage

The physician supervising thrombolytic therapy decides on the proper dose for each patient. He or she will take into account the type of drug, the purpose for which it is being used, and in some cases, the patient's weight.

KEY TERMS

Arteries—Blood vessels that carry blood away from the heart to the cells, tissues, and organs of the body.

Chemotherapy—Treatment of an illness with chemical agents. The term is usually used to describe the treatment of cancer with drugs that kill cancer cells.

Dialysis—A process used to separate waste products from the blood in people whose kidneys are not working well.

Hemorrhagic stroke—A disruption of the blood supply to the brain caused by bleeding into the brain.

Stent—A thin rodlike or tubelike device, inserted into a vein or artery to keep the vessel open.

Stroke—A serious medical event in which blood flow to the brain is stopped by a blood clot in an artery or because an artery has burst. Strokes may cause paralysis and changes in a person's speech, memory, and behavior.

Precautions

For thrombolytic therapy to be effective in treating stroke or heart attack, prompt medical attention is very important. The drugs must be given within a few hours of the beginning of a stroke or heart attack. This type of treatment is not right, however, for every patient who has a heart attack or a stroke. Only a qualified medical professional can decide whether a thrombolytic agent should be used. To increase the chance of survival and reduce the risk of serious permanent damage, anyone who has signs of a heart attack or stroke should get immediate medical help.

Thrombolytic therapy may cause bleeding in other parts of the body. This side effect is usually not serious, but severe bleeding does occur in some patients, especially older people. Some people have had minor hemorrhagic strokes in which there has been a small amount of bleeding into the brain. These hemorrhagic strokes have been blocked by clots that would be broken up by use of a thrombolytic agent, so that removal of the harmful clot would cause equally dangerous bleeding. To lower the risk of serious bleeding, people who are given thrombolytic medications should move around as little as possible and should not try to get up on their own unless told to do so by a health care professional. Following all the instructions of the health care providers in charge is very important.

Thrombolytic therapy may be more likely to cause serious bleeding in people who have certain medical conditions or have recently had certain procedures. Before being given a thrombolytic agent, anyone with any of these problems or conditions should tell the physician in charge:

- blood disease or current or past bleeding problems in any part of the body
- heart or blood vessel disease
- stroke (recent or in the past)
- high blood pressure
- brain tumor or other brain disease
- stomach ulcer or colitis
- severe liver disease
- active tuberculosis
- recent falls, injuries, or blows to the body or head
- recent injections into a blood vessel
- recent surgery, including dental surgery
- tubes recently placed in the body for any reason
- recent delivery of a baby

In addition, anyone who has had a recent streptococcal (strep) infection should tell the physician in charge. Some thrombolytic agents may not work properly in people who have just had a strep infection, so the physician may want to use a different drug.

People who take certain medicines may be at greater risk for severe bleeding when they are given a thrombolytic agent.

Women who are pregnant should tell the physician in charge before being given a thrombolytic agent. There is a slight chance that a woman who is given thrombolytic therapy during the first five months of pregnancy will have a miscarriage. Streptokinase and urokinase, however, have both been used without problems in pregnant women.

After being treated with thrombolytic therapy, women who are breastfeeding should check with their physicians before starting to breastfeed again.

Side effects

Anyone who has fever or who notices bleeding or oozing from their gums, from cuts, or from the site where the thrombolytic agent was injected should immediately tell their health care provider.

People who are given thrombolytic therapy should also be alert to the signs of bleeding inside the body and should check with a physician immediately if any of the following symptoms occur:

- blood in the urine
- blood in the stool, or black, tarry stools
- constipation
- coughing up blood
- vomiting blood or material that looks like coffee grounds
- nosebleeds
- unexpected or unusually heavy vaginal bleeding
- dizziness
- sudden, severe, or constant headaches
- pain or swelling in the abdomen or stomach
- back pain or backache
- severe or constant muscle pain or stiffness
- stiff, swollen, or painful joints

Other side effects of thrombolytic agents are possible. Anyone who has unusual symptoms during or after thrombolytic therapy should tell a health care professional.

Interactions

People who take certain medicines may be at greater risk for severe bleeding when they receive a thrombolytic agent. Anyone who is given a thrombolytic agent should tell the physician in charge about all other prescription or nonprescription (over-the-counter) medicines he or she is taking. Among the medicines that may increase the chance of bleeding are:

- aspirin and other medicines for pain and inflammation
- blood thinners (anticoagulants)
- antiseizure medicines, including divalproex (Depakote) and valproic acid (Depakene)
- cephalosporins, including cefamandole (Mandol), cefoperazone (Cefobid), and cefotetan (Cefotan)

In addition, anyone who has been treated with anistreplase or streptokinase within the past year should tell the physician in charge. These drugs may not work properly if they are given again, so the physician may want to use a different thrombolytic agent.

Patients who are taking thrombolytic medications should not take vitamin E supplements or certain herbal preparations without consulting their doctor. High doses of vitamin E can increase the risk of hemorrhagic stroke. Ginger, borage, angelica, dong quai, feverfew, and other herbs can intensify the anticlotting effect of thrombolytic medications and increase the risk of bleeding.

Resources

BOOKS

Brody, T. M., J. Larner, K. P. Minneman, and H. C. Neu. *Human Pharmacology: Molecular to Clinical*, 2nd ed. St. Louis: Mosby Year-Book, 1995.

Karch, A. M. *Lippincott's Nursing Drug Guide*. Springhouse, PA: Lippincott Williams & Wilkins, 2003.

Pelletier, Kenneth R., MD. *The Best Alternative Medicine*, Part I, Chapter 6, "Western Herbal Medicine." New York: Simon & Schuster, 2002.

Reynolds, J. E. F., ed. *Martindale: The Extra Pharmacopoeia*, 31st ed. London, UK: The Pharmaceutical Press, 1996.

Townsend, C. M., ed. *Sabiston Textbook of Surgery*, 16th ed. Philadelphia, PA: W. B. Saunders, 2001.

PERIODICALS

"Acute Myocardial Infarction: Clot-Busting Therapy May Reduce Death in Elderly Heart Attack Patients." *Heart Disease Weekly* May 18, 2003.

Dundar, Y., R. Hill, R. Dickson, and T. Walley. "Comparative Efficacy of Thrombolytics in Acute Myocardial Infarction: A Systematic Review." *QJM* 96 (February 2003): 103-113.

Marsh, P. "Clot-Bust' Drug Right On Target." *Birmingham Post and Mail Ltd*, February 6, 2003.

ORGANIZATIONS

American Society of Health-System Pharmacists (ASHP). 7272 Wisconsin Avenue, Bethesda, MD 20814. (301) 657-3000. www.ashp.org.

United States Food and Drug Administration (FDA). 5600 Fishers Lane, Rockville, MD 20857-0001. (888) INFO-FDA. www.fda.gov.

OTHER

Harvard Medical School. www.hms.harvard.edu/news/releases/0302soumerai.html.

University of Iowa. www.medicine.uiowa.edu/pharmacology/Lectures/Lecturenotes/111/RJH-Anticoagulants%20(Word).pdf.

Nancy Ross-Flanigan
Sam Uretsky, PharmD

Thyroid gland removal *see* **Thyroidectomy**

Thyroidectomy

Definition

Thyroidectomy is a surgical procedure in which all or part of the thyroid gland is removed. The thyroid gland is located in the forward (anterior) part of the neck just under the skin and in front of the Adam's apple. The thyroid is one of the body's endocrine glands, which means that it secretes its products inside the body, into the blood or lymph. The thyroid produces several hormones that have two primary functions: they increase the synthesis of proteins in most of the body's tissues, and they raise the level of the body's oxygen consumption.

Purpose

All or part of the thyroid gland may be removed to correct a variety of abnormalities. If a person has a goiter, which is an enlargement of the thyroid gland that causes swelling in the front of the neck, the swollen gland may cause difficulties with swallowing or breathing. Hyperthyroidism (overactivity of the thyroid gland) produces hypermetabolism, a condition in which the body uses abnormal amounts of oxygen, nutrients, and other materials. A thyroidectomy may be performed if the hypermetabolism cannot be adequately controlled by medication, or if the condition occurs in a child or pregnant woman. Both cancerous and noncancerous tumors (frequently called nodules) may develop in the thyroid gland. These growths must be removed, in addition to some or all of the gland itself.

Demographics

Screening tests indicate that about 6% of the United States population has some disturbance of thyroid function, but many people with mildly abnormal levels of thyroid hormone do not have any disease symptoms. It is estimated that between 12 and 15 million people in the United States and Canada received treatment for thyroid disorders as of 2002. In 2001, there were approximately 34,500 thyroidectomies performed in the United States. Females are somewhat more likely than males to require a thyroidectomy.

Description

A thyroidectomy begins with **general anesthesia** administered by an anesthesiologist. The anesthesiologist injects drugs into the patient's veins and then places an airway tube in the windpipe to ventilate (provide air for) the person during the operation. After the patient has been anesthetized, the surgeon makes an incision in the front of the neck at the level where a tight-fitting necklace would rest. The surgeon locates and takes care not to injure the parathyroid glands and the recurrent laryngeal nerves, while freeing the thyroid gland from these surrounding

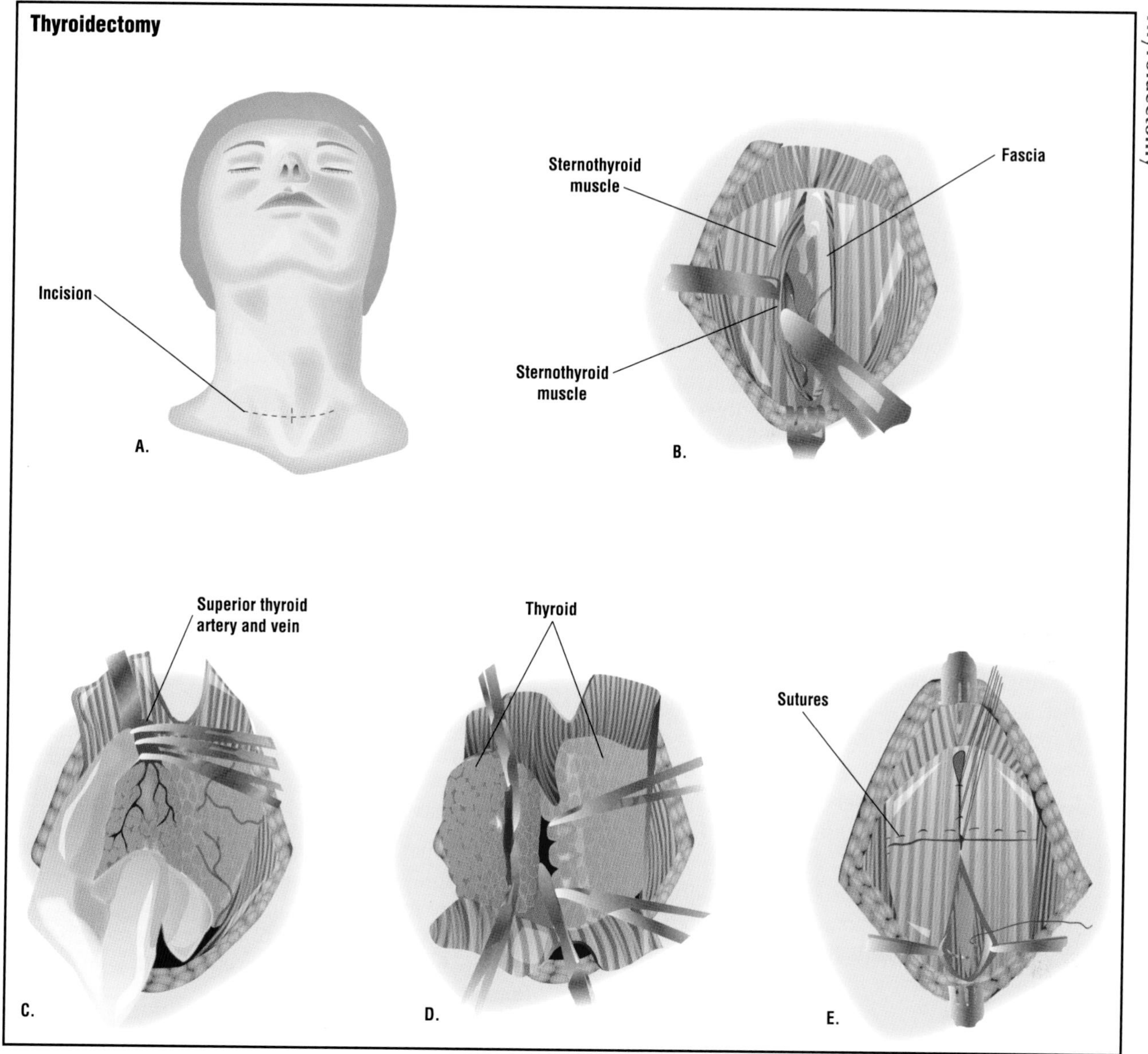

To remove the thyroid gland, an incision is made at the front of the neck (A). Muscles and connecting tissue, or fascia, are divided (B). The veins and arteries above and below the thyroid are severed (C), and the gland is removed in two parts (D). The tissues and muscles are repaired before the skin incision is closed (E). *(Illustration by GGS Information Services. Cengage Learning, Gale.)*

structures. The next step is clamping off the blood supply to the portion of the thyroid gland that is to be removed. Next, the surgeon removes all or part of the gland. If cancer has been diagnosed, all or most of the gland is removed. If other diseases or nodules are present, the surgeon may remove only part of the gland. The total amount of glandular tissue removed depends on the condition being treated. The surgeon may place a drain, which is a soft plastic tube that allows tissue fluids to flow out of an area, before closing the incision. The incision is closed with either sutures (**stitches**) or metal clips. A dressing is placed over the incision and the drain, if one has been placed.

People generally stay in the hospital one to four days after a thyroidectomy.

Diagnosis/Preparation

Thyroid disorders do not always develop rapidly; in some cases, the patient's symptoms may be subtle or difficult to distinguish from the symptoms of other disorders. Patients suffering from hypothyroidism

KEY TERMS

Endocrine—A type of organ or gland that secretes hormones or other products inside the body, into the bloodstream or the lymphatic system. The thyroid is an endocrine gland.

Endocrinologist—A physician who specializes in treating persons with diseases of the thyroid, parathyroid, adrenal glands, and the pancreas.

Goiter—An enlargement of the thyroid gland due to insufficient iodine in the diet.

Hyperthyroidism—Abnormal overactivity of the thyroid gland. People with hyperthyroidism are hypermetabolic, lose weight, exhibit nervousness, have muscular weakness and fatigue, sweat heavily, and have increased urination and bowel movements. This condition is also called thyrotoxicosis.

Hypothyroidism—Abnormal underfunctioning of the thyroid gland. People with hypothyroidism have a lowered body metabolism, gain weight, and are sluggish.

Parathyroid glands—Two pairs of smaller glands that lie close to the lower surface of the thyroid gland. They secrete parathyroid hormone, which regulates the body's use of calcium and phosphorus.

Recurrent laryngeal nerve—A nerve which lies very near the parathyroid glands and serves the larynx or voice box.

Thyroid storm—An unusual complication of thyroid function that is sometimes triggered by the stress of thyroid surgery. It is a medical emergency.

are sometimes misdiagnosed as having a psychiatric depression. Before a thyroidectomy is performed, a variety of tests and studies are usually required to determine the nature of the thyroid disease. Laboratory analysis of blood determines the levels of active thyroid hormones circulating in the body. The most common test is a blood test that measures the level of thyroid-stimulating hormone (TSH) in the bloodstream. Sonograms and computed tomography scans **(CT scans)** help to determine the size of the thyroid gland and location of abnormalities. A nuclear medicine scan may be used to assess thyroid function or to evaluate the condition of a thyroid nodule, but it is not considered a routine test. A needle biopsy of an abnormality or aspiration (removal by suction) of fluid from the thyroid gland may also be performed to help determine the diagnosis.

If the diagnosis is hyperthyroidism, a person may be asked to take antithyroid medication or iodides before the operation. Continued treatment with antithyroid drugs may be the treatment of choice. Otherwise, no other special procedure must be followed prior to the operation.

Aftercare

A thyroidectomy incision requires little to no care after the dressing is removed. The area may be bathed gently with a mild soap. The sutures or the metal clips are removed three to seven days after the operation.

Risks

There are definite risks associated with the procedure. The thyroid gland should be removed only if there is a pressing reason or medical condition that requires it.

As with all operations, people who are obese, smoke, or have poor nutrition are at greater risk for developing complications related to the general anesthetic itself.

Hoarseness or voice loss may develop if the recurrent laryngeal nerve is injured or destroyed during the operation. Nerve damage is more apt to occur in people who have large goiters or cancerous tumors.

Hypoparathyroidism (underfunctioning of the parathyroid glands) can occur if the parathyroid glands are injured or removed at the time of the thyroidectomy. Hypoparathyroidism is characterized by a drop in blood calcium levels resulting in muscle cramps and twitching.

Hypothyroidism (underfunctioning of the thyroid gland) can occur if all or nearly all of the thyroid gland is removed. Complete removal, however, may be intentional when the patient is diagnosed with cancer. If a person's thyroid levels remain low, thyroid replacement medications may be required for the rest of his or her life.

A hematoma is a collection of blood in an organ or tissue, caused by a break in the wall of a blood vessel. The neck and the area surrounding the thyroid gland have a rich supply of blood vessels. Bleeding in the area of the operation may occur and be difficult to control or stop. If a hematoma occurs in this part of the body, it may be life-threatening. As the hematoma enlarges, it may obstruct the airway and cause a person to stop breathing. If a hematoma does develop in the neck, the surgeon may need to perform drainage to clear the airway.

WHO PERFORMS THE PROCEDURE AND WHERE IS IT PERFORMED?

Thyroidectomies are usually performed by surgeons with specialized training in otolaryngology, head and neck surgery. Occasionally, a general surgeon will perform a thyroidectomy. The procedure is performed in a hospital under general anesthesia.

QUESTIONS TO ASK THE DOCTOR

- Which parts of the thyroid will be removed?
- What will my neck look like after surgery?
- Is the surgeon a board certified otolaryngologist?
- How many radical neck procedures has the surgeon performed?
- What is the surgeon's complication rate?
- Will I need any medications after surgery?

Wound infections can occur. If they do, the incision is drained, and there are usually no serious consequences.

Normal results

Most patients are discharged from the hospital one to four days after a thyroidectomy. Most resume their normal activities two weeks after the operation. People who have cancer may require subsequent treatment by an oncologist or endocrinologist.

Morbidity and mortality rates

The mortality of thyroidectomy is essentially zero. Hypothyroidism is thought to occur in 12–50% of persons in the first year after a thyroidectomy. Late-onset hypothyroidism develops among an additional 1–3% of persons each year. Although hypothyroidism may recur many years after a partial thyroidectomy, 43% of recurrences occur within five years.

Mortality from thyroid storm, an uncommon complication of thyroidectomy, is in the range of 20–30%. Thyroid storm is characterized by fever, weakness and wasting of the muscles, enlargement of the liver, restlessness, mood swings, change in mental status, and in some cases, coma. *Thyroid storm is a medical emergency requiring immediate treatment.* After a partial thyroidectomy, thyroid function returns to normal in 90–98% of persons.

Alternatives

Injections of radioactive iodine were used to destroy thyroid tissue in the past. This alternative is rarely performed in 2003.

Resources

BOOKS

Bland, K. I., W. G. Cioffi, and M. G. Sarr. *Practice of General Surgery*. Philadelphia, PA: Saunders, 2001.

Ruggieri, P. *A Simple Guide to Thyroid Disorders: From Diagnosis to Treatment*. Omaha, NE: Addicus Books, 2003.

Saheen, O. H. *Thyroid Surgery*. Boca Raton, FL: CRC Press, 2002.

Schwartz, S. I., J. E. Fischer, F. C. Spencer, et al. *Principles of Surgery*, 7th ed. New York: McGraw-Hill, 1998.

Townsend, C., K. L. Mattox, R. D. Beauchamp, et al. *Sabiston's Review of Surgery*, 3rd ed. Philadelphia, PA: Saunders, 2001.

PERIODICALS

Bellantone, R., C. P. Lombardi, M. Raffaelli, et al. "Is Routine Supplementation Therapy (Calcium and Vitamin D) Useful After Total Thyroidectomy?" *Surgery* 132 (December 2002): 1109-1113.

Dror, A., M. Salim, and R. Yoseph. "Sutureless Thyroidectomy Using Electrothermal System: A New Technique." *Journal of Laryngology and Otology* 117 (March 2003):198-201.

Ikeda, Y., H. Takami, Y. Sasaki. "Clinical Benefits in Endoscopic Thyroidectomy by the Axillary Approach." *Journal of the American College of Surgery* 196 (February 2003): 189-195.

Oey, I. F., B. D. Richardson, and D. A. Waller. "Video-Assisted Thoracoscopic Thyroidectomy for Obstructive Sleep Apnoea." *Respiratory Medicine* 97 (February 2003): 192-193.

ORGANIZATIONS

American Academy of Otolaryngology-Head and Neck Surgery. One Prince St., Alexandria, VA 22314-3357. (703) 836-4444. www.entnet.org/index2.cfm.

American College of Surgeons. 633 North St. Clair Street, Chicago, IL 60611-3231. (312) 202-5000. Fax: (312) 202-5001. www.facs.org.

American Medical Association. 515 N. State Street, Chicago, IL 60610. (312) 464-5000. www.ama-assn.org.

American Osteopathic College of Otolaryngology-Head and Neck Surgery. 405 W. Grand Avenue, Dayton, OH 45405. (937) 222-8820 or (800) 455-9404. Fax: (937) 222-8840. Email: info@aocoohns.org.

Association of Thyroid Surgeons. 717 Buena Vista St., Ventura, CA 93001, FAX: (509) 479-8678. www.thyroidsurgery.org.

OTHER

Beth Israel Deaconess Medical Center/Harvard University. [cited April 3, 2003]. www.bidmc.harvard.edu/thyroidcenter/edu-thysur.asp.

Columbia University School of Medicine. [cited April 3, 2003]. www.cpmcnet.columbia.edu/dept/thyroid/surgeryHP.html.

Cornell University Medical College. [cited April 3, 2003]. www.med.cornell.edu/surgery/endocrine/thyroid.html.

University of California-San Diego School of Medicine. [cited April 3, 2003]. www.surgery.ucsd.edu/ent/PatientInfo/th_thyroid.html.

L. Fleming Fallon, Jr., MD, DrPH

Tissue plasminogen activator *see* **Thrombolytic therapy**

Tissue typing *see* **Human leukocyte antigen test**

Tongue removal *see* **Glossectomy**

Tonsil removal *see* **Tonsillectomy**

Tonsillectomy

Definition

Tonsillectomy is a surgical procedure to remove the tonsils. The tonsils are part of the lymphatic system, which is responsible for fighting infection.

Purpose

Tonsils are removed when a person, most often a child, has any of the following conditions:

- obstruction
- sleep apnea (a condition in which an individual snores loudly and stops breathing temporarily at intervals during sleep)
- inability to swallow properly because of enlarged tonsils
- a breathy voice or other speech abnormality due to enlarged tonsils
- recurrent or persistent abscesses or throat infections

Physicians are not in complete agreement on the number of sore throats that necessitate a tonsillectomy. Most would agree that four cases of strep throat in any one year; six or more episodes of tonsillitis in one year; or five or more episodes of tonsillitis per year for two years indicate that the tonsils should be removed.

Demographics

A tonsillectomy is one of the most common surgical procedures among children. It is uncommon among adults. More than 400,000 tonsillectomies are performed each year in the United States. Approximately 70% of surgical candidates are under age 18.

Description

A tonsillectomy is usually performed under **general anesthesia**, although adults may occasionally receive a local anesthetic. The surgeon depresses the tongue in order to see the throat, and removes the tonsils with an instrument resembling a scoop or scissors.

Alternate methods for removing tonsils are being investigated, including lasers and other electronic devices.

Diagnosis/Preparation

Tonsillectomy procedures are not performed as frequently today as they once were. One reason for a more conservative approach is the risk involved when a person is put under general anesthesia.

In some cases, a tonsillectomy may need to be modified or postponed:

- Bleeding disorders must be adequately controlled prior to surgery.
- Acute tonsillitis should be successfully treated prior to surgery. Treatment may postpone the surgery three to four weeks.

Aftercare

Persons are turned on their side after the operation to prevent the possibility of blood being drawn into the lungs (aspirated). **Vital signs** are monitored. Patients can drink water and other non-irritating liquids when they are fully awake.

Adults are usually warned to expect a very sore throat and some bleeding after the operation. They are given **antibiotics** to prevent infection, and some receive pain-relieving medications. For at least the first 24 hours, individuals are instructed to drink fluids and eat soft, pureed foods.

People are usually sent home the day of surgery. They are given instructions to call their surgeon if there is bleeding or earache, or fever that lasts longer than three days. They are told to expect a white scab to

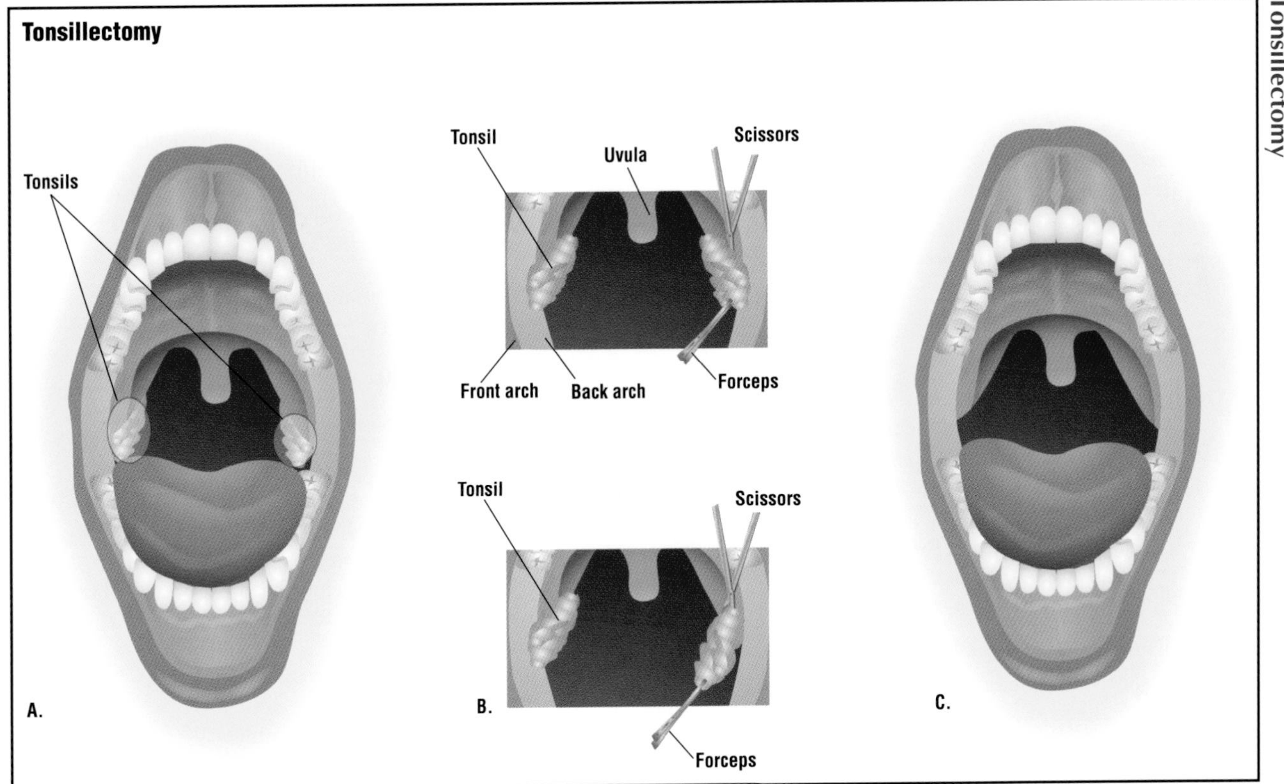

Tonsils are removed through the mouth (A). The surgeon uses a scissors to cut away the tonsils, and a forceps to pull them away (B). *(Illustration by GGS Information Services. Cengage Learning, Gale.)*

KEY TERMS

Abscess—A localized area of tissue destruction and pus formation.

Sleep apnea—A condition marked by loud snoring during sleep and periodic episodes of suspended breathing.

Tonsils—Oval masses of lymphoid tissue on each side of the throat.

form in the throat between five and 10 days after surgery.

Risks

There is a chance that children with previously normal speech will develop a nasal-sounding voice. In addition, children younger than five years may be emotionally upset by the hospital experience. There are risks associated with any surgical procedure, including post-operative infection and bleeding.

Normal results

Normal results include the correction of the condition for which the surgery was performed.

Morbidity and mortality rates

Morbidity other than minor post-surgical infection is uncommon. About one in every 15,000 tonsillectomies ends in **death**, either from the anesthesia or bleeding five to seven days after the operation.

Alternatives

There are no alternatives to surgical removal of the tonsils. Drug therapy may be used for recurrent infections involving the tonsils.

Resources

BOOKS

Bland, K.I., W.G. Cioffi, M.G. Sarr. *Practice of General Surgery*. Philadelphia: Saunders, 2001.

Braunwald, E., D.L. Longo, J.L. Jameson. *Harrison's Principles of Internal Medicine*, 15th ed. New York: McGraw-Hill, 2001.

WHO PERFORMS THE PROCEDURE AND WHERE IS IT PERFORMED?

A tonsillectomy is performed in an outpatient facility associated with a hospital by a general surgeon or otolaryngologist (physician who specializes in treating disorders of the ear, nose, and throat).

Goldman, L. & J.C. Bennett. *Cecil Textbook of Medicine,* 21st ed. Philadelphia: Saunders, 1999.

Schwartz, S.I., J.E. Fischer, F.C. Spencer, G.T. Shires, J.M. Daly. *Principles of Surgery,* 7th ed. New York: McGraw Hill, 1998.

Townsend, C., K.L. Mattox, R.D. Beauchamp, B.M. Evers, D.C. Sabiston. *Sabiston's Review of Surgery,* 3rd ed. Philadelphia: Saunders, 2001.

PERIODICALS

Remacle, M., J. Keghian, G. Lawson, J. Jamart. "Carbon-dioxide Laser-assisted Tonsil Ablation for Adults with Chronic Tonsillitis: A 6-month Follow-up Study." *European Archives of Otorhinolaryngology* 260, no.4 (2003): 243-6.

Silveira, H., J.S. Soares, H.A. Lima. "Tonsillectomy: Cold Dissection Versus Bipolar Electrodissection." *International Journal of Pediatric Otorhinolaryngology* 67, no.4 (2003): 345-51.

Werle, A.H., P.J. Nicklaus, D.J. Kirse, D.E. Bruegger. "A Retrospective Study of Tonsillectomy in the Under 2-Year-Old Child: Indications, Perioperative Management, and Complications." *International Journal of Pediatric Otorhinolaryngology* 67, no.5 (2003): 453-60.

Yaremchuk, K. "Tonsillectomy by Plasma-Mediated Ablation." *Archives of Otolaryngology Head and Neck Surgery* 129, no.4 (2003): 498-9.

ORGANIZATIONS

American College of Surgeons. 633 North St. Clair Street, Chicago, IL 60611-32311. (312) 202-5000. Fax: (312) 202-5001. E-mail: postmaster@facs.org. http://www.facs.org.

American Academy of Otolaryngology-Head and Neck Surgery. One Prince St., Alexandria, VA 22314-3357. (703) 836-4444. http://www.entnet.org/index2.cfm.

American Cancer Society. 1599 Clifton Road NE, Atlanta, GA 30329. (800) 227-2345. http://www.cancer.org.

American Osteopathic College of Otolaryngology-Head and Neck Surgery. 405 W. Grand Avenue, Dayton, OH 45405. (937) 222-8820 or (800) 455-9404, fax (937) 222-8840. Email: info@aocoohns.org.

OTHER

Columbia University School of Medicine. [cited May 5, 2003] http://www.entcolumbia.org/t-aproc.htm.

QUESTIONS TO ASK THE DOCTOR

What will be the resulting functional status of the body after the operation?

Is the surgeon board certified in head and neck surgery?

How many tonsillectomy procedures has the surgeon performed?

What is the surgeon's complication rate?

Has the surgeon operated on children?

Eastern Virginia Medical School. [cited May 5, 2003] http://www.evmsent.org/ped_ops/tonsillectomy.html.

National Library of Medicine. [cited May 5, 2003] http://www.nlm.nih.gov/medlineplus/ency/article/003013.htm.

University of California-San Diego. [cited May 5, 2003] <http://www-surgery.ucsd.edu/ent/PatientInfo/instructions_tonsillectomy.html>.

University of Florida. [cited May 5, 2003] http://www.ent.health.ufl.edu/patient%20info/T&A.htm.

L. Fleming Fallon, Jr., MD, Dr.PH.

Tooth extraction

Definition

Tooth extraction is the removal of a tooth from its socket in the bone.

Purpose

Extraction is performed for positional, structural, or economic reasons. Teeth are often removed because they are impacted. Teeth become impacted when they are prevented from growing into their normal position in the mouth by gum tissue, bone, or other teeth. Impaction is a common reason for the extraction of wisdom teeth. Extraction is the only known method that will prevent further problems with impaction.

Teeth may also be extracted to make more room in the mouth prior to straightening the remaining teeth (orthodontic treatment), or because they are so badly positioned that straightening is impossible. Extraction may be used to remove teeth that are so badly decayed or broken that they cannot be restored. In addition,

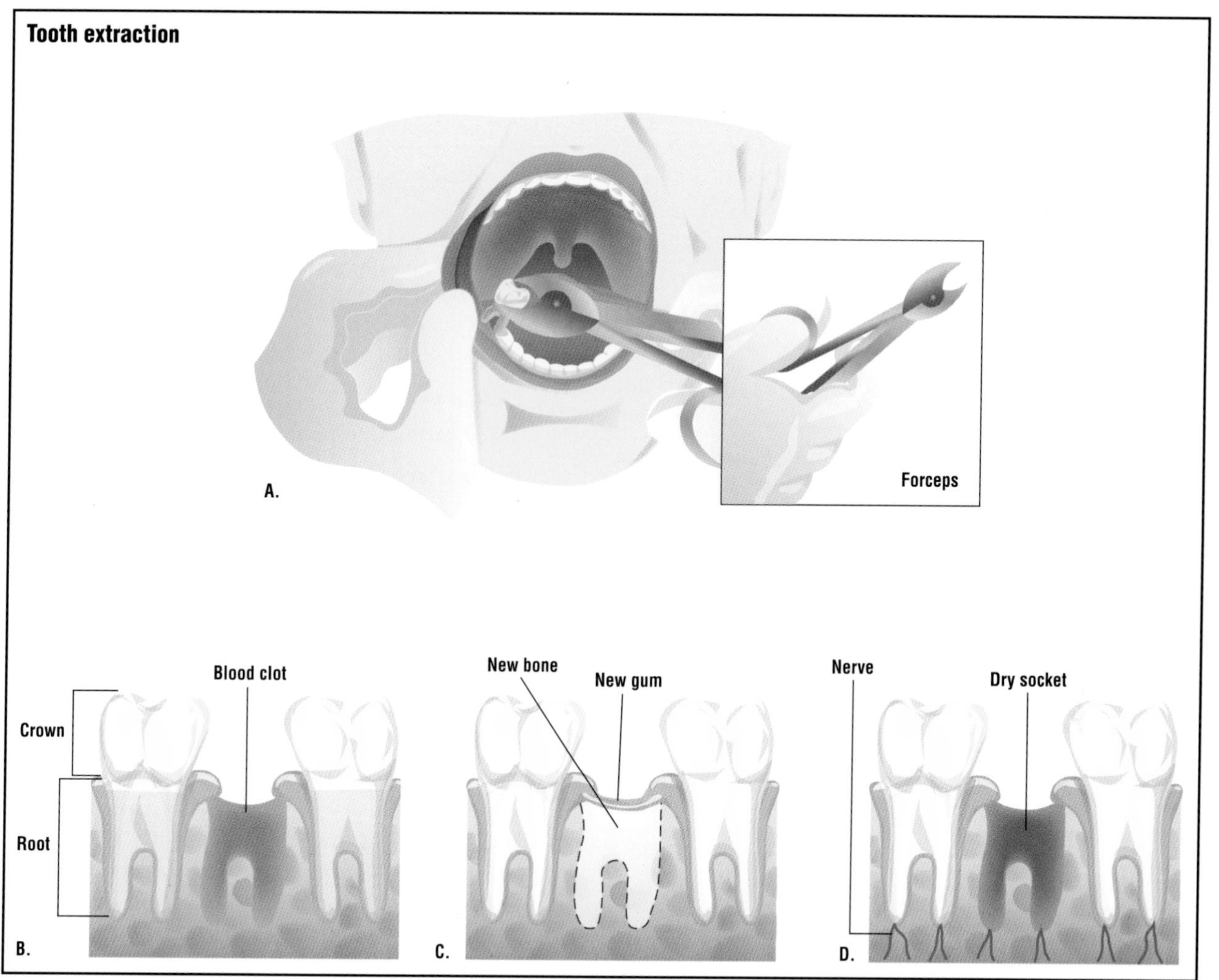

A dental surgeon uses special forceps to pull out a tooth (A). In its place, a blood clot forms (B), which becomes new bone with gum tissue over the top (C). If the blood clot does not form or falls out, a dry socket occurs (D). No new bone forms, and the nerves are exposed, causing pain. *(Illustration by GGS Information Services. Cengage Learning, Gale.)*

some patients choose extraction as a less expensive alternative to filling or placing a crown on a severely decayed tooth.

Demographics

Exact statistics concerning tooth extraction are not available. Experts estimate that over 20 million teeth are extracted each year in the United States. Many of these are performed in conjunction with orthodontic procedures. Some extractions are due to tooth decay.

Description

Tooth extraction can be performed with **local anesthesia** if the tooth is exposed and appears to be easily removable in one piece. The dentist or oral surgeon uses an instrument called an elevator to luxate, or loosen, the tooth; widen the space in the underlying bone; and break the tiny elastic fibers that attach the tooth to the bone. Once the tooth is dislocated from the bone, it can be lifted and removed with forceps.

If the extraction is likely to be difficult, a general dentist may refer the patient to an oral surgeon. Oral surgeons are specialists who are trained to administer nitrous oxide (laughing gas), an intravenous sedative, or a general anesthetic to relieve pain. Extracting an impacted tooth or a tooth with curved roots typically requires cutting through gum tissue to expose the tooth. It may also require removing portions of bone to free the tooth. Some teeth must be cut and removed in sections. The extraction site may or may not require one or more **stitches** (sutures) to close the incision.

KEY TERMS

Dry socket—A painful condition following tooth extraction in which a blood clot does not properly fill the empty socket. Dry socket leaves the underlying bone exposed to air and food particles.

Extraction site—The empty tooth socket following removal of a tooth.

Impacted tooth—A tooth that is growing against another tooth, bone, or soft tissue.

Luxate—To loosen or dislocate a tooth from its socket.

Nitrous oxide—A colorless, sweet-smelling gas used by dentists for mild anesthesia. It is sometimes called laughing gas because it makes some people feel giddy or silly.

Oral surgeon—A dentist who specializes in surgical procedures of the mouth, including extractions.

Orthodontic treatment—The process of realigning and straightening teeth to correct their appearance and function.

Diagnosis/Preparation

In some situations, tooth extractions may be temporarily postponed. These situations include:

- Infection that has progressed from the tooth into the bone. Infections may complicate administering anesthesia. They can be treated with antibiotics before the tooth is extracted.
- Use of drugs that thin the blood (anticoagulants). These medications include warfarin (Coumadin) and aspirin. The patient should stop using these medications for three days prior to extraction.
- People who have had any of the following procedures in the previous six months: heart valve replacement, open heart surgery, prosthetic joint replacement, or placement of a medical shunt. These patients may be given antibiotics to reduce the risk of bacterial infection spreading from the mouth to other parts of the body.

Before extracting a tooth, the dentist will take the patient's medical history, noting allergies and other prescription medications that the patient is taking. A dental history is also recorded. Particular attention is given to previous extractions and reactions to anesthetics. The dentist may then prescribe **antibiotics** or recommend stopping certain medications prior to the extraction. The tooth is x-rayed to determine its full shape and position, especially if it is impacted.

WHO PERFORMS THE PROCEDURE AND WHERE IS IT PERFORMED?

Teeth are most often extracted by maxillofacial or oral surgeons. Occasionally, a general dentist will extract a tooth. Teeth are most commonly removed in an outpatient facility adjacent to a hospital under general anesthesia.

Patients scheduled for deep anesthesia should wear loose clothing with sleeves that are easily rolled up to allow the dentist to place an intravenous line. They should not eat or drink anything for at least six hours before the procedure. Arrangements should be made for a friend or relative to drive them home after the surgery.

Aftercare

An important aspect of aftercare is encouraging a clot to form at the extraction site. The patient should put pressure on the area by biting gently on a roll or wad of gauze for several hours after surgery. Once the clot is formed, it should not be disturbed. The patient should not rinse, spit, drink with a straw, or smoke for at least 24 hours after the extraction and preferably longer. He or she should also avoid vigorous **exercise** for the first three to five days after the extraction.

For the first two days after the procedure, the patient should drink liquids without using a straw and eat soft foods. Any chewing must be done on the side away from the extraction site. Hard or sticky foods should be avoided. The mouth may be gently cleaned with a toothbrush, but the extraction area should not be scrubbed.

Wrapped ice packs can be applied to reduce facial swelling. Swelling is a normal part of the healing process; it is most noticeable in the first 48–72 hours after surgery. As the swelling subsides, the patient's jaw muscles may feel stiff. Moist heat and gentle exercise will restore normal jaw movement. The dentist or oral surgeon may prescribe medications to relieve postoperative pain.

Risks

Potential complications of tooth extraction include postoperative infection, temporary numbness

QUESTIONS TO ASK THE DOCTOR

- Why are you suggesting a tooth extraction?
- What will my mouth look like after surgery?
- Is the oral surgeon board certified in maxillofacial surgery?
- How many teeth extractions has the oral surgeon performed?
- What is the oral surgeon's complication rate?
- Will I need medication after surgery?

from nerve irritation, jaw fracture, and jaw joint pain. An additional complication is called dry socket. When a blood clot does not properly form in the empty tooth socket, the bone beneath the socket is exposed to air and contamination by food particles; as a result, the extraction site heals more slowly than is normal or desirable.

Normal results

The wound usually closes in about two weeks after a tooth extraction, but it takes three to six months for the bone and soft tissue to be restructured. Such complications as infection or dry socket may prolong the healing process.

Morbidity and mortality rates

Mortality from tooth extraction is very rare. Complications include a brief period of pain and swelling; post-extraction infections; and migration of adjacent teeth into the empty space created by an extraction. Most people experience some pain and swelling after having a tooth extracted. With the exception of removing wisdom teeth, migration into the empty space is common. Braces or orthodontic appliances usually control this problem.

Alternatives

Alternatives to tooth extraction depend on the reason for the extraction. Postponing or canceling an extraction to correct tooth crowding will cause malocclusion and an undesirable appearance. Not removing an impacted wisdom tooth may cause eventual misalignment, although it may have no impact. Not removing a decayed or abscessed tooth may lead to septicemia and other complications.

Resources

BOOKS

Harris, N. O., and F. Garcia-Godoy. *Primary Preventative Dentistry*, 6th ed. Englewood Cliffs, NJ: Prentice Hall, 2003.

Peterson, L. J. *Contemporary Oral and Maxillofacial Surgery*, 4th ed. Amsterdam: Elsevier Science, 2002.

Scully, C. *Oral and Maxillofacial Medicine: A Practical Guide*. London, UK: Butterworth-Heinemann, 2003.

Tronstad, L. *Clinical Endodontics*. New York: Thieme Medical Publishers, 2003.

PERIODICALS

Devlin, H., and P. Sloan. "Early Bone Healing Events in the Human Extraction Socket." *International Journal of Oral and Maxillofacial Surgery* 31 (December 2002): 641-645.

Magheri, P., S. Cambi, and R. Grandini. "Restorative Alternatives for the Treatment of an Impacted Canine: Surgical and Prosthetic Considerations." *Practical Procedures and Aesthetic Dentistry* 14 (October 2002): 659-664.

Moscovich, H. "Fitting Restorations from Extracted Teeth." *Journal of the South African Dental Association* 55 (August 2000): 411-412.

Rosted, P., and V. Jorgensen. "Acupuncture Treatment of Pain Dysfunction Syndrome After Dental Extraction." *Acupuncture in Medicine* 20 (December 2002): 191-192.

ORGANIZATIONS

American Association of Oral and Maxillofacial Surgeons. 9700 West Bryn Mawr Ave., Rosemont, IL 60018-5701. (847) 678-6200. www.aaoms.org.

American Board of Oral and Maxillofacial Surgery. 625 North Michigan Avenue, Suite 1820, Chicago, IL 60611. (312) 642-0070; FAX: (312) 642-8584. www.aboms.org.

American Dental Association. 211 E. Chicago Avenue, Chicago, IL 60611. (312) 440-2500. www.ada.org.

British Association of Oral and Maxillofacial Surgeons, Royal College of Surgeons. 35–43 Lincoln's Inn Fields, London, UK WC2A 3PN. www.baoms.org.uk.

OTHER

American Dental Association. [cited April 3, 2003]. www.ada.org/public/topics/extractions.html.

Bristol Biomed. [cited April 3, 2003]. www.brisbio.ac.uk/ROADS/subject-listing/toothextraction.html.

Dental Review Online. [cited April 3, 2003]. www.dentalreview.com/Tooth_Extraction.htm.

Emory University. [cited April 3, 2003]. www.emory.edu/COLLEGE/CULPEPER/RAVINA/PROJECT/Ancient_pages/Tooth_extraction.html.

L. Fleming Fallon, Jr., MD, DrPH

Tooth replantation

Definition

Tooth replantation is the reinsertion and splinting of a tooth that has been avulsed (knocked or torn out) of its socket.

Purpose

Teeth are replanted to prevent permanent loss of the tooth, and to restore the landscape of the mouth so that the patient can eat and speak normally.

Demographics

According to the National Center for Health Statistics, about 5 million teeth are accidentally avulsed in the United States each year. Most teeth that are replanted are lost through trauma, usually falls and other types of accidents. The most common traumata resulting in tooth avulsion are sports accidents that result in falls or blows to the head. The mandatory use of mouth guards, which are plastic devices that protect the upper teeth, has prevented approximately 200,000 oral injuries each year in football alone. The American Dental Association recommends the use of mouth guards for any sport that involves speed, contact, or the potential for falls. These categories include not only contact sports like football, wrestling, and boxing, but also gymnastics, baseball, hockey, bicycling, skateboarding, and skiing. Without a mouth guard, a person is 60 times more likely to experience dental trauma if he or she participates in these sports.

Other common causes of trauma to the mouth resulting in avulsed teeth include motor vehicle accidents, criminal assaults, and fist fights. Domestic violence is the most common cause of avulsed teeth in women over the age of 21.

Description

In most cases, only permanent teeth are replanted. Primary teeth (baby teeth) do not usually have long enough roots for successful replantation. The only exception may be the canine teeth, which have longer roots and therefore a better chance of staying in place. In some cases, however, the dentist may choose to replant a child's primary tooth because there is risk to the permanent tooth that has not yet emerged.

To replant a tooth, the dentist or oral surgeon will first administer a local anesthetic to numb the patient's gums. He or she will then reinsert the avulsed tooth in its socket and anchor it within the mouth by installing a splint made of wire and composite resin. Some dentists remove the root canal nerve of the tooth and replace it with a plastic material before reinserting the tooth. The splint holds the tooth in place for two to six weeks. At that time, the splint can be removed and the tooth examined for stability.

KEY TERMS

Avulsion—A ripping out or tearing away of a tooth or other body part.

Canine tooth—In humans, the tooth located in the mouth next to the second incisor. The canine tooth has a pointed crown and the longest root of all the teeth.

Crown—The top part of the tooth.

Endodontist—A dentist who specializes in the diagnosis and treatment of disorders affecting the pulp of a tooth, the root of the tooth, or the tissues surrounding the root. Some patients with avulsed teeth may be treated by an endodontist.

Eruption—The emergence of a tooth through the gum tissue.

Fibroblasts—Connective tissue cells that help to hold the teeth in their sockets in the jawbone.

Mouth guard—A plastic device that protects the upper teeth from injury during athletic events.

Primary teeth—A child's first set of teeth, sometimes called baby teeth.

Diagnosis/Preparation

When a tooth is dislodged, it is critical to recover the tooth, preserve it under proper conditions, and get the patient to a dentist immediately. The tooth should be handled carefully; it should be picked up or touched by its crown (the top part of the tooth), not by its root. The tooth should be rinsed and kept moist, but not cleaned or brushed. The use of toothpaste, soap, mouthwash, or other chemicals can remove the fibroblasts clinging to the root of the tooth. Fibroblasts are connective tissue cells that act as a **glue** between teeth and the underlying bone.

The avulsed tooth can be placed in milk or a special Save-a-Tooth (R) kit, which is a tooth-preserving cup that contains a medium for preserving the fibroblasts around the tooth. The tooth and the patient should go to the dentist within 30 minutes of the accident since fibroblasts begin to die within that time. Rapid treatment improves the chances for successful

WHO PERFORMS THE PROCEDURE AND WHERE IS IT PERFORMED?

Tooth replantations are performed by general dentists, endodontists, and oral surgeons, usually as office or outpatient procedures. In some cases, the patient may be treated in the emergency room of a hospital.

QUESTIONS TO ASK THE DOCTOR

- How should I take care of the replanted tooth?
- How long will it take to assess the results of treatment?
- What can be done if the tooth cannot be replanted?
- Where can I be fitted for a mouth guard?

replantation. In some cases, artificial fibroblasts can be substituted for the patient's own connective tissue cells.

If the tooth is a primary tooth, it should be rinsed and kept moist also. The dentist should be consulted to determine whether the tooth should be replanted by examining the gums and the emergent tooth. The dentist will take a set of x rays to determine how soon the permanent tooth is likely to emerge. Sometimes an artificial spacer is placed where the primary tooth was lost until the permanent tooth comes in.

Any injury to the gum is treated before the tooth is replanted. The dentist may give the patient an antibiotic medication to reduce the risk of infection. Cold compresses can reduce swelling. **Stitches** may be necessary if the gum is lacerated. The dentist may also take x rays of the mouth to see if there are other injuries to the jawbone or nearby teeth.

Aftercare

The patient may take **aspirin** or **acetaminophen** for pain. **Antibiotics** may also be given for infection. The patient should avoid rinsing the mouth, spitting, or smoking for the first 24 hours after surgery. He or she should limit food to a soft diet for the next few days.

Beginning 24 hours after surgery, the patient should rinse the mouth gently with a solution of salt and lukewarm water every one to two hours. The salt helps to reduce swelling in the tissues around the tooth.

Any kind of traumatic injury always carries the risk of infection. Patients with heart disease or disorders of the immune system should be monitored following tooth replantation. Dentists recommend consulting a physician within 48 hours of the dental surgery to determine the risk of tetanus, particularly if the patient has not received a tetanus booster within the past five years.

Adults with replanted teeth should have periodic checkups. According to the American Association of Endodontists, it takes about two to three years after replantation before the dentist can fully evaluate the outcome of treatment.

Risks

In addition to infection, tooth replantation carries the risks of excessive bleeding and rejection of the tooth. Rejection is a rare complication. An additional risk is that the root of the tooth may become fused to the underlying bone.

Normal results

Most permanent tooth replantations are successful when the patient acts quickly (within two hours). If the tooth is rejected, the dentist may attach the tooth to the bone with tissue glue.

Morbidity and mortality rates

Mortality following tooth replantation is almost unheard of. The rate of complications varies according to the circumstances of the injury, the patient's age, and his or her general health. A history of smoking increases the risk of rejection of the tooth, as well as infection.

Alternatives

There are no effective medical alternatives to oral surgery for replanting an avulsed tooth. Over-the-counter **analgesics** (pain relievers), prescription antibiotics, and some herbal preparations may be useful in relieving pain, reducing swelling, or preventing infection.

Herbal preparations that have been found useful as mouthwashes following oral surgery include calendula (*Calendula officinalis*) and clove (*Eugenia caryophyllata*).

Resources

BOOKS

Marx, John A., et al. *Rosen's Emergency Medicine*, 6th ed. St. Louis, MO: Mosby, Inc., 2006.

Roberts, J. R., et al. *Clinical Procedures in Emergency Medicine*, 6th ed. Philadelphia: Saunders, Inc., 2004.

PERIODICALS

Douglass, Alan B., MD, and Joanna M. Douglass, DDS. "Common Dental Emergencies." *American Family Physician* 67 (February 1, 2003): 511–516.

American Academy of Pediatric Dentistry Council on Clinical Affairs. "Guideline on management of acute dental trauma." *Pediatric Dentistry* 27 (January 1, 2005): 135–142.

Lin, S. "New emphasis in the treatment of dental trauma: avulsion and luxation." *Dental Traumatology* 23 (October 2007): 297–303.

ORGANIZATIONS

American Academy of Pediatric Dentistry. 211 East Chicago Avenue, Ste. 700, Chicago, IL 60611-2616. (312) 337- 2169. http://www.aapd.org (accessed April 11, 2008).

American Association of Endodontists. 211 East Chicago Avenues, Ste. 1100, Chicago, IL 60611-2691. (312) 266-7255. http://www.aae.org (accessed April 11, 2008).

American Association of Oral and Maxillofacial Surgeons. 9700 West Bryn Mawr Avenue, Rosemont, IL 60018-5701. (847) 678-6200. http://www.aaoms.org (accessed April 11, 2008).

American Dental Association. 211 East Chicago Avenue, Chicago, IL 60611. (312) 440-2500. http://www.ada.org (accessed April 11, 2008).

Janie Franz

Topical antibiotics *see* **Antibiotics, topical**

Total hip replacement *see* **Hip replacement**

Total knee replacement *see* **Knee replacement**

Total shoulder replacement *see* **Shoulder joint replacement**

Total wrist replacement *see* **Wrist replacement**

Trabeculectomy

Definition

Trabeculectomy is a surgical procedure that removes part of the trabeculum in the eye to relieve pressure caused by glaucoma.

Purpose

Glaucoma is a disease that injures the optic nerve, causing progressive vision loss. Glaucoma is a major cause of blindness in the United States. If caught early, glaucoma-related blindness is easily prevented. However, because it does not produce symptoms until late in its cycle, periodic tests for the disease are necessary.

Glaucoma is usually associated with an increase in the pressure inside the eye, called intraocular pressure (IOP). This increase occurs in front of the iris in a fluid called the aqueous humor. Aqueous humor exits through tiny channels between the iris and the cornea, in an area called the trabeculum. When the trabeculum is blocked, pressure from the build up of aqueous humor either increases rapidly with pain and redness, or builds slowly with no symptoms until there is a significant loss of vision. Trabeculectomy is the last treatment employed for either type of glaucoma. It is used only after medications and laser trabeculoplasty have failed to alleviate IOP.

Demographics

Glaucoma can develop at any age, but people over 45 are at higher risk. African Americans are more likely to develop glaucoma, especially primary open-angle glaucoma. Other factors, such as a family history of glaucoma, greatly increase the risk of contracting the disease. Diabetes and previous eye injury also increase chances of developing glaucoma.

Description

The procedure is performed in an **operating room**, usually under local anesthetic. However, some ophthalmologists give patients only a topical anesthetic. A trabeculectomy involves removing a tiny piece of the eyeball, where the cornea connects to the sclera, to create a flap that allows fluid to escape the anterior chamber without deflating the eye. The area is called the trabeculum. After the procedure, fluid can flow out onto the eye's surface, where it is absorbed by the conjunctiva, the transparent membrane that lines the sclera and the eyelids.

Sometimes, an additional piece is taken from the iris so that anterior chamber fluid can also flow backward into the vitreous. This procedure is called an **iridectomy**.

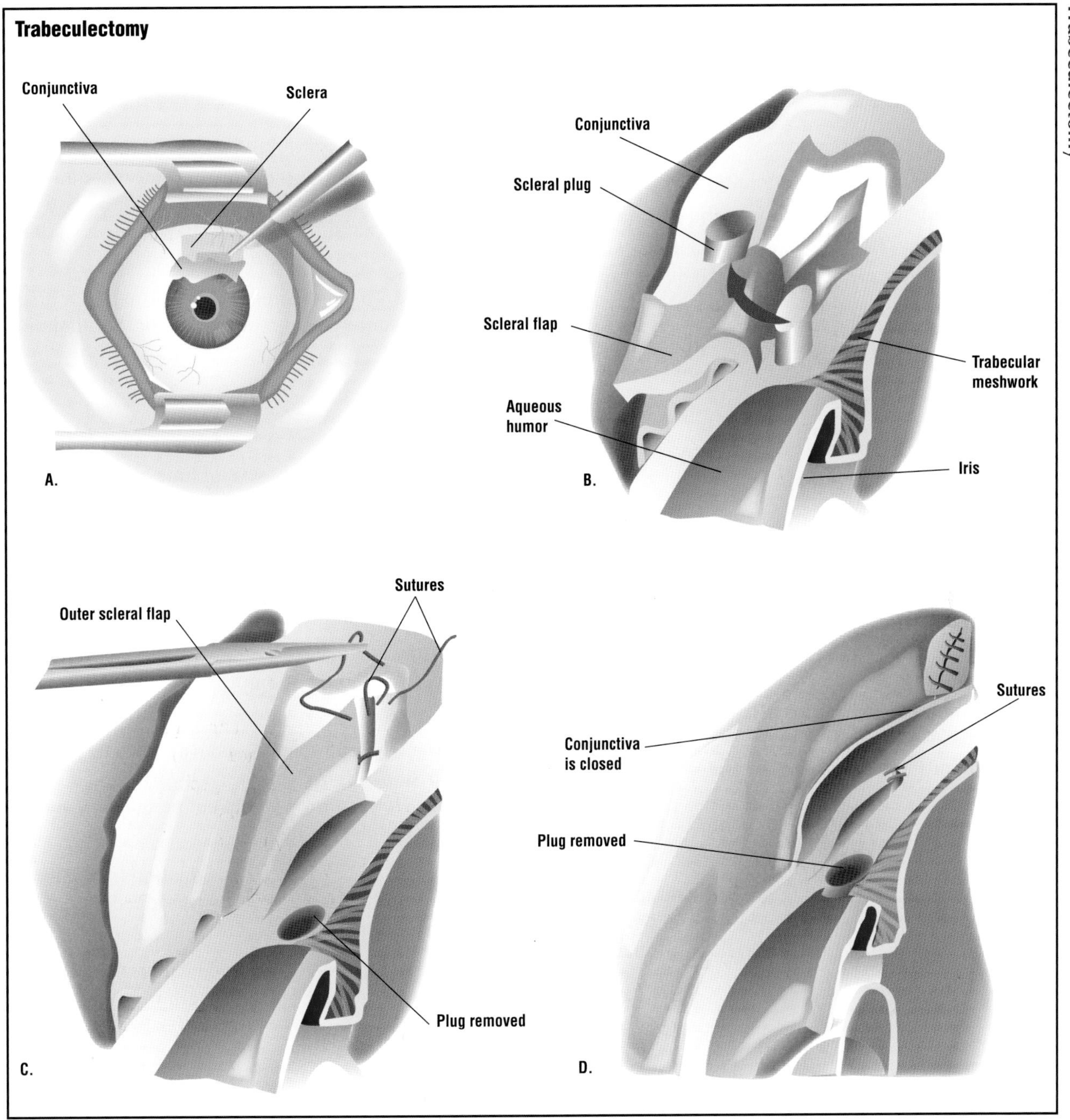

During a trabeculectomy, the patient's eye is held open with a speculum (A). The outer layer, or conjunctiva, and the white of the eye, or sclera, are cut open (A). A superficial scleral flap is created and a plug of sclera and underlying trabecular network is removed (B). This allows the fluid in the eye to circulate, relieving pressure. The scleral flap is closed and sutured (C). The conjunctiva is closed (D). *(Illustration by GGS Information Services. Cengage Learning, Gale.)*

Diagnosis/Preparation

The procedure is fully explained and any alternative methods to control intraocular pressure are discussed. Antiglaucoma drugs are prescribed before surgery. Added pressure on the eye caused from coughing or sneezing should be avoided.

Several eye drops are applied immediately before surgery. The eye is sterilized, and the patient draped. A

KEY TERMS

Cornea—Transparent film that covers the iris and pupil.

Iris—Colored part of the eye, which is suspended in aqueous humor and perforated by the pupil.

Sclera—White, outer coating of the eyeball.

Trabeculoplasty—Laser surgery that creates perforations in the trabeculum, to drain built-up aqueous humor and relieve pressure.

WHO PERFORMS THE PROCEDURE AND WHERE IS IT PERFORMED?

Ophthalmologists and optometrists may detect and treat glaucoma; however, only ophthalmologists can perform surgery. Ophthalmologists who are glaucoma subspecialists may have an additional two years of fellowship training.

The outpatient surgery is performed in a hospital or surgery suite designed for ophthalmic surgery.

speculum is inserted to keep the eyelids apart during surgery.

Aftercare

Eye drops, and perhaps patching, will be needed until the eye is healed. Driving should be restricted until the ophthalmologist grants permission. The patient may experience blurred vision. Severe eye pain, light sensitivity, and vision loss should be reported to the physician.

Antibiotic and anti-inflammatory eye drops must be used for at least six weeks after surgery. Additional medicines may be prescribed to reduce scarring.

Risks

Infection and bleeding are risks of any surgery. Scarring can cause the drainage to stop. One-third of trabeculectomy patients will develop cataracts.

Normal results

Trabeculectomy will delay the progression of glaucoma. In many cases, people still require medication to lower IOP.

Morbidity and mortality rates

Trabeculectomy is considered a safe procedure. Infection is a complication that could lead to more serious medical problems; however, it is controllable with eye drops.

Alternatives

Physicians will first try to lower IOP with glaucoma medications. Several types of eye drops are effective for this use. Sometimes a patient must instill more than one eye drop, several times a day. Compliance is very important when using these eye drops; missed dosages will raise IOPs.

Lasers are now used to treat both closed-angle and open-angle glaucoma. Peripheral iridectomy is used for people with acute angle-closure glaucoma attacks and chronic closed-angle glaucoma. The procedure creates a hole to improve the flow of aqueous humor.

Laser trabeculoplasty uses an argon laser to create tiny burns on the trabecular meshwork, which lowers IOP. The effects, however, are not permanent, and the patient must be retreated.

Transscleral cyclophotocoagulation treats the ciliary body with a laser to decrease production of aqueous humor, which reduces IOP.

A tube shunt might be implanted to create a drainage pathway in patients who are not candidates for trabeculectomy.

Resources

BOOKS

Cassel, Gary H., M.D., Michael D. Billig, O.D., and Harry G. Randall, M.D. *The Eye Book: A Complete Guide to Eye Disorders and Health.* Baltimore, MD: Johns Hopkins University Press, 1998.

Daly, Stephen, ed. *Everything You Need to Know About Medical Treatments.* Springhouse, PA: Springhouse Corp., 1996.

Sardegna, Jill, et. al. *The Encyclopedia of Blindness and Vision Impairment*, 2nd ed. New York: Facts on File, Inc., 2002.

Vaughan, Daniel, Ed. *General Ophthalmology*, 13th ed. Stamford, CT: Appleton & Lange, 1993.

QUESTIONS TO ASK THE DOCTOR

Will IOP-lowering medication be needed after the surgery?

How long will it take to determine if the surgery was a success?

Can cataracts be treated in conjunction with glaucoma surgery?

When will vision return to normal?

ORGANIZATIONS

The Glaucoma Foundation. 116 John Street, Suite 1605 New York, NY 10038. (212) 285-0080. E-mail: info@glaucomafoundation.org. www.glaucomafoundation.org

OTHER

"Glaucoma Filtration Procedure." *EyeMdLink.com*. [cited May 18, 2003] www.eyemdlink.com/EyeProcedure.aspEyeProcedureID = 44.

J. Ricker Polsdorfer, M.D.
Mary Bekker

Tracheoesophageal fistula repair *see* **Esophageal atresia repair**

Tracheostomy *see* **Tracheotomy**

Tracheotomy

Definition

A tracheotomy is a surgical procedure that opens up the windpipe (trachea). It is performed in emergency situations, in the **operating room**, or at bedside of critically ill patients. The term tracheostomy is sometimes used interchangeably with tracheotomy. Strictly speaking, however, tracheostomy usually refers to the opening itself while a tracheotomy is the actual operation.

Purpose

A tracheotomy is performed if enough air is not getting to the lungs, if the person cannot breathe without help, or is having problems with mucus and other secretions getting into the windpipe because of difficulty swallowing. There are many reasons why air cannot get to the lungs. The windpipe may be blocked by a swelling; by a severe injury to the neck, nose, or mouth; by a large foreign object; by paralysis of the throat muscles; or by a tumor. The patient may be in a coma, or need a ventilator to pump air into the lungs for a long period of time.

Demographics

Emergency tracheotomies are performed as needed in any person requiring one.

Description

Emergency tracheotomy

There are two different procedures that are called tracheotomies. The first is done only in emergency situations and can be performed quite rapidly. The emergency room physician or surgeon makes a cut in a thin part of the voice box (larynx) called the cricothyroid membrane. A tube is inserted and connected to an oxygen bag. This emergency procedure is sometimes called a **cricothyroidotomy**.

Surgical tracheotomy

The second type of tracheotomy takes more time and is usually done in an operating room. The surgeon first makes a cut (incision) in the skin of the neck that lies over the trachea. This incision is in the lower part of the neck between the Adam's apple and top of the breastbone. The neck muscles are separated and the thyroid gland, which overlies the trachea, is usually cut down the middle. The surgeon identifies the rings of cartilage that make up the trachea and cuts into the tough walls. A metal or plastic tube, called a tracheotomy tube, is inserted through the opening. This tube acts like a windpipe and allows the person to breathe. Oxygen or a mechanical ventilator may be hooked up to the tube to bring oxygen to the lungs. A dressing is placed around the opening. Tape or **stitches** (sutures) are used to hold the tube in place.

After a nonemergency tracheotomy, the patient usually stays in the hospital for three to five days, unless there is a complicating condition. It takes about two weeks to recover fully from the surgery.

Diagnosis/Preparation

Emergency tracheotomy

In the emergency tracheotomy, there is no time to explain the procedure or the need for it to the patient. The patient is placed on his or her back with face upward (supine), with a rolled-up towel between the shoulders. This positioning of the patient makes it easier for the doctor to feel and see the structures in

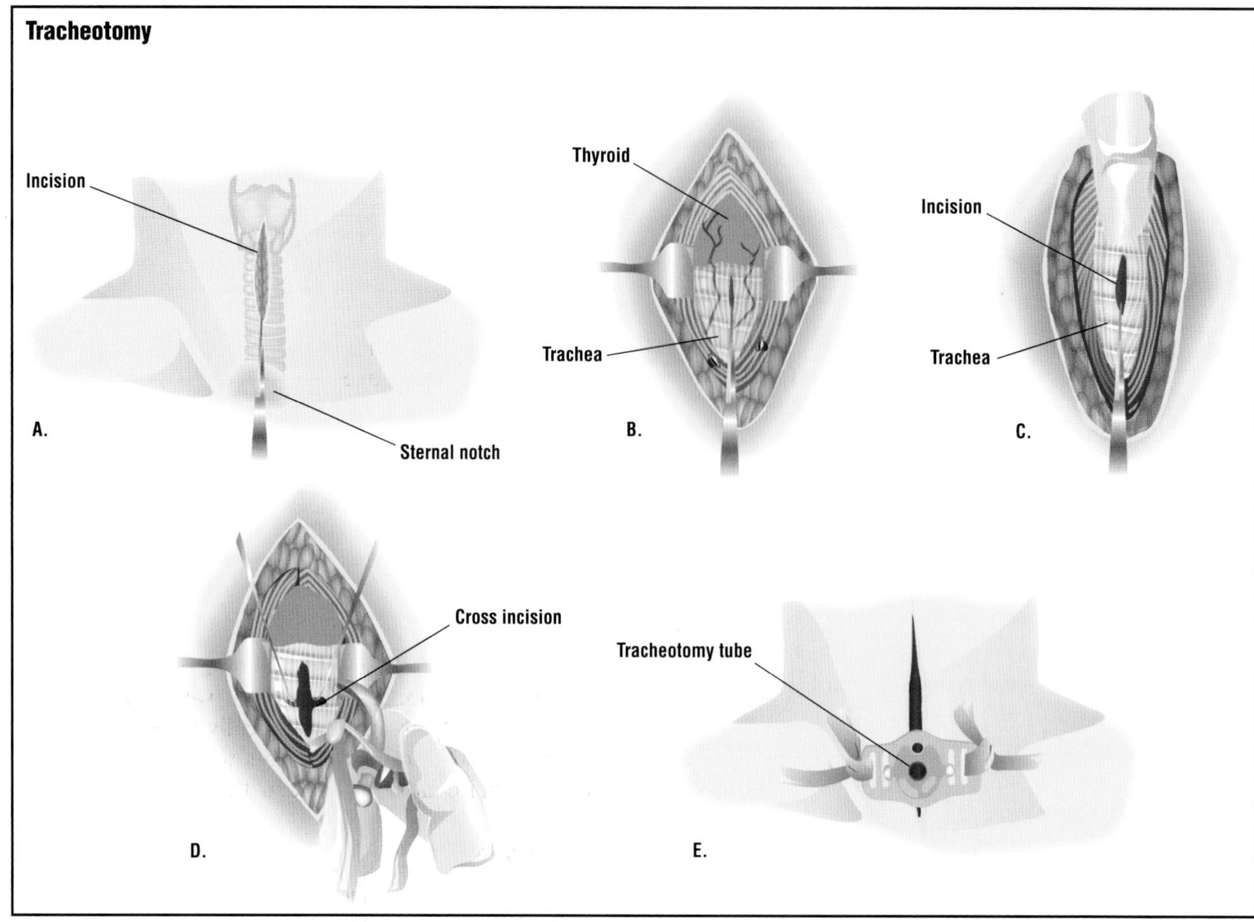

For a tracheotomy, an incision is made in the skin just above the sternal notch (A). Just below the thyroid, the membrane covering the trachea is divided (B), and the trachea itself is cut (C). A cross incision is made to enlarge the opening (D), and a tracheostomy tube may be put in place (E). *(Illustration by GGS Information Services. Cengage Learning, Gale.)*

the throat. A local anesthetic is injected across the cricothyroid membrane.

Nonemergency tracheotomy

In a nonemergency tracheotomy, there is time for the doctor to discuss the surgery with the patient, to explain what will happen and why it is needed. The patient is then put under **general anesthesia**. The neck area and chest are then disinfected and surgical drapes are placed over the area, setting up a sterile surgical field.

Aftercare

Postoperative care

A **chest x ray** is often taken, especially in children, to check whether the tube has become displaced or if complications have occurred. The doctor may prescribe **antibiotics** to reduce the risk of infection. If the patient can breathe without a ventilator, the room is humidified; otherwise, if the tracheotomy tube is to remain in place, the air entering the tube from a ventilator is humidified. During the hospital stay, the patient and his or her family members will learn how to care for the tracheotomy tube, including suctioning and clearing it. Secretions are removed by passing a smaller tube (catheter) into the tracheotomy tube.

It takes most patients several days to adjust to breathing through the tracheotomy tube. At first, it will be hard even to make sounds. If the tube allows some air to escape and pass over the vocal cords, then the patient may be able to speak by holding a finger over the tube. Special tracheostomy tubes are also available that facilitate speech.

The tube will be removed if the tracheotomy is temporary. Then the wound will heal quickly and only a small scar may remain. If the tracheotomy is permanent, the hole stays open and, if it is no longer needed, it will be surgically closed.

KEY TERMS

Cartilage—A tough, fibrous connective tissue that forms various parts of the body, including the trachea and larynx.

Cricothyroidotomy—An emergency tracheotomy that consists of a cut through the cricothyroid membrane to open the patient's airway as fast as possible.

Larynx—A structure made of cartilage and muscle that connects the back of the throat with the trachea. The larynx contains the vocal cords.

Trachea—The tube that leads from the larynx or voice box to two major air passages that bring oxygen to each lung. The trachea is sometimes called the windpipe.

Ventilator—A machine that helps patients to breathe. It is sometimes called a respirator.

Home care

After the patient is discharged, he or she will need help at home to manage the tracheotomy tube. Warm compresses can be used to relieve pain at the incision site. The patient is advised to keep the area dry. It is recommended that the patient wear a loose scarf over the opening when going outside. He or she should also avoid contact with water, food particles, and powdery substances that could enter the opening and cause serious breathing problems. The doctor may prescribe pain medication and antibiotics to minimize the risk of infections. If the tube is to be kept in place permanently, the patient can be referred to a speech therapist in order to learn to speak with the tube in place. The tracheotomy tube may be replaced four to 10 days after surgery.

Patients are encouraged to go about most of their normal activities once they leave the hospital. Vigorous activity is restricted for about six weeks. If the tracheotomy is permanent, further surgery may be needed to widen the opening, which narrows with time.

Risks

Immediate risks

There are several short-term risks associated with tracheotomies. Severe bleeding is one possible complication. The voice box or esophagus may be damaged during surgery. Air may become trapped in the surrounding tissues or the lung may collapse. The tracheotomy tube can be blocked by blood clots, mucus, or the pressure of the airway walls. Blockages can be prevented by suctioning, humidifying the air, and selecting the appropriate tracheotomy tube. Serious infections are rare.

WHO PERFORMS THE PROCEDURE AND WHERE IS IT PERFORMED?

Tracheotomy is performed by a surgeon in a hospital. In an emergency, a tracheotomy may be performed on the scene by another medical professional.

Long-term risks

Over time, other complications may develop following a tracheotomy. The windpipe itself may become damaged for a number of reasons, including pressure from the tube, infectious bacteria that forms scar tissue, or friction from a tube that moves too much. Sometimes the opening does not close on its own after the tube is removed. This risk is higher in tracheotomies with tubes remaining in place for 16 weeks or longer. In these cases, the wound is surgically closed. Increased secretions may occur in patients with tracheostomies, which require more frequent suctioning.

High-risk groups

The risks associated with tracheotomies are higher in the following groups of patients:

- children, especially newborns and infants
- smokers
- alcoholics
- obese adults
- persons over 60
- persons with chronic diseases or respiratory infections
- persons taking muscle relaxants, sleeping medications, tranquilizers, or cortisone

Normal results

Normal results include uncomplicated healing of the incision and successful maintenance of long-term tube placement.

Morbidity and mortality rates

The overall risk of **death** from a tracheotomy is less than 5%.

Alternatives

For most patients, there is no alternative to emergency tracheotomy. Some patients with pre-existing neuromuscular disease (such as ALS or muscular

QUESTIONS TO ASK THE DOCTOR

- How do I take care of my tracheostomy?
- How many of your patients use noninvasive ventilation?
- Am I a candidate for noninvasive ventilation?

dystrophy) can be sucessfully managed with emergency noninvasive ventilation via a face mask, rather than with tracheotomy. Patients who receive nonemergency tracheotomy in preparation for **mechanical ventilation** may often be managed instead with noninvasive ventilation, with proper planning and education on the part of the patient, caregiver, and medical staff.

Resources

BOOKS

Bach, John R. *Noninvasive Mechanical Ventilation*. NJ: Hanley and Belfus, 2002.

Fagan, Johannes J., et al. *Tracheotomy*. Alexandria, VA: American Academy of Otolaryngology-Head and Neck Surgery Foundation, Inc., 1997.

"Neck Surgery." In *The Surgery Book: An Illustrated Guide to 73 of the Most Common Operations*, ed. Robert M. Younson, et al. New York: St. Martin's Press, 1993.

Schantz, Nancy V. "Emergency Cricothyroidotomy and Tracheostomy." In *Procedures for the Primary Care Physician*, ed. John Pfenninger and Grant Fowler. New York: Mosby, 1994.

OTHER

"Answers to Common Otolaryngology Health Care Questions." Department of Otolaryngology–Head and Neck Surgery Page. University of Washington School of Medicine [cited July 1, 2003]. http://weber.u.washington.edu/~otoweb/trach.html.

Sicard, Michael W. "Complications of Tracheotomy." The Bobby R. Alford Department of Otorhinolaryngology and Communicative Sciences. December 1, 1994 [cited July 1, 2003]. http:www.bcm.tmc.edu/oto/grand/12194.html.

Jeanine Barone, Physiologist
Richard Robinson

Traction

Definition

Traction is force applied by weights or other devices to treat bone or muscle disorders or injuries.

Purpose

Traction treats fractures, dislocations, or muscle spasms in an effort to correct deformities and promote healing.

Description

Traction is referred to as a pulling force to treat muscle or skeletal disorders. There are two major types of traction: skin and skeletal traction, within which there are a number of treatments.

Skin traction

Skin traction includes weight traction, which uses lighter weights or counterweights to apply force to fractures or dislocated joints. Weight traction may be employed short-term, (e.g., at the scene of an accident) or on a temporary basis (e.g., when weights are connected to a pulley located above the patient's bed). The weights, typically weighing five to seven pounds, attach to the skin using tape, straps, or boots. They bring together the fractured bone or dislocated joint so that it may heal correctly.

In obstetrics, weights pull along the pelvic axis of a pregnant woman to facilitate delivery. In elastic traction, an elastic device exerts force on an injured limb.

Skin traction also refers to specialized practices, such as Dunlop's traction, used on children when a fractured arm must maintain a flexed position to avoid circulatory and neurological problems. Buck's skin traction stabilizes the knee, and reduces muscle spasm for knee injuries not involving fractures. In addition, splints, surgical collars, and corsets also may be used.

Skeletal traction

Skeletal traction requires an invasive procedure in which pins, screws, or wires are surgically installed for use in longer term traction requiring heavier weights. This is the case when the force exerted is more than skin traction can bear, or when skin traction is not appropriate for the body part needing treatment. Weights used in skeletal traction generally range from 25–40 lb (11–18 kg). It is important to place the pins correctly because they may stay in place for several months, and are the hardware to which weights and pulleys are attached. The pins must be clean to avoid infection. Damage may result if the alignment and weights are not carefully calibrated.

Other forms of skeletal traction are tibia pin traction, for fractures of the pelvis, hip, or femur; and overhead arm traction, used in certain upper arm

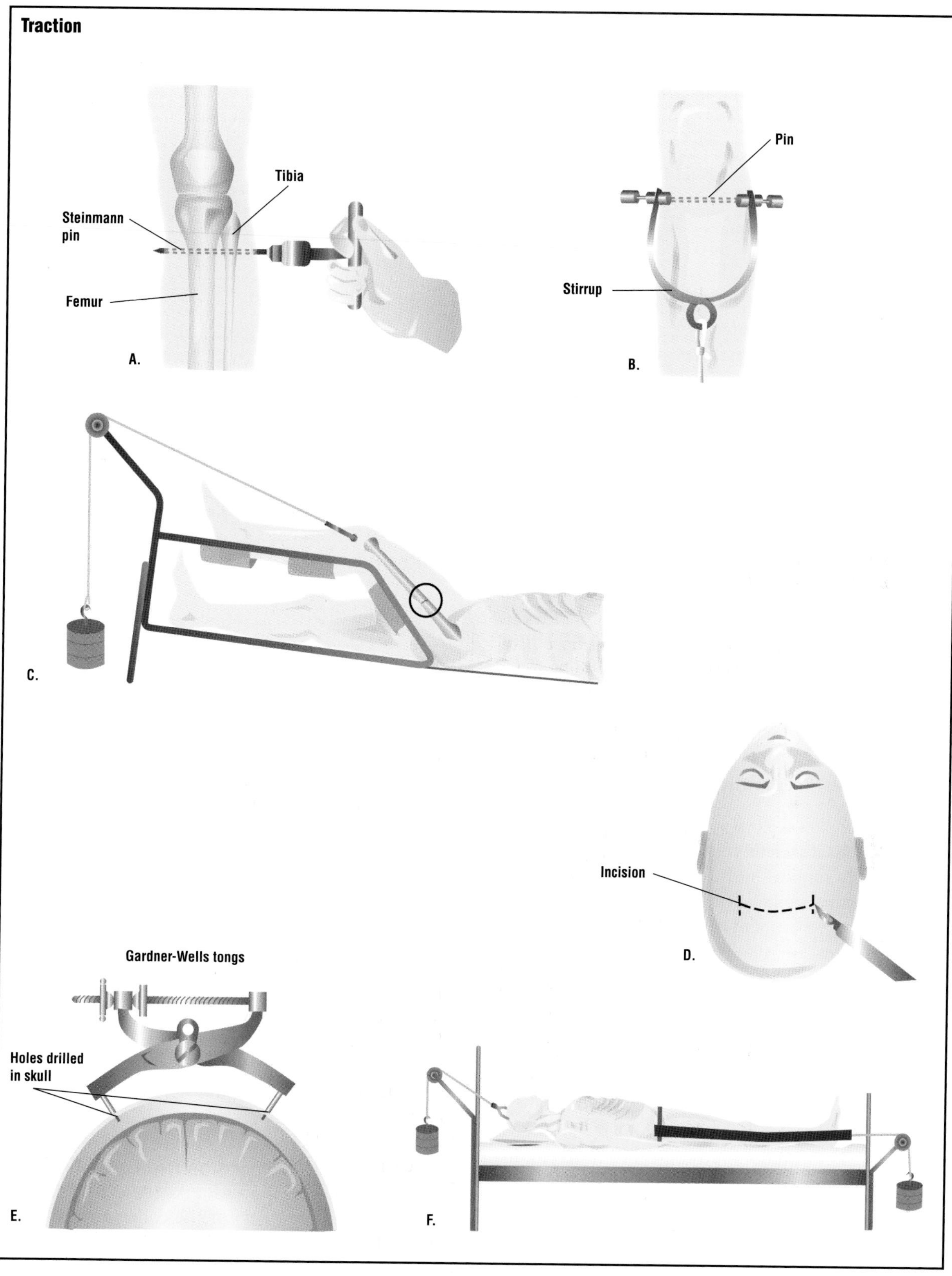

For tibial traction, a pin is surgically placed in the lower leg (A). The pin is attached to a stirrup (B), and weighted (C). In cervical traction, an incision is made into the head (D). Holes are drilled into the skull, and a halo or tongs are applied (E). Weights are added to pull the spine into place (F). *(Illustration by GGS Information Services. Cengage Learning, Gale.)*

KEY TERMS

Skeletal traction—Traction in which pins, screws, or wires are surgically connected to bone to which weights or pulleys are attached to exert force.

Skin traction—Traction in which weights or other devices are attached to the skin.

Weight traction—Sometimes used interchangeably with skin traction.

QUESTIONS TO ASK THE DOCTOR

How long will traction be required?

What are the risks and benefits?

What is the goal of traction?

What is the chance of complications?

fractures. Cervical traction is used when the neck vertebrae are fractured.

Proper care is important for patients in traction. Prolonged immobility should be avoided because it may cause **bedsores** and possible respiratory, urinary, or circulatory problems. Mobile patients may use a trapeze bar, giving them the option of controlling their movements. An **exercise** program instituted by caregivers will maintain the patient's muscle and joint mobility. Traction equipment should be checked regularly to ensure proper position and exertion of force. With skeletal traction, it is important to check for inflammation of the bone, a sign of foreign matter introduction (potential source of infection at the screw or pin site).

Diagnosis/Preparation

Both skin and skeletal traction require x rays prior to application. If skeletal traction is required, standard preoperative surgical tests are conducted, such as blood and urine studies. X rays may be repeated over the course of treatment to insure that alignment remains correct, and that healing is proceeding.

Normal results

There have been few scientific studies on the effects of traction. Criteria (such as randomized controlled trials and monitored compliance) do exist, but an outcome study incorporating all of them has not yet been done. Some randomized controlled trials emphasize that traction does not significantly influence long-term outcomes of neck pain or lower back pain.

Resources

BOOKS

"Cervical Spine Traction." In *Noble: Textbook of Primary Care Medicine,* 3rd ed.Mosby, Inc., (2001): 1132.

PERIODICALS

Glick, J.M. "Hip Arthroscopy. The Lateral Approach." *Clinics in Sports Medicine* 20, no.4 (October 1, 2001): 733-41.

Overly, M.D., Frank and Dale W. Steele, M.D. "Common Pediatric Fractures and Dislocations." *Clinical Pediatric Emergency Medicine* 3, no.2 (June 2002).

Nancy McKenzie, Ph.D.

Tranquilizers *see* **Antianxiety drugs**

Transfusion

Definition

Transfusion is the process of transferring whole blood or blood components from a donor to a recipient.

Purpose

Transfusions are given to restore lost blood, to improve clotting time, and to improve the ability of the blood to deliver oxygen to the body's tissues. About 32,000 pints of donated blood are transfused each day in the United States.

In the United States, blood collection is strictly regulated by the Food and Drug Administration (FDA), which has rules for the collection, processing, storage, and transportation of blood and blood products. In addition, the American Red Cross, the American Association of Blood Banks (AABB), and most states have specific rules for the collection and processing of blood. The main purpose of regulation is to ensure the quality of transfused blood and to prevent the transmission of infectious diseases through donated blood. Before blood and blood products are used, they are extensively tested for such infectious

KEY TERMS

ABO blood groups—A system in which human blood is classified according to the A and B antigens found in red blood cells. Type A blood has the A antigen, type B has the B antigen, AB has both, and O has neither.

Antibody—A simple protein produced by the body to destroy bacteria, viruses, or other foreign bodies. The production of each antibody is triggered by a specific antigen.

Antigen—A substance that stimulates the immune system to manufacture antibodies (immunoglobulins). The function of antibodies is to fight off such intruder cells as bacteria or viruses. Antigens stimulate the blood to fight other blood cells that have the wrong antigens. If a person with blood type A is given a transfusion with blood type B, the A antigens will fight the foreign blood cells as though they were an infectious agent.

Apheresis—A procedure in which whole blood is withdrawn from a donor, a specific blood component is separated and collected, and the remainder is reinfused into the patient.

Autologous blood—The patient's own blood, drawn and set aside before surgery for use during surgery in case a transfusion is needed.

Fractionation—The process of separating the various components of whole blood.

Hemoglobin—The red pigment in red blood cells that transports oxygen.

Hemolysis—The destruction of red blood cells through disruption of the cell membrane, resulting in the release of hemoglobin. A hemolytic transfusion reaction is one that results in the destruction of red blood cells.

Immunoglobulin—An antibody.

Infusion—Introduction of a substance directly into a vein or tissue by gravity flow.

Injection—Forcing a fluid into the body by means of a needle and syringe.

Plasma—The liquid portion of blood, as distinguished from blood cells. Plasma constitutes about 55% of blood volume.

Platelets—Disk-shaped structures found in blood that play an active role in blood clotting. Platelets are also known as thrombocytes.

Rh (rhesus) factor—An antigen present in the red blood cells of 85% of humans. A person with Rh factor is Rh positive (Rh+); a person without it is Rh negative (Rh-). The Rh factor was first identified in the blood of a rhesus monkey.

Serum (plural, sera)—The clear fluid that separates from blood when the blood is allowed to clot completely. Blood serum can also be defined as blood plasma from which fibrinogen has been removed.

agents as hepatitis and human immunodeficiency virus (HIV).

Blood and its components

Either whole blood or its components can be used for transfusion. Most blood collected from donors is broken down (fractionated) into components that are used to treat specific problems or diseases. Treating patients with fractionated blood is the most efficient way to use the blood supply.

WHOLE BLOOD. Whole blood is used exactly as received from the donor. Blood components are parts of whole blood, such as red blood cells (RBCs), white blood cells (WBCs), plasma, platelets, clotting factors, and immunoglobulins. Whole blood is used only when needed or when fractionated components are not available, because too much whole blood can raise the recipient's blood pressure. Use of blood components is a more efficient way to use the blood supply, because blood that has been fractionated can be used to treat more than one person.

Whole blood is generally used when a person has lost a large amount of blood. Such blood loss can be caused by injury or surgical procedures. Whole blood is given to help restore the blood volume, which is essential for maintaining blood pressure. It is also given to ensure that the body's tissues are receiving enough oxygen. Whole blood is occasionally given when a required blood fraction is unavailable in isolated form.

RED BLOOD CELLS. Red blood cells (RBCs) carry oxygen throughout the body. They pick up oxygen as they pass through the lungs, and give up oxygen to the other tissues of the body as they are pumped through the arteries and veins. When patients do not have enough RBCs to properly oxygenate their bodies, they can be given a transfusion with RBCs obtained from donors. This type of transfusion will increase the amount of oxygen carried to the tissues of the body. RBCs are recovered from whole blood after donation. They are then typed, removed from the watery blood plasma to minimize their volume (packed), and stored. RBCs are given to people with anemia (including thalassemia), whose bone marrow does not make enough RBCs, or who have other conditions that decrease the number of RBCs in the blood. Occasionally, red blood cells from rare blood types are frozen. Once frozen, RBCs can survive for as long as 10 years. Packed RBCs are given in the same manner as whole blood.

WHITE BLOOD CELLS. White blood cells (WBCs) are another infection-fighting blood component. On rare occasions, white blood cells are given by transfusion to treat life-threatening infections. Such transfusions are given when the WBC count is very low or when the patient's WBCs are not functioning normally. Most of the time, however, **antibiotics** are used in these cases.

PLASMA. Plasma is the clear yellowish liquid portion of blood. It contains many useful proteins, especially clotting factors and immunoglobulins. After plasma or plasma factors are processed, they are usually frozen. Some plasma fractions are freeze-dried. These fractions include clotting factors I through XIII. Some people have an inherited disorder in which the body produces too little of the clotting factors VIII (hemophilia A) or IX (hemophilia B). Transfusions of these clotting factors help to stop bleeding in people with hemophilia. Frozen plasma must be thawed before it is used; freeze-dried plasma must be mixed with liquid (reconstituted). In both cases, these blood fractions are usually small in volume and can be injected with a **syringe and needle**.

PLATELETS. Platelets are small disk-shaped structures in the blood that are essential for clotting. People who do not have enough platelets (a condition called thrombocytopenia) have bleeding problems. People who have lymphoma or leukemia and people who are receiving cancer therapy do not make enough platelets. Platelets have a very short shelf life; they must be used within five days of **blood donation**. After a unit of blood has been donated and processed, the platelets in it are packed into bags. A platelet transfusion is given in the same manner as whole blood.

IMMUNOGLOBULINS. Immunoglobulins are the infection-fighting fractions in blood plasma. They are also known as gamma globulin, antibodies, and immune sera. Immunoglobulins are given to people who have difficulty fighting infections, especially people whose immune systems have been depressed by such diseases as AIDS. Immunoglobulins are also used to prevent tetanus after a cut has been contaminated; to treat animal bites when rabies is suspected; or to treat severe childhood diseases. Generally, the volume of immunoglobulins used is small, and it can be injected.

Demographics

In order to donate blood, an individual must be at least 17 years old, weigh at least 110 lb (50 kg), and be in generally good health. The average blood donor is a white, married, college-educated male between the ages of 30 and 50. Twenty-five percent of people receiving blood transfusions are over the age of 65, although the elderly constitute only 13% of the population. Fewer than 5% of Americans donate blood each year.

Description

Blood is collected from the donor by inserting a large needle into a vein in the arm, usually one of the larger veins near the inside of the elbow. A tourniquet is placed on the upper arm to increase the pressure in the arm veins, which makes the veins swell and become more accessible. Once the nurse or technician has identified a suitable vein, she or he sterilizes the area where the needle will be inserted by scrubbing the skin with a soap solution or an antiseptic that contains iodine. Sometimes both solutions are used. The donor lies on a bed or cot during the procedure, which usually takes between 10 and 20 minutes. Generally, an 18-gauge needle is used. This size of needle fits easily into the veins and yet is large enough to allow blood to flow easily. Human blood will sometimes clot in a smaller needle and stop flowing. The donor's blood is collected in a sterile plastic bag that holds one pint (450 ml). The bags contain an anticoagulant to prevent clotting and preservatives to keep the blood cells alive. A sample of the donator's blood is collected at the time of donation and tested for infectious diseases. The blood is not used until the test results confirm that it is safe. Properly handled and refrigerated, whole blood can last for 42 days.

The recipient of a transfusion is prepared in much the same way as the blood donor. The site for the needle insertion is carefully washed with a soap-based solution followed by an antiseptic containing iodine. The skin is then dried and the transfusion needle inserted into the vein. During the early stages of a transfusion, the recipient is monitored closely to detect any adverse reactions. If no signs of adverse reaction are evident, the patient is monitored occasionally for the duration of the transfusion period. Upon completion of the transfusion, a compress is placed over the needle insertion site to prevent extensive bleeding.

Blood typing

All donated blood is typed, which means that it is analyzed to determine which of several major and minor blood types (also called blood groups) it belongs to. Blood types are genetically determined. The major types are classified by the ABO system. This system groups blood with reference to two substances in the red blood cells called antigen A and antigen B. The four ABO blood types are A, B, AB, and O. Type A blood has the A antigen, type B has the B antigen, type AB has both, and type O has neither. These four types of blood are further classified by the Rh factor. The Rh, or rhesus factor, is also an antigen in the red blood cells. A person who has the Rh factor is Rh positive; a person who does not have the factor is Rh negative. If a person has red blood cells with both the B and the Rh antigens, that person is said to have a B positive (B+) blood type. Blood types determine which kinds of donated blood a patient can receive. Generally, patients are limited to receiving only blood of the exact same ABO and Rh type as their own. For example, a person with B+ blood can receive blood or blood cells only from another person with B+ blood. An exception is blood type O. Individuals with type O blood are called universal donors, because people of all blood types can accept their blood.

Blood can also be typed with reference to several other minor antigens, such as Kell, Kidd, Duffy, and Lewis. These minor antigens can become important when a patient has received many transfusions. These patients tend to build up an immune response to the minor blood groups that do not match their own. They may have an adverse reaction upon receiving a transfusion with a mismatched minor blood group. A third group of antigens that may cause a reaction are residues from the donor's plasma attached to the RBCs. To eliminate this problem, the RBCs are rinsed to remove plasma residues. These rinsed cells are called washed RBCs.

Other transfusion procedures

Autologous transfusion is a procedure in which patients donate blood for their own use. Patients who are to undergo surgical procedures requiring a blood transfusion may choose to donate several units of blood ahead of time. The blood is stored at the hospital for the patient's exclusive use. Autologous donation assures that the blood type is an exact match. It also assures that no infection will be transmitted through the blood transfusion. Autologous donation accounts for 5% of blood use in the United States each year.

Directed donors are family or friends of the patient who needs a transfusion. Some people think that family and friends provide a safer source of blood than the general blood supply. Studies do not show that directed donor blood is any safer. Blood that is not used for the identified patient becomes part of the general blood supply.

Apheresis is a special procedure in which only certain specific components of a donor's blood are collected. The remaining blood fractions are returned to the donor. A special blood-processing instrument is used in apheresis. It fractionates the blood, saves the desired component, and pumps all the other components back into the donor. Because donors give only part of their blood, they can donate more frequently. For example, people can give almost 10 times as many platelets by apheresis as they could give by donating whole blood. The donation process takes about one to two hours.

Preparation

The first step in blood donation is the taking of the donor's medical history. Blood donors are questioned about their general health, their lifestyle, and any medical conditions that might disqualify them. These conditions include hepatitis, AIDS, cancer, heart disease, asthma, malaria, bleeding disorders, and high blood pressure. Screening prevents people from donating who might transmit diseases or whose medical condition would place them at risk if they donated blood. Some geographical areas or communities have a high rate of hepatitis or AIDS. Blood collection in most of these areas has been discontinued indefinitely.

The blood pressure, temperature, and pulse of donors are taken to ensure that they are physically able to donate blood. One pint (450 mL) of blood is usually withdrawn, although it is possible to donate smaller amounts. The average adult male has 10–12 pints of blood in his body; the average adult female has 8–9 pints in hers. Within hours after donating, most people's bodies have replaced the fluid lost with the donated blood, which brings their blood volume back to normal. Replacement of the blood cells and platelets, however, can take several weeks. Pregnant women and people with low blood pressure or anemia should not donate blood or should limit the amount of blood they give. Generally, people are allowed to donate blood only once every two months. This restriction ensures the health of the donor and discourages people from selling their blood. The former practice of paying donors for blood has essentially stopped. Donors who sell blood tend to be at high risk for the transmission of blood-borne diseases.

Aftercare

Recipients of blood transfusion are monitored during and after the transfusion for signs of an adverse reaction. Blood donors are generally given fluids and light refreshments to prevent such possible side effects as dizziness and nausea. They are also asked to remain in the donation area for 15–20 minutes after giving blood to make sure that they are not likely to faint when they leave.

Risks

Risks for donors

For donors, the process of giving blood is very safe. Only sterile equipment is used and there is no chance of catching an infection from the equipment. There is a slight chance of infection at the puncture site if the skin is not properly washed before the collection needle is inserted. Some donors feel lightheaded when they sit up or stand for the first time after donating. Occasionally, a donor will faint. Donors are encouraged to drink plenty of liquids to replace the fluid lost with the donated blood. It is important to maintain the fluid volume of the blood so that the blood pressure will remain stable. Strenuous **exercise** should be avoided for the rest of the day. It is normal to feel some soreness or to find a small bluish bruise at the site of the needle insertion. Most donors have very slight symptoms or no symptoms at all after giving blood.

Risks for recipients

A number of precautions must be taken for transfusion recipients. Donated blood must be matched with the recipient's blood type, as incompatible blood types can cause a serious adverse reaction (transfusion reaction). Blood is introduced slowly by gravity flow directly into the veins (intravenous infusion) so that medical personnel can observe the patient for signs of adverse reactions. People who have received many transfusions may develop an immune response to some factors in foreign blood cells. This immune reaction must be evaluated before the patient is given new blood.

Adverse reactions to mismatched blood (transfusion reaction) is a major risk of blood transfusion. Transfusion reaction occurs when antibodies in the recipient's blood react to foreign blood cells introduced by the transfusion. The antibodies bind to the foreign cells and destroy them. This destruction is called a hemolytic reaction. In addition, a transfusion reaction may also cause a hypersensitivity of the immune system that may in turn result in tissue damage within the patient's body. The patient may also have an allergic reaction to mismatched blood.

The first symptoms of transfusion reaction are a feeling of general discomfort and anxiety. Breathing difficulties, flushing, and a sense of pressure in the chest or back pain may also be present. Evidence of a hemolytic reaction can be seen in the urine, which will be colored from the hemoglobin leaking from the destroyed red blood cells. Severe hemolytic reactions are occasionally fatal. Reactions to mismatches of minor factors are milder. These symptoms include itchiness, dizziness, fever, headache, rash, and swelling. Sometimes the patient will experience breathing difficulties and muscle spasms. Most adverse reactions from mismatched blood are not life-threatening.

Infectious diseases can also be transmitted through donated blood and constitute another major risk of blood transfusion. The infectious diseases most often acquired from blood transfusion in the United States are hepatitis and HIV.

Patients who are given too much blood can develop high blood pressure, a concern for people who have heart disease. Very rarely, an air embolism is created when air is introduced into a patient's veins through the tubing used for intravenous infusion. The danger of embolism is greatest when infusion is begun or ended. Care must be taken to ensure that all air is bled out of the tubing before infusion begins, and that the infusion is stopped before air can enter the patient's blood system.

Normal results

Most individuals will feel only a slight sting from the needle used during the blood donation process, and will not experience any side effects after the procedure is over. Plasma is regenerated by the body

WHO PERFORMS THE PROCEDURE AND WHERE IS IT PERFORMED?

Blood may be donated at hospital donor centers, Red Cross chapter houses, or other locations where special blood drives have been organized (churches, places of business, schools, colleges, etc.). The procedure of blood donation is generally performed by a nurse or phlebotomist (a person who has been trained to draw blood). Blood transfusions are generally administered in a hospital or emergency center with a blood bank.

QUESTIONS TO ASK THE DOCTOR

- Why is a transfusion recommended for my condition?
- Do I have the option of donating my own blood for future use?
- Will I need a transfusion of whole blood or blood components?
- What alternatives to blood transfusion are available to me?

within 24 hours, and red blood cells within a few weeks. Patients who receive a blood transfusion will usually experience mild or no side effects.

Morbidity and mortality rates

The risk of acquiring an infectious disease from a blood transfusion is very low. The risk of HIV transmission is one in 2,135,000 units of blood; hepatitis B virus (HBV), one in 205,000 units; and hepatitis C virus (HCV), one in 1,935,000 units. Bacterial contamination (a cause of infection) is identified in one in 500,000 for red blood cell units and one in 15,400 for apheresis platelet units. In about 1 in 600,000 to 800,000 transfusions a "fatal misidentification error" occurs; and in about 1 in 12,000 to 19,000 cases a nonfatal error occurs.

Alternatives

There are several alternatives to blood transfusion. These include:

- Volume expanders. Certain fluids (saline, Ringer's lactate solution, dextran, etc.) may be used to increase the patient's blood volume without adding additional blood cells.
- Blood substitutes. Much research is currently being done into compounds that can replace some or all of the functions of blood components. One such compound, called HBOC-201 or Hemopure, is hemoglobin derived from bovine (cow) blood. Hemopure shows promise as a substitute for red blood cell transfusion.
- Bloodless surgery. It may be possible to avoid excessive blood loss through careful planning prior to surgery. Specialized instruments can minimize the amount of blood lost during a procedure. It is also possible to collect some of the blood lost during surgery and reinfuse it into the patient at the end of the operation.

Resources

BOOKS

Hoffman, R., et al. *Hematology: Basic Principles and Practice*, 4th ed. Philadelphia: Elsevier, 2005.

Khatri, V. P., and J. A. Asensio. *Operative Surgery Manual*, 1st ed. Philadelphia: Saunders, 2003.

McPherson, R. A., et al. *Henry's Clinical Diagnosis and Management By Laboratory Methods*, 21st ed. Philadelphia: Saunders, 2007.

Miller, R. D. *Miller's Anesthesia*, 6th ed. Philadelphia: Elsevier, 2005.

ORGANIZATIONS

American Association of Blood Banks (AABB). 8101 Glenbrook Road, Bethesda, MD 20814-2749. (301) 907-6977. http://www.aabb.org (accessed April 11, 2008).

American Red Cross (ARC) National Headquarters. 431 18th Street, NW. Washington, DC 20006. (202) 303-4498. http://www.redcross.org (accessed April 11, 2008).

America's Blood Centers. 725 15th St., NW, Suite 700, Washington, DC 20005. (202) 393-5725. http://www.americasblood.org (accessed April 11, 2008).

National Blood Data Resource Center (NBDRC). 8101 Glenbrook Road, Bethesda, MD 20814-2749. (301) 215-6506. http://www.nbdrc.org (accessed April 11, 2008).

OTHER

"Hemopure (HBOC-201) Shows Promise as Alternative to Red Blood Cell Transfusion in Elective Orthopedic Surgery." *Doctor's Guide*, January 28, 2002 [cited February 27, 2003]. http://www.pslgroup.com/dg/21371a.htm (accessed April 11, 2008).

John T. Lohr, PhD
Stephanie Dionne Sherk

Transplant surgery

Definition

Transplant surgery is the surgical removal of organs, tissue, or blood products from a donor and surgically placing or infusing them into a recipient. There are four categories of transplantation, classified by tissue origin: autograft (donor and recipient are the same person); isograft or syngeneic graft (donor and recipient are genetically identical, as in identical twins); allograft or homograft (donor and recipient are genetically unrelated but belong to the same species, i.e., both are human beings) and xenograft or heterograft (donor and recipient belong to different species, i.e., chimpanzee or rabbit tissues have been used in humans on an experimental basis).

KEY TERMS

Antibody—A substance produced by the immune system in response to specific antigens, thereby helping the body fight infection and foreign substances. An antibody screen involves mixing the white blood cells of the donor with the serum of the recipient to determine if antibodies in the recipient react with the antigens of the donor.

Autologous blood—The patient's own blood, drawn and set aside for use during surgery in case a transfusion is needed.

Bone densitometry test—A test that quickly and accurately measures the density of bone.

Brain death—Irreversible cessation of brain function. Patients with brain death have no potential capacity for survival or for recovery of any brain function.

Cadaveric donor—An organ donor who has recently died of causes not affecting the organ intended for transplant.

Compatible donor—A person whose tissue and blood type are the same as the recipient's.

Confirmatory typing—Repeat tissue typing to confirm the compatibility of the donor and patient before transplant

Donor—A person who supplies organ(s), tissue or blood to another person for transplantation.

Harvesting—The process of removing tissues or organs from a donor and preserving them for transplantation.

Hemodilution—A technique in which the fluid content of the blood is increased without increasing the number of red blood cells.

Human leuckocyte antigen (HLA)—A group of protein molecules located on bone marrow cells that can provoke an immune response. A donor's and a recipient's HLA types should match as closely as possible to prevent the recipient's immune system from attacking the donor's marrow as a foreign material that does not belong in the body.

Immunosuppression—The use of medications to suppress the immune system to prevent organ rejection.

Organ procurement—The process of donor screening, and the evaluation, removal, preservation, and distribution of organs for transplantation.

Pulmonary function test—A test that measures the capacity and function of the lungs as well as the blood's ability to carry oxygen. During the test, the patient breathes into a device called a spirometer.

Rejection—An immune response that occurs when a transplanted organ is viewed as a foreign substance by the body. If left untreated, rejection can lead to organ failure and even death.

Purpose

Transplant surgery is a treatment option for diseases or conditions that have not improved with other medical treatments and have led to organ failure or injury. Transplant surgery is generally reserved for people with end-stage disease who have no other options.

The decision to perform transplant surgery is based on the patient's age, general physical condition, specific diagnosis, and stage of the disease. Transplant surgery is not recommended for patients who have liver, lung, or kidney problems; poor leg circulation; cancer; or chronic infections.

Demographics

The typical cut-off age for a transplant recipient ranges between 40 and 55 years; however, a person's general health is usually a more important factor. In addition, the percentage of transplant recipients over age 50 has increased since 1996.

On average, 66 people receive transplants every day from either a living or deceased donor. Between January and October 2007, 23,703 transplants were performed in the United States; 18,388 organs came from deceased donors, while 5,315 came from living donors.

The national waiting list for most transplanted organs continues to grow every year, even though the number of recipients waiting for a heart transplant has leveled off in recent years, and the waiting list for heart-lung transplants has decreased over the past few years. As of January 2008, there were about 98,000 eligible recipients waiting for an organ transplant in the United States.

Description

Organ donors

Organ donors are classified as living donors or cadaveric (non-living) donors. All donors are carefully screened to make sure there is a suitable blood type match and to prevent any transmissible diseases or other complications.

LIVING DONORS. Living donors may be family members or biologically unrelated to the recipient. From 1992 to 2001, the number of biologically unrelated living donors increased tenfold. Living donors must be physically fit, in good general health, and have no existing disorders such as diabetes, high blood pressure, cancer, kidney disease, or heart disease. Of all the organs transplanted in 2007, about 23% came from living donors. Organs that can be donated from living donors include:

- Single kidneys. In 2002, 52% of all kidney transplants came from living donors. There is little risk in living with one kidney because the remaining kidney compensates for and performs the work of both.
- Liver. Living donors can donate segments of the liver because the organ can regenerate and regain full function. The number of living donor liver transplants has doubled since 1999.
- Lung. Living donors can donate lobes of the lung although lung tissue does not regenerate.
- Pancreas. Living donors can donate a portion of the pancreas even though the gland does not regenerate.

Organs donated from living donors eliminate the need to place the recipient on the national waiting list. Transplant surgery can be scheduled at a mutually acceptable time rather than performed under emergency conditions. In addition, the recipient can begin taking immunosuppressant medications two days before the transplant surgery to prevent the risk of rejection. Living donor transplants are often more successful than cadaveric donor transplants because there is a better tissue match between the donor and recipient. The living donor's medical expenses are usually covered by the organ recipient's insurance company, but the amount of coverage may vary.

CADAVERIC OR DECEASED DONORS. Organs from cadaveric donors come from people who have recently died and have willed their organs before **death** by signing an organ donor card, or are brain-dead. The donor's family must give permission for organ donation at the time of death or diagnosis of brain death. Cadaveric donors may be young adults with traumatic head injuries, or older adults suffering from a stroke. The majority of deceased donors are older than the general population.

Transplant procedures

ORGAN HARVESTING. Harvesting refers to the process of removing cells or tissues from the donor and preserving them until they are transplanted. If the donor is deceased, the organ or tissues are harvested in a sterile **operating room**. They are packed carefully for transportation and delivered to the recipient via ambulance, helicopter, or airplane. Organs from deceased donors should be transplanted within a few hours of harvesting. After the recipient is notified that an organ has become available, he or she should not eat or drink anything.

When the organ is harvested from a living donor, the recipient's transplant surgery follows immediately after the donor's surgery. The recipient and the donor should not eat or drink anything after midnight the evening before the scheduled operation.

PREOPERATIVE PROCEDURES. After arriving at the hospital, the recipient will have a complete physical and such other tests as a **chest x ray**, blood tests, and an **electrocardiogram** (EKG) to evaluate his or her fitness for surgery. If the recipient has an infection or major medical problem, or if the donor organ is found to be unacceptable, the operation will be canceled.

The recipient will be prepared for surgery by having the incision site shaved and cleansed. An intravenous tube (IV) will be placed in the arm to deliver medications and fluids, and a sedative will be given to help the patient relax.

TRANSPLANT SURGERY. After the patient has been brought to the operating room, the anesthesiologist will administer a general anesthetic. A central venous catheter may be placed in a vein in the patient's arm or groin. A breathing tube will be placed in the patient's throat. The breathing tube is attached to a mechanical ventilator that expands the lungs during surgery.

The patient will then be connected to a heart-lung bypass machine, also called a cardiopulmonary bypass pump, which takes over for the heart and lungs during the surgery. The heart-lung machine removes carbon dioxide from the blood and replaces it with oxygen. A tube is inserted into the patient's aorta to carry the oxygenated blood from the bypass machine back to the heart for circulation to the body. A nasogastric tube is placed to drain stomach secretions, and a urinary catheter is inserted to drain urine during the surgery.

The surgeon carefully removes the diseased organ and replaces it with the donor organ. The blood vessels of the donated organ are connected to the patient's blood vessels, allowing blood to flow through the new organ.

Diagnosis/Preparation

Pre-transplant evaluation

Several tests are performed before the transplant surgery to make sure that the patient is eligible to receive the organ and to identify and treat any problems ahead of time. The more common pre-transplant tests include:

- tissue typing
- blood tests
- chest x ray
- pulmonary function tests
- computed tomography (CT) scan
- heart function tests (electrocardiogram, echocardiogram, and cardiac catheterization)
- sigmoidoscopy
- bone densitometry test

The pre-transplant evaluation usually includes a dietary and social work assessment. In addition, the patient must undergo a complete dental examination to reduce the risk of infection from bacteria in the mouth.

Insurance considerations

Organ transplantation is an expensive procedure. Insurance companies and health maintenance organizations (HMOs) may not cover all costs. Many insurance companies require precertification letters of medical necessity. As soon as transplantation is discussed as a treatment option, the patient should contact his or her insurance provider as soon as possible to determine what costs will be covered. In the United States as of early 2008, a kidney transplant may cost as much as $100,000, a liver transplant $250,000, and a heart transplant $860,000. There are, however, organizations that can assist with raising funds to cover the cost of transplantation, such as the National Foundation for Transplants and the National Transplant Assistance Fund and Catastrophic Injury Program.

Patient education and lifestyle changes

Before undergoing transplant surgery, the transplant team will ensure that the patient understands the potential benefits and risks of the procedure. In addition, a team of health care providers will review the patient's social history and psychological test results to ensure that he or she is able to comply with the regimen that is needed after transplant surgery. An organ transplant requires major lifestyle changes, including dietary adjustments, complex drug treatments, and frequent examinations. The patient must be committed to making these changes in order to become a candidate for transplant. Most transplant centers have extensive patient education programs.

Smoking cessation is an important consideration for patients who use tobacco. Many transplant programs require the patient to be a nonsmoker for a certain amount of time (usually six months) before he or she is eligible to participate in the pre-transplant screening evaluation. The patient must also be committed to avoid tobacco products after the transplant.

Informed consent

Patients are legally required to sign an **informed consent** form prior to transplant surgery. Informed consent signifies that the patient is a knowledgeable participant in making healthcare decisions. The doctor will discuss all of the following with the patient before he or she signs the form: the nature of the surgery; reasonable alternatives to the surgery; and the risks, benefits, and uncertainties of each option. Informed consent also requires the doctor to make sure that the patient understands the information that has been given.

Finding a donor

After the patient has completed the pre-transplant evaluation and has been approved for transplant surgery, the next step is locating a donor. Organs from cadaveric donors are located through a computerized national waiting list maintained by the United Network for Organ Sharing (UNOS) to assure equal access to and fair distribution of organs. When a deceased organ donor is identified, a transplant coordinator from an organ procurement organization enters the donor's data in the UNOS computer. The computer then generates a list of potential recipients. This list is called a match run. Factors affecting a potential organ recipient's ranking on the match run list include: tissue match, blood type, size of the organ, length of time on the waiting list, immune status, and the geographical distance between the recipient and donor. For some transplants, such as heart, liver, and intestinal segments, the degree of medical urgency is also taken into consideration.

The organ is offered to the transplant team of the first person on the ranked waiting list. The recipient must be healthy enough to undergo surgery, available, and willing to receive the organ transplant immediately. The matching process involves cross matching, performing an antibody screen and a host of other tests.

Donor searching can be a long and stressful process. A supportive network of friends and family is important to help the patient cope during this time. The healthcare provider or social worker can also put the patient in touch with support groups for transplant patients.

Contact and travel arrangements

The patient must be ready to go to the hospital as soon as possible after being notified that an organ is available. A suitcase should be kept packed at all times. Transportation arrangements should be made ahead of time. If the recipient lives more than a 90-minute drive from the transplant center, the transplant coordinator will help make transportation arrangements for the recipient and one friend or family member.

Because harvested organs cannot be preserved for more than a few hours, the transplant team must be able to contact the patient at all times. Some transplant programs offer a pager rental service, to be used only for receiving the call from the transplant center. The patient should clear travel plans with the transplant coordinator before taking any trips.

Blood donation and conservation

Some transplant centers allow patients to donate their own blood before surgery, which is known as autologous donation. Autologous blood is the safest blood for **transfusion**, since there is no risk of disease transmission. Preoperative donation is an option for patients receiving an organ from a living donor, since the surgery can be scheduled in advance. In autologous donation, the patient donates blood once a week for one to three weeks before surgery. The blood is separated and the blood components needed are reinfused during the operation.

In addition to preoperative donation, there are several techniques for minimizing the patient's blood loss during surgery:

- Intraoperative blood collection. The blood lost during surgery is processed, and the red blood cells are reinfused during or immediately after surgery.
- Immediate preoperative hemodilution. The patient donates blood immediately before surgery to decrease the loss of red blood cells during the operation. The patient is then given fluids to restore the volume of the blood.
- Postoperative blood collection. The blood lost from the incision following surgery is collected and reinfused after the surgical site has been closed.

Aftercare

Inpatient recovery

A transplant recipient can expect to spend three to four weeks in the hospital after surgery. Immediately following the operation, the patient is transferred to an **intensive care unit** (ICU) for close monitoring of his or her **vital signs**. When the patient's condition is stable, he or she is transferred to a hospital room, usually in a specialized transplant unit. The IV in the patient's arm, the urinary catheter, and a dressing over the incision remain in place for several days. A chest tube may be placed to drain excess fluids. Special stockings may be placed on the patient's legs to prevent blood clots in the deep veins of the legs. A breathing aid called an incentive spirometer is used to help keep the patient's lungs clear and active after surgery.

Medications to relieve pain will be given every three to four hours, or through a device known as a PCA (patient-controlled anesthesia). The PCA is a small pump that delivers a dose of medication into the IV when the patient pushes a button. The transplant recipient will also be given immunosuppressive medications to prevent the risk of organ rejection. These medications are typically taken by the recipient for the rest of his or her life.

A 2–4 week waiting period is necessary before the transplant team can evaluate the success of the procedure. Visitors are limited during this time to minimize the risk of infection. The patient will be given intravenous antibiotic, antiviral and antifungal medications, as well as blood and platelet transfusions to help fight off infection and prevent excessive bleeding. Blood tests are performed daily to monitor the patient's kidney and liver function, as well as his or her nutritional status. Other tests are performed as needed.

Outpatient recovery

After leaving the hospital, the transplant recipient will be monitored through home or outpatient visits for as long as a year. Medication adjustments are often necessary, but barring complications, the recipient can return to normal activities about 6–8 months after the transplant.

Proper outpatient care includes:

- taking medications exactly as prescribed
- attending all scheduled follow-up visits
- contacting the transplant team at the first signs of infection or organ rejection
- having blood drawn regularly
- following dietary and exercise recommendations
- avoiding rough contact sports and heavy lifting
- taking precautions against infection
- avoiding pregnancy for at least a year

Risks

Short-term risks following an organ transplant include pneumonia and other infectious diseases;

excessive bleeding; and liver disorders caused by blocked blood vessels. In addition, the new organ may be rejected, which means that the patient's immune system is attacking the new organ. Characteristic signs of rejection include fever, rash, diarrhea, liver problems, and a compromised immune system. Transplant recipients are given immunosuppressive medications to minimize the risk of rejection. In most cases, the patient will take these medications for the rest of his or her life.

Long-term risks include an elevated risk of cancer, particularly skin cancer. An estimated 6–8% of transplant patients develop cancer over their lifetime as compared to less than 1% in the general population.

There is a very small risk of infection from a transplanted organ, even though donors in the United States and Canada are carefully screened. In 2007, the Centers for Disease Control and Prevention (CDC) reported a case in which four organ recipients in the Chicago area developed hepatitis C and HIV infection from a high-risk donor. The diseases did not show up on screening tests because the donor contracted them about three weeks before his death, when there were not enough antibodies in his blood to be detected by present tests.

Normal results

In a successful organ transplant, the patient returns to a more nearly normal lifestyle with increased strength and stamina.

Morbidity and mortality rates

Mortality figures for transplant surgery include recipients who die before a match with a suitable donor can be found. About 17 patients die every day in the United States waiting for a transplant. In 2001, over 6,000 patients died because the organ they needed was not donated in time.

The Scientific Registry of Transplant Recipients gives the first-year survival rates for transplant surgery as follows:

- 97% of pancreas transplant recipients
- 95% of kidney transplant and kidney/pancreas recipients
- 90% of autologous bone marrow transplant patients
- 86% of liver transplant patients
- 85% of heart transplant patients
- 77% of lung transplant patients
- 70% of allogeneic bone marrow transplant patients

WHO PERFORMS THIS PROCEDURE AND WHERE IS IT PERFORMED?

A transplant surgeon, along with a multidisciplinary team of transplant specialists, should perform the transplant surgery. Transplant surgeons are usually board-certified by the American Board of Surgery, as well as certified by the medical specialty board or boards related to the type of organ transplant performed. Members of transplant teams include infectious disease specialists, pharmacologists, psychiatrists, advanced care registered nurses, and transplant coordinators in addition to the surgeons and anesthesiologists.

Organ transplants are performed in special transplant centers, which should be members of the United Network for Organ Sharing (UNOS) as well as of state-level accreditation organizations.

Three-year survival rates are:

- 91% for kidney transplant patients
- 87% for pancreas and kidney/pancreas transplant patients
- 80% for liver transplant patients
- 79% for heart transplant patients
- 59% for lung transplant patients

As of early 2008, about 180,000 Americans are living with a transplanted organ.

Alternatives

Clinical trials

Available alternatives to transplant surgery depend upon the individual patient's diagnosis and severity of illness. Some patients may be eligible to participate in clinical trials, which are research programs that evaluate a new medical treatment, drug or device. As of early 2008, the NIH has 1,092 studies of organ transplantation that are seeking new volunteers.

Complementary and alternative (CAM) therapies

Complementary therapies can be used along with standard treatments to help alleviate the patient's pain; strengthen muscles; and decrease depression, anxiety, and stress. Before trying a complementary treatment, however, patients should check with their doctors to make sure that it will not interfere with standard therapy

QUESTIONS TO ASK THE DOCTOR

- Who performs the transplant surgery? How many other transplant surgeries has this surgeon performed?
- Where will my organ come from?
- What is the typical waiting period before a donor is found?
- Will my insurance provider cover the expenses of my transplant?
- What types of precautions must I follow before and after my transplant?
- What are the signs of infection and rejection, and what types of symptoms should I report to my doctor?
- When will I find out if the transplant was successful?

or cause harm. Alternative approaches that have helped transplant recipients maintain a positive mental attitude both before and after surgery include meditation, **biofeedback**, and various relaxation techniques. Massage therapy, music therapy, aromatherapy, and hydrotherapy are other types of treatment that can offer patients some pleasant sensory experiences as well as relieve pain. Acupuncture has been shown in a number of NIH-sponsored studies to be effective in relieving nausea and headache, as well as chronic muscle and joint pain. Some insurance carriers cover the cost of acupuncture treatments.

Resources

BOOKS

Farndon, John. *From Laughing Gas to Face Transplants: Discovering Transplant Surgery*. Chicago: Heinemann Library, 2006.

Hoffman, Nancy. *Heart Transplants*. Farmington Hills, MI: Lucent Books, 2003.

Morris, Peter J., and Stuart J. Knechtle. *Kidney Transplantation: Principles and Practice*, 6th ed. Philadelphia: Saunders/Elsevier, 2008.

PERIODICALS

Axelrod, D. A., M. K. Guidinger, S. Finlayson, et al. "Rates of Solid-Organ Wait-Listing, Transplantation, and Survival among Residents of Rural and Urban Areas." *Journal of the American Medical Association* 299 (January 9, 2008): 202–207.

Fishman, J. A. "Infection in Solid-Organ Transplant Recipients." *New England Journal of Medicine* 357 (December 20, 2007): 2601–2614.

Morris, P. J. "Transplantation—A Medical Miracle of the 20th Century." *New England Journal of Medicine* 351 (December 23, 2004): 2761–2766.

Williams, S. G. "A Piece of My Mind: Giving Back." *Journal of the American Medical Association* 298 (December 19, 2007): 2723–2724.

ORGANIZATIONS

American Society of Transplant Surgeons (ASTS). 2461 South Clark St., Suite 640, Arlington, VA 22202. (703) 414-7870. http://www.asts.org (accessed April 12, 2008).

Children's Organ Transplant Association, Inc. 2501 West COTA Drive, Bloomington, IN 47403. (800) 366-2682. http://www.cota.org (accessed April 12, 2008).

Coalition on Donation. 700 North 4th Street, Richmond, VA 23219. (804)782-4920. http://www.organtransplants.org/donor/coalition/ (accessed April 12, 2008).

Division of Transplantation, Health Resources and Services Administration (HRSA). 5600 Fishers Lane, Rm. 14-45, Rockville, MD 20857. 301-443-3376. http://www.organdonor.gov/ (accessed April 12, 2008).

National Foundation for Transplants. 5350 Poplar Avenue, Suite 430, Memphis, TN 38119. (800) 489-3863 or (901) 684-1697. http://www.transplants.org (accessed April 12, 2008).

National Heart, Lung and Blood Institute (NHLBI) Information Center. P. O. Box 30105, Bethesda, MD 20824-0105. (301) 251-2222. http://www.nhlbi.nih.gov (accessed April 12, 2008).

National Transplant Assistance Fund and Catastrophic Injury Program. 150 N. Radnor Chester Road, Suite F-120, Radnor, PA 19087. (800) 642-8399. http://www.transplantfund.org/ (accessed April 12, 2008).

Partnership for Organ Donation. Two Oliver Street, Boston, MA 02109. (617) 482-5746. http://www.transweb.org/partnership/ (accessed April 12, 2008).

Transplant Foundation, Inc. 701 SW 27th Ave, Suite 705, Miami, FL 33135. (305) 817-5645 or (866) 900-3172. http://www.transplantfoundation.org/.

Transplant Recipients International Organization (TRIO). International Headquarters: 1000 16th Street, NW, Suite 602, Washington, DC 20036-5705. (800) TRIO-386. http://www.transweb.org/people/recips/resources/support/bkuptrio_main.html (accessed April 12, 2008).

United Network for Organ Sharing (UNOS). P.O. Box 2484, Richmond, VA 23218. (804) 782-4800. http://www.unos.org (accessed April 12, 2008).

OTHER

CenterSpan. http://www.centerspan.org (accessed April 12, 2008).

Scientific Registry of Transplant Recipients. http://www.ustransplant.org (accessed April 12, 2008).

Sharma, Sat, and Helmut Unruh. "History of Adult Transplantation." *eMedicine*, June 1, 2006 [cited January 14, 2008]. http://www.emedicine.com/med/topic3497.htm (accessed April 12, 2008).

TransWeb. http://www.transweb.org (accessed April 12, 2008).

United Press International. "Patients Receive HIV-Infected Transplants," November 13, 2007. http://www.earthtimes.org/articles/show/141348.html [cited January 15, 2008, accessed April 12, 2008].

Angela M. Costello
Rebecca Frey, PhD

Transposition of the great arteries *see* **Heart surgery for congenital defects**

Transurethral bladder resection

Definition

Transurethral bladder resection is a surgical procedure used to view the inside of the bladder, remove tissue samples, and/or remove tumors. Instruments are passed through a cystoscope (a slender tube with a lens and a light) that has been inserted through the urethra into the bladder.

Purpose

Transurethral resection is the initial form of treatment for bladder cancers. The procedure is performed to remove and examine bladder tissue and/or a tumor. It may also serve to remove lesions, and it may be the only treatment necessary for noninvasive tumors. This procedure plays both a diagnostic and therapeutic role in the treatment of bladder cancers.

Demographics

Bladder cancer is the sixth most commonly diagnosed malignancy in the United States. According to the American Cancer Society, about 67,160 new cases of bladder cancer were projected to be diagnosed in the United States in 2007.

Industrialized countries such as the United States, Canada, France, Denmark, Italy, and Spain have the highest incidence rates for bladder cancer. Rates are lower in England, Scotland, and Eastern Europe. The lowest rates occur in Asia and South America.

Smoking is a major risk factor for bladder cancer; it increases one's risk by two to five times and accounts for approximately 50% of bladder cancers found in men and 30% found in women. If cigarette smokers quit, their risk declines in two to four years. Exposure to a variety of industrial chemicals also increases the risk of developing this disease. Occupational exposures may account for approximately 25% of all urinary bladder cancers.

Men have a 1-in-30 chance of developing bladder cancer; women have a 1-in-90 chance of developing bladder cancer. The incidence of bladder cancer in the white population is almost twice that of the black population. For other ethnic and racial groups in the United States, the incidence of bladder cancer falls between that of whites and blacks.

There is a greater incidence of bladder cancer with advancing age. Of newly diagnosed cases in both men and women, approximately 80% occur in people aged 60 years and older.

Description

Cancer begins in the lining layer of the bladder and grows into the bladder wall. Transitional cells line the inside of the bladder. Cancer can begin in these lining cells.

During transurethral bladder resection, a cystoscope is inserted through the urethra into the bladder. A clear solution is infused to maintain visibility and the tumor or tissue to be examined is cut away using an electric current. A biopsy is taken of the tumor and muscle fibers in order to evaluate the depth of tissue involvement, while avoiding perforation of the bladder wall. Every attempt is made to remove all visible tumor tissue, along with a small border of healthy tissue. The resected tissue is examined under the microscope for diagnostic purposes. An indwelling catheter may be inserted to ensure adequate drainage of the bladder postoperatively. At this time, interstitial radiation therapy may be initiated, if necessary.

Diagnosis/Preparation

If there is reason to suspect a patient may have bladder cancer, the physician will use one or more methods to determine if the disease is actually present. The doctor first takes a complete medical history to check for risk factors and symptoms, and does a **physical examination**. An examination of the rectum and vagina (in women) may also be performed to determine the size of a bladder tumor and to see if and how far it has spread. If bladder cancer is suspected, the following tests may be performed, including:

- biopsy
- cystoscopy
- urine cytology
- bladder washings
- urine culture
- intravenous pyelogram

KEY TERMS

Biopsy—The removal and microscopic examination of a small sample of body tissue to see whether cancer cells are present.

Bladder irrigation—To flush or rinse the bladder with a stream of liquid (as in removing a foreign body or medicating).

Bladder washings—A procedure in which bladder washing samples are taken by placing a salt solution into the bladder through a catheter (tube) and then removing the solution for microscopic testing.

Bladder tumor marker studies—A test to detect specific substances released by bladder cancer cells into the urine using chemical or immunologic (using antibodies).

Chemotherapy—The treatment of cancer with anti-cancer drugs.

Cystoscopy—A procedure in which a slender tube with a lens and a light is placed into the bladder to view the inside of the bladder and remove tissue samples.

Immunotherapy—A method of treating allergies in which small doses of substances that a person is allergic to are injected under the skin.

Interstitial radiation therapy—The process of placing radioactive sources directly into the tumor. These radioactive sources can be temporary (removed after the proper dose is reached) or permanent.

Intravenous pyelogram—An x ray of the urinary system after injecting a contrast solution that enables the doctor to see images of the kidneys, ureters, and bladder.

Metastatic—A change of position, state, or form; as a transfer of a disease-producing agency from the site of disease to another part of the body; a secondary growth of a cancerous tumor.

Noninvasive tumors—Tumors that have not penetrated the muscle wall and/or spread to other parts of the body.

Radiation therapy—The use of high-dose x rays to destroy cancer cells.

Retrograde pyelography—A test in which dye is injected through a catheter placed with a cystoscope into the ureter to make the lining of the bladder, ureters, and kidneys easier to see on x rays.

Urine culture—A test which tests urine samples in the lab to see if bacteria are present.

Ureters—Two thin tubes that carry urine downward from the kidneys to the bladder.

Urethra—The small tube-like structure that allows urine to empty from the bladder.

Urine cytology—The examination of the urine under a microscope to look for cancerous or precancerous cells.

- retrograde pyelography
- bladder tumor marker studies

Most of the time, the cancer begins as a superficial tumor in the bladder. Blood in the urine is the usual warning sign. Based on how they look under the microscope, bladder cancers are graded using Roman numerals 0 through IV. In general, the lower the number, the less the cancer has spread. A higher number indicates greater severity of cancer.

Because it is not unusual for people with one bladder tumor to develop additional cancers in other areas of the bladder or elsewhere in the urinary system, the doctor may biopsy several different areas of the bladder lining. If the cancer is suspected to have spread to other organs in the body, further tests will be performed.

Because different types of bladder cancer respond differently to treatment, the treatment for one patient could be different from that of another person with bladder cancer. Doctors determine how deeply the cancer has spread into the layers of the bladder in order to decide on the best treatment.

Aftercare

As with any surgical procedure, blood pressure and pulse will be monitored. Urine is expected to be blood-tinged in the early postoperative period. Continuous bladder irrigation (rinsing) may be used for approximately 24 hours after surgery. Most operative sites should be completely healed in three months. The patient is followed closely for possible recurrence with visual examination, using a special viewing device (cystoscope) at regular intervals. Because bladder cancer has a high rate of recurrence, frequent screenings are recommended. Normally, screenings would be needed every three to six months for the first three years, and every year after that, or as the physician considers necessary. **Cystoscopy** can catch a recurrence before it progresses to invasive cancer, which is difficult to treat.

Risks

All surgery carries some risk due to heart and lung problems or the anesthesia itself, but these risks are generally extremely small. The risk of **death** from **general anesthesia** for all types of surgery, for example, is only about one in 1,600. Bleeding and infection are other risks of any surgical procedure. If bleeding becomes a complication, bladder irrigation may be required postoperatively, during which time the patient's activity is limited to bed rest. Perforation of the bladder is another risk, in which case the urinary catheter is left in place for four to five days postoperatively. The patient is started on antibiotic therapy preventively. If the bladder is lacerated accompanied by spillage of urine into the abdomen, an abdominal incision may be required.

WHO PERFORMS THIS PROCEDURE AND WHERE IS IT PERFORMED?

Transurethral bladder resections are usually performed in a hospital by a urologist, a medical doctor who specializes in the diagnosis and treatment of diseases of the urinary systems in men and women and also treats structural problems and tumors or stones in the urinary system. Urologists can prescribe medications and perform surgery. If a transurethral bladder resection is required by a female patient, and there are complicating factors, an urogynecologist may perform the surgery. Urogynecologists treat urinary problems involving the female reproductive system.

Normal results

The results of transurethral bladder resection will depend on many factors, including the type of treatment used, the stage of the patient's cancer before surgery, complications during and after surgery, the age and overall health of the patient, as well as the recurrence of the disease at a later date. The chances for survival are improved if the cancer is found and treated early.

Morbidity and mortality rates

After a diagnosis of bladder cancer, up to 95% of patients with superficial tumors survive for at least five years. Patients whose cancer has grown into the lining of the bladder but not into the muscle itself, and is not in any lymph nodes or distant sites, have a five year survival rate as high as 85%. The five-year survival rate may be as high as 55% for patients whose tumors have invaded the bladder muscle, but not spread through the muscle into the surrounding fatty tissue. When the cancer has grown totally through the bladder muscle into the surrounding fatty tissue, and perhaps into nearby tissues such as the prostate, uterus, or vagina, the five-year survival rate is about 38%. For patients whose cancer has spread through the bladder wall to the pelvis or abdominal wall or has spread distantly to lymph nodes or other organs (such as the bones, liver, or lungs), the five-year survival rate is 16%.

The five-year survival rate refers to the percentage of patients who live at least five years after their cancer is found, although many people live much longer. Five-year relative survival rates do not take into account patients who die of other diseases. Every person's situation is unique and the statistics cannot predict exactly what will happen in every case; these numbers provide an overall picture.

Mortality rates are two to three times higher for men than women. Although the incidence of bladder cancer in the white population exceeds those of the black population, black women die from the disease at a greater rate. This is due to a larger proportion of these cancers being diagnosed and treated at an earlier stage in the white population. The mortality rates for Hispanic and Asian men and women are only about one-half those for whites and blacks. Over the past 30 years, the age-adjusted mortality rate has decreased in both races and genders. This may be due to earlier diagnosis, better therapy, or both.

About 67,160 cases of bladder cancer were projected to be diagnosed in 2007 in the United States. There are over 500,000 bladder cancer survivors in the United States, and approximately 13,750 will die of the disease in 2007.

Alternatives

Surgery, radiation therapy, immunotherapy, and chemotherapy are the main types of treatment for cancer of the bladder. One type of treatment or a combination of these treatments may be recommended, based on the stage of the cancer.

After the cancer is found and staged, the cancer care team discusses the treatment options with the patient. In choosing a treatment plan, the most significant factors to consider are the type and stage of the cancer. Other factors to consider include the patient's overall physical health, age, likely side effects of the treatment, and the personal preferences of the patient.

QUESTIONS TO ASK THE DOCTOR

- What benefits can I expect from this operation?
- What are the risks of this operation?
- What are the normal results of this operation?
- What happens if this operation does not go as planned?
- Are there any alternatives to this surgery?
- What is the expected recovery time?

In considering treatment options, a **second opinion** may provide more information and help the patient feel more confident about the treatment plan chosen.

Alternative methods are defined as unproved or disproved methods, rather than evidence-based or proven methods to prevent, diagnose, and treat cancer. For some cancer patients, conventional treatment is difficult to tolerate and they may decide to seek a less unpleasant alternative. Others are seeking ways to alleviate the side effects of conventional treatment without having to take more drugs. Some do not trust traditional medicine, and feel that with alternative medicine approaches, they are more in control of making decisions about what is happening to their bodies.

A cancer patient should talk to the doctor or nurse before changing the treatment or adding any alternative methods. Some methods can be safely used along with standard medical treatment. Others may interfere with standard treatment or cause serious side effects.

The American Cancer Society (ACS) encourages people with cancer to consider using methods that have been proven effective or those that are currently under study. They encourage people to discuss all treatments they may be considering with their physician and other health care providers. The ACS acknowledges that more research is needed regarding the safety and effectiveness of many alternative methods. Unnecessary delays and interruptions in standard therapies could be detrimental to the success of cancer treatment.

At the same time, the ACS acknowledges that certain complementary methods such as aromatherapy, **biofeedback**, massage therapy, meditation, tai chi, or yoga may be very helpful when used in conjunction with conventional treatment.

Resources

BOOKS

Hicks, M. *Bladder Cancer*, Cambridge, UK: Cambridge University Press, 2004.

Miller, R. D. *Miller's Anesthesia*, 6th ed. Philadelphia: Elsevier, 2005.

Wein, A. J., et al. *Campbell-Walsh Urology*, 9th ed. Philadelphia: Saunders, 2007.

ORGANIZATIONS

American Cancer Society. 1599 Clifton Road, N.E., Atlanta, GA 30329-4251. (800) 227-2345. http://www.cancer.org (accessed April 12, 2008).

American Foundation for Urologic Disease. 1128 North Charles St., Baltimore, MD 21201. (410) 468-1800. (800) 242-2383. Fax: (410) 468-1808. E-Mail: admin@afud.org. http://www.afud.org/ (accessed April 12, 2008).

National Cancer Institute Public Inquiries Office. Suite 3036A. 6116 Executive Boulevard, MSC8322. Bethesda, MD 20892-8322. (800) 422-6237. http://www.nci.nih.gov (accessed April 12, 2008).

National Comprehensive Cancer Network. 50 Huntingdon Pike, Suite 200, Rockledge PA 19046. (215) 728-4788. Fax: (215) 728-3877. Email: information@nccn.org. http://www.nccn.org/ (accessed April 12, 2008).

National Institutes of Health (NIH), Department of Health and Human Services. 9000 Rockville Pike. Bethesda, MD 20892.

OTHER

Aetna InteliHealth Inc. *Bladder Cancer*, 2003 [cited April 24, 2003]. http://www.intelihealth.com/IH/ihtIH?t=31066&p=∼br,IHW|~st,24479|~r,WSIHW000|~b,*| (accessed April 12, 2008).

American Cancer Society, Inc. (ACS) *Cancer Reference Information*, 2003 [cited April 24, 2003]. http://www.cancer.org/cancerinfo (accessed April 12, 2008).

Kathleen D. Wright, RN
Crystal H. Kaczkowski, MSc
Rosalyn Carson-DeWitt, MD

Transurethral resection of the prostate

Definition

Transurethral resection of the prostate (TURP) is a surgical procedure in which portions of the prostate gland are removed through the urethra.

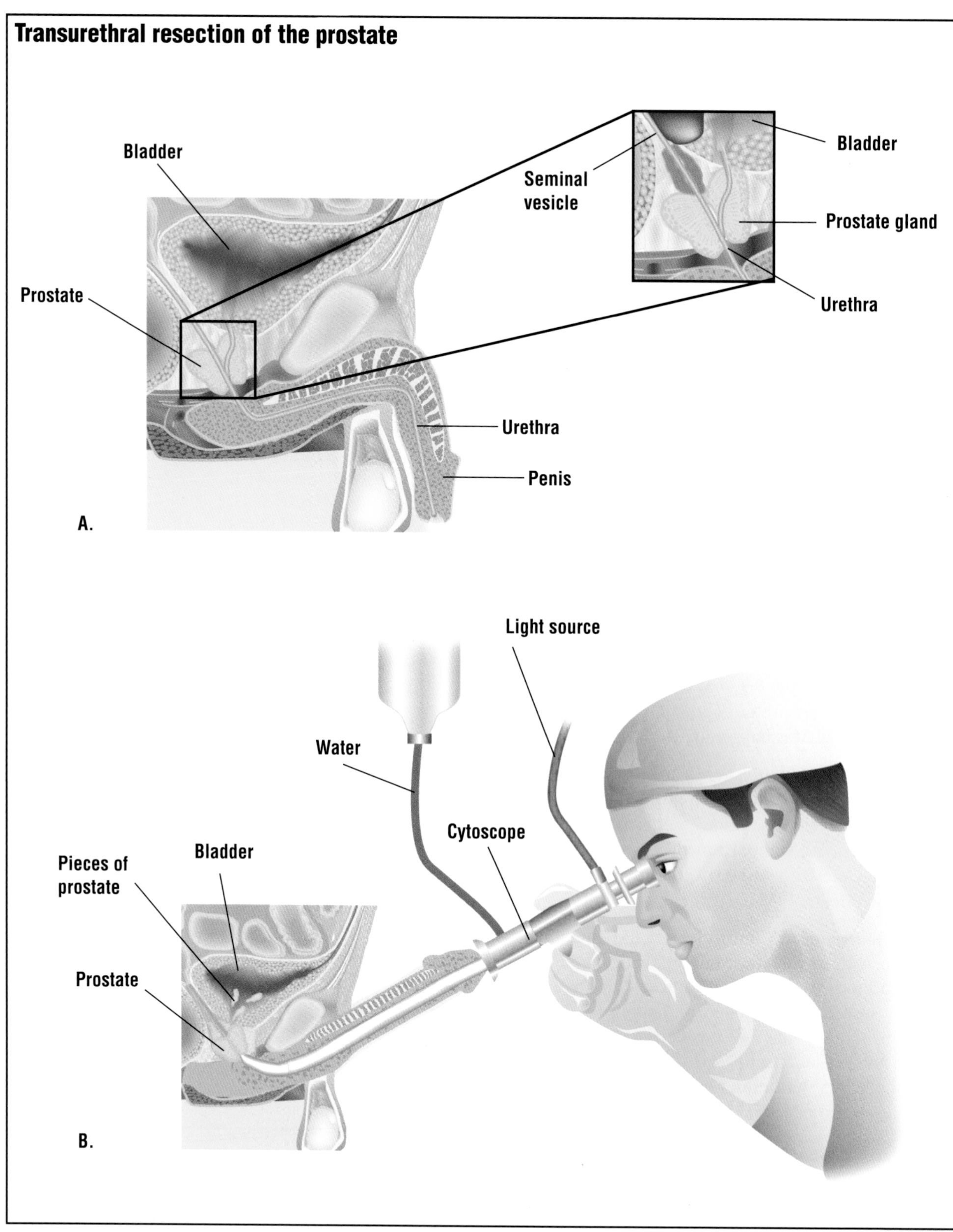

An enlarged prostate can cause urinary problems due to its location around the male urethra (A). In TURP, the physician uses a cystoscope to gain access to the prostate through the urethra (B). The prostate material that has been restricting urine flow is cut off in pieces, which are washed into the bladder with water from the scope (B). *(Illustration by GGS Information Services. Cengage Learning, Gale.)*

Purpose

The prostate is a gland that is part of the male reproductive system. It consists of three lobes and surrounds the neck of the bladder and urethra (a tube that channels urine from the bladder to the outside through the tip of the penis). The prostate weighs approximately 1 oz (28 g) and is walnut-shaped. It is partly muscular and partly glandular, with ducts opening into the urethra. It secretes an antigen called prostate-specific antigen (PSA), and a slightly alkaline fluid that forms part of the seminal fluid (semen) that carries sperm.

The prostate gland undergoes several changes as a man ages. The pea-size gland at birth grows only slightly during puberty and reaches its normal adult shape and size when a male is in his early 20s. The prostate gland remains stable until the mid-40s. At that time, in most men, the number of cells begins to multiply and the gland starts to enlarge.

Enlargement of the prostate causes a common disorder called benign (i.e., non-cancerous) prostatic hyperplasia (BPH) or benign prostatic enlargement (BPE). BPH occurs due to hormonal changes in the prostate, and is characterized by the enlargement or overgrowth of the gland because of an increase in the number of its constituent cells. BPH can raise PSA levels two to three times higher than normal. Men with increased PSA levels have a higher chance of developing prostate cancer.

BPH usually affects the innermost part of the prostate first, and enlargement frequently results in a gradual squeezing of the urethra at the point where it runs through the prostate. The squeezing sometimes causes urinary symptoms (referred to as lower urinary tract symptoms, LUTS), which often include:

- straining when urinating
- hesitation before urine flow starts
- dribbling at the end of urination or leakage afterward
- weak or intermittent urinary stream
- painful urination
- inability to completely empty the bladder

Other symptoms (called storage symptoms) sometime appear, and may include:

- urgent need to urinate
- bladder pain when urinating
- increased frequency of urination, especially at night
- bladder irritation during urination

The cause of BPH is not fully understood. As of 2008, it was thought to be caused by a hormone that the prostate gland synthesizes from testosterone called dihydrotestosterone (DHT).

Until the mid 1980s, transurethral resection of the prostate was the treatment of choice for BPH, and the most common surgery performed by urologists. By the mid-2000s, TURP surgery was being performed less frequently because of less invasive alternatives such as microwave therapy and prostatic **laser surgery**. Transurethral refers to the procedure being performed through the urethra. Resection means surgical removal.

Demographics

Before age 40, a small amount of prostatic hyperplasia is present in 80% of males, and about 10% of males under age 40 have fully developed BPH. Approximately 8–31% of males experience moderate to severe LUTS in their fifties. By age 80, about 80% of men have LUTS. A risk factor is the presence of normally functioning testicles; research indicates that castration can minimize prostatic enlargement. It appears that the glandular tissues that multiply abnormally use male hormones produced in the testicles differently than the normal tissues do.

Approximately 10 million American men and 30 million men worldwide have symptoms of BPH. It is more prevalent in the United States and Europe, and less common among Asians. BPH is more common in men who are married rather than single, and there is a strong inherited component to the disorder. A man's chance for developing BPH is greater if three of more family members have the condition. The average age of men having TURP surgery is 69.

Description

TURP is a type of surgery that does not involve an external incision. The surgeon reaches the prostate by inserting an instrument through the urethra. In addition to TURP, two other types of transurethral surgery are commonly performed: transurethral incision of the prostate (TUIP), and transurethral laser incision of the prostate (TULIP). The TUIP procedure widens the urethra by making small cuts in the bladder neck (where the urethra and bladder meet), and in the prostate gland itself. In TULIP, a laser beam directed through the urethra melts the tissue.

The actual TURP procedure is simple. It is performed under general or **local anesthesia**. After an intravenous line (IV) is inserted, the surgeon examines the patient with a cystoscope, an instrument that allows him or her to see inside the bladder. The surgeon then inserts a device up the urethra via the penis

KEY TERMS

Benign prostatic hyperplasia (BPH)—Also called benign prostatic enlargement (BPE). Non-cancerous enlargement of the prostate gland as a result of an increase in the number of its constituent cells.

Benign tumor—An abnormal growth that is not cancerous (malignant), and does not spread to other areas of the body.

Cryoprostatectomy—Freezing of the prostate through the use of liquid nitrogen probes guided by transrectal ultrasound of the prostate.

Digital rectal exam (DRE)—Procedure in which the physician inserts a gloved finger into the rectum to examine the rectum and the prostate gland for signs of cancer.

Prostate gland—A gland in the male that surrounds the neck of the bladder and urethra. The prostate contributes to the seminal fluid.

Prostatitis—Inflammation of the prostate gland that may be accompanied by discomfort, pain, frequent urination, infrequent urination, and sometimes fever.

Protozoan—A single-celled, usually microscopic organism that is eukaryotic and, therefore, different from bacteria (prokaryotic).

Transurethral surgery—Surgery in which no external incision is needed. For prostate transurethral surgery, the surgeon reaches the prostate by inserting an instrument through the urethra.

Urethra—The tube that channels urine from the bladder to the outside. In the female, it measures 1–1.5 in (25–38 mm); in the male, 9.8 in (25 cm).

opening, and removes the excess capsule material that has been restricting the flow of urine. The density of the normal prostate differs from that of the restricting capsule, making it relatively easy for the surgeon to tell exactly how much to remove. After excising the capsule material, the surgeon inserts a catheter into the bladder through the urethra for the subsequent withdrawal of urine.

Diagnosis/Preparation

Common BPH symptoms include:

- increase in urination frequency
- the need to urinate during the night
- difficulty starting urine flow
- a slow, interrupted flow and dribbling after urinating
- sudden, strong urges to pass urine
- a sensation that the bladder is not completely empty
- pain or burning during urination

In evaluating the prostate gland for BPH, the physician usually performs a complete **physical examination** as well as the following procedures:

- Digital rectal examination (DRE). Recommended annually for men over age 50, the DRE is an examination performed by a physician who feels the prostate through the wall of the rectum. Hard or lumpy areas may indicate the presence of cancer.
- Prostate-specific antigen (PSA) test. Also recommended annually for men over the age of 50, the PSA test measures the levels of prostate-specific antigen secreted by the prostate. It is normal to observe small quantities of PSA in the blood. PSA levels vary with age, and tend to increase gradually in men over age 60. They also tend to rise as a result of infection (prostatitis), BPH, or cancer.

If the results of the DRE and PSA tests suggest a significant prostate disorder, the examining physician usually refers the patient to a urologist, a medical doctor who specializes in diseases of the urinary tract and male reproductive system. The urologist performs additional tests, including blood and urine studies, to establish a diagnosis.

Patients should select an experienced TURP surgeon to perform the procedure.

Aftercare

When the patient awakens in the **recovery room** after the procedure, he already has a catheter in his penis, and is receiving pain medication via the IV line inserted prior to surgery. The initial recovery period lasts approximately one week, and includes some pain and discomfort from the urinary catheter. Spastic convulsions of the bladder and prostate are expected as they respond to the surgical changes.

The following medications or ones similar in function may be prescribed after TURP:

- B&O suppository (belladonna and opium). This medication has the dual purpose of providing pain relief and reducing the ureter and bladder spasms that follow TURP surgery. It is a strong medication that must be used only as prescribed.
- Bulk-forming laxative. Because of the surgical trauma and large quantities of liquids that patients are required to drink, they may need some form of laxative to promote normal bowel movements.

- Detrol. This pain reliever is not as strong as B&O. There may be wide variations in its effectiveness and the patient's response. It also controls involuntary bladder contractions.
- Macrobid. This antibiotic helps prevent urinary tract infections.
- Pyridium. This medication offers symptomatic relief from pain, burning, urgency, frequency, and other urinary tract discomfort.

When discharged from the hospital, patients are advised to avoid weight lifting or strenuous **exercise**. They should check their temperature and report any fever to the physician, and drink plenty of liquids.

Risks

Serious complications have become less common for prostate surgery patients because of advances in operative methods. Nerve-sparing surgical procedures help prevent permanent injury to the nerves that control erection, as well as injury to the opening of the bladder. However, there are risks associated with prostate surgery. The first is the possible development of incontinence (the inability to control urination), which may result in urine leakage or dribbling, especially immediately after surgery. Normal control usually returns within several weeks, but 3% of patients still experience incontinence three months after surgery. There is also a risk of impotence. For a month or so after surgery, most men are not able to become erect. Eventually, approximately 90% of men who were able to have an erection before surgery will be able to have an erection sufficient for sexual intercourse.

Other risks associated with TURP include blood loss requiring **transfusion**, and postoperative urinary tract infections.

TUR syndrome effects about 2% of TURP patients. Symptoms may include temporary blindness due to irrigation fluid entering the bloodstream. On very rare occasions, this can lead to seizures, coma, and even **death**. The syndrome may also include toxic shock due to bacteria entering the bloodstream, as well as internal hemorrhage.

Normal results

TURP patients usually notice urine flow improvement as soon as the catheter is removed. Other improvements depend on the condition of the patient's prostate before TURP, his age, and overall health status. Patients are told to expect the persistence of some pre-surgery symptoms. In fact, some new symptoms may appear following TURP, such as occasional blood and tissue in the urine, bladder spasms, pain when urinating, and difficulty judging when to urinate. TURP represents a major adaptation for the body, and healing requires some time. Full recovery may take up to one year. Patients are almost always satisfied with their TURP outcome, and the adaptation to new symptoms is offset by the disappearance of previous problems. For example, most patients no longer have to take daily prostate medication and quickly learn to gradually increase the time between urinating while enjoying uninterrupted and more restful sleep at night.

Normal postoperative symptoms, some of which are often temporary, include:

- urination at night and reduced flow
- mild burning and stinging sensation while urinating
- reduced semen at ejaculation
- bladder control problems
- mild bladder spasm
- fatigue
- urination linked to bowel movements

To eliminate these symptoms, patients are advised to exercise, retrain their bladders, take all medications that were prescribed, and get plenty of rest to facilitate the post-surgery healing process.

Morbidity and mortality rates

TURP improves symptoms in about 90% of BPH patients. Overall, 90-day TURP mortality rates are less than 1.5%. The most common cause of death is an overwhelming systemic infection (sepsis). Following surgery, inadequate relief of BPH symptoms occurs in 20–25% of patients, and 15–20% require another operation within 10 years. Urinary incontinence affects about 3%, and about 10% of TURP patients become impotent.

Alternatives

Conventional surgical alternatives for BPH patients include:

- Interstitial laser coagulation. In this procedure, a laser beam inserted in the urethra via a catheter heats and destroys the extra prostate capsule tissue.
- Transurethral needle ablation (TUNA). It uses radio waves to heat and destroy the enlarged prostate through needles positioned in the gland. It is generally less effective than TURP for reducing symptoms and increasing urine flow.
- Transurethral electrovaporization. This procedure is a modified version of TURP, and uses a device that

WHO PERFORMS THE PROCEDURE AND WHERE IS IT PERFORMED?

Transurethral resection of the prostate is performed in hospitals by experienced urologic surgeons who specialize in prostate disorders and in performing the TURP procedure.

QUESTIONS TO ASK THE DOCTOR

- What are the alternative treatments for benign prostatic hyperplasia?
- What are the risks involved with TURP?
- How long will it take to recover from the surgery?
- How painful is the TURP surgery?
- When and how often will the catheter require flushing?
- How long will it take to feel improvement?
- What are the postoperative problems?
- How will the surgery affect the ability to achieve erection?
- How many TURP procedures does the surgeon perform in a year?
- Will the surgery have to be repeated?

produces electronic waves to vaporize the enlarged prostate.

- Photoselective vaporization of the prostate (PVP). This procedure uses a strong laser beam to vaporize the tissue in a 20–50 minute outpatient operation.
- Transurethral incision of the prostate (TUIP). In this procedure, a small incision is made in the bladder, followed by a few cuts into the sphincter muscle to release some of the tension.
- Transurethral microwave thermotherapy (TUMT). TUMT uses microwave heat energy to shrink the enlarged prostate through a probe inserted into the penis to the level of the prostate. This outpatient procedure takes about one hour. The patient can go home the same day, and is able to resume normal activities within a day or two. TUMT does not lead to immediate improvement, and it usually takes up to four weeks for urinary problems to completely resolve.
- Water-induced thermotherapy (WIT). WIT is administered via a closed-loop catheter system, through which heated water is maintained at a constant temperature. WIT is usually performed using only a local anesthetic gel to anesthetize the penis, and is very well tolerated. The procedure is FDA approved.
- Balloon dilation. In this procedure, a balloon is inserted in the urethra up to where the restriction occurs. At that point, the balloon expands to push out the prostate tissue and widen the urinary path. Improvements with this technique may only last a few years.

Some BPH patients have experienced improved prostate health from the following:

- Zinc supplements. This mineral plays an important role in prostate health because it decreases prolactin secretion and protects against heavy metals such as cadmium. Both prolactin and cadmium have been associated with BPH.
- Saw palmetto. Saw palmetto has long been used by Native Americans to treat urinary tract disturbances without causing impotence. It shows no significant side effects. A number of recent European clinical studies have also shown that fat soluble extracts of the berry help increase urinary flow and relieve other urinary problems resulting from BPH.
- Garlic. Garlic is believed to contribute to overall body and prostate health.
- Pumpkin seed oil. This oil contains high levels of zinc and has been shown to help most prostate disorders. Eating raw pumpkin seeds each day has long been a folk remedy for urinary problems, but German health authorities have recently recognized pumpkin seeds as a legitimate BPH treatment.
- Pygeum bark. The bark of the *Pygeum africanus* tree has been used in Europe since early times in the treatment of urinary problems. In France, 81% of BPH prescriptions are for Pygeum bark extract.

Resources

BOOKS

Blute, Michael, ed. *Mayo Clinic on Prostate Health*, 2nd ed. Rochester, MN: Mayo Clinic, 2003.

Katz, Aaron E. *Dr. Katz's Guide to Prostate Health: From Conventional to Holistic Therapies*, Topanga, CA: Freedom Press, 2006.

Scardino, Peter T. and Judith Kelman. *Dr. Peter Scardino's Prostate Book: The Complete Guide to Overcoming Prostate Cancer, Prostatitis, and BPH*, New York : Avery, 2005.

ORGANIZATIONS

American Urological Association (AUA). 1000 Corporate Boulevard, Linthicum, MD 21090. Toll Free (U.S. only): (866) 746-4282 or 410-689-3700. http://www.auanet.org (accessed April 14, 2008).

OTHER

Leslie, Stephen W. "Transurethral Resection of the Prostate." *eMedicine.com*, October 3, 2006 [cited January 29, 2008]. http://www.emedicine.com/MED/topic 3071.htm (accessed April 14, 2008).

"Prostate Health." *University of Maryland Medicine*, [cited January 29, 2008]. http://www.umm.edu/prostate/ (accessed April 14, 2008).

"Transurethral Resection of the Prostate." *WebMD*, March 31, 2006 [cited January 29, 2008]. http://men.webmd.com/prostate-enlargement-bph/transurethral-resection-of-the-prostate-turp-for-benign-prostatic-hyperplasia (accessed April 14, 2008).

Monique Laberge, PhD
Tish Davidson, AM

Treadmill stress test *see* **Stress test**

Tremor reduction surgery *see* **Pallidotomy; Deep brain stimulation**

Triglyceride test *see* **Lipid tests**

Trisegmentectomy *see* **Hepatectomy**

Trocars

Definition

A trocar is a surgical instrument. It is a hollow cylinder into which fits another piece called an obturator with a pointed or blunt end. It is used to insert various surgical implements into a blood vessel or body cavity. Trocars were originally three-sided pointed instruments, but are now made in multiple designs with varying degrees of sharpness. Sometimes only the obturator portion is referred to as the trocar and the entire apparatus is referred to as trocar and cannula.

Procedures Using Trocars

Trocars may be used to insert **surgical instruments** during a **laparoscopy**, a procedure that allows for examination of the peritoneal cavity with minimal cutting of the body wall. Laparoscopic procedures in which trocars are used include **hysterectomy**, endometriosis ablation, and salpingectomy. Trocars can be used to help insert an intravenous cannula (flexible tube) into a blood vessel to allow for the administration of fluids or medication. Trocars may also be used on human cadavers during the embalming procedure to assist in draining bodily fluids in a process known as aspiration.

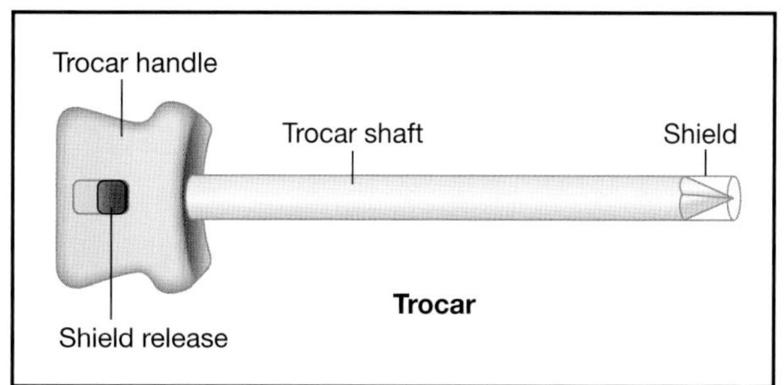

(Illustration by Electronic Illustrators Group.)

Description of Trocar Usage

Laparoscopy

The first trocar used in a laparoscopic procedure is called the primary trocar. A primary trocar is inserted into the peritoneal cavity, and the obturator portion is withdrawn. The insertion of the primary trocar into the peritoneal cavity requires enough force to penetrate the body wall with the obturator, while avoiding damage to the underlying structures. Appropriate training and skill is required to properly insert the primary trocar with guided force known as a "controlled jab". The cannula remains in the insertion site and is used as an access port through which to put other instruments in place. Through the cannula, a laparoscope (camera), or other surgical tool may be inserted into the body cavity. Once the laparoscope is inserted, the surgeon can see the internal structures of the body. However, when the primary trocar is inserted, it is usually done without being able to view the structures lying just underneath it. Hence insertion of the primary trocar is sometimes referred to as a "blind jab". Potential for damage to internal organs is decreased by inflating the abdominal cavity with carbon dioxide gas before trocar insertion, to hold the body wall away from the organs. Multiple trocars may be used for each procedure. Laparoscopies commonly require two to five trocars for completion. Insertion of each trocar carries the risk for a life threatening injury.

Embalming

Trocars are used during the embalming of human cadavers to insert tubes for drainage of bodily fluids. Once the blood has been replaced with embalming chemicals, the trocar is inserted and attached to a suction hose for aspiration. The insertion is made near the umbilicus in order to aspirate the main body cavities. Once the fluid is drained the trocar is detached from the aspirating hose and attached to a bottle of cavity-embalming fluid. The trocar is then used to fill

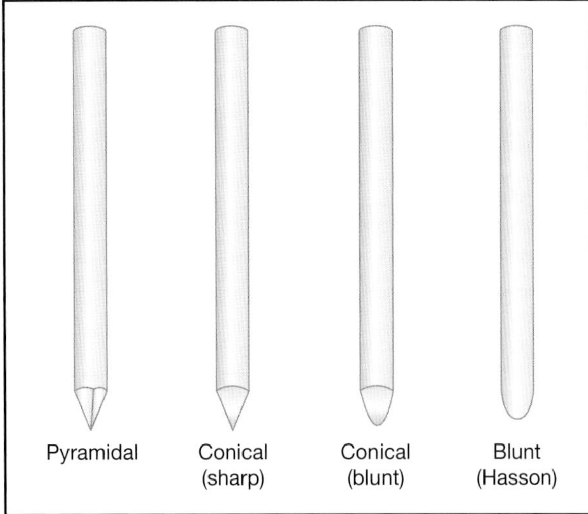

(Illustration by Electronic Illustrators Group.)

the body cavities with the fluid. The trocar puncture is sealed with a plastic plug called a trocar button.

Description of Trocar Designs

Trocars have evolved from one to two basic designs to many. According to the last trocar review done by the FDA, in 2003 there were greater than 100 different brand names being produced from greater than 20 different manufacturers. Trocars may be pointed with a cutting blade at the tip, blunt and bladeless, fitted with a protective shield, or contain a tiny camera for guided, optical entry into the body.

Cutting Trocars

Cutting trocars have been designed with sharp tips in order to create an incision in the body wall and facilitate insertion of the cannula into the peritoneal cavity. Sharp trocar ends may be three-sided and pyramidal, or conical. Multiple types of cutting trocars exist, most of which require blind entry into the peritoneal cavity. Cutting trocars require the least amount of force to insert into the body cavity. However, they cause the greatest amount of postsurgical insertion site pain, scarring, and sometimes hernia formation. Cutting trocars pose the greatest risk for damage to a major blood vessel or puncture of internal organs such as the intestines. Cutting trocars are associated with the greatest number of life threatening injuries, especially in patients for whom trocar insertion is difficult to perform.

Shielded Cutting Trocars

Trocars have been designed with a retractable, protective shield that covers the pointed tip before and after insertion into the peritoneal cavity. The shield was added to trocar designs in 1984 in an attempt to protect the abdominal and pelvic blood vessels and organs from accidental puncture with the trocar tip. For this reason shielded tips were originally called "safety trocars". However, whether or not the shielded tip actually warrants the term "safety trocar" is controversial. Serious injuries as well as deaths have both been associated with shielded trocars. According to trocar safety reviews done by the FDA, shielded trocars may have a somewhat improved safety profile if used properly. However, a general concern for the use of shielded trocars is a mistaken sense of security on the part of the surgeon, leading to inadvertent injury despite the shield. The shield itself has been shown to damage blood vessels, and shielded trocars can still cause life-threatening injury. Because of a lack of data proving shielded trocars as "safe" and concern for the issues previously described, in 1996 the FDA asked manufacturers to stop using the term "safety trocars" when describing a shielded trocars.

Bladeless Trocars

Trocars have also been designed in varying degrees of bluntness to help prevent accidental damage to blood vessels or internal organs when inserted into the peritoneal cavity. A Hasson trocar is very blunt and pushes through the layers of the abdominal wall instead of cutting them. The tissue fibers are merely separated instead of sliced, and can reposition naturally after the trocar is removed. Compared with cutting trocars, the blunt trocars require more force to insert into the peritoneal cavity. However, they create smaller trocar insertion tissue defects that take less time to heal, decrease the incidence of hernia formation, cause less scarring, and less postsurgical trocar insertion site pain. Bladeless trocars were designed in an attempt to minimize trocar-related injury or puncture of internal structures.

A Hasson trocar is implemented using the Hasson "cut-down" or "open" technique. Hasson trocars are so blunt-ended that they can only be inserted into the peritoneal cavity after the surgeon makes a small 2 to 3 cm incision through which to push the trocar (hence the term "cut-down" technique). The surgeon can see the area through which the trocar is penetrating and so the procedure does not require blind insertion (hence the term "open" technique). The Hasson trocar can then be used along with retractors to introduce other tools such as a laparoscope into the body cavity. The Hasson technique offers the advantage over traditional cutting trocars of being an open technique (as opposed to blind), and so may further minimize risk to blood vessels and internal organs. Whether or not the Hasson technique has succeeded as such is a matter of controversy, with studies especially differing on whether there is any real advantage regarding organ injury. Some types of blunt trocars are radially-expanding upon entry of the abdominal cavity to lift the abdominal wall up and away from the internal structures. Whether this design of trocar confers greater safety margins and reduces risk of injury is also controversial.

Optical Trocars

Each of the trocars discussed so far offer only blind access into the peritoneal cavity, potentially resulting in inadvertent, life threatening injury. In 1994, trocars were developed that have a tiny viewing "window" positioned at their tip for a laparoscope. This design of trocar enables the surgeon to observe the primary trocar insertion through the laparoscope and removes the necessity of a blind initial puncture. The surgeon can actually view each tissue layer being penetrated by the trocar device, as well as the underlying abdominal cavity and internal structures. While this design is an improvement over blind insertion trocars, injuries are still reported with optical trocars.

Risks

Trocar use is associated with risk of life-threatening injury. Injuries most commonly occur during the initial insertion of the primary trocar, often a blind insertion of the trocar before the laparoscope can be inserted. The risk is that the force being applied to penetrate the abdominal wall may accidentally propel the trocar into a blood vessel or puncture an internal organ such as the large intestine. Blood vessel hemorrhage or life-threatening bacterial infections may result. Each patient and circumstance requires a different amount of force to be applied for trocar insertion. It requires skill and experience on the part of the surgeon to insert the trocar with sufficient force to penetrate the abdominal cavity, while still maintaining enough control to stop the movement of the trocar once the abdominal wall has been traversed. The safety margin between the force required for trocar insertion and trocar injury is very slim, especially for children and small, thin adults. Blunt trocars require more force for insertion than cutting trocars. Despite the blunt edges of these trocars, the extra force required for penetration contributes to risk of propelling the trocar into and injuring the bowels. Additionally, the larger a trocar is, the greater the risk of injury to the patient. For each patient, surgeons use the smallest trocar possible.

Patients who have had prior abdominal surgery have a higher risk of trocar injury. After abdominal surgery, the internal organs and other structures of the abdominal cavity sometimes develop scar tissue that causes them to adhere to the abdominal wall. If internal structures are attached to the site of trocar entry, even filling the abdomen with carbon dioxide gas is not sufficient to keep them out of the path of injury upon primary trocar insertion. For this reason, blind insertion trocars should not be used on patients with a history of abdominal surgery. If lower abdominal surgery is included in patient history, there is a location that may be safely used for trocar insertion known as Palmer's Point. Palmer's Point is located in the upper left quadrant of the abdomen, and usually does not contain internal structures that may be injured upon trocar insertion.

Morbidity and mortality rates

The most common types of trocar injury are blood vessel damage leading to hemorrhage and bowel injury leading to peritoneal infection. The morbidity and mortality of trocar-related injuries increases when not caught early on. A delay in recognition or treatment of trocar injuries can be fatal for the patient. Injuries occur most frequently with insertion of the primary trocar, which may be the step in laparoscopies associated with the greatest risk.

Trocar use requires extensive training, experience, manual skill, muscular strength, control, and knowledge of the associated risks for each type of patient. Morbidity and mortality are due to a combination of the surgeon's skill level, the type of trocar, and patient-based risk factors. Whether on the part of the patient or the doctor, the failure of recognition of the symptoms of injury in a timely manner contribute much to the morbidity and mortality of trocar usage.

Patient-based risk factors for injury with blind trocar insertion

- Prior abdominal surgery
- Children
- Small, thin body type
- Alterations in abdomen skin due to multiple pregnancies
- Atrophied abdominal musculature

Alternatives to procedures with blind trocar insertion

- Laparotomy
- Hasson open technique
- Radially-expanding and optical-access trocars

KEY TERMS

Atrophy—Wasting of body tissues.

Cadaver—A dead body.

Cannula—A tube inserted into a body cavity.

Endometriosis Ablation—Procedure of removing endometrial tissue from deposition on structures within the abdominal cavity.

Embalming—Process of treating a dead body with chemicals to preserve it from decay.

Hemorrhage—Excessive blood loss through blood vessel walls.

Hernia—Protrusion of a structure through the tissues normally containing it.

Hysterectomy—Removal of the uterus.

Laparoscope—Tiny camera inserted into the body and used in surgical procedures called laparoscopies.

Laparoscopy—A type of minimally invasive surgery performed in the peritoneal cavity.

Laparotomy—Incision into the loin.

Morbidity—A state of disease or illness.

Obturator—Any structure that occludes an opening. A trocar obturator has a tip used to penetrate the body wall while being held in the cannula of the trocar apparatus.

Peritoneal Cavity—Part of the abdominal cavity holding many organs.

Retractor—Surgical tool used to hold structures away from the surgical field.

Salpingectomy—Removal of the uterine tube.

- Use of Palmer's point for trocar insertion (for patients with a history of prior abdominal surgery)

Potential signs and symptoms of internal hemorrhage into abdominal cavity

- Anemia, fatigue, and pallor
- Low-grade fever
- Increased heart rate
- Low blood pressure
- Shoulder pain
- Dizziness
- Faintness
- Nausea
- Lack of appetite

Potential signs and symptoms of untreated bowel injury

- Tender abdomen
- Pain
- Fever and chills
- Loss of appetite
- Nausea and vomiting
- Increased breathing rate
- Increased heart rate
- Low blood pressure
- Decreased urine production
- Inability to pass gas or feces

Resources

PERIODICALS

Fuller J, Scott W, Ashar B, Corrado J. Laparoscopic Trocar Injuries: A report from a U.S. Food and Drug Administration (FDA) Center for Devices and Radiological Health (CDRH) Systematic Technology Assessment of Medical Products (STAMP) Committee. FDA: Nov. 2003.

Maria Basile, PhD

Troponins test *see* **Cardiac marker tests**

Tubal ligation

Definition

Tubal ligation is a permanent voluntary form of birth control (contraception) in which a woman's fallopian tubes are surgically cut, tied, or blocked off to prevent pregnancy.

Purpose

Tubal ligation is performed in women who want to prevent future pregnancies. It is frequently chosen by women who do not want more children, but who are still sexually active and potentially fertile, and want to be free of the limitations of other types of birth control. Women who should not become pregnant for health concerns or other reasons may also choose this birth control method.

Demographics

Tubal ligation is one of the leading methods of contraception. This form of contraception is chosen by about 650,000–700,000 annually in the United

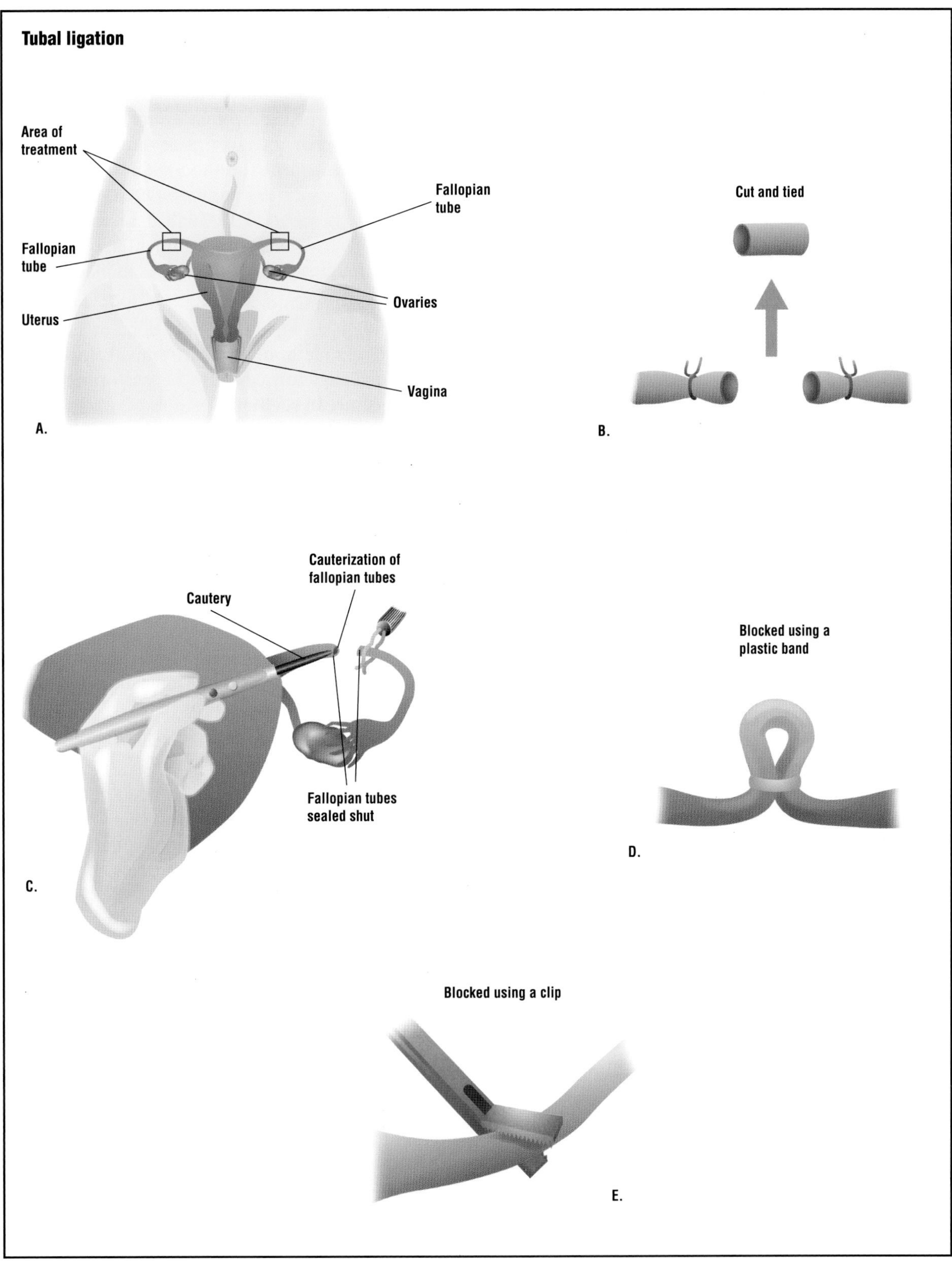

In a tubal ligation, a woman's reproductive organs are accessed by abdominal incision or laparoscopy (A). The fallopian tubes are cut and tied (B), cauterized (C), blocked with a silicone band (D), or clipped (E) to ensure sperm is not able to fertilize an egg. *(Illustration by GGS Information Services. Cengage Learning, Gale.)*

KEY TERMS

Contraception—The prevention of the union of the male's sperm with the female's egg.

Ectopic pregnancy—The implantation of a fertilized egg in a fallopian tube instead of the uterus.

Electrocoagulation—The coagulation or destruction of tissue through the application of a high-frequency electrical current.

Female sterilization—The process of permanently ending a woman's ability to conceive by tying off or cutting apart the fallopian tubes.

Laparoscopy—Abdominal surgery performed through a laparoscope, which is a thin telescopic instrument inserted through an incision near the navel.

Laparotomy—A procedure in which the surgeon opens the abdominal cavity to inspect the patient's internal organs.

Vasectomy—Surgical sterilization of the male, done by removing a portion of the tube that carries sperm to the urethra.

States. The typical tubal ligation patient is over age 30, is married, and has had two or three children.

Description

Tubal ligation, or getting one's "tubes tied," refers to female sterilization, the surgery that ends a woman's ability to conceive. The operation is performed on the patient's fallopian tubes. These tubes, which are about 4 in (10 cm) long and 0.2 in (0.5 cm) in diameter, are found on the upper outer sides of the uterus. They open into the uterus through small channels. It is within the fallopian tube that fertilization, the joining of the egg and the sperm, takes place. During tubal ligation, the tubes are cut or blocked in order to close off the sperm's access to the egg.

Normally, tubal ligation takes about 20–30 minutes, and is performed under **general anesthesia**, spinal anesthesia, or **local anesthesia** with sedation. The surgery can be performed on either hospitalized patients within 24 hours after childbirth or on outpatients. The woman can usually leave the hospital the same day.

Tubal ligation should be postponed if the woman is unsure about her decision. While the procedure is sometimes reversible, it should be considered permanent and irreversible. As many as 10% of sterilized women regret having had the surgery, and about 1% seek treatment to restore their fertility.

The most common surgical approaches to tubal ligation include **laparoscopy** and mini-laparotomy. In a laparoscopic tubal ligation, a long, thin telescope-like surgical instrument called a laparoscope is inserted into the pelvis through a small cut about 0.5 in (1 cm) long near the navel. Carbon dioxide gas is pumped in to help move the abdominal wall to give the surgeon easier access to the tubes. Often, the **surgical instruments** are inserted through a second incision near the pubic hair line. An instrument may be placed through the vagina to hold the uterus in place.

In a mini-laparotomy, a 1.2–1.6 in (3–4 cm) incision is made just above the pubic bone or under the navel. A larger incision, or laparotomy, is rarely used today. Tubal ligation can also be performed at the time of a **cesarean section**.

The tubal ligation itself is performed in several ways, including:

- Electrocoagulation. A heated needle connected to an electrical device is used to cauterize or burn the tubes. Electrocoagulation is the most common method of tubal ligation.
- Falope ring. In this technique, an applicator is inserted through an incision above the bladder and a plastic ring is placed around a loop of the tube.
- Hulka clip. The surgeon places a plastic clip across a tube held in place by a steel spring.
- Silicone rubber bands. A band placed over a tube forms a mechanical block to sperm.

Tubal ligation costs between $2,000 and $2,500 when performed by a private physician, but is less expensive when performed at a family planning clinic. Most insurance plans cover treatment costs.

Diagnosis/Preparation

Preparation for tubal ligation includes patient education and counseling. Before surgery, it is important that the woman understand the permanent nature of tubal ligation as well as the risks of anesthesia and surgery. Her medical history is reviewed, and a **physical examination** and laboratory testing are performed. The patient is not allowed to eat or drink for several hours before surgery.

Aftercare

After surgery, the patient is monitored for several hours before she is allowed to go home. She is instructed on care of the surgical wound, and what signs to watch for, such as fever, nausea, vomiting, faintness, or pain. These signs could indicate that complications have occurred.

WHO PERFORMS THE PROCEDURE AND WHERE IS IT PERFORMED?

Tubal ligation is generally performed by an obstetrician/gynecologist, a medical doctor who has completed specialized training in the areas of women's general health, pregnancy, labor and childbirth, prenatal testing, and genetics. The procedure is performed in a hospital or family planning clinic, and usually as an outpatient procedure.

QUESTIONS TO ASK THE DOCTOR

- How many tubal ligations do you perform each year?
- What method of ligation will you use?
- What form of anesthesia will be used?
- How long will the procedure take?
- What side effects or complications might I expect?
- What is your failure rate?

Risks

While major complications are uncommon after tubal ligation, there are risks with any surgical procedure. Possible side effects include infection and bleeding. After laparoscopy, the patient may experience pain in the shoulder area from the carbon dioxide used during surgery, but the technique is associated with less pain than mini-laparotomy, as well as a faster recovery period. Mini-laparotomy results in a higher incidence of pain, bleeding, bladder injury, and infection compared with laparoscopy. Patients normally feel better after three to four days of rest, and are able to resume sexual activity at that time.

The possibility for treatment failure is very low—about five women per 1,000 will become pregnant during the first year after sterilization. The failure rate increases over time, so that 10 years after the procedure, the failure rate is 18 women per 1,000. Failure can happen if the cut ends of the tubes grow back together; if the tube was not completely cut or blocked off; if a plastic clip or rubber band has loosened or come off; or if the woman was already pregnant at the time of surgery.

Normal results

After having her tubes tied, a woman does not need to use any form of birth control to avoid pregnancy. Tubal ligation is almost 100% effective for the prevention of conception.

Morbidity and mortality rates

About 1–4% of patients experience complications following tubal ligation. There is a low risk (less than 1%, or seven per 1,000 procedures) of a later ectopic pregnancy. Ectopic pregnancy is a condition in which the fertilized egg implants in a place other than the uterus, usually in one of the fallopian tubes. Ectopic pregnancies are more likely to happen in younger women, and in women whose tubes were closed off by electrocoagulation.

Rarely, **death** may occur as a complication of general anesthesia if a major blood vessel is cut. The mortality rate of tubal ligation is about 4-in-100,000 sterilizations.

Alternatives

There are numerous options available to women who wish to prevent pregnancy. Oral contraceptives are the second most common form of contraception—the first being female sterilization—and have a success rate of 95–99.5%. Other methods of preventing pregnancy include **vasectomy** (99.9% effective) for the male partner; the male condom (86–97% effective); the diaphragm or cervical cap (80–94% effective); the female condom (80–95% effective); and abstinence.

Resources

BOOKS

Gabbe, S. G., et al. *Obstetrics: Normal and Problem Pregnancies*, 5th ed. London: Churchill Livingstone, 2007.

Katz, V. L., et al. *Comprehensive Gynecology*, 5th ed. St. Louis: Mosby, 2007.

Khatri, V. P., and J. A. Asensio. *Operative Surgery Manual*, 1st ed. Philadelphia: Saunders, 2003.

Townsend, C. M., et al. *Sabiston Textbook of Surgery*, 17th ed. Philadelphia: Saunders, 2004.

PERIODICALS

Baill, I. C., V. E. Cullins, and S. Pati. "Counseling Issues in Tubal Sterilization." *American Family Physician* 67 (March 15, 2003): 1287–1294.

Kariminia, A., D. M. Saunders, and M. Chamberlain. "Risk Factors for Strong Regret and Subsequent IVF Request After Having Tubal Ligation." *Australian and New Zealand Journal of Obstetrics and Gynaecology* 42 (November 2002): 526–529.

ORGANIZATIONS

American College of Obstetricians and Gynecologists. 409 12th St., SW, P. O. Box 96920, Washington, DC 20090-6920. http://www.acog.org (accessed April 14, 2008).

Planned Parenthood Federation of America, Inc. 810 Seventh Ave., New York, NY, 10019. (800) 669-0156. http://www.plannedparenthood.org (accessed April 14, 2008).

OTHER

Centers for Disease Control and Prevention. *Risk of Ectopic Pregnancy after Tubal Sterilization*, August 6, 2002 [cited March 1, 2003]. http://www.cdc.gov/reproductive health/UnintendedPregnancy/EctopicPreg_fact sheet.htm (accessed April 14, 2008).

Planned Parenthood Federation of America. http://www.plannedparenthood.org (accessed April 14, 2008).

Mercedes McLaughlin
Stephanie Dionne Sherk
Rosalyn Carson-DeWitt, MD

Tube-shunt surgery

Definition

Tube-shunt surgery, or Seton tube shunt glaucoma surgery, is a surgical method to treat glaucoma. Glaucoma is a potentially blinding disease affecting 2–3% of the United States population. The major known cause of glaucoma is a relative increase in intraocular pressure, or IOP. The purpose of glaucoma treatment, whether medical or surgical, is to lower the IOP.

Aqueous fluid is made continuously, and circulates throughout the eye before draining though channels in the eye's anterior chamber. When too much fluid is made, or it is not drained sufficiently, the IOP rises. This fluid build-up can lead to glaucoma. Normal intraocular pressure is under 21 mm/Hg. Glaucoma develops at IOPs higher than 21mm/Hg. However, approximately 20% of glaucoma patients never have pressures higher than 21 mm/Hg.

Seton tube implants are also called glaucoma drainage tubes or implants. The Seton implant is comprised of two parts:

- Tubing, a portion of which is implanted along the inside of the front of the eye. The distal (furthest from the center) end of the tubing protrudes through the anterior (front) or less commonly, the posterior (rear), chamber of the eye.
- An attached reservoir, called a plate, is placed under the conjunctiva of the eye at its equator, or midpoint.

Purpose

The function of the implant is to lower the intraocular pressure by filtering excess aqueous fluid out of the eye. During the first few weeks after surgery, a bleb of fibrous tissue and collagen forms around the plate of the implant. The formation of a filtration bleb is essential for filtering the excessive aqueous fluid. The thickness of the bleb, as well as the size or number of plates, determines the rate at which aqueous flows out of the anterior chamber of the eye. The excess aqueous fluid is shunted through the tubing of the implant, and passes through the space that develops between the bleb and the plate. By diffusion, the fluid flows into the capillaries where it exits the eye and enters general circulation. The IOP is lowered as a result of this decrease in fluid.

There are various types of implants used in glaucoma surgery. They fall into two categories: the non-valved (free flow implants) and valved (resisted-flow implants). One of the first free-flow implants was the Molteno implant, which consists of one or two polypropylene reservoirs connected to a silicone tube. The non-valved Baerveldt implant is larger than the Molteno, and is available in three sizes.

The restrictive implants, which include the Krupin and Ahmed implant, have valves that automatically close if the intraocular pressure is too low. This is important because in the first few weeks after surgery (before the bleb forms), the aqueous fluid can flow unimpeded through the implant. As a result, hypotony (low level of fluid in the eye) can develop.

Newer implants such as the Express shunt and the Gore-Tex tube shunt are in early stages of use.

Demographics

Seton tube implants are employed to treat all forms of glaucoma, but are primarily used in patients with elevated IOP despite aggressive medical treatment. They are also used when other types of surgery, such as conventional filtration, or **trabeculectomy**, have not been successful, or would not be recommended. A trabeculectomy should not be performed on patients with neovascular glaucoma, as well as those who have ocular complications caused by previous glaucoma surgeries.

Implants are often placed in the eyes of patients with uveitic glaucoma (fluctuating IOP). The surgeon implants a tube with a ligature, and manipulates the ligature to control pressure. Seton tubes are also used in young patients with aniridia, who often develop glaucoma. These tubes should not be used for patients

KEY TERMS

Anterior chamber—The front chamber of the eye bound by the cornea in front and the iris in the back. The anterior chamber is filled with aqueous humor. The drainage site for the aqueous fluid is in the anterior chamber.

Choroid—The middle, highly vascular layer of the eye that lies between the sclera and the retina.

Conjunctiva—A thin membrane covering the sclera (white of the eye).

Cornea—The clear part of the eye, surrounded by the sclera, through which light passes into the eye.

Glaucoma—A group of eye diseases, of which the primary feature is a relative elevation in the intraocular pressure, or IOP. The damage caused by pressure changes in the eye are potentially blinding.

IOP—A measure of the pressure in the eye. The gold standard for measurement of IOP is Goldmann tonometry.

Ophthalmologist—A physician with either an M.D. or D.O. degree, who has had residency training in the diagnosis and treatment of eye diseases.

Posterior chamber—The posterior part of the eye bound by the lens in front and the retina in back. The posterior chamber is filled with a jellylike substance called the vitreous.

Rectus muscles—The muscles responsible for movement of the eye.

Retina—The innermost layer in which the receptors for vision are located.

Sclera—The outer layer of the eye covering all of the front part of the eye, except for the cornea.

Seton tube—An implant placed in the eye that provides an alternative route for aqueous fluid drainage.

Strabismus—A condition in which the muscles of the eye do not work together, often causing double vision.

Vitrectomy—Removal of the vitreous jelly located in the posterior chamber.

who have silicon oil implants for the treatment of retinal detachment.

Description

A Seton implant is usually inserted under **local anesthesia**, but may be done under **general anesthesia** for an anxious patient or child. Since implantation may be painful for some children, drugs may be given intravenously during surgery.

After anesthesia is administered, the eye is draped and retractors are placed on the eye to hold it in place. An incision is made on the conjunctiva, a thin membrane layer that lies above the sclera (white of the eye). The implant plate is placed under the conjunctiva and sutured to the sclera, carefully avoiding damage to the recti muscles in the area. Incisions may be made in two quadrants of the eye if a double plate implant is inserted.

If the tubing is implanted into the anterior chamber, that portion of the eye is drained of excess fluid. If the tube is placed in the posterior chamber of the eye, all or part of the vitreous is removed. A needle puncture is made at the limbus where the cornea and the sclera meet, and the tubing is passed through this hole into one of the chambers of the eye. This opening is sealed with a donor scleral patch, which may be autologous (from the patient's own tissue). If a free-flow implant is used, the tubing is ligated with either a disposable suture, or the ligature is positioned such that it can be removed with a minor incision after a few weeks. As an alternative, the non-valved implant may be inserted in two stages. The plate is first implanted, and the tube is attached during a second surgery after the bleb has formed.

Diagnosis/Preparation

Prior to surgery, the patient's eye is examined with a slit-lamp biomicroscope. It is important that the conjunctiva in which the plate is placed is not scarred; that the cornea is clear; and that there are no attachments of the iris to the lens behind it or to the cornea in front of it. An **ultrasound** of pediatric patients is done to assess the size of the eye because not all implants are small enough to fit into a child's eye.

Antibiotic drops may be given for up to three days prior to surgery. The patient will continue most glaucoma medication until the day of surgery.

Informed consent must be given for the procedure. This includes consent for surgery and a list of risks for the Seton tube implant. It is important for the patient to understand that any vision loss acquired prior to surgery cannot be corrected.

Aftercare

For several weeks postoperatively, the patient is given **topical antibiotics** and steroids. In addition, oral steroids may be given to patients who had ocular inflammation prior to surgery. Some surgeons use atropine to maintain the eye in a temporary dilated state. Glaucoma medication may be continued for a few months due to possible IOP fluctuation during the early post-operative period. Follow-up visits are scheduled for one day after the surgery, weekly during the first month, twice a month during the second month, and again at three months. Patients can resume normal daily activities within a few days. The sutures may cause a foreign body sensation, which decreases as the **stitches** dissolve. This does not usually require treatment.

Aftercare in the surgeon's office involves monitoring for the signs of hypotony and lowered IOP. The treatment for post-operative hypotony is to tighten the tube of a non-valved implant. As the bleb forms, adjustments are made in the tubing ligature to increase flow through the ligature. If the pressure continues to rise, the tube may be blocked, and excess fluid may have to be tapped. Tube blockage may occasionally occur. Hypotony may also be caused by leakage from the conjunctival wound site.

Risks

This surgery has intraoperative and postoperative risks. During the procedure, an extraocular muscle can be severed. This is particularly true if the implant is placed in the inferior nasal section of the eye. Strabismus and double vision may follow. Also, the cornea may become scarred, hemorrhaging can occur within the eye, and the iris and lens can be damaged by the protruding tube.

Early post-operative complications include hyphema (blood clots in the anterior chamber of the eye), hypotony, tube obstruction, suture rupture with wound leakage, movement of the implanted plate, corneal edema, and detachment of the retina. Because of the position of the implant plate, retinal detachments are difficult to treat successfully if a Seton implant is present. Double vision during the early post-operative period may be due to swelling in the area, and often will resolve as the orbital edema decreases.

In the late post-surgical period, strabismus as well as orbital cellulitis, a condition that can spread to the central nervous system, can develop. Other long-term risks of glaucoma implant surgery include cataract formation, proptosis (bulging of the eye), and phthisis bulbi (a dangerous situation in which the eye is devoid of all fluid).

WHO PERFORMS THE PROCEDURE AND WHERE IS IT PERFORMED?

Tube implants are performed by ophthalmologists as outpatient procedures in a hospital operating room. The implantation of a Seton tube takes about two hours. An ophthalmologist is a physician with advanced training in the treatment of eye disease. If general anesthesia or extra pain medication is administered, an anesthesiologist may be present during surgery.

Surgical intervention is required for choroidal detachments, strabismus, and if tubing blocks or comes in contact with other structures of the eye, particularly the cornea. If the tube is blocked by blood clots, tissue plasminogen activator may dissolve them. A laser can cut strands of vitreous or iris that may clog the tubing. If bleb enlargement impinges on a muscle, causing strabismus, the implant may be removed and replaced with a smaller type. If the tubing continually rubs on the back or endothelium of the cornea, decomposition of the cornea is possible and a corneal transplant may be required if vision is comprised. In this case, the tubing will have to be relocated to the posterior chamber, and a vitrectomy performed.

Loss of vision is possible with this and all glaucoma surgery. For Seton tube implants, hypotony is the primary cause of vision loss. Other causes include retinal detachment, vitreous bleeding, and macular edema.

Normal results

Usually the IOP is lower within two weeks of Seton tube placement. At two months, the pressure is stabilized at 16–18 mm/Hg. Glaucoma medication must still be taken. The IOP in 85% of patients with a non-valved implant is lower than 21 mm/Hg without additional medication intervention. Only 50% of patients with a Krupin valve implant have an IOP lower than 21 mm/ Hg without added medical treatment.

Morbidity and mortality rates

For 70–90% of patients, the implant is functional one year after surgery. After three years, 60% remain functional. The failure rate for Seton implants is 4–8% per year, and differ for valved and non-valved implants. For the non-valved implants, the success rate is 90% at one year, but drops to 60% at two years. At least 66% of valved Seton tube implants

QUESTIONS TO ASK THE DOCTOR

Which implant will be used?

Is a tube implant the best surgical approach for this case?

How many of these procedures has the surgeon performed?

When will it be determined if the surgery has been successful?

What are the risks for this surgery?

Will glaucoma eye drops still be required after surgery?

are effective at one year, but this drops to 34% at six years. Choroidal detachment is a complication in one-third of these patients.

Strabismus is more common with the Krupin valve as opposed to the Ahmed valve, possibly because it is larger.

For high-risk glaucoma patients, the success rate for Seton tube surgery is approximately 50%. The rate of failure increases 10% with each year. High-risk patients include those who are aphakic (have no intraocular lens), have neovascular glaucoma (which develops from uncontrolled diabetes and hypertension), have congenital glaucoma, and who have had other unsuccessful glaucoma surgeries. Although the success rate for neovascular glaucoma is 56% at 18 months, eventually 31% of neovascular glaucoma patients will lose all vision except for light perception.

Alternatives

Trabeculectomy is another surgical filtration technique used to treat glaucoma. Trabeculectomy surgery is performed by making a flap in the sclera of the eye, which serves as an alternative drainage site for aqueous fluid. Patients who receive this treatment are not as high risk as those undergoing an implant procedure. Overall, they have a lower IOP, but may have more advanced glaucoma. If vascularization of the iris is present, as in neovascular glaucoma, a trabeculectomy is not performed. For patients who do not have neovascular glaucoma, the failure rate for trabeculotomy is similar to that of drainage tube implants.

Cyclodestruction is another alternative to Seton tube implants. Freezing temperatures or lasers are used to destroy the ciliary body, the part of the eye where the aqueous fluid is produced. When compared to the YAG laser cyclophotocoagulation, tube shunts are twice as successful.

Resources

BOOKS

Albert, Daniel M., M.D., M.S., et. al. *Ophthalmic Surgery Principles and Techniques* Malden, MA: Blackwell Science, 1999.

Albert, Daniel M., M.D., M.S., et. al. *Principles and Practice of Ophthalmology*, 2nd ed. Philadelphia, PA: W.B. Saunders Company, 2000.

Azuara-Blanco, Augusto, M.D., Ph.D., et. al. *Handbook of Glaucoma*. London, UK: Martin Dunitz Ltd., 2002.

Ritch, Robert, M.D., et. al. *The Glaucomas*. St Louis, MO: Mosby, 1996.

Shields, M. Bruce. M.D. *Textbook of Glaucoma*. Baltimore, MD: Williams and Wilkins, 1998.

Weinreb, Robert, et. al. *Glaucoma in the 21st Century*. London, UK: Mosby International, 2000.

PERIODICALS

Arroyave, Claudia P.,M.D., et. al. "Use of Glaucoma Drainage Devices in the Management of Glaucoma Associated with Aniridia."*American Journal of Ophthalmology* 135 (February 2003): 155-9.

Benz, Matthew S., M.D., et. al. "Retinal Detachment in Patients with a Preexisting Glaucoma Drainage Device." *Retina* 22 (June 2002): 283-7.

Garcia-Feijoo, J., M.D., Ph.D., et. al., "Peritubular Filtration as Cause of Severe Hypotony after Ahmed Valve Implantation for Glaucoma." *American Journal of Ophthalmology* 132 (October 2001): 571-2.

Nazemi, Paul P., et. al. "Migration of Intraocular Silicone Oil Into the Subconjunctival Space and Orbit Through an Ahmed Glaucoma Valve."*American Journal of Ophthalmology* 132 (December 2001): 929-31.

Netland, M.D. Peter A. and Lee, David A., M.D. "What's New in Glaucoma Research." *Review of Ophthalmology* (May 1999): 102-10.

OTHER

"Drainage Implants." *Glaucoma Associates of Texas*.http://www.glaucomaassociates.com/drainage-implants.html

Glaucoma Drainage Devices. http://www.eyelink.com/EyeProcedure.asp?EyeProcedureID=45

Martha Reilly, O.D.

Tube enterostomy

Definition

Tube enterostomy, or tube feeding, is a form of enteral or intestinal site feeding that employs a stoma or semi-permanent surgically placed tube to the small intestines.

Purpose

Many patients are unable to take in food by mouth, esophagus, or stomach. A number of conditions can render a person unable to take in nutrition through the normal pathways. Neurological conditions or injuries, injuries to the mouth or throat, obstructions of the stomach, cancer or ulcerative conditions of the gastrointestinal tract, and certain surgical procedures can make it impossible for a person to receive oral nutrition. Tube feeding is indicated for patients unable to ingest adequate nutrition by mouth, but who may have a cleared passage in the esophagus and stomach, and even partial functioning of the gastrointestinal tract. Enteral nutrition procedures that utilize the gastrointestinal tract are preferred over intravenous feeding or parenteral nutrition because they maintain the function of the intestines, provide for immunity to infection, and avoid complications related to intravenous feeding.

Tube enterostomy, a feeding tube placed directly into the intestines or jejunum, is one such enteral procedure. It is used if the need for enteral feeding lasts longer than six weeks, or if it improves the outcomes of drastic surgeries such as removal or resection of the intestines. Recently, it has become an important technique for use in surgery in which a gastroectomy—resection of the intestinal link to the esophagus—occurs. The procedure makes healing easier, and seeks to retain the patient's nutritional status and quality of life after **reconstructive surgery**. Some individuals have a tube enterostomy surgically constructed, and successfully utilize it for a long period of time.

There are a variety of enteral nutritional products, liquid feedings with the nutritional quality of solid food. Patients with normal gastrointestinal function can benefit from these products. Other patients must have nutritional counseling, monitoring, and precise nutritional diets developed by a health care professional.

Demographics

Tube enterostomy provides temporary enteral nutrition to patients with injuries as well as inflammatory, obstructive, and other intestinal, esophageal, and abdominal conditions. Other uses include patients with pediatric abnormalities, and those who have had surgery for cancerous tumors of the gastroesophageal junction (many of these cases are associated with Barrett's epithelium). Intestinal cancers in the United States have declined since the 1950s. However, this endemic form of gastric cancer is one of the most common causes of **death** from malignant disease, with an estimated 798,000 annual cases worldwide; 21,900 in the United States. As gastric cancer has declined, esophageal cancers have increased, requiring surgeries that resect and reconstruct the passage between the esophagus and intestine.

KEY TERMS

Enteral nutritional support—Nutrition utilizing an intact gastrointestinal tract, but bypassing another organ such as the stomach or esophagus.

Parenteral nutritional support—Intravenous nutrition that bypasses the intestines and its contribution to digestion.

Stoma—A portal fashioned from the side of the abdomen that allows for ingestion into or drainage out of the intestines or urinary tract.

Tube feeding—Feeding or nutrition through a tube placed into the body through the esophagus, nose, stomach, intestines, or via a surgically constructed artificial orifice called a stoma.

Description

Tube enterostomy refers to placement via a number of surgical approaches:

- laparoscopy
- esophagostomy (open surgery via the esophagus)
- stomach (gastrostomy or PEG)
- upper intestines or jejunum (jejunostomy)

The appropriate method depends on the clinical prognosis, anticipated duration of feeding, risk of aspirating or inhaling gastric contents, and patient preference. Whether through a standard operation or with laparascopic surgical techniques, the surgeon fashions a stoma or opening into the esophagus, stomach or intestines, and inserts a tube from the outside through which nutrition will be introduced. These tubes are made of silicone or polyurethane, and contain weighted tips and insertion features that facilitate placement. The surgery is fairly simple to perform, and most patients have good outcomes with stoma placement.

Diagnosis/Preparation

A number of conditions necessitate tube enterostomy for nutritional support. Many are chronic and require a complete medical evaluation including history, **physical examination**, and extensive imaging tests. Some conditions are critical or acute, and may emerge from injuries or serious inflammatory conditions in which the patient is not systematically prepared for the surgery. In many cases, the patient undergoing this type of surgery has been ill for a period of time. Sometimes the patient is a small child or adult who accidentally swallowed a caustic substance. Some are elderly patients who have obstructive carcinoma of the esophagus or stomach.

Optimal preparation includes an evaluation of the patient's nutritional status, and his or her potential requirement for blood transfusions and **antibiotics**. Patients who do not have gastrointestinal inflammatory or obstructive conditions are usually required to undergo bowel preparation that flushes the intestines of all material. The bowel preparation reduces the chances of infection.

The patient's acceptance of tube feeding as a substitute for eating is of paramount importance. Health care providers must be sensitive to these problems, and offer early assistance and feedback in the self-care that the tube enterostomy requires.

In preparation for surgery, patients learn that the tube enterostomy will be an artificial orifice placed outside the abdomen through which they will deliver their nutritional support. Patients are taught how to care for the stoma, cleaning and making sure it functions optimally. In addition, patients are prepared for the loss of the function of eating and its place in their lives. They must be made aware that their physical body will be altered, and that this may have social implications and affect their intimate activities.

Aftercare

Tube enterostomy requires monitoring the patient for infection or bleeding, and educating him or her on the proper use of the enterostomy. According to the type of surgery—minimally invasive or open surgery—it may take several days for the patient to resume normal functioning. Fluid intake and urinary output must be monitored to prevent dehydration.

Risks

Tube enterostomies are not considered high risk surgeries. Insertions have been completed in over 90% of attempts. Possible complications include diarrhea, skin irritation due to leakage around the stoma, and difficulties with tube placement.

Tube enterostomy is becoming more frequent due to great advances in minimally invasive techniques and new materials used for stoma construction.

WHO PERFORMS THE PROCEDURE AND WHERE IS IT PERFORMED?

Gastrointestinal surgeons and surgical oncologists perform this surgery in general hospital settings.

However, one recent radiograph study of 289 patients who had jejunostomy found that 14% of patients suffered one or more complications, 19% had problems related to the location or function of the tube, and 9% developed thickened small-bowel folds.

Normal results

Recovery without complications is the norm for this surgery. The greatest challenge is educating the patient on proper stoma usage and types of nutritional support that must be used.

Morbidity and mortality rates

Some feeding or tube stomas have the likelihood of complications. A review of 1,000 patients indicated that PEG tube placement has mortality in 0.5%, with major complications (stomal leakage, peritonitis [infection in the abdomen], traumatized tissue of the abdominal wall, and gastric [stomach] hemorrhage) in 1% of cases. Wound infection, leaks, tube movement or migration, and fever occurred in 8% of patients. In a review of seven published studies, researchers found that a single intravenous dose of a broad-spectrum antibiotic was very effective in reducing infections with the stoma. Open surgery always carries with it a small percentage of cardiac complications, blood clots, and infections. Many gastric stoma patients have complicated diseases that increase the likelihood of surgical complications.

Alternatives

Oral routes are always the preferred method of providing nutritional intake. Intravenous fluid intake can be used as an eating substitute, but only for a short period of time. It is the preferred alternative when adequate protein and calories cannot be provided by oral or other enteral routes, or when the gastrointestinal system is not functioning.

QUESTIONS TO ASK THE DOCTOR

How long will the tube enterostomy remain in place?

How much assistance will be given in adjusting to the stoma and the special diet?

If the condition does not improve, what other surgical alternatives are available?

How long can a person live safely and comfortably with a tube enterostomy?

Resources

BOOKS

Feldman, M.D., Mark. *Sleisenger & Fordtran's Gastrointestinal and Liver Disease*,7th ed. Elsevier, 2002.

Townsend, Courtney M. *Sabiston Textbook of Surgery*, 16th ed. W. B. Saunders Company, 2001.

PERIODICALS

ASPEN Board of Directors and the Clinical Guidelines Task Force. "Guidelines for the Use of Parenteral and Enteral Nutrition in Adult and Pediatric Patients." *Journal of Parenteral Enteral Nutrition* 26, no.1 (Suppl) (January/February 2002).

Chin, A. and N.J. Espat. "Total Gastrectomy: Options for the Restoration of Gastrointestinal Continuity." *The Lancet Oncology* 4, no.5 (May 2003).

Marik, P.E. and G.P. Zaloga. "Early Enteral Nutrition in Acutely Ill Patients: A Systematic Review." *Critical Care Medicine* 29, no.12 (December 2001).

Mentec, H., et.al. "Upper Digestive Intolerance During Enteral Nutrition in Critically Ill Patients: Frequency, Risk Factors, and Complications." *Critical Care Medicine* 29, no.10 (October 2001).

ORGANIZATIONS

American Society Parenteral and Enteral Nutrition. 8630 Fenton St., Suite 412, Silver Springs, Maryland 20910. (301) 587-6315. Fax: (301) 587-2365. www.clinnutr.org.

United Ostomy Association, Inc. 19772 MacArthur Blvd., Suite 200, Irvine, CA 92612-2405. (800) 826-0826. www.uoa.org.

OTHER

Tube Feeding. Patient Handout. MDConsult. www.MDConsult.com.

Nancy McKenzie, Ph.D.

Tube feeding *see* **Tube enterostomy**

Tummy tuck *see* **Abdominoplasty**

Tumor marker tests

Definition

Tumor markers are a group of proteins, hormones, enzymes, receptors, and other cellular products that are overexpressed (produced in higher than normal amounts) by malignant cells. Tumor markers are usually normal cellular constituents that are present at normal or very low levels in the blood of healthy persons. If the substance in question is produced by the tumor, its levels will be increased either in the blood or in the tissue of origin.

Purpose

The majority of tumor markers are used to monitor patients for recurrence of tumors following treatment. In addition, some markers are associated with a more aggressive course and higher relapse rate and have value in staging and prognosis of the cancer. Most tumor markers are not useful for screening because levels found in early malignancy overlap the range of levels found in healthy persons. The levels of most tumor markers are elevated in conditions other than malignancy, and are therefore not useful in establishing a diagnosis.

Precautions

Tumor markers are sometimes elevated in nonmalignant conditions. Not every tumor will cause a rise in the level of its associated marker, especially in the early stages of some cancers. When a marker is used for cancer screening or diagnosis, the physician must confirm a positive test result by using imaging studies, tissue biopsies, and other procedures. False positive results may occur in laboratory tests when the patient has cross-reacting antibodies that interfere with the test.

Description

Physicians use changes in tumor marker levels to follow the course of a patient's disease, to measure the effect of treatment, and to check for recurrence of certain cancers. Tumor markers have been identified in several types of cancer, including malignant melanoma; multiple myeloma; and bone, breast, colon, gastric, liver, lung, ovarian, pancreatic, prostate, renal, and uterine cancers. Serial measurements of a tumor marker are often an effective means to monitor the course of therapy. Some tumor markers can provide physicians with information used in staging cancers, and some help predict the response to treatment.

KEY TERMS

Analyte—A material or chemical substance subjected to analysis.

Antitrypsin—A substance that inhibits the action of trypsin.

Biopsy—The removal of living tissue from the body, done in order to establish a diagnosis.

Glycoprotein—Any of a group of complex proteins that consist of a carbohydrate combined with a simple protein. Some tumor markers are glycoproteins.

Immunoassay—A laboratory method for detecting the presence of a substance by using an antibody that reacts with it.

Multiple myeloma—An uncommon disease that occurs more often in men than in women and is associated with anemia, hemorrhage, recurrent infections and weakness. Ordinarily it is regarded as a malignant neoplasm that originates in bone marrow and involves mainly the skeleton.

Oncogene—A gene that is capable under certain conditions of triggering the conversion of normal cells into cancer cells.

Oncologist—A physician who specializes in the diagnosis and treatment of tumors.

Overexpression—Production in abnormally high amounts.

Serum (plural, sera)—The clear, pale yellow liquid part of blood that separates from a clot when the blood coagulates.

Staging—The classification of cancerous tumors according to the extent of the tumor.

Substrate—A substance acted upon by an enzyme.

A decrease in the levels of the tumor marker during treatment indicates that the therapy is having a positive effect on the cancer, while an increase indicates that the cancer is growing and not responding to the therapy.

Types of tumor markers

There are five basic types of tumor markers.

ENZYMES. Many enzymes that occur in certain tissues are found in blood plasma at higher levels when the cancer involves that tissue. Enzymes are usually measured by determining the rate at which they convert a substrate to an end product, while most tumor markers of other types are measured by a test called an immunoassay. Some examples of enzymes whose levels rise in cases of malignant diseases are acid phosphatase, alkaline phosphatase, amylase, creatine kinase, gamma glutamyl transferase, lactate dehydrogenase, and terminal deoxynucleotidyl transferase.

TISSUE RECEPTORS. Tissue receptors, which are proteins associated with the cell membrane, are another type of tumor marker. These substances bind to hormones and growth factors, and therefore affect the rate of tumor growth. Some tissue receptors must be measured in tissue samples removed for a biopsy, while others are secreted into the extracellular fluid (fluid outside the cells) and may be measured in the blood. Some important receptor tumor markers are estrogen receptor, progesterone receptor, interleukin-2 receptor, and epidermal growth factor receptor.

ANTIGENS. Oncofetal antigens are proteins made by genes that are very active during fetal development but function at a very low level after birth. The genes become activated when a malignant tumor arises and produce large amounts of protein. Antigens comprise the largest class of tumor marker and include the tumor-associated glycoprotein antigens. Important tumor markers in this class are alpha-fetoprotein (AFP), carcinoembryonic antigen (CEA), prostate specific antigen (PSA), cathespin-D, HER-2/neu, CA-125, CA-19-9, CA-15-3, nuclear matrix protein, and bladder tumor-associated antigen.

ONCOGENES. Some tumor markers are the product of oncogenes, which are genes that are active in fetal development and trigger the growth of tumors when they are activated in mature cells. Some important oncogenes are BRAC-1, myc, p53, RB (retinoblastoma) gene (RB), and Ph^1 (Philadelphia chromosome).

HORMONES. The fifth type of tumor marker consists of hormones. This group includes hormones that are normally secreted by the tissue in which the malignancy arises as well as those produced by tissues that do not normally make the hormone (ectopic production). Some hormones associated with malignancy are adrenal corticotropic hormone (ACTH), calcitonin, catecholamines, gastrin, human chorionic gonadotropin (hCG), and prolactin.

Tumor markers in clinical use

Currently, there are over 60 analytes that are used as tumor markers. All of the enzymes and hormones mentioned above have been approved as tumor markers by the Food and Drug Administration (FDA), but most of the others are not; they have been designated for investigation purposes only. The following list describes the most commonly used tumor markers approved by the FDA for screening, diagnosis, or monitoring of cancer.

- Alpha-fetoprotein (AFP): AFP is a glycoprotein produced by the developing fetus, but blood levels of alpha-fetoprotein decline after birth. Healthy adults who are not pregnant rarely have detectable levels of AFP in their blood. The maternal serum AFP test (AFP triple screen or AFP Tetra screen) is primarily used to screen for spina bifida and other open fetal abnormalities, such as an abdominal wall defect. Very rarely a very high level of alpha-fetoprotein may be associated with congenital Finnish nephrosis. Lower than average levels of AFP in maternal serum may increase the risk for fetal Down syndrome or other chromosome abnormalities. In adult males and nonpregnant females, an AFP above 300 ng/L is often associated with cancer, although levels in this range may be seen in nonmalignant liver diseases. Levels above 1000 ng/L are almost always associated with cancer. AFP has been approved by the FDA for the diagnosis and monitoring of patients with nonseminoma testicular cancer. It is elevated in almost all yolk sac tumors and 80% of malignant liver tumors. An elevated AFP level in the maternal circulation during pregnancy warrants further discussion and possible further testing, but usually is not an indication of fetal anomaly, as it can be elevated in normal pregnancies. An elevated level may indicate problems other than fetal anomalies, such as placental problems that may lead to premature delivery or low birth-weight.
- CA-125: Measurement of this tumor marker is FDA-approved for the diagnosis and monitoring of women with ovarian cancer. Approximately 75% of persons with ovarian cancer shed CA-125 into the blood and have elevated serum levels. This figure includes approximately 50% of persons with stage I disease and 90% with stage II or higher. Elevated levels of CA-125 are also found in approximately 20% of persons with pancreatic cancer. Other cancers detected by this marker include malignancies of the liver, colon, breast, lung, and digestive tract. Test results, however, are affected by pregnancy and menstruation. Benign diseases detected by the test include endometriosis, ovarian cysts, fibroids, inflammatory bowel disease, cirrhosis, peritonitis, and pancreatitis. CA-125 levels correlate with tumor mass; consequently, this test is used to determine whether recurrence of the cancer has occurred following chemotherapy. Some patients, however, have a recurrence of their cancer without a corresponding increase in the level of CA-125.
- Carcinoembryonic antigen (CEA): CEA is a glycoprotein that is part of the normal cell membrane. It is shed into blood serum and reaches very high levels in colorectal cancer. Over 50% of persons with breast, colon, lung, gastric, ovarian, pancreatic, and uterine cancer have elevated levels of CEA. CEA levels in plasma are monitored in patients with tumors that secrete this antigen to determine if second-look surgery should be performed. CEA levels may also be elevated in inflammatory bowel disease (IBD), pancreatitis, and liver disease. Heavy smokers and about 5% of healthy persons have elevated plasma levels of CEA.
- Prostate specific antigen (PSA): PSA is a small glycoprotein with protease activity that is specific for prostate tissue. The antigen is present in low levels in all adult males, which means that an elevated level may require additional testing to confirm that cancer is the cause. High levels are seen in prostate cancer, benign prostatic hypertrophy, and inflammation of the prostate. PSA is approved as a screening test for prostatic carcinoma. PSA has been found to be elevated in more than 60% of persons with Stage A and more than 70% with Stage B cancer of the prostate. It has replaced the use of prostatic acid phosphatase for prostate cancer screening because it is far more sensitive. Most PSA is bound to antitrypsins in plasma but some PSA circulates unbound to protein (free PSA). Persons with a borderline total PSA (4–10 ng/L), but who have a low free PSA are more likely to have malignant prostate disease.
- Estrogen receptor (ER): ER is a protein found in the nucleus of breast and uterine tissues. The level of ER in the tissue is used to determine whether a person with breast cancer is likely to respond to estrogen therapy with tamoxifen, which binds to the receptors blocking the action of estrogen. Women who are ER-negative have a greater risk of recurrence than women who are ER-positive. Tissue levels are measured using one of two methods. The tissue can be homogenized into a cytosol, and an immunoassay used to measure the concentration of ER receptor protein. Alternatively, the tissue is frozen and thin-sectioned. An immunoperoxidase stain is used to detect and measure the estrogen receptors in the tissue.
- Progesterone receptor (PR): PR consists of two proteins, like the estrogen receptor, which are located in the nuclei of both breast and uterine tissues. PR has the same prognostic value as ER, and is measured by similar methods. Tissue that does not express the PR receptors is less likely to bind estrogen analogs used to treat the tumor. Persons who test negative for both

ER and PR have less than a 5% chance of responding to endocrine therapy. Those who test positive for both markers have greater than a 60% chance of tumor shrinkage when treated with hormone therapy.

- Human chorionic gonadotropin (hCG): hCG is a glycoprotein produced by cells of the trophoblast and developing placenta. Very high levels are produced by trophoblastic tumors and choriocarcinoma, which is an aggressive tumor that arises from cells that help to attach the fetus to the uterine wall. About 60% of testicular cancers secrete hCG. hCG is also produced less frequently by a number of other tumors. Some malignancies cause an increase in alpha and/or beta hCG subunits in the absence of significant increases in intact hCG. For this reason, separate tests have been developed for alpha and beta hCG, and most laboratories use these assays as tumor marker tests. Most EIA tests for pregnancy are specific for hCG, but detect the whole molecule and are called intact hCG assays.
- Nuclear matrix protein (NMP22) and bladder tumor-associated analytes (BTA): NMP22 is a structural nuclear protein that is released into the urine when bladder carcinoma cells die. Approximately 70% of bladder carcinomas are positive for NMP22. BTA is comprised of type IV collagen, fibronectin, laminin, and proteoglycan, which are components of the basement membrane that are released into the urine when bladder tumor cells attach to the basement membrane of the bladder wall. These products can be detected in urine using a mixture of antibodies to the four components. BTA is elevated in about 30% of persons with low-grade bladder tumors and over 60% of persons with high-grade tumors.

Preparation

Determination of the circulating level of tumor markers requires a blood test performed by a laboratory scientist. A nurse or phlebotomist usually draws the patient's blood; he or she ties a tourniquet above the patient's elbow, locates a vein near the inner elbow, cleanses the skin overlying the vein with an antiseptic solution, and inserts a sterile needle into that vein. The blood is drawn through the needle into an attached vacuum tube. Collection of a blood sample takes only a few minutes.

Tissue samples are collected by a physician at the time of surgical or needle biopsy. A urine sample is collected by the patient, using the midstream void technique.

Aftercare

Aftercare following a blood test consists of routine care of the area around the puncture site. Pressure is applied for a few seconds and the wound is covered with a bandage. If a bruise or swelling develops around the puncture site, the area is treated with a moist warm compress.

Risks

The risks associated with drawing blood include dizziness, bruising, swelling, or excessive bleeding from the puncture site. As previously mentioned, the results of blood tests should be interpreted with caution. A single test result may not yield clinically useful information. Several laboratory reports over a period of months may be needed to evaluate treatment and identify recurrence. Positive results must be interpreted cautiously because some tumor markers are increased in nonmalignant diseases and in a small number of apparently healthy persons. In addition false negative results may occur because the tumor does not produce the marker, and because levels seen in healthy persons may overlap those seen in the early stages of cancer. A false positive result occurs when the value is elevated even though cancer is not present. A false negative result occurs when the value is normal but cancer is present.

Normal results

Reference ranges for tumor markers will vary from one laboratory to another because different antibodies and calibrators are used by various test systems. The values below are representative of normal values or cutoffs for commonly measured tumor markers.

- Alpha-fetoprotein (AFP): Less than 15 ng/L in men and nonpregnant women. Levels greater than 1,000 ng/L indicate malignant disease (except in pregnancy).
- CA125: Less than 35 U/mL.
- Carcinoembryonic antigen (CEA): Less than 3 μg/L for nonsmokers and less than 5 μg/L for smokers.
- Estrogen receptor: Less than 6 fmol/mg protein is negative; greater than 10 fmol/mg protein is positive.
- Human chorionic gonadotropin (HCG): Less than 20 IU/L for males and non-pregnant females. Greater than 100,00 IU/L indicates trophoblastic tumor.
- Progesterone receptor: Less than 6 fmol/mg protein is negative. Greater than 10 fmol/mg protein is positive.
- Prostate specific antigen (PSA): Less than 4 ng/L.

Resources

BOOKS

Burtis, C.A., and E.R. Ashwood, eds. *Tietz Fundamentals of Clinical Chemistry*, 5th ed. Philadelphia, PA: Saunders, 2001.

Henry, J.B., ed. *Clinical Diagnosis and Management by Laboratory Methods*, 20th ed. Philadelphia, PA: Saunders, 2001.

"Tumor Immunology." Section 11, Chapter 143 in *The Merck Manual of Diagnosis and Therapy*, edited by Mark H. Beers, MD, and Robert Berkow, MD. Whitehouse Station, NJ: Merck Research Laboratories, 1999.

Wallach, Jacques. *Interpretation of Diagnostic Tests*, 7th ed. Philadelphia, PA: Lippincott Williams & Wilkens, 2000.

ORGANIZATIONS

American Cancer Society. 1599 Clifton Rd. NE, Atlanta, GA 30329-4251. (800) 227-2345. www.cancer.org.

American Society of Clinical Oncology (ASCO). 1900 Duke Street, Suite 200, Alexandria, VA 22314. (703) 299-0150. www.asco.org.

National Cancer Institute (NCI). NCI Public Inquiries Office, Suite 3036A, 6116 Executive Boulevard, MSC8332, Bethesda, MD 20892-8322. (800) 4-CANCER or (800) 332-8615 (TTY). www.nci.nih.gov.

United States Food and Drug Administration (FDA). 5600 Fishers Lane, Rockville, MD 20857-0001. (888) INFO-FDA. www.fda.gov.

OTHER

National Institutes of Health. [cited April 5, 2003]. www.nlm.nih.gov/medlineplus/encyclopedia.html

Victoria E. DeMoranville
Mark A. Best
Renee Laux, M.S.

Tumor removal

Definition

A tumor is an abnormal growth in the body that is caused by the uncontrolled division of cells. Benign tumors do not have the potential to spread to other parts of the body (a process called metastasis) and are curable by surgical removal. Malignant or cancerous tumors, however, may metastasize to other parts of the body and will ultimately result in **death** if not successfully treated by surgery and/or other methods.

Purpose

Surgical removal is one of four main ways that tumors are treated; the other treatment options include chemotherapy, radiation therapy, and biological therapy. There are a number of factors used to determine which methods will best treat a tumor. Because benign tumors do not have the potential to metastasize, they are often treated successfully with surgical removal alone. Malignant tumors, however, are most often treated with a combination of surgery and chemotherapy and/or radiation therapy (in about 55% of cases). In some instances, non-curative surgery may make other treatments more effective. Debulking a cancer—making it smaller by surgical removal of a large part of it—is thought to make radiation and chemotherapy more effective.

Surgery is often used to accurately assess the nature and extent of a cancer. Most cancers cannot be adequately identified without examining a sample of the abnormal tissue under a microscope. Such tissue samples are procured during a surgical procedure. Surgery may also be used to determine exactly how far a tumor has spread.

There are a few standard methods of comparing one cancer to another for the purposes of determining appropriate treatments and estimating outcomes. These methods are referred to as staging. The most commonly used method is the TNM system, including:

- "T" stands for tumor, and reflects the size of the tumor.
- "N" represents the spread of the cancer to lymph nodes, largely determined by those nodes removed at surgery that contain cancer cells. Since cancers spread mostly through the lymphatic system, this is a useful measure of a cancer's ability to disperse.
- "M" refers to metastasis, and indicates if metastases are present and how far they are from the original cancer.

Staging is particularly important with such lymphomas as Hodgkin's disease, which may appear in many places in the lymphatic system. Surgery is a useful tool for staging such cancers and can increase the chance of a successful cure, since radiation treatment is often curative if all the cancerous sites are located and irradiated.

Demographics

The American Cancer Society estimates that approximately 1.45 million cases of cancer are diagnosed in the United States each year. Seventy-eight

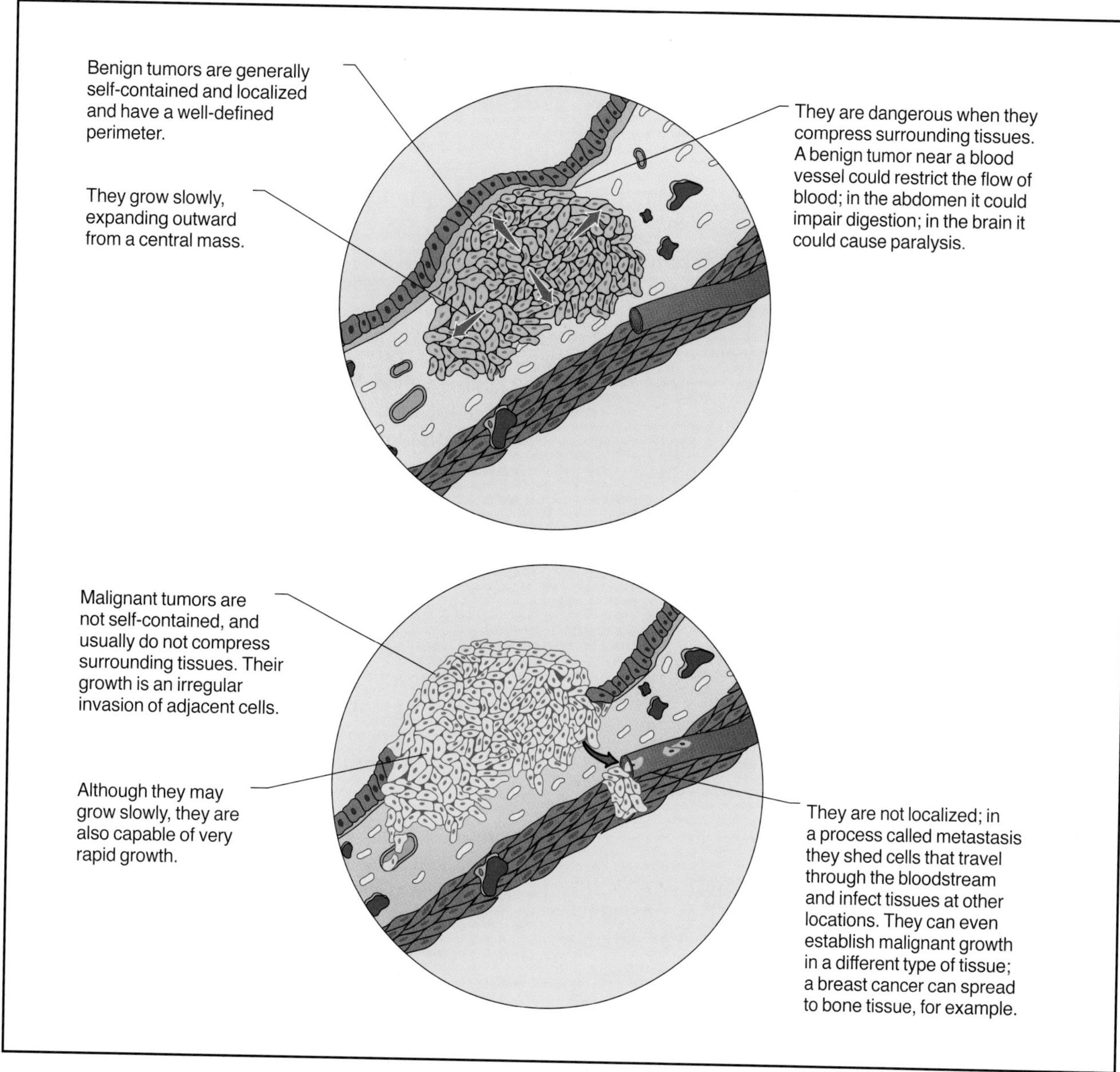

A comparison of benign (top of illustration) and malignant tumor characteristics. *(Illustration by Hans & Cassidy, Inc. Cengage Learning, Gale.)*

percent of cancers are diagnosed in men and women over the age of 55, although cancer may affect individuals of any age. Men develop cancer more often than women; one in two men will be diagnosed with cancer during his lifetime, compared to one in three women. Cancer affects individuals of all races and ethnicities, although incidence may differ among these groups by cancer type.

Description

Surgery may be used to remove tumors for diagnostic or therapeutic purposes.

Diagnostic tumor removal

A biopsy is a medical procedure that obtains a small piece of tissue for diagnostic testing. The sample is examined under a microscope by a doctor who specializes in the effects of disease on body tissues (a pathologist) to detect any abnormalities. A definitive diagnosis of cancer cannot be made unless a sample of the abnormal tissue is examined histologically (under a microscope).

There are four main biopsy techniques used to diagnose cancer, including:

KEY TERMS

Aspiration—A technique for obtaining a piece of tissue for biopsy by using suction applied through a needle attached to a syringe.

Biopsy—The removal of living tissue from the body, done in order to establish a diagnosis.

Debulking—Surgical removal of a major portion of a tumor so that there is less of the cancer left for later treatment by chemotherapy or radiation.

Mammogram—A set of x rays taken of the front and side of the breast; used to diagnose various abnormalities of the breast.

Metastasis (plural, metastases)—A growth of cancer cells at a site in the body distant from the primary tumor.

Oncologist—A physician who specializes in the diagnosis and treatment of tumors.

Palliative—Offering relief of symptoms, but not a cure.

Pap test—The common term for the Papanicolaou test, a simple smear method of examining stained cells to detect cancer of the cervix.

Staging—The classification of cancerous tumors according to the extent of the tumor.

- Aspiration biopsy. A needle is inserted into the tumor and a sample is withdrawn. This procedure may be performed under local anesthesia or with no anesthesia at all.
- Needle biopsy. A special cutting needle is inserted into the core of the tumor and a core sample is cut out. Local anesthesia is most often administered.
- Incisional biopsy. A portion of a large tumor is removed, usually under local anesthesia in an outpatient setting.
- Excisional biopsy. An entire cancerous lesion is removed along with surrounding normal tissue (called a clear margin). Local or general anesthesia may be used.

Therapeutic tumor removal

Once surgical removal has been decided, a surgical oncologist will remove the entire tumor, taking with it a large section of the surrounding normal tissue. The healthy tissue is removed to minimize the risk that abnormal tissue is left behind. Tumors may be removed by cutting with steel instruments, by the use of a laser beam, by radiofrequency ablation (the use of radiofrequency energy to destroy tissue), by cryoablation (the use of extreme cold to freeze and thus destroy the tumor), or by injecting alcohol into the tumor.

When surgical removal of a tumor is unacceptable as a sole treatment, a portion of the tumor is removed to debulk the mass; this process is called cytoreduction. Cytoreductive surgery aids radiation and chemotherapy treatments by increasing the sensitivity of the tumor and decreasing the number of necessary treatment cycles.

Certain types of skin tumors can be removed by a technique called Mohs micrographic surgery, developed in the late 1930s by Dr. Frederick E. Mohs. The Mohs method involves four steps: surgical removal of the tumor; making a slide of the removed tissue and examining it for cancer cells (called mapping the tissue); interpreting the microscope slides and removing more tissue if necessary until no more cancer cells are found; and performing **reconstructive surgery** to cover the wound.

A newer technique for removing some tumors of the spinal cord involves the use of a suction tip rather than a scalpel. The newer technique appears to have a wider margin of safety when working around the delicate structures of the central nervous system.

In some instances, the purpose of tumor removal is not to cure the cancer, but to relieve the symptoms of a patient who cannot be cured. This approach is called palliative surgery. For example, a patient with advanced cancer may have a tumor causing significant pain or bleeding; in such a case, the tumor may be removed to ease the patient's pain or other symptoms even though a cure is not possible.

Seeding

The surgical removal of malignant tumors demands special considerations. There is a danger of spreading cancerous cells during the process of removing abnormal tissue (called seeding). Presuming that cancer cells can implant elsewhere in the body, the surgeon must minimize the dissemination of cells throughout the operating field or into the bloodstream.

Special techniques called block resection and no-touch are used. Block resection involves taking the entire specimen out as a single piece. The no-touch technique involves removing a specimen by handling only the normal tissue surrounding it; the cancer itself is never touched. These approaches prevent the spread of cancer cells into the general circulation. The surgeon takes great care to clamp off the blood supply

WHO PERFORMS THE PROCEDURE AND WHERE IS IT PERFORMED?

Tumors are usually removed by a general surgeon or surgical oncologist. The procedure is frequently done in a hospital setting, but specialized outpatient facilities may sometimes be used.

first, preventing cells from leaving by that route later in the surgery.

Diagnosis/Preparation

A tumor may first be palpated (felt) by the patient or by a healthcare professional during a **physical examination**. A tumor may be visible on the skin or protrude outward from the body. Still other tumors are not evident until their presence begins to cause such symptoms as weight loss, fatigue, or pain. In some instances, tumors are located during routine tests (e.g., a yearly mammogram or Pap smear).

Aftercare

Retesting and periodical examinations are necessary to ensure that a tumor has not returned or metastasized after total removal.

Risks

Each tumor removal surgery carries certain risks that are inherent to the procedure. There is always a risk of misdiagnosing a cancer if an inadequate sample was procured during biopsy, or if the tumor was not properly located. There is a chance of infection of the surgical site, excessive bleeding, or injury to adjacent tissues. The possibility of metastasis and seeding are risks that have to be considered in consultation with an oncologist.

Normal results

The results of a tumor removal procedure depend on the type of tumor and the purpose of the treatment. Most benign tumors can be removed successfully with no risk of the abnormal cells spreading to other parts of the body and little risk of the tumor returning. Malignant tumors are considered successfully removed if the entire tumor can be removed, if a clear margin of healthy tissue is removed with the tumor, and if there is no evidence of metastasis. The normal results of palliative tumor removal are a reduction in the patient's symptoms with no impact on length of survival.

QUESTIONS TO ASK THE DOCTOR

- What type of tumor do I have and where is it located?
- What procedure will be used to remove the tumor?
- Is there evidence that the tumor has metastasized?
- What diagnostic tests will be performed prior to tumor removal?
- What method of anesthesia/pain relief will be used during the procedure?

Morbidity and mortality rates

The recurrence rates of benign and malignant tumors after removal depend on the type of tumor and its location. The rate of complications associated with tumor removal surgery differs by procedure, but is generally very low.

Alternatives

If a benign tumor shows no indication of harming nearby tissues and is not causing the patient any symptoms, surgery may not be required to remove it. Chemotherapy, radiation therapy, and biological therapy are treatments that may be used alone or in conjunction with surgery.

Resources

BOOKS

Abeloff, Martin D., James O. Armitage, Allen S. Lichter, and John E. Niederhuber. "Cancer Management." *Clinical Oncology*, 3rd ed. Philadelphia, PA: Elsevier Churchill Livingstone, Inc., 2004.

"Principles of Cancer Therapy: Surgery." Section 11, Chapter 144 in *The Merck Manual of Diagnosis and Therapy*, edited by Mark H. Beers, MD, and Robert Berkow, MD. Whitehouse Station, NJ: Merck Research Laboratories, 1999.

Townsend, Courtney M., Jr., et al, eds. *Sabiston Textbook of Surgery: The Biological Basis of Modern Surgical Practice*, 18th ed. Philadelphia: Saunders/Elsevier, 2008.

PERIODICALS

Amersi, F. F., A. McElrath-Garza, A. Ahmad, et al. "Long-Term Survival after Radiofrequency Ablation of Complex Unresectable Liver Tumors." *Archives of Surgery* 141 (June 2006): 581–587.

Atwell, T. D., J. W. Charboneau, F. G. Que, et al. "Treatment of Neuroendocrine Cancer Metastatic to the Liver: The Role of Ablative Techniques." *Cardiovascular and Interventional Radiology* 28 (July–August 2005): 409–421.

Bachmann, A., and R. Ruszat. "The KTP-(Greenlight-) Laser—Principles and Experiences." *Minimally Invasive Therapy and Allied Technologies* 16 (2007): 5–10.

Fahrner, L. J., III. "Mohs Micrographic Surgery for Mucocutaneous Malignancies." *Oral and Maxillofacial Surgery Clinics of North America* 17 (May 2005): 161–171.

LeFranc, F., and J. Brotchi. "Performance of a New Type of Suction Tip Attachment during Intramedullary Tumor Dissection: Technical Note." *Neurosurgery* 61 (November 2007): E241.

Paleri, V., F. W. Stafford, and M. S. Sammut. "Laser Debulking in Malignant Upper Airway Obstruction." *Head and Neck* 27 (April 2005): 296–301.

ORGANIZATIONS

American Cancer Society. 1599 Clifton Rd. NE, Atlanta, GA 30329-4251. (800) 227-2345. http://www.cancer.org (accessed April 14, 2008).

National Cancer Institute (NCI). NCI Public Inquiries Office, Suite 3036A, 6116 Executive Boulevard, MSC8332, Bethesda, MD 20892-8322. (800) 4-CANCER or (800) 332-8615 (TTY). http://www.nci.nih.gov (accessed April 14, 2008).

Society of Surgical Oncology. 85 West Algonquin Rd., Suite 550, Arlington Heights, IL 60005. (847) 427-1400. http://www.surgonc.org (accessed April 14, 2008).

OTHER

American Cancer Society. *All About Cancer: Detailed Guide*, 2008 [cited January 14, 2008]. http://www.cancer.org/docroot/CRI/CRI_2_3x.asp?dt=72 (accessed April 14, 2008).

J. Ricker Polsdorfer, MD
Stephanie Dionne Sherk
Rebecca Frey, PhD

TURP *see* **Transurethral resection of the prostate**

Tylenol *see* **Acetaminophen**

Tympanoplasty

Definition

Tympanoplasty, also called eardrum repair, refers to surgery performed to reconstruct a perforated tympanic membrane (eardrum) or the small bones of the middle ear. Eardrum perforation may result from chronic infection or, less commonly, from trauma to the eardrum.

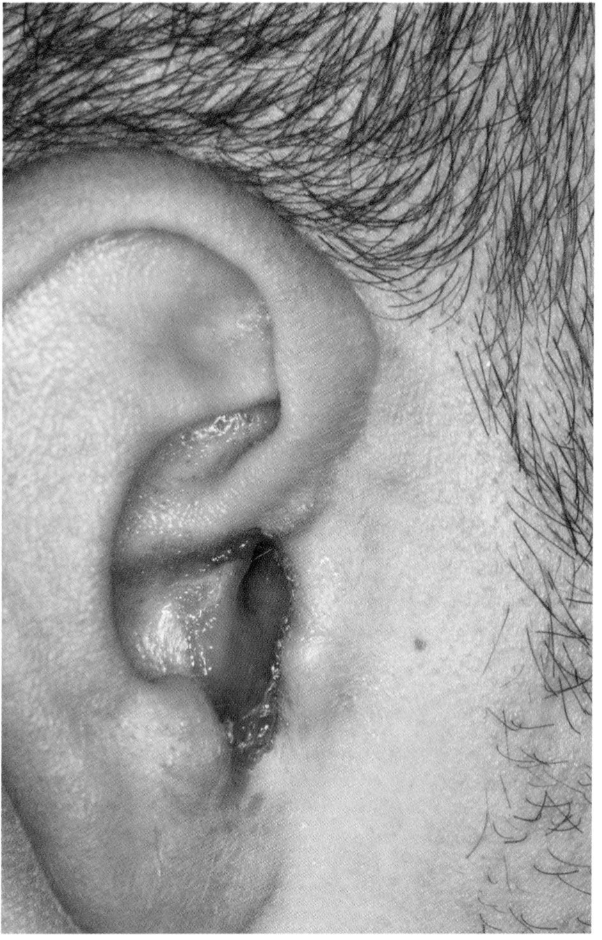

Yellowish discharge from the ear of an adult with past tympanoplasty. *(Pulse Picture Library/CMP Images/Phototake. Reproduced by permission.)*

Purpose

The tympanic membrane of the ear is a three-layer structure. The outer and inner layers consist of epithelium cells. Perforations occur as a result of defects in the middle layer, which contains elastic collagen fibers. Small perforations usually heal spontaneously. However, if the defect is relatively large, or if there is a poor blood supply or an infection during the healing process, spontaneous repair may be hindered. Eardrums may also be perforated as a result of trauma, such as an object in the ear, a slap on the ear, or an explosion.

The purpose of tympanoplasty is to repair the perforated eardrum, and sometimes the middle ear bones (ossicles) that consist of the incus, malleus, and stapes. Tympanic membrane grafting may be required. If needed, grafts are usually taken from a vein or fascia

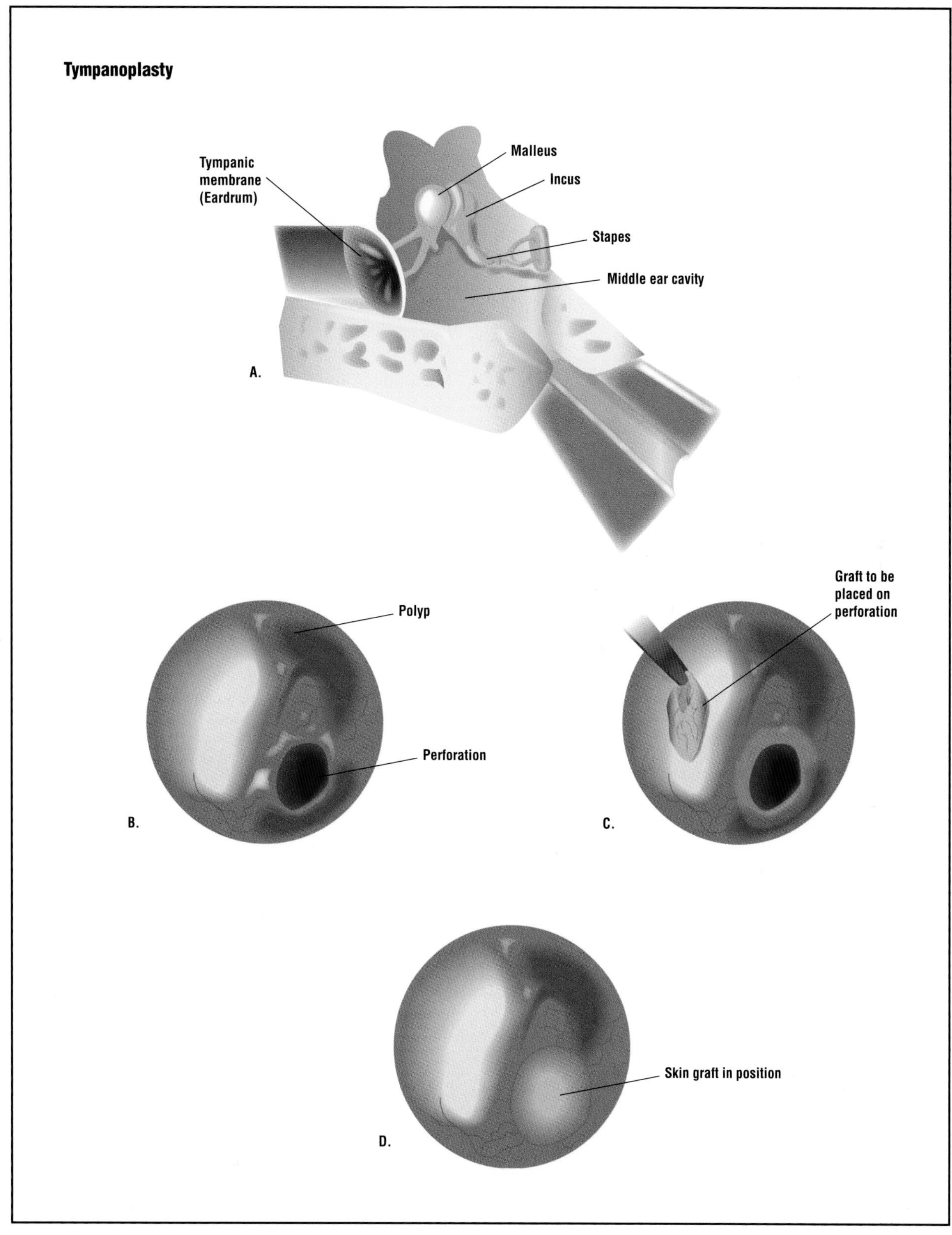

The tympanic membrane, or ear drum, may need surgical repair when punctured (A). During a type I tympanoplasty, a perforation in the eardrum is visualized (B). A tissue graft is placed over the perforation (C) and held in place by the existing eardrum (D) *(Illustration by GGS Information Services. Cengage Learning, Gale.)*

(muscle sheath) tissue on the lobe of the ear. Synthetic materials may be used if patients have had previous surgeries and have limited graft availability.

Demographics

In the United States, ear disorders leading to hearing loss affect all ages. Over 60% of the population with hearing loss is under the age of 65, although nearly 25% of those above age 65 have a hearing loss that is considered significant. Causes include: birth defect (4.4%), ear infection (12.2%), ear injury (4.9%), damage due to excessive noise levels (33.7%), advanced age (28%), and other problems (16.8%).

Description

There are five basic types of tympanoplasty procedures:

- Type I tympanoplasty is called myringoplasty and involves the restoration of the perforated eardrum by grafting.
- Type II tympanoplasty is used for tympanic membrane perforations with erosion of the malleus. It involves grafting onto the incus or the remains of the malleus.
- Type III tympanoplasty is indicated for destruction of two ossicles, with the stapes still intact and mobile. It involves placing a graft onto the stapes, and providing protection for the assembly.
- Type IV tympanoplasty is used for ossicular destruction, which includes all or part of the stapes arch. It involves placing a graft onto or around a mobile stapes footplate.
- Type V tympanoplasty is used when the footplate of the stapes is fixed.

Depending on its type, tympanoplasty can be performed under local or **general anesthesia**. In small perforations of the eardrum, Type I tympanoplasty can be easily performed under **local anesthesia** with intravenous sedation. An incision is made into the ear canal and the remaining eardrum is elevated away from the bony ear canal, and lifted forward. The surgeon uses an operating microscope to enlarge the view of the ear structures. If the perforation is very large or the hole is far forward and away from the view of the surgeon, it may be necessary to perform an incision behind the ear. This elevates the entire outer ear forward, providing access to the perforation. Once the hole is fully exposed, the perforated remnant is rotated forward, and the bones of hearing are inspected. If scar tissue is present, it is removed either with micro hooks or laser.

KEY TERMS

Audiogram—A test of hearing at a range of sound frequencies.

Epithelium—The covering of internal and external surfaces of the body, including the lining of vessels and other small cavities. It consists of cells joined by small amounts of cementing substances.

Fistula test—Compression or rarefaction of the air in the external auditory canal.

Mastoid process—The nipple-like projection of part of the temporal bone (the large irregular bone situated in the base and side of the skull).

Mastoidectomy—Hollowing out the mastoid process by curretting, gouging, drilling, or otherwise removing the bony partitions forming the mastoid cells.

Myringoplasty—Surgical restoration of a perforated tympanic membrane by grafting.

Ossicles—Small bones of the middle ear, called stapes, malleus, and incus.

Ossiculoplasty—Surgical insertion of an implant to replace one or more of the ear ossicles. Also called ossicular replacement.

Otoscopy—Examination of the ear with an otoscope, an instrument designed to evaluate the condition of the ear.

Tinnitus—Noises or ringing in the ear.

Tissue is then taken either from the back of the ear, the tragus (small cartilaginous lobe of skin in front the ear), or from a vein. The tissues are thinned and dried. An absorbable gelatin sponge is placed under the eardrum to support the graft. The graft is then inserted underneath the remaining eardrum remnant, which is folded back onto the perforation to provide closure. Very thin sheeting is usually placed against the top of the graft to prevent it from sliding out of the ear when the patient sneezes.

If it was opened from behind, the ear is then stitched together. Usually, the **stitches** are buried in the skin and do not have to be removed later. A sterile patch is placed on the outside of the ear canal and the patient returns to the **recovery room**.

Diagnosis/Preparation

The examining physician performs a complete physical with diagnostic testing of the ear, which includes an audiogram and history of the hearing loss, as well as any vertigo or facial weakness. A microscopic exam is also performed. Otoscopy is used to assess the mobility of the tympanic membrane and the malleus. A fistula test can be performed if there is a history of dizziness or a marginal perforation of the eardrum.

Preparation for surgery depends upon the type of tympanoplasty. For all procedures, however; blood and urine studies, and hearing tests are conducted prior to surgery.

Aftercare

Generally, the patient can return home within two to three hours. **Antibiotics** are given, along with a mild pain reliever. After 10 days, the packing is removed and the ear is evaluated to see if the graft was successful. Water is kept away from the ear, and nose blowing is discouraged. If there are allegies or a cold, antibiotics and a decongestant are usually prescribed. Most patients can return to work after five or six days, or two to three weeks if they perform heavy physical labor. After three weeks, all packing is completely removed under the operating microscope. It is then determined whether or not the graft has been completely successful.

Postoperative care is also designed to keep the patient comfortable. Infection is generally prevented by soaking the ear canal with antibiotics. To heal, the graft must be kept free from infection, and must not experience shearing forces or excessive tension. Activities that change the tympanic pressure are forbidden, such as sneezing with the mouth shut, using a straw to drink, or heavy nose blowing. A complete hearing test is performed four to six weeks after the operation.

Risks

Possible complications include failure of the graft to heal, causing recurrent eardrum perforation; narrowing (stenosis) of the ear canal; scarring or adhesions in the middle ear; perilymph fistula and hearing loss; erosion or extrusion of the prosthesis; dislocation of the prosthesis; and facial nerve injury. Other problems such as recurrence of cholesteatoma, may or may not result from the surgery.

Tinnitus (noises in the ear), particularly echo-type noises, may be present as a result of the perforation itself. Usually, with improvement in hearing and closure of the eardrum, the tinnitus resolves. In some cases, however, it may worsen after the operation. It is rare for the tinnitus to be permanent after surgery.

WHO PERFORMS THE PROCEDURE AND WHERE IS IT PERFORMED?

Tympanoplasty is usually performed on an outpatient basis by an otolaryngologist, a physician specialized in the diagnosis and treatment of disorders and diseases of the ears, nose, and throat. For most adults, Type I tympanoplasty is performed in the office of the otolaryngologist with topical anesthesia at the tympanic membrane site, and subcutaneous local anesthesia injection at the graft donor site. An overnight stay is recommended if the the tympanoplasty involves ossicular replacement.

Normal results

Tympanoplasty is successful in over 90% of cases. In most cases, the operation relieves pain and infection symptoms completely. Hearing loss is minor.

Morbidity and mortality rates

There can be imbalance and dizziness immediately after this procedure. Dizziness, however, is uncommon in tympanoplasties that only involve the eardrum. Besides failure of the graft, there may be further hearing loss due to unexplained factors during the healing process. This occurs in less than 5% of patients. A total hearing loss from tympanoplasty surgery is rare, occurring in less than 1% of operations. Mild postoperative dizziness and imbalance can persist for about a week after surgery. If the ear becomes infected after surgery, the risk of dizziness increases. Generally, imbalance and dizziness completely disappears after a week or two.

Alternatives

Myringoplasty is another operative procedure used in the reconstruction of a perforation of the tympanic membrane. It is performed when the middle ear space, its mucosa, and the ossicular chain are free of active infection. Unlike tympanoplasty, there is no direct inspection of the middle ear during this procedure.

Resources

BOOKS

Fisch, H. and J. May. *Tympanoplasty, Mastoidectomy, and Stapes Surgery*. New York: Thieme Medical Pub., 1994.

Roland, P. S. *Tympanoplasty: Repair of the Tympanic Membrane*. Continuing Education Program (American

QUESTIONS TO ASK THE DOCTOR

- Are there any other options aside from tympanoplasty?
- How will the surgery impact hearing?
- How long will it take to recover from the surgery?
- What are the possible complications?
- How many tympanoplasty surgeries does the surgeon perform each year?
- How successful is tympanoplasty in restoring normal hearing?

Academy of Otolaryngology-Head and Neck Surgery Foundation). Alexandria, VA: American Academy of Otolaryngology, 1994.

Tos, M. *Manual of Middle Ear Surgery: Approaches, Myringoplasty, Ossiculoplasty and Tympanoplasty*. New York: Thieme Medical Pub., 1993.

PERIODICALS

Downey, T. J., A. L. Champeaux, and A. B. Silva. "AlloDerm Tympanoplasty of Tympanic Membrane Perforations." *American Journal of Otolaryngology* 24 (January/February 2003): 6-13.

Duckert, L. G., K. H. Makielski, and J. Helms. "Prolonged Middle Ear Ventilation with the Cartilage Shield T-tube Tympanoplasty." *Otology & Neurotology* 24 (March 2003): 153-7.

Oshima, T., Y. Kasuya, Y. Okumura, E. Terazawa, and S. Dohi. "Prevention of Nausea and Vomiting with Tandospirone in Adults after Tympanoplasty." *Anesthesia & Analgesia* 95 (November 2002): 350-1.

Sheahan, P., T. O'Dwyer, and A. Blayney. "Results of Type 1 Tympanoplasty in Children and Parental Perceptions of Outcome of Surgery." *Journal of Laryngology & Otology* 116 (June 2002): 430-4.

Uzun, C., M. Velepic, D. Manestar, D. Bonifacic, and T. Braut. "Cartilage Palisade Tympanoplasty, Diving and Eustachian Tube Function." *Otology & Neurotology* 24 (March 2003): 350-1.

ORGANIZATIONS

American Hearing Research Foundation. 55 E. Washington St., Suite 2022, Chicago, IL 60602. (312) 726-9670. http://www.american-hearing.org/

American Academy of Otolaryngology - Head and Neck Surgery. One Prince Street, Alexandria, VA 22314. (703) 806-4444. www.entnet.org.

OTHER

"Perforated Ear Drums." *Audiology Net*. www.voice-center.com/tmperf.html.

Tympanoplasty animation. *Otolaryngology Houston:* www.ghorayeb.com/TympanoplastyPictures.html.

"What is Tympanoplasty?" *PennHealth*. www.pennhealth.com/health/hi_files/balance/hi13.html.

Monique Laberge, Ph.D.

Type and screen

Definition

Blood typing is a laboratory test that identifies blood group antigens (substances that stimulate an immune response) belonging to the ABO blood group system. The test classifies blood into four groups designated A, B, AB, and O. Antibody screening is a test to detect atypical antibodies in the serum that may have been formed as a result of **transfusion** or pregnancy. An antibody is a protein produced by lymphocytes (nongranular white blood cells) that binds to an antigen, facilitating its removal by phagocytosis (or engulfing by macrophages) or lysis (cell rupture or decomposition). The type and screen (T&S) is performed on persons who may need a transfusion of blood products. These tests are followed by the compatibility test (cross-match). This test insures that no antibodies are detected in the recipient's serum that will react with the donor's red blood cells.

Purpose

Blood typing and screening are most commonly performed to ensure that a person who needs a transfusion will receive blood that matches (is compatible with) his or her own; and that clinically significant antibodies are identified if present. People must receive blood of the same blood type; otherwise, a severe transfusion reaction may result.

Prenatal care

Parents who are expecting a baby have their blood typed to diagnose and prevent hemolytic disease of the newborn (HDN), a type of anemia also known as erythroblastosis fetalis. Babies who have a blood type different from their mother's are at risk for developing this disease.

Determination of paternity

A child inherits factors or genes from each parent that determine his or her blood type. This fact makes blood typing useful in paternity testing. The blood

KEY TERMS

ABO blood type—Blood type based on the presence or absence of the A and B antigens on the red blood cells. There are four types: A, B, AB, and O.

Acute hemolytic transfusion reaction (AHTR)—A severe transfusion reaction with abrupt onset, most often caused by ABO incompatibility. Symptoms include difficulty breathing, fever and chills, pain, and sometimes shock.

Antibody—A protein produced by B-lymphocytes that binds to an antigen facilitating its removal by phagocytosis or lysis.

Antigen—Any substance that stimulates the production of antibodies and combines specifically with them.

Autologous donation—Donation of the patient's own blood, made several weeks before elective surgery.

Blood bank—A laboratory that specializes in blood typing, antibody identification, and transfusion services.

Blood type—Any of various classes into which human blood can be divided according to immunological compatibility based on the presence or absence of certain antigens on the red blood cells. Blood types are sometimes called blood groups.

Cross-match—A laboratory test done to confirm that blood from a donor and blood from the recipient are compatible. Serum from each is mixed with red blood cells from the other and observed for hemagglutination.

Ectopic pregnancy—The implantation of a fertilized egg in a woman's fallopian tube instead of the uterus.

Gene—A piece of DNA, located on a chromosome, that determines how such traits as blood type are inherited and expressed.

Hemagglutination—The clumping of red blood cells due to blood type incompatibility.

Hematocrit—The proportion of the volume of a blood sample that consists of red blood cells. It is expressed as a percentage.

Indirect Coombs' test—A test used to screen for unexpected antibodies against red blood cells. The patient's serum is mixed with reagent red blood cells, incubated, washed, tested with antihuman globulin, and observed for clumping.

Lysis—Destruction or decomposition.

Pathologist—A doctor who specializes in the study of diseases. The ABO blood groups were discovered by an Austrian pathologist.

Rh blood type—In general, refers to the blood type based on the presence or absence of the D antigen on the red blood cells. There are, however, other antigens in the Rh system.

Serum (plural, sera)—The clear, pale yellow liquid that separates from a clot when blood coagulates.

Tourniquet—A thin piece of tubing or other device used to stop bleeding or control circulation by compressing the blood vessels in an arm or leg. Health care professionals apply a tourniquet before drawing blood.

Transfusion—The therapeutic introduction of blood or a blood component into a patient's bloodstream.

types of the child, mother, and alleged father are compared to determine paternity.

Forensic investigations

Legal investigations may require typing of blood or such other body fluids as semen or saliva to identify criminal suspects. In some cases typing is used to identify the victims of crime or major disasters.

Description

Blood typing and screening tests are performed in a blood bank laboratory by technologists trained in blood bank and transfusion services. The tests are performed on blood after it has been separated into cells and serum (the yellow liquid left after the blood cells are removed). Costs for both tests are covered by insurance when the tests are determined to be medically necessary.

Blood bank laboratories are usually located in blood center facilities, such as those operated by the American Red Cross, that collect, process, and supply blood that is donated. Blood bank laboratories are also found in most hospitals and other facilities that prepare blood for transfusion. These laboratories are regulated by the United States Food and Drug Administration (FDA) and are inspected and accredited by a professional association such as the American Association of Blood Banks (AABB).

Blood typing and screening tests are based on the reaction between antigens and antibodies. An antigen can be anything that triggers the body's immune response. The body produces a special protein called an antibody that has a uniquely shaped site that combines with the antigen to neutralize it. A person's body normally does not produce antibodies against its own antigens.

The antigens found on the surface of red blood cells are important because they determine a person's blood type. When red blood cells having a certain blood type antigen are mixed with serum containing antibodies against that antigen, the antibodies combine with and stick to the antigen. In a test tube, this reaction is visible as clumping or aggregating.

Although there are over 600 known red blood cell antigens organized into 22 blood group systems, routine blood typing is usually concerned with only two systems: the ABO and Rh blood group systems. Antibody screening helps to identify antibodies against several other groups of red blood cell antigens.

Blood typing

THE ABO BLOOD GROUP SYSTEM. In 1901, Karl Landsteiner, an Austrian pathologist, randomly combined the serum and red blood cells of his colleagues. From the reactions he observed in test tubes, he developed the ABO blood group system, which earned him the 1930 Nobel Prize in Medicine. A person's ABO blood type—A, B, AB, or O—is based on the presence or absence of the A and B antigens on his red blood cells. The A blood type has only the A antigen and the B blood type has only the B antigen. The AB blood type has both A and B antigens, and the O blood type has neither the A nor the B antigen.

By the time a person is six months old, he or she will have developed antibodies against the antigens that his or her red blood cells lack. That is, a person with A blood type will have anti-B antibodies, and a person with B blood type will have anti-A antibodies. A person with AB blood type will have neither antibody, but a person with O blood type will have both anti-A and anti-B antibodies. Although the distribution of each of the four ABO blood types varies among racial groups, O is the most common and AB is the least common in all groups.

FORWARD AND REVERSE TYPING. ABO typing is the first test done on blood when it is tested for transfusion. A person must receive ABO-matched blood because ABO incompatibilities are the major cause of fatal transfusion reactions. To guard against these incompatibilities, typing is done in two steps. In the first step, called forward typing, the patient's blood is mixed with serum that contains antibodies against type A blood, then with serum that contains antibodies against type B blood. A determination of the blood type is based on whether or not the blood clots in the presence of these sera.

In reverse typing, the patient's blood serum is mixed with blood that is known to be type A and type B. Again, the presence of clotting is used to determine the type.

An ABO incompatibility between a pregnant woman and her baby is a common cause of HDN but seldom requires treatment. This is because the majority of ABO antibodies are IgM, which are too large to cross the placenta. It is the IgG component that may cause HDN, and this is most often present in the plasma of group O mothers.

Paternity testing compares the ABO blood types of the child, mother, and alleged father. The alleged father cannot be the biological father if the child's blood type requires a gene that neither he nor the mother have. For example, a child with blood type B whose mother has blood type O requires a father with either AB or B blood type; a man with blood type O cannot be the biological father.

In some people, ABO antigens can be detected in body fluids other than blood, such as saliva, sweat, or semen. People whose body fluids contain detectable amounts of antigens are known as secretors. ABO typing of these fluids provides clues in legal investigations.

THE RH BLOOD GROUP SYSTEM. The Rh, or Rhesus, system was first detected in 1940 by Landsteiner and Wiener when they injected blood from rhesus monkeys into guinea pigs and rabbits. More than 50 antigens have since been discovered that belong to this system, making it the most complex red blood cell antigen system.

In routine blood typing and cross-matching tests, only one of these 50 antigens, the D antigen, also known as the Rh factor or Rh_o[D], is tested for. If the D antigen is present, that person is Rh-positive; if the D antigen is absent, that person is Rh-negative.

Other important antigens in the Rh system are C, c, E, and e. These antigens are not usually tested for in routine blood typing tests. Testing for the presence of these antigens, however, is useful in paternity testing, and in cases in which a technologist screens blood to identify unexpected Rh antibodies or find matching blood for a person with antibodies to one or more of these antigens.

Unlike the ABO system, antibodies to Rh antigens don't develop naturally. They develop only as an immune response after a transfusion or during pregnancy. The incidence of the Rh blood types varies between racial groups, but not as widely as the ABO blood types: 85% of whites and 90% of blacks are Rh-positive; 15% of whites and 10% of blacks are Rh-negative.

The distribution of ABO and Rh blood groups in the overall United States population is as follows:

- O Rh-positive, 38%
- O Rh-negative, 7%
- A Rh-positive, 34%
- A Rh-negative, 6%
- B Rh-positive, 9%
- B Rh-negative, 2%
- AB Rh-positive, 3%
- AB Rh-negative, 1%

In transfusions, the Rh system is next in importance after the ABO system. Most Rh-negative people who receive Rh-positive blood will develop anti-D antibodies. A later transfusion of Rh-positive blood may result in a severe or fatal transfusion reaction.

Rh incompatibility is the most common and severe cause of HDN. This incompatibility may occur when an Rh-negative mother and an Rh-positive father have an Rh-positive baby. Cells from the baby can cross the placenta and enter the mother's bloodstream, causing the mother to make anti-D antibodies. Unlike ABO antibodies, the structure of anti-D antibodies makes it likely that they will cross the placenta and enter the baby's bloodstream. There, they can destroy the baby's red blood cells, causing a severe or fatal anemia.

The first step in preventing HDN is to find out the Rh types of the expectant parents. If the mother is Rh-negative and the father is Rh-positive, the baby is at risk for developing HDN. The next step is performing an antibody screen of the mother's serum to make sure she doesn't already have anti-D antibodies from a previous pregnancy or transfusion. Finally, the Rh-negative mother is given an injection of Rh immunoglobulin (RhIg) at 28 weeks of gestation and again after delivery, if the baby is Rh positive. The RhIg attaches to any Rh-positive cells from the baby in the mother's bloodstream, preventing them from triggering anti-D antibody production in the mother. An Rh-negative woman should also receive RhIg following a miscarriage, abortion, or ectopic pregnancy.

OTHER BLOOD GROUP SYSTEMS. Several other blood group systems may be involved in HDN and transfusion reactions, although they are much less common than ABO and Rh incompatibilities. Some of the other groups are the Duffy, Kell, Kidd, MNS, and P systems. Tests for antigens from these systems are not included in routine blood typing, but they are commonly used in paternity testing.

Like Rh antibodies, antibodies in these systems do not develop naturally, but as an immune response after transfusion or during pregnancy. An antibody screening test is done before a cross-match to check for unexpected antibodies to antigens in these systems. A person's serum is mixed in a test tube with commercially prepared cells containing antigens from these systems. If hemagglutination, or clumping, occurs, the antibody is identified.

Antibody screening

Antibody screening is done to look for unexpected antibodies to other blood groups, such as certain Rh (e.g. E, e, C, c), Duffy, MNS, Kell, Kidd, and P system antigens. The recipient's serum is mixed with screening reagent red blood cells. The screening reagent red blood cells are cells with known antigens. This test is sometimes called an indirect antiglobulin or Coombs test. If an antibody to an antigen is present, the mixture will cause agglutination (clumping) of the red blood cells or cause hemolysis (breaking of the red cell membrane). If an antibody to one of these antigens is found, only blood without that antigen will be compatible in a cross-match. This sequence must be repeated before each transfusion a person receives.

Testing for infectious disease markers

As of 2003, pretransfusion testing includes analyzing blood for the following infectious disease markers:

- Hepatitis B surface antigen (HBsAg). This test detects the outer envelope of the heptatitis B virus.
- Antibodies to the core of the hepatitis B virus (Anti-HBc). This test detects an antibody to the hepatitis B virus that is produced during and after an infection.
- Antibodies to the hepatitis C virus (Anti-HCV).
- Antibodies to human immunodeficiency virus, types 1 and 2 (Anti-HIV-1, -2).
- HIV-1 p24 antigen. This test screens for antigens of HIV-1. The advantage of this test is that it can detect HIV-1 infection a week earlier than the antibody test.
- Antibodies to human T-lymphotropic virus, types I and II (Anti-HTLV-I, -II). In the United States, HTLV infection is most common among intravenous drug users.
- Syphilis. This test is performed to detect evidence of infection with the spirochete *Treponema pallidum*.

- Nucleic acid amplification testing (NAT). NAT uses a new form of blood testing technology that directly detects the genetic material of the HCV and HIV viruses.
- Confirmatory tests. These are done to screen out false positives.

Cross-matching

Cross-matching is the final step in pretransfusion testing. It is commonly referred to as compatibility testing, or "type and cross." Before blood from a donor and the recipient are cross-matched, both are ABO and Rh typed. To begin the cross-match, a unit of blood from a donor with the same ABO and Rh type as the recipient is selected. Serum from the patient is mixed with red blood cells from the donor. The cross-match can be performed either as a short (5–10 min) incubation intended only to verify ABO compatibility or as a long (45 min) incubation with an antihuman globulin test intended to verify compatibility for all other red cell antigens. If clumping occurs, the blood is not compatible; if clumping does not occur, the blood is compatible. If an unexpected antibody is found in either the patient or the donor, the blood bank does further testing to ensure that the blood is compatible.

In an emergency, when there is not enough time for blood typing and cross-matching, O red blood cells may be given, preferably Rh-negative. O-type blood is called the universal donor because it has no ABO antigens for a patient's antibodies to combine with. In contrast, AB blood type is called the universal recipient because it has no ABO antibodies to combine with the antigens on transfused red blood cells. If there is time for blood typing, red blood cells of the recipient type (type-specific cells) are given. In either case, the cross-match is continued even though the transfusion has begun.

Autologous donation

The practice of collecting a patient's own blood prior to **elective surgery** for later transfusion is called autologous donation. Since the safest blood for transfusion is the patient's own, autologous donation is particularly useful for patients with rare blood types. Two to four units of blood are collected several weeks before surgery, and the patient is given iron supplements to build up his or her hemoglobin levels.

Preparation

To collect the 10 mL of blood needed for these tests, a healthcare worker ties a tourniquet above the patient's elbow, locates a vein near the inner elbow, cleans the skin overlying the vein, and inserts a needle into that vein. The blood is drawn through the needle into an attached vacuum tube. Collection of the sample takes only a few minutes.

Blood typing and screening must be done three days or less before a transfusion. A person does not need to change diet, medications, or activities before these tests. Patients should tell their health care provider if they have received a blood transfusion or a plasma substitute during the last three months, or have had a radiology procedure using intravenous contrast media. These can give false clumping reactions in both typing and cross-matching tests.

Aftercare

The possible side effects of any blood collection are discomfort, bruising, or excessive bleeding at the site where the needle punctured the skin, as well as dizziness or fainting. Bruising and bleeding is reduced if pressure is applied with a finger to the puncture site until the bleeding stops. Discomfort can be treated with warm packs to the puncture site.

Risks

Aside from the rare event of infection or bleeding, there are no risks from blood collection. Blood transfusions, however, always have the risk of an unexpected transfusion reaction. These complications may include an acute hemolytic transfusion reaction (AHTR), which is most commonly caused by ABO incompatibility. The patient may complain of pain, difficult breathing, fever and chills, facial flushing, and nausea. Signs of shock may appear, including a drop in blood pressure and a rapid but weak pulse. If AHTR is suspected, the transfusion should be stopped at once.

Other milder transfusion reactions include a delayed hemolytic transfusion reaction, which may occur one to two weeks after the transfusion. It consists of a slight fever and a falling **hematocrit**, and is usually self-limited. Patients may also have allergic reactions to unknown components in donor blood.

Normal results

The blood type is labeled as A+, A–, B+, B–, O+, O–, AB+, or AB–, based on both the ABO and Rh systems. If antibody screening is negative, only a cross-match is necessary. If the antibody screen is positive, then blood that is negative for those antigens must be identified. The desired result of a cross-match is that compatible donor blood is found. Compatibility testing procedures are designed to provide the safest blood product possible for the recipient, but a compatible cross-match is no guarantee that an unexpected adverse reaction will not appear during the transfusion.

Except in an emergency, a person cannot receive a transfusion without a compatible cross-match result. In rare cases, the least incompatible blood has to be given.

Resources

BOOKS

Beadling, Wendy V., Laura Cooling, and John B. Henry. "Immunohematology." In *Clinical Diagnosis and Management by Laboratory Methods*, 20th ed., edited by John B. Henry. Philadelphia: W. B. Saunders Company, 2001.

Boral, Leonard I., Edward D. Weiss, and John B. Henry. "Transfusion Medicine." In *Clinical Diagnosis and Management by Laboratory Methods*, 20th ed. Edited by John B. Henry. Philadelphia: W. B. Saunders Company, 2001.

Daniels, Geoff. *Human Blood Groups*. Oxford, UK: Blackwell, 1995.

Issitt, Peter D. and David J. Anstee *Applied Blood Group Serology*, 4th ed. Durham, NC: Montgomery Scientific Publications, 1998.

Triulzi, Darrell J., ed. *Blood Transfusion Therapy: A Physician's Handbook*, 7th ed. Bethesda: American Association of Blood Banks, 2002.

ORGANIZATIONS

American Association of Blood Banks (AABB). 8101 Glenbrook Road, Bethesda, MD 20814. (301) 907-6977. www.aabb.org.

American College of Obstetricians and Gynecologists. 409 12th Street SW, Washington, DC 20024-2188. (202) 638-5577. www.acog.org.

American Red Cross Blood Services. 430 17th Street NW, Washington, DC 20006. (202) 737-8300. www.redcross.org.

OTHER

All About Blood. American Association of Blood Banks. June 2002. [cited April 7, 2003]. www.aabb.org/All_About_Blood/FAQs/aabb_faqs.htm.

Mark A. Best

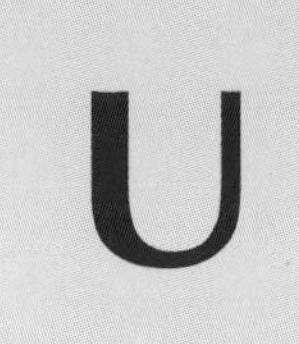

U

UGI *see* **Upper GI exam**

Ulcer surgery *see* **Vagotomy**

Ultrasonic lithotripsy *see* **Lithotripsy**

Ultrasound

Definition

Medical ultrasound imaging involves the use of high frequency sound waves to produce pictures of different parts of the inside of the body. This medical procedure is painless, safe, and non-invasive. Ultrasound imaging is not an X-ray as it uses sound waves and not ionizing radiation. Ultrasound images are unlike x-rays also in that they are done in "real time" and not just a picture taken at a single moment. Therefore, ultrasound imaging can help to show movement inside of body organs as well as the structure of the organs. Most people are familiar with ultrasound imaging being used during pregnancy to look safely and carefully at the developing fetus. There are also many other uses in medicine for ultrasound imaging.

The following are some other uses for medical ultrasound imaging:

- Cardiac ultrasound is used to diagnose problems with the heart and major blood vessels surrounding the heart.
- Ultrasound imaging in gynecology is used to diagnose problems with the female reproductive tract including being used to diagnose problems associated with infertility. Ultrasound is also used to monitor infertility treatments.
- Ultrasound imaging is used to look for problems with other internal organs, such as the gallbladder, bladder, testicles, liver, spleen, kidneys, and pancreas.
- Ultrasound imaging is also used to look for problems with glands, such as the thyroid.
- Vascular ultrasound imaging is used to watch the blood flow in blood vessels or blood flow to tumors. Ultrasound doppler imaging and color flow mapping can show the flow of blood.
- Ultrasound imaging is also used during medical procedures such as needle biopsies or egg retrieval during in vitro fertilization.

Purpose

The purpose of ultrasound imaging in medicine is to help the physician diagnose, monitor and treat medical conditions.

Precautions

The greatest precaution that should be taken when using ultrasound imaging to diagnose medical problems is the over and under diagnosing of problems by staff that is not properly trained, using poor equipment or not adequately supervised. This is especially true in the obstetrical setting where it is important to have properly trained ultrasound technicians (sonographers) to perform routine and advanced diagnostic ultrasound on a pregnant woman. The Society of Diagnostic Medical Sonography and the American Institute for Ultrasound in Medicine are great resources for helping to find certified sonographers from accredited programs.

Description

Ultrasound imaging is performed by using a transducer, which is a small device that the technician holds in his/her hand and is attached to a cord that connects to the ultrasound machine. The ultrasound machine has a keyboard, a computer, and a display screen. The patient is usually lying down on an examination table and clear gel (cold or warm) is applied to the area of the body that is to be imaged or scanned so that the transducer makes easy contact with the body and can easily be slid back and forth during the ultrasound. As the transducer is moved over that part of the body, it sends out high frequency sound waves, looks for the returning echo and instantly puts that image up onto the screen. An ultrasound examination is usually painless, however, on occasion, discomfort from the pressure being pressed on the body may occur, especially if the patient's bladder is full, or if the area being scanned is injured or tender. Sometimes ultrasound imaging is performed by using an ultrasound probe that is inserted into an area of the body, such as the vagina. Vaginal ultrasounds are used to scan for early pregnancy or to look carefully at the ovaries or guide the physician during procedures such as egg retrieval for in vitro fertilization. This ultrasound is not usually painful, but to some may be uncomfortable.

Preparation

Preparation for an ultrasound examination depends upon the area of the body that is to be scanned. For example during pregnancy, a patient may be instructed to drink water and not to empty her bladder prior to the ultrasound examination to help with visualization during the ultrasound. Other procedures may require no eating or drinking prior to the ultrasound examination. Comfortable, loose clothing should be worn, although a gown may be provided to be worn for the ultrasound examination. It is important to ask for and follow the instructions that are given prior to the ultrasound examination so that the procedure does not need to be rescheduled.

Aftercare

After the ultrasound, the gel is wiped off and the patient is usually able to return to normal activity. Usually, after the examination, the technician has the images reviewed by the physician and the physician may then speak to the patient at that time. Otherwise, the results are called to the patient or discussed at a later visit. On occasion, especially during pregnancy, the technician or physician will discuss the results of the ultrasound while the ultrasound is being performed. If an ultrasound examination shows abnormal results, those results may need to be followed-up with other tests or consultations to discuss possible treatment.

Risks

For routine diagnostic ultrasound imaging, there are no known risks to humans and therefore, if necessary it is safe to repeat the procedure as often as needed to monitor a particular health concern or treatment. For over 30 years, diagnostic ultrasound imaging has been used on pregnant women. A multitude of studies on the effects of ultrasound use during pregnancy have been reported and although there have been a number of small studies citing possible hearing problems, low birth-weight and left handedness, these studies have not been verified by larger studies. Overall, there has been no evidence that ultrasound is harmful to a developing fetus, however, the medical community should be diligent about preventing unnecessary use of ultrasound in pregnancy.

Resources

BOOKS

Nyberg, David A., JP McGahan, D. Pretorius, G. Pilu. *Diagnostic Imaging of Fetal Anomalies*. 2 Sub ed.: Lippincott, Williams and Wilkins, 2002.

ORGANIZATIONS

American Institute of Ultrasound in Medicine, 14750 Sweitzer Lane, Suite 100, Laurel, MD 20707. (301)498-4100. http://www.aium.org/.

Society of Diagnostic Medical Sonography, 2745 Dallas Parkway Suite 350, Plano, TX 75093. (214)-473-8057. http://www.sdms.org/.

OTHER

Medline Plus, a service of the National Library of Medicine and the National Institutes of Health, 8600 Rockville Pike, Bethesda, MD 20894. http://www.nlm.nih.gov/medlineplus/ency/article/003336.htm

Renee Laux, M.S.

Umbilical hernia repair

Definition

An umbilical hernia repair is a surgical procedure performed to fix a weakness in the abdominal wall or to close an opening near the umbilicus (navel) that has allowed abdominal contents to protrude. The abdominal contents may or may not be contained within a membrane or sac. The medical name for a hernia repair is herniorraphy.

Purpose

Umbilical hernias are usually repaired either to relieve discomfort or to prevent complications. It is not always necessary to fix an umbilical hernia. If the person is not in pain, the hernia is often not repaired. Complications may develop if pressure inside the abdomen resulting from daily activity pushes the abdominal contents further through the opening. They may then become twisted or strangulated. Strangulation is a condition in which the circulation to a section of the intestine

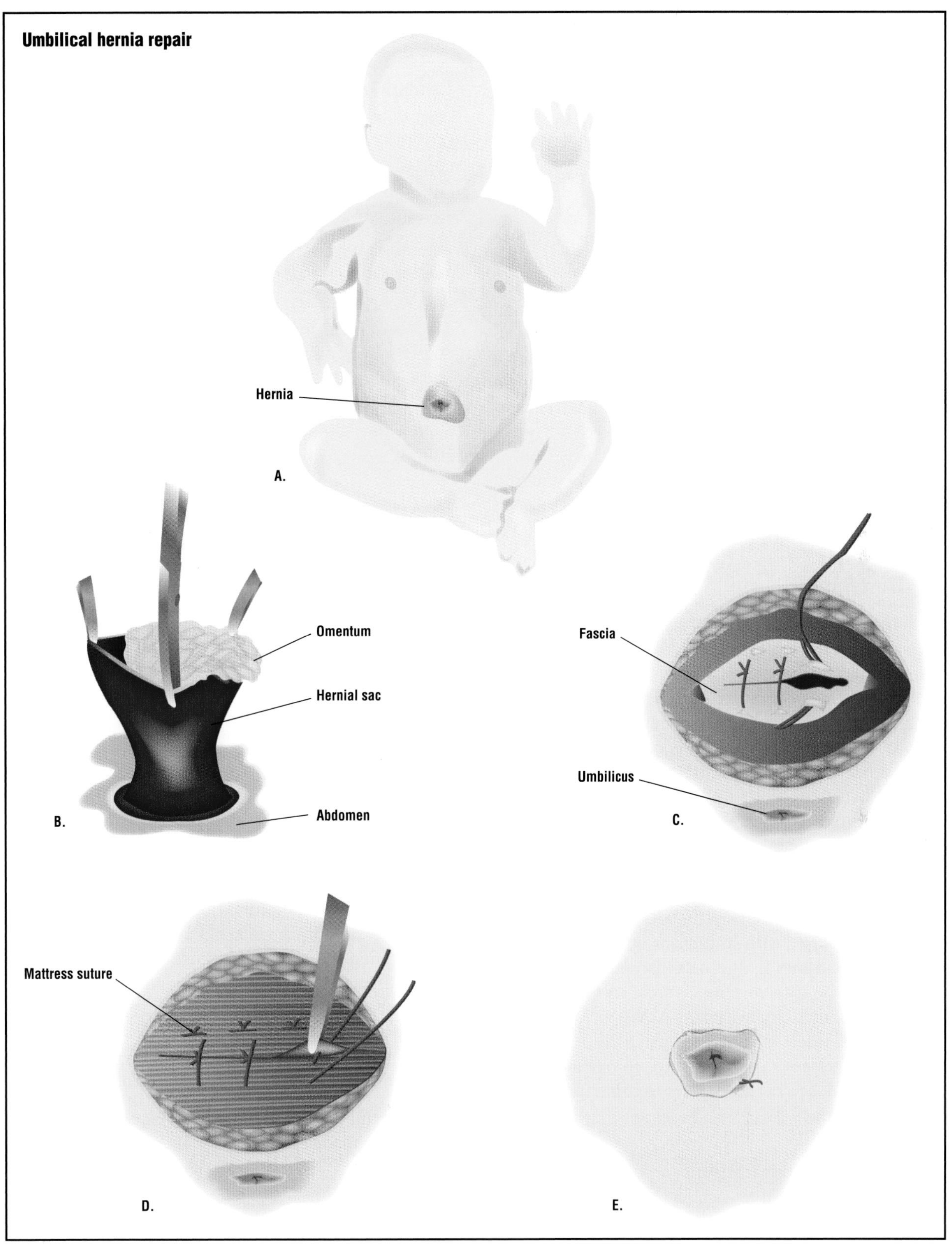

Baby with an umbilical hernia (A). To repair, the hernia is cut open (B), and the contents replaced in the abdomen. Connecting tissues, or fascia, are sutured closed (D), and the skin is repaired (D). *(Illustration by GGS Information Services. Cengage Learning, Gale.)*

(or other part of the body) is cut off by compression or constriction; it can cause extreme pain. If the strangulation persists, the tissue can die from lack of blood supply and lead to an infection.

Demographics

An umbilical hernia can occur in both men and women, and can occur at any age, although it is often present at birth. Umbilical hernias are found in about 20% of newborns, especially in premature infants. Umbilical hernias are more common in male than in female infants; with regard to race, they are eight times more common in African Americans than in Caucasians or Hispanics. While umbilical hernia is not a genetically determined condition, it tends to run in families. In the adult population, umbilical hernias are more common in overweight persons with weak abdominal muscles, and in women who are either pregnant or have borne many children. People with liver disease or fluid in the abdominal cavity are also at higher risk of developing an umbilical hernia.

Description

Repair of an abdominal hernia involves a cut, or incision, in the umbilical area. Most herniorrhaphies take about two hours to complete. After the patient has been given a sedative, the anesthesiologist will administer a local, spinal, or general anesthetic. The type of anesthesia used depends on the patient's age, general health, and complexity of the procedure. The incision is usually made underneath the belly button. The herniated tissues are isolated and pushed back inside the abdominal cavity. A hernia repair may be done using traditional open surgery or with a laparoscope. A laparoscopic procedure is performed through a few very small incisions. The hole in the abdominal wall may be closed with sutures, or by the use of a fine sterile **surgical mesh**. The mesh provides additional strength. Some surgeons may choose to use the mesh when repairing a larger hernia. A hernia repair done with a mesh insert is called a tension-free procedure because the surgeon does not have to put tension on the layer of muscle tissue in order to bring the edges of the hole together.

Diagnosis/Preparation

Diagnosis

In children, umbilical hernias are often diagnosed at birth, usually when the doctor feels a lump in the area around the belly button. The hernia may also be diagnosed if the child is crying from pain, because the crying will increase the pressure inside the abdomen and make the hernia more noticeable.

Umbilical hernias in adults occur more often in pregnant women and obese persons with weak stomach muscles. They may develop gradually without producing any discomfort, but the patient may see a bulge in the abdomen while bathing or getting dressed. Other patients consult their doctor because they have felt the tissues in the abdomen suddenly give way when they are having a bowel movement. In an office examination, the patient may be asked to lie down, lift the head, and cough. This action increases pressure inside the abdomen and causes the hernia to bulge outward.

A hernia that has become incarcerated or strangulated is a medical emergency. Its symptoms include:

- nausea
- vomiting
- abdominal swelling or distension
- pale complexion
- weakness or dizziness
- extreme pain

KEY TERMS

Abdominal distension—Swelling of the abdominal cavity, which creates painful pressure on the internal organs.

Hernia—The protrusion of a loop or piece of tissue through an incision or abnormal opening in other tissues.

Herniorraphy—The medical name for a hernia repair procedure.

Incarceration—The abnormal confinement of a section of the intestine or other body tissues. An umbilical hernia may lead to incarceration of part of the intestine.

Intra-abdominal pressure—Pressure that occurs within the abdominal cavity. Pressure in this area builds up with coughing, crying, and the pressure exerted when bearing down with a bowel movement.

Strangulation—A condition in which a vessel, section of the intestine, or other body part is compressed or constricted to the point that blood cannot circulate.

Umbilicus—The area where the umbilical cord was attached; also known as the navel or belly button.

When a hernia is present at birth, some surgeons may opt for a "wait and see" approach, as umbilical hernias in children often close by themselves with time. If the hernia has not closed by the time the child is three or four years old, then surgery is usually considered. If the hernia is very large, surgery may be recommended.

Repair of an umbilical hernia in an adult is usually considered **elective surgery**. The patient's surgeon may recommend the procedure, however, on the grounds that hernias in adults do not close by themselves and tend to grow larger over time.

Preparation

Adults scheduled for a herniorraphy are given standard blood tests and a **urinalysis**. They should not eat breakfast on the morning of the procedure, and they should wear loose-fitting, comfortable clothing that they can easily pull on after the surgery without straining their abdomen.

Aftercare

Aftercare will depend in part on the invasiveness of the surgery, whether laparoscopic or open; the type of anesthesia; the patient's age; and his or her general medical condition. Immediately after the procedure, the person will be taken to the recovery area of the surgical center, where nurses will monitor the patient for signs of excessive bleeding, infection, uncontrolled pain, or shock. Hernia repairs are usually performed on an outpatient basis, which means that the patient can expect to go home within a few hours of the surgery. Adult patients, however, should arrange to have a friend or relative drive them home. If possible, someone should stay with them for the first night.

The nurses will provide the patient with instructions on **incision care**. The specific instructions will depend on the type of surgery and the way in which the incision was closed. Sometimes a see-through dressing is placed on the wound that the patient can remove about three days after the procedure. It may be necessary to keep the dressing dry until some healing has taken place. Very small incisions may be closed with Steri-strips rather than sutures.

Risks

There are surgical and anesthesia-related risks with all surgical procedures. The primary surgical risks include bleeding and infection. Anesthesia-related risks include reactions to the specific anesthetic agents that are used; interactions with over-the-counter and herbal preparations; and respiratory problems. The greatest risk associated with umbilical hernia is missing the diagnosis. Additional risks include the formation of scar tissue and recurrence of the hernia.

WHO PERFORMS THE PROCEDURE AND WHERE IS IT PERFORMED?

This procedure is performed by a general surgeon or a pediatric surgeon. It is usually performed on an outpatient, or ambulatory, basis in a hospital. After a few hours of recovery in the surgical center, the patient is able to return home.

Normal results

Umbilical hernia repair is usually considered an uncomplicated procedure with a relatively short recovery period. A study reported in the December 2002 issue of the *American Journal of Surgery* found that patients who had laparoscopic surgery with the use of a surgical mesh had fewer complications and reoccurrences of a hernia than those with the traditional open surgery. However, laparoscopic surgery took somewhat longer to perform, possibly because the laparoscopic approach is often used for larger repairs.

Morbidity and mortality rates

In general, there are few complications with hernia repair in children. The most serious complication is surgical injury to the bladder or intestine; fortunately, this complication is very rare—about one in 1,000 patients. The recurrence rate is between 1% and 5%; recurrence is more likely in patients with very large hernias. The rate of infection is less than 1%. In the adult population, a November 2001 study reported in the *American Journal of Surgery* found a 5% mortality in elderly patients undergoing emergency hernia repairs.

Alternatives

There are no medical or surgical alternatives to an umbilical hernia repair other than watchful waiting. Since umbilical hernias present at birth often close on their own, intervention can often be delayed until the child is several years old. There is some risk that the hernia will enlarge, however, which increases the risk of incarceration or strangulation.

QUESTIONS TO ASK THE DOCTOR

- How soon can my child return to normal activities?
- How soon can I return to work and my other normal activities?
- When can I drive?
- What should I do to take care of the incision?
- How many times have you performed this surgery?
- What kinds of complications are there to this procedure?
- What kinds of complications have your patients experienced?

Resources

BOOKS

"Congenital Anomalies: Gastrointestinal Defects." Section 19, Chapter 261 in *The Merck Manual of Diagnosis and Therapy*, edited by Mark H. Beers, MD, and Robert Berkow, MD. Whitehouse Station, NJ: Merck Research Laboratories, 1999.

Delvin, David. *Coping with a Hernia*. London, UK: Sheldon Press, 1998.

PERIODICALS

Wright, B.E., et al. "Is Laparoscopic Umbilical Hernia Repair with Mesh a Reasonable Alternative to Conventional Repair?" *American Journal of Surgery* 184 (December 2002): 505-508.

ORGANIZATIONS

American Academy of Family Physicians. 11400 Tomahawk Creek Parkway, Leawood, KS 66211-2672. (913) 906-6000. E-mail: fp@aafp.org. www.aafp.org.

American Academy of Pediatrics. 141 Northwest Point Boulevard, Elk Grove Village, IL 60007-1098. (847) 434-4000. Fax: (847) 434-8000. E-mail: kidsdoc@aap.org. www.aap.org.

American College of Surgeons. 633 North St. Clair Street, Chicago, IL 60611-3231. (312) 202-5000. Fax: (312) 202-5001. www.facs.org.

OTHER

American College of Surgeons. *About Hernia Repair*. www.facs.org/public_info/operation/hernrep.pdf.

Manthey, David, MD. "Hernias." *eMedicine*, June 22, 2001 [June 6, 2003]. www.emedicine.com/EMERG/topic251.htm.

Esther Csapo Rastegari, R.N., B.S.N., Ed.M.

Undescended testicle repair *see* **Orchiopexy**

Upper GI exam

Definition

An upper GI examination is a fluoroscopic examination (a type of x-ray imaging) of the upper gastrointestinal tract, including the pharynx (throat), esophagus, stomach, and upper small intestine (duodenum). An x-ray examination that evaluates only the pharynx and esophagus is called a barium swallow.

Purpose

An upper GI series is frequently requested when a patient experiences unexplained symptoms of abdominal pain, difficulty in swallowing (dysphagia), regurgitation (reflux), diarrhea, unexplained vomiting, blood in the stool, or unexplained weight loss. It is used to help diagnose disorders and diseases of, or related to, the upper gastrointestinal tract. Some of these conditions are: **hiatal hernia**, diverticula, tumors, obstruction, gastroesophageal reflux disease (GERD), pulmonary aspiration, and inflammation (e.g., ulcers, enteritis, and Crohn's disease).

Glucagon, a medication sometimes given prior to an upper GI procedure, may cause nausea and dizziness. It is used to relax the natural movements of the stomach, which will enhance the overall study.

Description

An upper GI series takes place in a hospital or clinic setting, and is performed by an x-ray technologist and a radiologist. Before the test begins, the patient is sometimes given a glucagon injection, a medication that slows stomach and bowel activity, to provide the radiologist with a clear picture of the gastrointestinal tract. In order to further improve the upper GI picture clarity, the patient may be given a cup of fizzing baking soda crystals to swallow, which distends the esophagus and stomach by producing gas. This procedure is called a double-contrast or air-contrast upper GI.

Once these preparatory steps are complete, the patient stands against an upright x-ray table, and a fluoroscopic screen is placed in front of him or her. The patient will be asked to drink from a cup of flavored barium sulfate, a thick and chalky-tasting liquid, while the radiologist views the esophagus, stomach, and duodenum on the fluoroscopic screen. The patient will be asked to change positions frequently to coat the entire surface of the gastrointestinal tract with barium, move overlapping loops of bowel to isolate each segment, and provide multiple

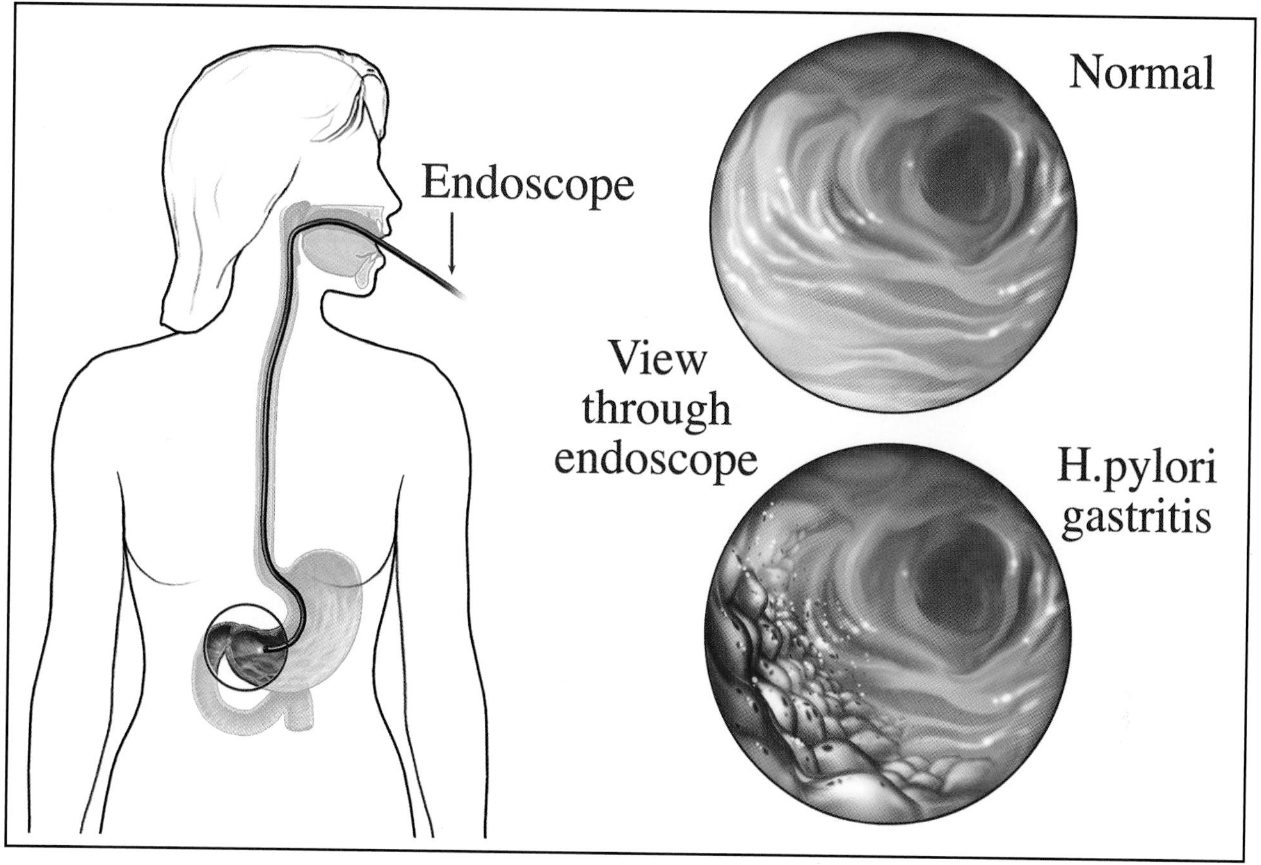

Illustration of endoscope placement in upper GI tract. *(Nucleus Medical Art, Inc./Phototake. Reproduced by permission.)*

views of each segment. The technician or radiologist may press on the patient's abdomen to spread the barium throughout the folds within the lining of the stomach. The x-ray table will also be moved several times throughout the procedure. The radiologist will ask the patient to hold his or her breath periodically while exposures are taken. After the radiologist completes his or her portion of the exam, the technologist takes three to six additional films of the GI tract. The entire procedure takes approximately 15–30 minutes.

In addition to the standard upper GI series, a physician may request a detailed small bowel follow-through (SBFT), which is a timed series of films. After the preliminary upper GI series is complete, the patient will drink additional barium sulfate, and will be escorted to a waiting area while the barium moves through the small intestines. X rays are initially taken at 15-minute intervals until the barium reaches the colon (the only way to be sure the terminal ileum is fully seen is to see the colon or ileocecal valve). The interval may be increased to 30 minutes, or even one hour if the barium passes slowly. Then the radiologist will obtain additional views of the terminal ileum (the most distal segment of the small bowel, just before the colon). This procedure can take from one to four hours.

Esophageal radiography, also called a barium esophagram or a barium swallow, is a study of the esophagus only, and is usually performed as part of the upper GI series (sometimes only a barium swallow is done). It is commonly used to diagnose the cause of difficulty in swallowing (dysphagia), and to detect a hiatal hernia. The patient drinks a barium sulfate liquid, and sometimes eats barium-coated food while the radiologist examines the swallowing mechanism on a fluoroscopic screen. The test takes approximately 30 minutes.

Preparation

Patients must not eat, drink, chew gum, or smoke for eight hours prior to undergoing an upper GI examination. Longer dietary restrictions may be required, depending on the type and diagnostic purpose of the test. Patients undergoing a small-bowel

KEY TERMS

Contrast medium—Any substance that is swallowed or injected in order to increase the visibility of body structures or fluids.

Crohn's disease—A chronic, inflammatory bowel disease usually affecting the ileum, colon, or both.

Diverticula (singular, diverticulum)—Pouch-like herniations through the muscular wall of an organ such as the stomach, small intestine, or colon.

Enteritis—Inflammation of the mucosal lining of the small intestine.

Gastroesophageal reflux disease (GERD)—A painful, chronic condition in which stomach acid flows back into the esophagus causing heartburn and, in time, erosion of the esophageal lining.

Hiatal hernia—Protrusion of the stomach up through the diaphragm.

follow-through exam may be asked to take **laxatives** the day before the test. Patients are required to wear a hospital gown, or similar attire, and to remove all jewelry, to provide the camera with an unobstructed view of the abdomen.

Aftercare

No special aftercare treatment or regimen is required for an upper GI series. The patient may eat and drink as soon as the test is completed. The barium sulfate may make the patient's stool white for several days, and can cause constipation; therefore, patients are encouraged to drink plenty of water to eliminate it from their system.

Risks

Because the upper GI series is an x-ray procedure, it does involve minor exposure to ionizing radiation. Unless the patient is pregnant, or multiple radiological or fluoroscopic studies are required, the small dose of radiation incurred during a single procedure poses little risk. However, multiple studies requiring fluoroscopic exposure that are conducted in a short time period have been known, on very rare occasions, to cause skin **death** (necrosis) in some individuals. This risk can be minimized by careful monitoring and documentation of cumulative radiation doses.

Some patients find the barium liquid unpleasant to the taste or difficult to swallow. The radiologist may be able to provide a strawberry- or chocolate-flavored version. In addition, some patients feel gassy, bloated, or nauseated while they are being tilted on the examination table or having their abdomen pressed.

A few patients are allergic to barium and other contrast materials. Patients should inform the radiologist of any known allergies.

Normal results

A normal upper GI series shows a healthy, normally functioning, and unobstructed digestive tract. Hiatal hernia, obstructions, inflammation (including ulcers or polyps of the esophagus, stomach, or small intestine), or irregularities in the swallowing mechanism are just a few of the possible abnormalities that may appear on an upper GI series. Additionally, abnormal peristalsis, or digestive movements of the esophagus, stomach, and small intestine can often be visualized on the fluoroscopic part of the exam, and in the interpretation of the SBFT.

Resources

BOOKS

Brant, William E., and Clyde A. Helms. *Fundamentals of Diagnostic Radiology*, 3rd ed. Philadelphia: Lippincott Williams and Wilkins, 2006.

PERIODICALS

Nandurkar, S., G. R. Locke, III, J. A. Murray, et al. "Rates of Endoscopy and Endoscopic Findings among People with Frequent Symptoms of Gastroesophageal Reflux in the Community." *American Journal of Gastroenterology* 100 (July 2005): 1459–1465.

"Patient Page: Upper GI Series." *Radiologic Technology* 77 (May–June 2006): 415–416.

ORGANIZATIONS

American College of Gastroenterology (ACG). P.O. Box 342260, Bethesda, MD 20827-2260. (301) 263-9000. http://www.acg.gi.org/ (accessed April 14, 2008).

American College of Radiology (ACR). 1891 Preston White Drive, Reston, VA 20191. (703) 648-8900. http://www.acr.org/ (accessed April 14, 2008).

Radiological Society of North America (RSNA). 820 Jorie Blvd., Oak Brook, IL 60523-2251. (630) 571-2670. http://www.rsna.org/ (accessed April 14, 2008).

OTHER

Kefalas, Costas H. *Commonly Performed Radiographic Tests in Gastroenterology*. http://www.acg.gi.org/patients/gihealth/radiographic.asp [cited January 14, 2008; accessed April 14, 2008].

Radiological Society of North America (RSNA). *Upper Gastrointestinal (GI) Tract X-ray (Radiography)*. http://www.radiologyinfo.org/en/info.cfm?pg = uppergi&bhcp = 1 [cited January 14, 2008; accessed April 14, 2008].

Sawyer, Michael A. J., and Tarak H. Patel. "Gastroesophageal Reflux." *eMedicine*, December 15, 2005 [cited January 14, 2008]. http://www.emedicine.com/radio/topic300.htm (accessed April 14, 2008).

Debra Novograd, BS, RT(R)(M)
Lee A. Shratter, MD
Rebecca Frey, PhD

Ureteral stenting

Definition

A ureteral stent is a thin, flexible tube threaded into the ureter to help urine drain from the kidney to the bladder or to an external collection system.

Purpose

Urine is normally carried from the kidneys to the bladder via a pair of long, narrow tubes called ureters (each kidney is connected to one ureter). A ureter may become obstructed as a result of a number of conditions including kidney stones, tumors, blood clots, postsurgical swelling, or infection. A ureteral stent is placed in the ureter to restore the flow of urine to the bladder. Ureteral stents may be used in patients with active kidney infection or with diseased bladders (e.g., as a result of cancer or radiation therapy). Alternatively, ureteral stents may be used during or after urinary tract surgical procedures to provide a mold around which healing can occur, to divert the urinary flow away from areas of leakage, to manipulate kidney stones or prevent stone migration prior to treatment, or to make the ureters more easily identifiable during difficult surgical procedures. The stent may remain in place on a short-term (days to weeks) or long-term (weeks to months) basis.

Demographics

Chronic blockage of a ureter affects approximately five individuals out of every 1,000; acute blockage affects one out of every 1,000. Bilateral obstruction (blockage to both ureters) is more rare; chronic blockage affects one individual per 1,000 people, and acute blockage affects five per 10,000.

Description

The size, shape, and material of the ureteral stent to be used depends on the patient's anatomy and the reason why the stent is required. Most stents are 5–12 inches (12–30 cm) in length, and have a diameter of 0.06–0.2 inches (1.5–6 mm). One or both ends of the stent may be coiled (called a pigtail stent) to prevent it from moving out of place; an open-ended stent is better suited for patients who require temporary drainage. In some instances, one end of the stent has a thread attached to it that extends through the bladder and urethra to the outside of the body; this aids in stent removal. The stent material must be flexible, durable, non-reactive, and radiopaque (visible on an x ray).

The patient is usually placed under **general anesthesia** for stent insertion; this ensures the physician that the patient will remain relaxed and will not move during the procedure. A cystoscope (a thin, telescope-like instrument) is inserted into the urethra to the bladder, and the opening to the ureter to be stented is identified. In some instances, a guide wire is inserted into the ureter under the aid of a fluoroscope (an imaging device that uses x rays to visualize structures on a fluorescent screen). The guide wire provides a path for the placement of the stent, which is advanced over the wire. Once the stent is in place, the guide wire and cystoscope are removed. Patients who fail this method of ureteral stenting may have the stent placed percutaneously (through the skin), into the kidney, and subsequently into the ureter.

A stent that has an attached thread may be pulled out by a physician in an office setting. **Cystoscopy** may also be used to remove a stent.

Diagnosis/Preparation

A number of different technologies aid in the diagnosis of ureteral obstruction. These include:

- cystoscopy (a procedure in which a thin, tubular instrument is used to visualize the interior of the bladder)
- ultrasonography (an imaging technique that uses high-frequency sound waves to visualize structures inside the body)

KEY TERMS

Acute—A condition that has a short but severe course.

Chronic—A condition that is persistent or recurs frequently.

Cystoscopy—Examination or treatment of the interior of the urinary bladder by looking through a special instrument with reflected light.

Kidney stones—Small, solid masses that form in the kidney.

Urethra—The tube through which urine travels from the bladder to the outside of the body.

WHO PERFORMS THE PROCEDURE AND WHERE IS IT PERFORMED?

Ureteral stenting is typically performed in a hospital by an interventional radiologist (a physician who specializes in the treatment of medical disorders using specialized imaging techniques) or a urologist (a physician who specializes in the diagnosis and treatment of diseases of the urinary tract and genital organs).

QUESTIONS TO ASK THE DOCTOR

- Why is ureteral stenting recommended?
- What diagnostic tests will be performed prior to the stenting procedure?
- What technique will be used to place the stent?
- What type of stent will be used, and when will it be removed?
- Are there any alternatives to ureteral stenting?

- computed tomography (an imaging technique that uses x rays to produce two-dimensional cross-sections on a viewing screen)
- pyelography (x rays taken of the urinary tract after a contrast dye has been injected into a vein or into the kidney, ureter, or bladder)

Prior to ureteral stenting, the procedure should be thoroughly explained by a medical professional. No food or drink is permitted after midnight the night before surgery. The patient wears a hospital gown during the procedure. If the stent insertion is performed with the aid of a cystoscope, the patient will assume a position that is typically used in a gynecological exam (lying on the back, with the legs flexed and supported by stirrups).

Aftercare

Stents must be periodically replaced to prevent fractures within the catheter wall or build-up of encrustation. Stent replacement is recommended approximately every six months; more often in patients who form stones.

Risks

Complications associated with ureteral stenting include:

- bleeding (usually minor and easily treated, but occasionally requiring transfusion)
- catheter migration or dislodgement (may require readjustment)
- coiling of the stent within the ureter (may cause lower abdominal pain or flank pain on urination, urinary frequency, or blood in the urine)
- introduction or worsening of infection
- penetration of adjacent organs (e.g., bowel, gallbladder, or lungs)

Normal results

Normally, a ureteral stent re-establishes the flow of urine from the kidney to the bladder. Postoperative urine flow will be monitored to ensure the stent has not been dislodged or obstructed.

Morbidity and mortality rates

Serious complications occur in approximately 4% of patients undergoing ureteral stenting, with minor complications in another 10%.

Alternatives

If a ureter is obstructed and ureteral stenting is not possible, a **nephrostomy** may be performed. During this procedure, a tube is placed through the skin on the patient's back, into the area of the kidney that collects urine. The tube may be connected to an external drainage bag. In other cases, the tube is connected directly from the kidney to the bladder.

Resources

BOOKS

Su, Li-Ming & R. Ernest Sosa. "Ureteroscopy and Retrograde Ureteral Access." (Chapter 97) In *Campbell's Urology*, 8th ed., edited by Patrick C. Walsh. Philadelphia: Elsevier Science, 2002.

ORGANIZATIONS

American Urological Association. 1120 North Charles Street, Baltimore, MD 21201. (410) 727-1100. http://www.auanet.org.

OTHER

"Extrinsic Obstruction of the Ureter." *UrologyHealth.org*. [cited May 19, 2003] http://www.urologyhealth.org/adult/index.cfm?cat=01&topic=93.

Sutherland, Suzette E. and Martin I. Resnick. "Urinary Tract Obstruction." *eMedicine*. May 6, 2002 [cited May 19, 2003] http://www.emedicine.com/med/topic2782.htm.

Kathleen D. Wright, R.N.
Stephanie Dionne Sherk

Ureterosigmoidoscopy

Definition

Ureterosigmoidoscopy is a surgical procedure that treats urinary incontinence by joining the ureters to the lower colon, thereby allowing urine to evacuate through the rectum.

Purpose

The surgery is indicated when there is resection (surgical removal), malformation, or injury to the bladder. The bladder disposes of wastes passed to it from the kidneys, which is the organ that does most of the blood filtering and retention of needed glucose, salts, and minerals.

Wastes from the kidneys drip through the ureters to the bladder, and on to the urethra where they are expelled via urination. Waste from the kidneys is slowed or impaired when the bladder is diseased because of ulcerative, inflammatory, or malignant conditions; is malformed; or if it has been removed. In these cases, the kidney is unable to get rid of the wastes, resulting in hydronephrosis (distention of the kidneys). Over time, this leads to kidney deterioration. Saving the kidneys by bladder diversion is as important as restoring urinary continence.

The surgical techniques for urinary and fecal diversion fall into two categories: continent diversion and conduit diversion. In continent diversion, an internal reservoir for urine or feces is created, allowing natural evacuation from the body. In urinary and fecal conduit diversion, a section of existing tissue is altered to serve as a passageway to an external reservoir or ostomy. Both continent and conduit diversions reproduce bladder or colon function that was impaired due to surgery, obstruction, or a neurogenically (nerve dysfunction) created condition. Both the continent and conduit diversion methods have been used for years, with advancements in minimally invasive surgical techniques and biochemical improvements in conduit materials and ostomy appliances.

Catheterization was the original solution for urinary incontinence, especially when major organ failure or removal was involved. But catherization was found to have major residual back flow of urine into the kidneys over the long term. With the advent of surgical anatomosis—the grafting of vascularizing tissue for the repair and expansion of organ function—and with the ability to include flap-type valves to prevent back-up into the kidneys, major continent restoring procedures have become routine in **urologic surgery**. Catherization has been replaced as a permanent remedy for persistent incontinence. Continent surgical procedures developed since the 1980s offer the possibility of safely retaining natural evacuation functions in both colonic (intestinal) and urinary systems.

KEY TERMS

Bladder exstrophy—One of many bladder and urinary congenital abnormalities. Occurs when the wall of the bladder fails to close in embryonic development and remains exposed to the abdominal wall.

Conduit diversion— A surgical procedure that restores urinary and fecal continence by diverting these functions through a constructed conduit leading to an external waste reservoir (ostomy).

Cystectomy—The surgical resection of part or all of the bladder.

Urinary continent diversion—A surgical procedure that restores urinary continence by diverting urinary function around the bladder and into the intestines, thereby allowing for natural evacuation through the rectum or an implanted artificial sphincter.

Quality of life issues associated with urinary diversion are increasingly important to patients and, along with medical requirements, put an optimal threshold on the requirements for the surgical procedure. The bladder substitute or created reservoir must offer the following advantages:

- maintain continence
- maintain sterile urine
- empty completely
- protect the kidneys
- prevent absorption of waste products
- maintain quality of life

Ureterosigmoidoscopy is one of the earliest continent diversions for a resected bladder, bladder abnormalities, and dysfunction. It is one of the more difficult surgeries, and has significant complications. Ureterosigmoidoscopy does have a major benefit; it allows the natural expelling of wastes without the construction of a stoma—an artificial conduit—by using the rectum as a urinary reservoir. When evacuation occurs, the urine is passed along with the fecal matter.

Ureterosigmoidoscopy is a single procedure, but there are additional refinements that allow rectal voiding of urine. A procedure known as the Mainz II pouch has undergone many refinements in attempts to lessen the complications that have traditionally accompanied uretersigmoidoscopy. This surgery is indicated for significant and serious conditions of the urinary tract including:

- Cancer or ulceration of the bladder that necessitates a radical cystectomy or removal of the bladder, primarily occurring in adults, particularly those of advanced age.
- Various congential abnormalities of the bladder in infants, especially eversion of part or all of the bladder. Eversion (or exotrophy) is a malformation of the bladder in which the wall adjacent to the abdomen fails to close. In some children, the bladder plate may be too small to fashion a closure.

Demographics

Bladder cancer affects over 50,000 people annually in the United States. The average age at diagnosis is 68 years. It accounts for approximately 10,000 deaths per year. Bladder cancer is the fifth leading cause of cancer deaths among men older than 75 years. Male bladder cancer is three times more prevalent than female bladder cancer.

In the United States, radical **cystectomy** (total removal of the bladder) is the standard treatment for muscle-invading bladder cancer. The operation usually involves removal of the bladder (with oncology staging) and pelvic lymph node, and prostate and seminal conduits with a form of urinary diversion. Uretersigmoscopy is one option that restores continence.

Pediatric ureterosigmoidoscopy is performed primarily for bladder abnormalities occuring at birth. Classic bladder exstrophy occurs in 3.3 per 100,000 births, with a male to female ratio of 3:1 (6:1 in some studies).

Description

The most basic ureterosigmoidoscopy modification is the Mainz II pouch. There is a 2.4 in (6 cm) cut along antimesenteric border of the colon, both on the proximal and distal sides of the rectum/sigmoid colon junction. The ureters are drawn down into the colon. A special flap technique is applied by folding the colon to stop urine from refluxing back to the kidneys. After the colon is closed, the result is a small rectosigmoid reservoir that holds urine without refluxing it back to the upper urinary tract. Some variations of the Mainz II pouch include the construction of a valve, as in the Kock pouch, that confines urine to the distal segment of the colon.

Ureterosigmoidoscopy is typically performed in patients with complex medical problems, often those who have had numerous surgeries. Ureterosigmoidoscopy as a continent diversion technique relies heavily upon an intact and functional rectal sphincter. The treatment of pediatric urinary incontinence due to bladder eversion or other anatomical anomalies is a technical challenge, and is not always the first choice of surgeons. In Europe, early urinary diversion with ureterosigmoidoscopy is used widely for most exstrophy patients. Its main advantage is the possibility for spontaneous emptying by evacuation of urine and stool.

Diagnosis/Preparation

A number of tests are performed as part of the pre-surgery diagnostic workup for bladder conditions such as cancer, ulcerative or inflammatory disease, or pediatric abnormalities. Tests may include:

- cystoscopy (bladder inspection with a laparoscope)
- CT scan
- liver function
- renal function
- rectal sphincter function evaluation (The rectal sphincter will be a critical ingredient in urination after the surgery, and it is important to determine its ability to function. Adult patients are often asked to have an oatmeal enema and sit upright for a period of time to test sphincter function.)

In adult patients, a discussion of continent diversion is conducted early in the diagnostic process. Patients are asked to consider the possibility of a conduit urinary diversion if the ureterosigmoidoscopy proves impossible to complete. Educational sessions on specific conduit alternatives take place prior to surgery. Topics include options for placement of a stoma, and appliances that may be a part of the daily voiding routine after surgery. Many doctors provide a stomal therapist to consult with the patient.

Aftercare

After surgery, patients may remain in the hospital for a few days to undergo blood, renal, and liver tests, and monitoring for fever or other surgical complications. In pediatric patients, a cast keeps the legs abducted (apart) and slightly elevated for three weeks. Bladder and kidneys are fully drained via multiple catheters during the first few weeks after surgery. **Antibiotics** are continued after surgery. Permanent

WHO PERFORMS THE PROCEDURE AND WHERE IS IT PERFORMED?

Uretersigmoidoscopy is usually performed by a urological surgeon with advanced training in urinary continent surgeries, often in consultation with a neonatalist (in newborn patients) or an oncological surgeon. The surgery takes place in a general hospital.

QUESTIONS TO ASK THE DOCTOR

How many times has the surgeon performed this operation?

Is conduit surgery the best route for protecting renal function?

What is the surgeon's complication rate?

follow-up with the urologist is essential for proper monitoring of kidney function.

Normal results

Good results have been reported, especially in children; however, ureterosigmoidoscopy offers some severe morbid complications. Post-surgical bladder function and continence rates are very high. However, many newly created reservoirs do not function normally; some deteriorate over time, creating a need for more than one diversion surgery. Many patients have difficulty voiding after surgery. Five-year survival rates for bladder surgery patients are 50–80%, depending on the grade, depth of bladder penetration, and nodal status.

Morbidity and mortality rates

The continence success rate with ureterosigmoidoscopy and its variants is higher than 95% for exstrophy; however, long-term malignancy rates are quite high. Adenocarcinoma is the most common of these malignancies, and may be caused by chronic irritation and inflammation of exposed mucosa of the exostrophic bladder. In one series of studies, adenocarcinoma was reported in more than 10% of patients. However, the malignancy is actually higher in untreated patients whose bladders are left exposed for years before surgery.

Upper urinary tract deterioration is a potential complication, caused by reflux of urine back to the kidneys, resulting in febrile infections.

Alternatives

Other options include construction of a full neobladder in certain carefully defined circumstances, and bladder enhancement for congenitally shortened or abnormal bladders. Surgical bladder resection is often followed by continent operations using other parts of the colon, and by various conduit surgeries that utilize an external ostomy appliance.

Resources

BOOKS

"Continent Urinary Diversion." In Walsh, P. *Campbell's Urology,* 8th ed. Elsevier, 2002.

"Pediatric Urology: Continent Urinary Diversion." In Walsh, P. *Campbell's Urology,* 8th ed. Elsevier, 2002.

PERIODICALS

Stehr, M. "Selected Secondary Reconstructive Procedures for Improvement of Urinary Incontinence in Bladder Exstrophy and Neurogenic Bladder Dysfunction in Childhood." *Wiener Medizinische Wochenschr* 150, no.11 (January 1, 2000): 245-8.

Yerkes, B. and H.M. Snyder, H.M. "Exstrophy and Epispadias." *Pediatrics/Urology* 3, no.5 (May 6, 2002). www.author.eMedicine.com.

ORGANIZATIONS

American Academy of Pediatrics. 141 Northwest Point Boulevard; Elk Grove Village, IL 60007-1098. (847) 434-4000. Fax: (847) 434-8000. www.aap.org.

National Institutes of Diabetes & Digestive & Kidney Disease. www.niddk.nih.gov/tools/mail.htm.

OTHER

Girgin, C., et. al. "Comparison of Three Types of Continent Urinary Diversions in a Single Center." *Digital Urology Journal* www.duj.com.

Nancy McKenzie, Ph.D.

Ureterostomy, cutaneous

Definition

A cutaneous ureterostomy, also called ureterocutaneostomy, is a surgical procedure that detaches one or both ureters from the bladder, and brings them to the surface of the abdomen with the formation of an opening (stoma) to allow passage of urine.

Purpose

The bladder is the membranous pouch that serves as a reservoir for urine. Contraction of the bladder results in urination. A ureterostomy is performed to divert the flow of urine away from the bladder when the bladder is not functioning or has been removed. The following conditions may result in a need for ureterostomy.

- bladder cancer
- spinal cord injury
- malfunction of the bladder
- birth defects, such as spina bifida

Demographics

Bladder disorders afflict millions of people in the United States. According to the American Cancer Society (ACS), there were 54,200 new cases of bladder cancer in 1999, with approximately 12,100 deaths from the disease. Bladder cancer incidence is steadily rising, and by 2010 it is projected to increase by 28% for both men and women.

Description

Urostomy is the generic name for any surgical procedure that diverts the passage of urine by redirecting the ureters (fibromuscular tubes that carry the urine from the kidney to the bladder). There are two basic types of urostomies. The first features the creation of a passage called an "ileal conduit." In this procedure, the ureters are detached from the bladder and joined to a short length of the small intestine (ileum). The other type of urostomy is cutaneous ureterostomy. With this technique, the surgeon detaches the ureters from the bladder and brings one or both to the surface of the abdomen. The hole created in the abdomen is called a stoma, a reddish, moist abdominal protrusion. The stoma is not painful; it has no sensation. Since it has no muscles to regulate urination, urine collects in a bag.

There are four common types of ureterostomies:

- Single ureterostomy. This procedure brings only one ureter to the surface of the abdomen.
- Bilateral ureterostomy. This procedure brings the two ureters to the surface of the abdomen, one on each side.

KEY TERMS

Anastomosis—An opening created by surgical, traumatic, or pathological means between two separate spaces or organs.

Cecum—The pouch-like start of the large intestine (colon) at the end of the small intestine.

Gastrointestinal (GI) tract—The entire length of the digestive tract, from the stomach to the rectum.

Ileum—The last portion of the small intestine that communicates with the large intestine.

Large intestine—Also called the colon, this structure has six major divisions: cecum, ascending colon, transverse colon, descending colon, sigmoid colon, and rectum.

Ostomy—General term meaning a surgical procedure in which an artificial opening is formed to either allow waste (stool or urine) to pass from the body, or to allow food into the GI tract. An ostomy can be permanent or temporary, as well as single-barreled, double-barreled, or a loop.

Small intestine—The small intestine consists of three sections: duodenum, jejunum, and ileum.

Spina bifida—A congenital defect in the spinal column, characterized by the absence of the vertebral arches through which the spinal membranes and spinal cord may protrude.

Stent—A tube made of metal or plastic that is inserted into a vessel or passage to keep it open and prevent closure.

Stoma—A surgically created opening in the abdominal wall.

Ureter—The fibromuscular tube that transports the urine from the kidney to the bladder.

- Double-barrel ureterostomy. In this approach, both ureters are brought to the same side of the abdominal surface.
- Transuretero ureterostomy (TUU). This procedure brings both ureters to the same side of the abdomen, through the same stoma.

Diagnosis/Preparation

Ureterostomy patients may have the following tests and procedures as part of their diagnostic work-up:

- Renal function tests; blood, urea, nitrogen (BUN); and creatinine.

- Blood tests, complete blood count (CBC), and electrolytes.
- Imaging studies of the ureters and renal pelvis. These studies characterize the ureters, and define the surgery required to obtain adequate ureteral length.

The quality, character, and usable length of the ureters is usually assessed using any of the following tests:

- Intravenous pyelogram (IVP). A special diagnostic test that follows the time course of excretion of a contrast dye through the kidneys, ureters, and bladder after it is injected into a vein.
- Retrograde pyelogram (RPG). X-ray study of the kidney, focusing on the urine-collecting region of the kidney and ureters.
- Antegrade nephrostogram.
- CT scan. A special imaging technique that uses a computer to collect multiple x-ray images into a two-dimentional cross-sectional image.
- MRI with intravenous gadolinium. A special technique used to image internal stuctures of the body, particularly the soft tissues. An MRI image is often superior to a routine x-ray image.

The presurgery evaluation also includes an assessment of overall patient stability. The surgery may take from two to six hours, depending on the health of the ureters, and the experience of the surgeon.

Aftercare

After surgery, the condition of the ureters is monitored by IVP testing, repeated postoperatively at six months, one year, and then yearly.

Following ureterostomy, urine needs to be collected in bags. Several designs are available. One popular type features an open bag fitted with an anti-reflux valve, which prevents the urine from flowing back toward the stoma. A urostomy bag connects to a night bag that may be attached to the bed at night. Urostomy bags are available as one- and two-piece bags:

- One-piece bags: The adhesive and the bag are sealed together. The advantage of using a one-piece appliance is that it is easy to apply, and the bag is flexible and soft.
- Two-piece bags: The bag and the adhesive are two separate components. The adhesive does not need to be removed frequently from the skin, and can remain in place for several days while the bag is changed as required.

WHO PERFORMS THE PROCEDURE AND WHERE IS IT PERFORMED?

Ureterostomy is performed in a hospital setting by experienced surgeons trained in urology, the branch of medicine concerned with the diagnosis and treatment of diseases of the urinary tract and urogenital system. Specially trained nurses called wound ostomy continence nurses (WOCN) are commonly available for consultation in most major medical centers.

Risks

The complication rate associated with ureterostomy procedures is less than 5–10%. Risks during surgery include heart problems, pulmonary (lung) complications, development of blood clots (thrombosis), blocking of arteries (embolism), and injury to adjacent structures, such as bowel or vascular entities. Inadequate ureteral length may also be encountered, leading to ureteral kinking and subsequent obstruction. If plastic tubes need inserting, their malposition can lead to obstruction and eventual breakdown of the opening (anastomosis). Anastomotic leak is the most frequently encountered complication.

Normal results

Normal results for a ureterostomy include the successful diversion of the urine pathway away from the bladder, and a tension-free, watertight opening to the abdomen that prevents urinary leakage.

Morbidity and mortality rates

The outcome and prognosis for ureterostomy patients depends on a number of factors. The highest rates of complications exist for those who have pelvic cancer or a history of radiation therapy.

In one study, a French medical team followed 69 patients for a minimum of one year (an average of six years) after TUU was performed. They reported one complication per four patients (6.3%), including a case requiring open drainage, prolonged urinary leakage, and common ureteral **death** (necrosis). Two complications occurred three and four years after surgery. The National Cancer Institute performed TUU for pelvic malignancy in 10 patients. Mean follow-up was 6.5 years. Complications include common ureteral narrowing (one patient); subsequent kidney removal, or

QUESTIONS TO ASK THE DOCTOR

- Why is ureterostomy required?
- What type will be performed?
- How long will it take to recover from the surgery?
- When can normal activities be resumed?
- How many ureterostomies does the surgeon perform each year?
- What are the possible complications?

nephrectomy (one patient); recurrence of disease with ureteral obstruction (one patient); and disease progression in a case of inflammation of blood vessels, or vasulitis (one patient). One patient died of sepsis (infection in the bloodstream) due to urine leakage at the anastomosis, one died after a heart attack, and three died from metastasis of their primary cancer.

Alternatives

There are several alternative surgical procedures available:

- Ileal conduit urostomy, also known as "Bricker's loop." The two ureters that transport urine from the kidneys are detached from the bladder, and then attached so that they will empty through a piece of the ileum. One end of the ileum piece is sealed off and the other end is brought to the surface of the abdomen to form the stoma. It is the most common technique used for urinary diversion.
- Cystostomy. The flow of urine is diverted from the bladder to the abdominal wall. It features placement of a tube through the abdominal wall into the bladder, and is indicated in cases of blockage or stricture of the ureters. It can be temporary or permanent.
- Indiana pouch. A pouch is constructed using the end part of the ileum and the first part of the large intestine (cecum). The remaining ileum is first attached to the large intestine to maintain normal digestive flow. A pouch is then created from the removed cecum, and the attached ileum is brought to the surface of the abdominal wall to create a stoma.
- Percutaneous nephrostomy. A nephrostomy is created when the flow of urine is diverted directly from the kidneys to the abdominal wall. Tubes are placed within the kidney to collect the urine as it is generated, and transport it to the abdominal wall. This procedure is usually temporary; however, it may be permanent for cancer patients.

Resources

BOOKS

Door Mullen, B. & K. A. McGinn. *The Ostomy Book: Living Comfortably With Colostomies, Ileostomies, and Urostomies.* Boulder, CO: Bull Publishing Co., 1992.

Jeter, K. F. *Urostomy Guide.* Irvine, CA: American Urological Association, code 05-006.

PERIODICALS

Cedillo, U., C. Gracida, R. Espinoza, and J. Cancino. "Vesical Augmentation and Continent Ureterostomy in Kidney Transplant Patients." *Transplant Proceedings* 34 (November 2002): 2541-2.

Hiratsuka, Y., T. Ishii, H. Taira, and A. Okadome. "Simple Correction of Ureteral Stomal Stenosis for Cutaneous Ureterostomy." *International Journal of Urology* 10 (March 2003): 180-1.

Purohit, R. S., and P. N. Bretan, Jr. "Successful Long-term Outcome Using Existing Native Cutaneous Ureterostomy for Renal Transplant Drainage." *Journal of Urology* 163 (February 2000): 446-9.

Yoshimura, K., S. Maekawa, K. Ichioka, N. Terada, Y. Matsuta, K. Okubo, and Y. Arai. "Tubeless Cutaneous Ureterostomy: The Toyoda Method Revisited." *Journal of Urology* 165 (March 2001): 785-8.

ORGANIZATIONS

American Urological Association (AUA). 1120 North Charles Street, Baltimore, MD 21201. (410) 727-1100. www.auanet.org.

United Ostomy Association (UOA). 19772 MacArthur Blvd., #200, Irvine, CA 92612-2405. (800) 826-0826. www.uoa.org.

Monique Laberge, Ph.D.

Uric acid tests *see* **Kidney function tests**

Urinalysis

Definition

A urinalysis is a group of manual and/or automated qualitative and semi-quantitative tests performed on a urine sample. A routine urinalysis usually includes the following tests: color, transparency, specific gravity, pH, protein, glucose, ketones, blood, bilirubin, nitrite, urobilinogen, and leukocyte esterase. Some laboratories include a microscopic examination of urinary sediment with all routine urinalysis tests. If not, it is customary to perform the microscopic exam, if transparency, glucose, protein, blood, nitrite, or leukocyte esterase is abnormal.

Purpose

Routine urinalyses are performed for several reasons:

- general health screening to detect renal and metabolic diseases
- diagnosis of diseases or disorders of the kidneys or urinary tract
- monitoring of patients with diabetes

In addition, quantitative urinalysis tests may be performed to help diagnose many specific disorders, such as endocrine diseases, bladder cancer, osteoporosis, and porphyrias (a group of disorders caused by chemical imbalance). Quantitative analysis often requires the use of a timed urine sample. The urinary microalbumin test measures the rate of albumin excretion in the urine using laboratory tests. This test is used to monitor kidney function of persons with diabetes mellitus. In diabetics, the excretion of greater than 200 μg/mL albumin is predictive of impending kidney disease.

Precautions

Voided specimens

All patients should avoid intense athletic training or heavy physical work before the test, as these activities may cause small amounts of blood to appear in the urine. Many urinary constituents are labile, and samples should be tested within one hour of collection or refrigerated. Samples may be stored at 36–46°F (2–8°C) for up to 24 hours for chemical urinalysis tests; however, the microscopic examination should be performed within four hours of collection, if possible. To minimize sample contamination, women who require a urinalysis during menstruation should insert a fresh tampon before providing a urine sample.

Over two dozen drugs are known to interfere with various chemical urinalysis tests. These include:

- ascorbic acid
- chlorpromazine
- L-dopa
- nitrofurantoin (Macrodantin, Furadantin)
- penicillin
- phenazopyridine (Pyridium)
- rifampin (Rifadin)
- tolbutamide

The preservatives that are used to prevent loss of glucose and cells may affect biochemical test results. The use of preservatives should be avoided whenever possible in urine tests.

Description

Routine urinalysis consists of three testing groups: physical characteristics, biochemical tests, and microscopic evaluation.

Physical tests

The physical tests measure the color, transparency (clarity), and specific gravity of a urine sample. In some cases, the volume (daily output) may be measured. Color and transparency are determined from visual observation of the sample.

COLOR. Normal urine is straw yellow to amber in color. Abnormal colors include bright yellow, brown, black (gray), red, and green. These pigments may result from medications, dietary sources, or diseases. For example, red urine may be caused by blood or hemoglobin, beets, medications, and some porphyrias. Black-gray urine may result from melanin (melanoma) or homogentisic acid (alkaptonuria, a rare metabolic disorder). Bright yellow urine may be caused by bilirubin (a bile pigment). Green urine may be caused by a bile pigment or certain medications. Orange urine may be caused by some medications or excessive urobilinogen (a chemical produced in the intestines). Brown urine may be caused by excessive amounts of prophobilin or urobilin (chemical relatives of urobilinogen).

TRANSPARENCY. Normal urine is transparent. Turbid (cloudy) urine may be caused by either normal or abnormal processes. Normal conditions giving rise to turbid urine include precipitation of crystals, mucus, or vaginal discharge. Abnormal causes of turbidity include the presence of blood cells, yeast, and bacteria.

SPECIFIC GRAVITY. The specific gravity of urine is a measure of the concentration of dissolved solutes (substances in a solution), and it reflects the ability of the kidneys to concentrate the urine (conserve water). Specific gravity is usually measured by determining the refractive index of a urine sample (refractometry) or by chemical analysis. Specific gravity varies with fluid and solute intake. It will be increased (above 1.035) in persons with diabetes mellitus and persons taking large amounts of medication. It will also be increased after radiologic studies of the kidney owing to the excretion of x-ray contrast dye. Consistently low specific gravity (1.003 or less) is seen in persons with diabetes insipidus. In renal (kidney) failure, the specific gravity remains equal to that of blood plasma (1.008–1.010) regardless of changes in the patient's salt and water intake. Urine volume below 400 mL per day is considered oliguria (low urine production), and may occur in persons who are dehydrated and

KEY TERMS

Acidosis—A condition of the blood in which bicarbonate levels are below normal.

Alkalosis—A condition of the blood and other body fluids in which bicarbonate levels are higher than normal.

Bilirubin—A yellow bile pigment found as sodium (soluble) bilirubinate, or as an insoluble calcium salt found in gallstones.

Biliverdin—A green bile pigment formed from the oxidation of heme, which is a bilin with a structure almost identical to that of bilirubin.

Cast—An insoluble gelled protein matrix that takes the form of the renal tubule in which it was deposited. Casts are washed out by normal urine flow.

Catheter—A thin flexible tube inserted through the urethra into the bladder to allow urine to flow out.

Clean-catch specimen—A urine specimen that is collected from the middle of the urine stream after the first part of the flow has been discarded.

Cystine—An amino acid normally reabsorbed by the kidney tubules. Cystinuria is an inherited disease in which cystine and some other amino acids are not reabsorbed by the body in normal amounts. Cystine crystals then form in the kidney, which leads to obstructive renal failure.

Epithelium—A general term for the layer of cells that lines blood vessels or small body cavities.

Ketones—Substances produced during the breakdown of fatty acids. They are produced in excessive amounts in diabetes and certain other abnormal conditions.

pH—A chemical symbol that denotes the acidity or alkalinity of a fluid, ranging from 1 (more acid) to 14 (more alkaline).

Meatus—A general term for an opening or passageway in the body. The urethral meatus should be cleansed before a urine sample is collected.

Porphyrias—A group of disorders involving heme biosynthesis, characterized by excessive excretion of polyphrins. The porphyrias may be either inherited or acquired (usually from the effects of certain chemical agents).

Trichomonads—Parasitic protozoa commonly found in the digestive and genital tracts of humans and other animals. Some species cause vaginal infections in women characterized by itching and a frothy discharge.

Turbidity—The degree of cloudiness of a urine sample (or other solution).

Urethra—The tube that carries urine from the bladder to the outside of the body.

Urinalysis (plural, urinalyses)—The diagnostic testing of a urine sample.

Voiding—The medical term for emptying the bladder or urinating.

those with some kidney diseases. A volume in excess of 2 liters (slightly more than 2 quarts) per day is considered polyuria (excessive urine production); it is common in persons with diabetes mellitus and diabetes insipidus.

Biochemical tests

Biochemical testing of urine is performed using dry reagent strips, often called dipsticks. A urine dipstick consists of a white plastic strip with absorbent microfiber cellulose pads attached to it. Each pad contains the dried reagents needed for a specific test. The person performing the test dips the strip into the urine, lets it sit for a specified amount of time, and compares the color change to a standard chart.

Additional tests are available for measuring the levels of bilirubin, protein, glucose, ketones, and urobilinogen in urine. In general, these individual tests provide greater sensitivity; they therefore permit detection of a lower concentration of the respective substance. A brief description of the most commonly used dry reagent strip tests follows.

pH: A combination of pH indicators (methyl red and bromthymol blue) react with hydrogen ions (H^+) to produce a color change over a pH range of 5.0 to 8.5. pH measurements are useful in determining metabolic or respiratory disturbances in acid-base balance. For example, kidney disease often results in retention of H^+ (reduced acid excretion). pH varies with a person's diet, tending to be acidic in people who eat meat but more alkaline in vegetarians. pH testing is also useful for the classification of urine crystals.

Protein: Based upon a phenomenon called the "protein error of indicators," this test uses a pH indicator, such as tetrabromphenol blue, that changes color (at constant pH) when albumin is present in the urine. Albumin is important in determining the presence of glomerular damage. The glomerulus is the network of capillaries in the kidneys that filters low molecular weight solutes such as urea, glucose, and salts, but normally prevents passage of protein or cells from blood into filtrate. Albuminuria occurs when the glomerular membrane is damaged, a condition called glomerulonephritis.

Glucose (sugar): The glucose test is used to monitor persons with diabetes. When blood glucose levels rise above 160 mg/dL, the glucose will be detected in urine. Consequently, glycosuria (glucose in the urine) may be the first indicator that diabetes or another hyperglycemic condition is present. The glucose test may be used to screen newborns for galactosuria and other disorders of carbohydrate metabolism that cause urinary excretion of a sugar other than glucose.

Ketones: Ketones are compounds resulting from the breakdown of fatty acids in the body. These ketones are produced in excess in disorders of carbohydrate metabolism, especially Type 1 diabetes mellitus. In diabetes, excess ketoacids in the blood may cause life-threatening acidosis and coma. These ketoacids and their salts spill into the urine, causing ketonuria. Ketones are also found in the urine in several other conditions, including fever; pregnancy; glycogen storage diseases; and weight loss produced by a carbohydrate-restricted diet.

Blood: Red cells and hemoglobin may enter the urine from the kidney or lower urinary tract. Testing for blood in the urine detects abnormal levels of either red cells or hemoglobin, which may be caused by excessive red cell destruction, glomerular disease, kidney or urinary tract infection, malignancy, or urinary tract injury.

Bilirubin: Bilirubin is a breakdown product of hemoglobin. Most of the bilirubin produced in humans is conjugated by the liver and excreted into the bile, but a very small amount of conjugated bilirubin is reabsorbed and reaches the general circulation to be excreted in the urine. The normal level of urinary bilirubin is below the detection limit of the test. Bilirubin in the urine is derived from the liver, and a positive test indicates hepatic disease or hepatobiliary obstruction.

Specific gravity: Specific gravity is a measure of the ability of the kidneys to concentrate urine by conserving water.

Nitrite: Some disease bacteria, including the lactose-positive *Enterobactericeae, Staphylococcus, Proteus, Salmonella,* and *Pseudomonas* are able to reduce nitrate in urine to nitrite. A positive test for nitrite indicates bacteruria, or the presence of bacteria in the urine.

Urobilinogen: Urobilinogen is a substance formed in the gastrointestinal tract by the bacterial reduction of conjugated bilirubin. Increased urinary urobilinogen occurs in prehepatic jaundice (hemolytic anemia), hepatitis, and other forms of hepatic necrosis that impair the circulation of blood in the liver and surrounding organs. The urobilinogen test is helpful in differentiating these conditions from obstructive jaundice, which results in decreased production of urobilinogen.

Leukocytes: The presence of white blood cells in the urine usually signifies a urinary tract infection, such as cystitis, or renal disease, such as pyelonephritis or glomerulonephritis.

Microscopic examination

A urine sample may contain cells that originated in the blood, the kidney, or the lower urinary tract. Microscopic examination of urinary sediment can provide valuable clues regarding many diseases and disorders involving these systems.

The presence of bacteria or yeast and white blood cells helps to distinguish between a urinary tract infection and a contaminated urine sample. White blood cells are not seen if the sample has been contaminated. The presence of cellular casts (casts containing RBCs, WBCs, or epithelial cells) identifies the kidneys, rather than the lower urinary tract, as the source of such cells. Cellular casts and renal epithelial (kidney lining) cells are signs of kidney disease.

The microscopic examination also identifies both normal and abnormal crystals in the sediment. Abnormal crystals are those formed as a result of an abnormal metabolic process and are always clinically significant. Normal crystals are formed from normal metabolic processes; however, they may lead to the formation of renal calculi, or kidney stones.

Preparation

A urine sample is collected in an unused disposable plastic cup with a tight-fitting lid. A randomly voided sample is suitable for routine urinalysis, although the urine that is first voided in the morning is preferable because it is the most concentrated. The best sample for analysis is collected in a sterile container after the external genitalia have been cleansed using the midstream void (clean-catch) method. This sample may be cultured if the laboratory findings indicate bacteruria.

To collect a sample using the clean-catch method:

- Females should use a clean cotton ball moistened with lukewarm water (or antiseptic wipes provided with collection kits) to cleanse the external genital area before collecting a urine sample. To prevent contamination with menstrual blood, vaginal discharge, or germs from the external genitalia, they should release some urine before beginning to collect the sample.
- Males should use a piece of clean cotton moistened with lukewarm water or antiseptic wipes to cleanse the head of the penis and the urethral meatus (opening). Uncircumcised males should draw back the foreskin. After the area has been thoroughly cleansed, they should use the midstream void method to collect the sample.
- For infants, a parent or health care worker should cleanse the baby's outer genitalia and surrounding skin. A sterile collection bag should be attached to the child's genital area and left in place until he or she has urinated. It is important to not touch the inside of the bag, and to remove it as soon as a specimen has been obtained.

Urine samples can also be obtained via bladder catheterization, a procedure used to collect uncontaminated urine when the patient cannot void. A catheter is a thin flexible tube that a health care professional inserts through the urethra into the bladder to allow urine to flow out. To minimize the risk of infecting the patient's bladder with bacteria, many clinicians use a Robinson catheter, which is a plain rubber or latex tube that is removed as soon as the specimen is collected. If urine for culture is to be collected from an indwelling catheter, it should be aspirated (removed by suction) from the line using a syringe and not removed from the bag in order to avoid contamination.

Suprapubic bladder aspiration is a collection technique sometimes used to obtain urine from infants younger than six months or urine directly from the bladder for culture. The doctor withdraws urine from the bladder into a syringe through a needle inserted through the skin.

Aftercare

The patient may return to normal activities after collecting the sample and may start taking any medications that were discontinued before the test.

Risks

There are no risks associated with voided specimens. The risk of bladder infection from catheterization with a Robinson catheter is about 3%.

Normal results

Normal urine is a clear straw-colored liquid, but may also be slightly hazy. It has a slight odor, and some laboratories will note strong or atypical odors on the urinalysis report. A normal urine specimen may contain some normal crystals as well as squamous or transitional epithelial cells from the bladder, lower urinary tract, or vagina. Urine may contain transparent (hyaline) casts, especially if it was collected after vigorous **exercise**. The presence of hyaline casts may be a sign of kidney disease, however, when the cause cannot be attributed to exercise, running, or medications. Normal urine contains a small amount of urobilinogen, and may contain a few RBCs and WBCs. Normal urine does *not* contain detectable amounts of glucose or other sugars, protein, ketones, bilirubin, bacteria, yeast cells, or trichomonads. Normal values used in many laboratories are given below:

- Glucose: negative (quantitative less than 130 mg/day or 30 mg/dL).
- Bilirubin: negative (quantitative less than 0.02 mg/dL).
- Ketones: negative (quantitative 0.5–3.0 mg/dL).
- pH: 5.0–8.0.
- Protein: negative (quantitative 15–150 mg/day, less than 10 mg/dL).
- Blood: negative.
- Nitrite: negative.
- Specific gravity: 1.015–1.025.
- Urobilinogen: 0–2 Ehrlich units (quantitative 0.3–1.0 Ehrlich units).
- Leukocyte esterase: negative.
- Red blood cells: 0–2 per high power field.
- White blood cells: 0–5 per high power field (0–10 per high power field for some standardized systems).

Resources

BOOKS

Chernecky, Cynthia C, and Barbara J. Berger. *Laboratory Tests and Diagnostic Procedures*, 3rd ed. Philadelphia, PA: W. B. Saunders Company, 2001.

Henry, J.B. *Clinical Diagnosis and Management by Laboratory Methods*, 20th ed. Philadelphia, PA: W.B. Saunders Company, 2001.

Kee, Joyce LeFever. *Handbook of Laboratory and Diagnostic Tests*, 4th ed. Upper Saddle River, NJ: Prentice Hall, 2001.

Wallach, Jacques. *Interpretation of Diagnostic Tests*, 7th ed. Philadelphia, PA: Lippincott Williams & Wilkens, 2000.

ORGANIZATIONS

American Association of Kidney Patients. 100 S. Ashley Drive, Suite 280, Tampa, FL 33260. (800) 749-2257. www.aakp.org.

American Kidney Fund. 6110 Executive Blvd., Suite 1010, Rockville, MD 20852. (301) 881-3052. www.akfinc.org.

American Medical Technologists. 710 Higgins Road, Park Ridge, IL 60068-5765. (847) 823-5169. www.amt1.com.

American Society for Clinical Pathology (ASCP). 2100 West Harrison Street, Chicago, Il 60612-3798. (312) 738-1336. www.ascp.org.

National Kidney and Urologic Diseases Information Clearinghouse. 3 Information Way, Bethesda, MD 20892-3580.

OTHER

National Institutes of Health. [cited April 4, 2003]. www.nlm.nih.gov/medlineplus/encyclopedia.html.

Victoria E. DeMoranville
Mark A. Best

Urinary anti-infectives

Definition

Urinary anti-infectives are medicines used to treat or prevent infections of the urinary tract, which is the passage through which urine flows from the kidneys out of the body.

Purpose

Normally, no bacteria or other disease-causing organisms live in the bladder. Likewise, the urethra—the tube-like structure that carries urine from the bladder to the outside of the body—usually does not contain any bacteria, or not enough to cause problems. But the bladder, urethra, and other parts of the urinary tract may become infected when disease-causing organisms enter it from other body regions or from outside the body. Urinary anti-infectives are used to treat such infections.

Although many **antibiotics** and some **sulfonamides** are equally effective in treating urinary tract infections, urinary anti-infectives have the advantage of being active only in the urinary tract. This means they are less likely to cause development of resistant microorganisms, or cause diarrhea by destroying the bacteria in the large intestine.

Some urinary anti-infectives have been used to prevent urinary tract infections, but the evidence that they are effective for this purpose is limited.

Description

Commonly used urinary anti-infectives include methenamine (Urex, Hiprex, Mandelamine); nalidixic acid (NegGram); and nitrofurantoin (Macrobid, Furatoin, and other brands). Nalidixic acid belongs to a group of synthetic antibacterial drugs known as quinolones. The first quinolone to be approved for clinical use, nalidixic acid, has been used to treat urinary tract infections since 1967. Nitrofurantoin is also a synthetic antibacterial medication.

Urinary anti-infectives are available only with a physician's prescription. They come in capsule, tablet, granular, and liquid forms.

Recommended dosage

Methenamine

For adults and children 12 years and over, the usual dosage is 1 gram, taken either twice a day or four times a day, depending on the form of the medication that the doctor prescribes. For children aged six to 12 years, the dosage ranges from 500 mg taken two to four times a day to 1 gram taken twice a day, again depending on the form of the drug. A physician must determine the dose for children under six years.

Urinary anti-infectives will not work properly unless the urine is acidic, with a pH reading of 5.5 or lower. The physician who prescribes the medicine will explain how to test the urine's acidity. He or she may suggest dietary changes that will make the urine more acidic, such as eating more protein; drinking cranberry juice; eating plums and prunes while avoiding most other fruits; and cutting down on milk and other dairy products. The patient should also avoid taking antacids.

Nalidixic acid

The recommended dosage of this drug for adults and children 12 years and older is 1 gram every six hours. If the medicine is taken for more than one or two weeks, the dosage may be decreased to 500 mg every six hours. A physician must determine the correct dosage for children three months to 12 years old. Children under three months should not take nalidixic acid because it causes bone problems in young animals and could have the same effect in young children.

Nitrofurantoin

CAPSULES, TABLETS, OR LIQUID. The usual dose for adults and adolescents is 50–100 mg every six hours.

KEY TERMS

Altitude sickness—A set of symptoms that people who normally live at low altitudes may have when they climb mountains or travel to high altitudes. The symptoms include nosebleed, nausea, and shortness of breath.

Anemia—A low level of hemoglobin in the blood.

Anticoagulant—A type of medication given to prevent the formation of blood clots. Anticoagulants are sometimes called blood thinners.

Bacteria—Microscopically small one-celled forms of life that cause many diseases and infections.

Glaucoma—A condition in which fluid pressure in the eye is abnormally high. If not treated, glaucoma may lead to blindness.

Glucose-6-phosphate dehydrogenase (G6PD) deficiency—An inherited disorder in which the body lacks an enzyme that normally protects red blood cells from toxic chemicals. Certain drugs can cause patients' red blood cells to break down, resulting in anemia. This may also happen when they have a fever or an infection. The condition usually occurs in males. About 10% of black males have it, as do a small percentage of people from the Mediterranean region.

Granule—A small grain or pellet. Medicines that come in granule form are usually mixed with liquids or sprinkled on food before they are taken.

Hemoglobin—The reddish-colored compound in blood that carries oxygen from the lungs throughout the body and brings waste carbon dioxide from the cells to the lungs, where it is released

pH—A measure of the acidity or alkalinity of a substance or compound. The pH scale ranges from 0 to 14. Values below 7 are acidic; values above 7 are alkaline.

Psyllium—A herb whose seeds contain a water-soluble fiber that adds bulk to the contents of the digestive tract. The bulk helps to prevent constipation. Laxatives containing psyllium may interfere with the body's absorption of urinary anti-infectives.

Quinolones—A group of synthetic antibacterial drugs originally derived from quinine. Nalidixic acid is the first quinolone that was approved for clinical use.

Seizure—A sudden attack, spasm, or convulsion.

EXTENDED-RELEASE CAPSULES. For adults and children 12 years and older, the usual dosage is 100 mg every 12 hours for seven days.

A physician must determine the correct dose of all forms of nitrofurantoin for children one month and older according to the child's body weight. Children under one month should not be given this medicine.

Precautions

Methenamine

Methenamine may produce adverse effects in some patients with systemic disorders. For example, it may worsen the symptoms of people with severe liver disease. People who are dehydrated or who have severe kidney disease may be more likely to have side effects that affect the kidneys.

Nalidixic acid

Some people feel drowsy, dizzy, or less alert than usual when using this drug. Nalidixic acid may also cause blurred vision or other visual problems. Because of these possible side effects, anyone who takes nalidixic acid should not drive, operate machinery, or do anything else that might be dangerous until they have found out how the drugs affect them.

Nalidixic acid may increase sensitivity to sunlight. Even brief exposure to sunlight may cause severe sunburn or a rash. Patients treated with this medication should avoid sun exposure, especially during high sun (between 10 A.M. and 3 P.M.). They should wear a hat or scarf and tightly woven clothing that covers the arms and legs; use a sunscreen with a sun protection factor (SPF) of at least 15; protect the lips with a lip balm containing sun block; and avoid the use of tanning beds, tanning booths, and sunlamps.

Diabetic patients should be aware that nalidixic acid may cause false results on some urine sugar tests. They should check with a physician before making any changes in their diet or diabetes medicine based on the results of a urine test.

In laboratory studies, nalidixic acid has been found to interfere with bone development in young animals. The drug's effects have not been studied in pregnant women, but because of its effects in animals, it is not recommended for use during pregnancy.

This medicine does not cause problems in most nursing babies whose mothers are taking it during lactation. However, nursing babies with glucose-6-phosphate dehydrogenase (G6PD) deficiency (an inherited disorder that affects mainly black males) may have blood problems if their mothers take nalidixic acid.

People with certain medical conditions may be more likely to have particular side effects if they take this medicine. For example, people with a history of seizures or severe hardening of the arteries in the brain may be more likely to have side effects that affect the nervous system. People with glucose-6-phosphate dehydrogenase (G6PD) deficiency are more likely to have side effects that affect the blood. In addition, people with liver disease or severe kidney disease are at increased risk of having any of the drug's possible side effects.

Nitrofurantoin

Pregnant women should not take this medicine within two weeks of their delivery date. They should not use it during labor and delivery, as this could cause problems in the baby.

Women who are breastfeeding should check with their physicians before using this medicine. It passes into breast milk and could cause problems in nursing babies whose mothers take it. This is especially true of babies with glucose-6-phosphate dehydrogenase (G6PD) deficiency. The medicine also should not be given directly to babies up to one month of age, as they are particularly sensitive to its effects.

Older people may be more likely to have side effects when taking nitrofurantoin, because they are more sensitive to the drug's effects.

Taking nitrofurantoin may cause problems for people with certain medical conditions. Side effects may be greater, for example, in people with lung disease or nerve damage. In people with kidney disease, the medicine may not work as well as it should, but may cause more side effects. Those with glucose-6-phosphate dehydrogenase (G6PD) deficiency who take nitrofurantoin may develop anemia.

Diabetic patients should be aware that this medicine may cause false results on some urine sugar tests. They should check with a physician before making any changes in diet or diabetes medicine based on the results of a urine test.

General precautions for all urinary anti-infectives

The symptoms of a urinary tract infection should improve within a few days of starting to take a urinary anti-infective. If they do not, or if they become worse, the patient should consult a physician right away. Patients who need to take this medicine for long periods should see their doctors regularly, so that their improvement and any side effects can be monitored.

Anyone who has had unusual reactions to urinary anti-infectives in the past should let his or her physician know before taking the drugs again. The physician should also be told about any allergies to foods, dyes, preservatives, or other substances. Patients taking nalidixic acid should tell their physicians if they have ever had reactions to such other quinolones as cinoxacin (Cinobac), ciprofloxacin (Cipro), enoxacin (Penetrex), norfloxacin (Noroxin), or ofloxacin (Floxin), all of which are also used to treat or prevent infections. Anyone taking nitrofurantoin should let the physician know if he or she has had an unusual reaction to such drugs as furazolidone (Furoxone) or nitrofurazone (Furacin).

Side effects

Methenamine

Nausea and vomiting are not common, but may occur. These side effects do not need medical attention unless they are severe. One side effect that should be brought to a physician's attention immediately is a skin rash.

Nalidixic acid

Some side effects are fairly minor and are likely to go away as the body adjusts to the drug. These include dizziness, drowsiness, headache, nausea or vomiting, stomach pain, and diarrhea. Unless these problems continue or are bothersome, they do not need medical attention.

Other side effects, however, should have prompt medical attention. Anyone who has such visual symptoms as blurred vision, double vision, decreased vision, changes in color vision, seeing halos around lights, or increased glare from lights should consult a physician immediately.

Nitrofurantoin

This medicine may discolor the urine, causing it to turn reddish-yellow or brown. Patients should not be concerned about this change in color. Other possible side effects that do not need medical attention, unless they are severe, include pain in the stomach or abdomen, stomach upset, diarrhea, loss of appetite, and nausea or vomiting.

Anyone who has chest pain, breathing problems, fever, chills, or a cough while taking nitrofurantoin should consult their physician immediately.

General advice on side effects for all urinary anti-infectives

Other side effects are possible when taking any urinary anti-infective. Anyone who has unusual symptoms while taking this type of medication should contact his or her physician.

Interactions

Methenamine

Certain medicines may make methenamine less effective. These include thiazide **diuretics** (water pills) and medicines that make the urine less acid, such as antacids, bicarbonate of soda (baking soda), and the drugs acetazolamide (Diamox), dichlorphenamide (Daranide), and methazolamide (Neptazane), which are used to treat glaucoma, epilepsy, altitude sickness, and other conditions.

Nalidixic acid

People who are taking blood thinners (anticoagulants) may be more likely to have bleeding problems if they take this medicine.

Nitrofurantoin

Nitrofurantoin may interact with many other medicines. For example, taking nitrofurantoin with certain drugs that include methyldopa (Aldomet), sulfonamides (sulfa drugs), vitamin K, and diabetes medicines taken by mouth may increase the chance of side effects that affect the blood. General side effects are more likely in people who take nitrofurantoin with the gout drugs probenecid (Benemid) or sulfinpyrazone (Anturane). The risk of side effects that involve the nervous system is higher in people who take nitrofurantoin with such drugs as lithium (Lithane); disulfiram (Antabuse); other anti-infectives; and the cancer drugs cisplatin (Platinol) and vincristine (Oncovin). Patients who have been vaccinated with DPT (diphtheria, tetanus, and pertussis) within the last 30 days or are vaccinated after taking nitrofurantoin are also more likely to have side effects that affect the nervous system. Because of the many possible interactions, anyone taking nitrofurantoin should be sure to consult a physician before combining it with any other medicine.

Laxatives containing psyllium and other bulk-forming substances may interfere with the body's absorption of nitrofurantoin. Patients with constipation who are taking nitrofurantoin should consult their doctor before taking an over-the-counter laxative.

General advice about drug interactions

Patients should check with a physician or pharmacist before combining a urinary anti-infective with any other prescription or nonprescription (over-the-counter) medicine.

Patients who are taking any kind of herbal preparation or other alternative medicine should give their doctor and pharmacist a list of all the compounds that they use on a regular basis. Most of these preparations are unlikely to interact with urinary anti-infectives, but there is much that is still unknown about possible interactions between standard prescription medications and alternative medicines.

Resources

BOOKS

Mandell, G. L., et al. *Principles and Practice of Infectious Diseases*, 6th ed. London: Churchill Livingstone, 2005.

Wein, A. J., et al. *Campbell-Walsh Urology*, 9th ed. Philadelphia: Saunders, 2007.

PERIODICALS

Chang, S. L. "Pediatric urinary tract infections." *Pediatric Clinics of North America* 53 (June 2006): 379–400.

Emmerson, A. M., and A. M. Jones. "The Quinolones: Decades of Development and Use." *Journal of Antimicrobial Chemotherapy* 51 (May 2003): Supplement 1, 13–20.

Juthani-Mehta, M. "Asymtpomatic Bacteriuria and Urinary Tract Infections in Older Adults." *Clinics of Geriatric Medicine* 23 (August 2007): 585–594.

ORGANIZATIONS

American Society of Health-System Pharmacists (ASHP). 7272 Wisconsin Avenue, Bethesda, MD 20814. (301) 657-3000. http://www.ashp.org (accessed April 15, 2008).

United States Food and Drug Administration (FDA). 5600 Fishers Lane, Rockville, MD 20857-0001. (888) INFO-FDA. http://www.fda.gov (accessed April 15, 2008).

Nancy Ross-Flanigan
Sam Uretsky, PharmD

Urinary artificial sphincter *see* **Artificial sphincter insertion**

Urinary catheterization, female *see* **Catheterization, female**

Urinary catheterization, male *see* **Catheterization, male**

Urinary diversion *see* **Ureterostomy, cutaneous**

Urinary diversion surgery *see* **Ileal conduit surgery**

Urine culture

Definition

A urine culture is a diagnostic laboratory test performed to detect the presence of bacteria in the urine (bacteriuria).

Purpose

Culture of the urine is a method of diagnosis for urinary tract infection that determines the number of microorganisms present in a given quantity of urine.

Precautions

If delivery of the urine specimen to the laboratory within one hour of collection is not possible, it should be refrigerated. The healthcare provider should be informed of any **antibiotics** currently or recently taken.

Description

There are several different methods for collection of a urine sample. The most common is the midstream clean-catch technique. Hands should be washed before beginning. For females, the external genitalia (sex organs) are washed two or three times with a cleansing agent and rinsed with water. In males, the external head of the penis is similarly cleansed and rinsed. The patient is then instructed to begin to urinate, and the urine is collected midstream into a sterile container. In infants, a urinary collection bag (plastic bag with an adhesive seal on one end) is attached over the labia in girls or a boy's penis to collect the specimen.

Another method is the catheterized urine specimen in which a lubricated catheter (thin rubber tube) is inserted through the urethra (tube-like structure in which urine is expelled from the bladder) into the bladder. This avoids contamination from the urethra or external genitalia. If the patient already has a urinary catheter in place, a urine specimen may be collected by clamping the tubing below the collection port and using a sterile needle and syringe to obtain the urine sample; urine cannot be taken from the drainage bag, as it is not fresh and has had an opportunity to grow bacteria at room temperature. On rare occasions, the healthcare provider may collect a urine sample by inserting a needle directly into the bladder (suprapubic tap) and draining the urine; this method is used only when a sample is needed quickly.

Negative culture results showing no bacterial growth are available after 24 hours. Positive results require 24–72 hours to complete identification of the number and type of bacteria found.

KEY TERMS

Bacteriuria—The presence of bacteria in the urine.

Preparation

Drinking a glass of water 15–20 minutes before the test is helpful if there is no urge to urinate. There are no other special preparations or aftercare required for the test.

Aftercare

No aftercare is required for a urine culture.

Risks

There are no risks associated with the culture test itself. If insertion of a urinary catheter (thin rubber tube) is required to obtain the urine, there is a slight risk of introducing infection from the catheter.

Normal results

No growth of bacteria is considered the normal result, and this indicates absence of infection.

Abnormal results

Abnormal results, or a positive test, where bacteria are found in the specimen, may indicate a urinary tract infection. Contamination of the specimen from hair, external genitalia, or the rectum may cause a false-positive result. Identification of the number and type of bacteria, with consideration of the method used in obtaining the specimen, is significant in diagnosis.

Escherichia coli causes approximately 80% of infections in patients without catheters, abnormalities of the urinary tract, or calculi (stones). Other bacteria that account for a smaller portion of uncomplicated infections include *Proteus klebsiella* and *Enterobacter*.

Alternatives

There are no alternatives to a urine culture.

Precautions

Two precautions are needed. The first is to clean the urethral meatus by urinating and then stopping the stream before collecting a specimen. The second is to use a sterile container to collect the urine specimen.

Side effects

There are no known side effects associated with a urine culture.

Resources

BOOKS

Fischbach, F. T. and M. B. Dunning. *A Manual of Laboratory and Diagnostic Tests*, 8th ed. Philadelphia: Lippincott Williams & Wilkins, 2008.

McGhee, M. *A Guide to Laboratory Investigations*, 5th ed. Oxford, England: Radcliffe Publishing Ltd, 2008.

Price, C. P. *Evidence-Based Laboratory Medicine: Principles, Practice, and Outcomes*, 2nd ed. Washington, DC: AACC Press, 2007.

Scott, M.G., A. M. Gronowski, and C. S. Eby. *Tietz's Applied Laboratory Medicine*, 2nd ed. New York: Wiley-Liss, 2007.

Springhouse, A. M.. *Diagnostic Tests Made Incredibly Easy!*, 2nd ed. Philadelphia: Lippincott Williams & Wilkins, 2008.

PERIODICALS

Barrett, M., and V. L. Campbell. "Aerobic bacterial culture of used intravenous fluid bags intended for use as urine collection reservoirs." *Journal of the American Animal Hospital Association* 44, no. 1 (2008): 2–4.

Dalen, D.M., R. K. Zvonar, and P. G. Jessamine. "An evaluation of the management of asymptomatic catheter-associated bacteriuria and candiduria at The Ottawa Hospital." *Canadian Journal of Infectious Disease and Medical Microbiology* 16, no. 3 (2005): 166–170.

Mishriki, S. F., G. Nabi, and N. P. Cohen. "Diagnosis of urologic malignancies in patients with asymptomatic dipstick hematuria: prospective study with 13 years' follow-up." *Urology* 71, no. 1 (2008): 13–16.

Nicolle, L. "Complicated urinary tract infection in adults." *Canadian Journal of Infectious Disease and Medical Microbiology* 16, no. 6 (2005): 349–360.

ORGANIZATIONS

American Foundation for Urologic Disease. 300 West Pratt St., Suite 401, Baltimore, MD 21201.

American Society for Clinical Laboratory Science. http://www.ascls.org/ (accessed April 15, 2008).

American Society of Clinical Pathologists. http://www.ascp.org/ (accessed April 15, 2008).

College of American Pathologists. http://www.cap.org/apps/cap.portal (accessed April 15, 2008).

OTHER

American Clinical Laboratory Association. Information about clinical chemistry. 2008 [cited February 24, 2008]. http://www.clinical-labs.org/ (accessed April 15, 2008).

Clinical Laboratory Management Association. Information about clinical chemistry. 2008 [cited February 22, 2008]. http://www.clma.org/ (accessed April 15, 2008).

Lab Tests On Line, 2008. http://www.labtestsonline.org/ (accessed April 15, 2008).

National Accreditation Agency for Clinical Laboratory Sciences, 2008. http://www.naacls.org/ (accessed April 15, 2008).

L. Fleming Fallon, Jr, MD, DrPH

Urobilinogen test *see* **Urinalysis**

Urologic surgery

Definition

Urologic surgery is the integration of surgical activities for the pelvis—the colon, urogenital, and gynecological organs—primarily for the treatment of obstructions, dysfunction, malignancies, and inflammatory diseases. Common urologic operations include:

- renal (kidney) surgery
- kidney removal (nephrectomy)
- surgery of the ureters, including ureterolithotomy or removal of calculus (stones) in the ureters
- bladder surgery
- pelvic lymph node dissection
- prostatic surgery, removal of the prostate
- testicular (scrotal) surgery
- urethra surgery
- surgery to the penis

Purpose

Conditions that commonly dictate a need for urologic surgery include neurogenic sources like spinal cord injury; injuries to the pelvic organs; chronic digestive and urinary diseases; and prostate infections and inflammations. There are many other common chronic and malignant diseases that can benefit from resection, surgical augmentation, or surgery to clear obstructions. These conditions impact the digestive, renal, and reproductive systems.

Most organs are susceptible to cancer in the form of tumors and invasion of the surrounding tissue. Urologic malignancies are on the rise. Other conditions that are seen more frequently include kidney stones, diseases and infections; pancreatic diseases;

KEY TERMS

Genitourinary reconstruction—Surgery that corrects birth defects or the results of disease that involve the genitals and urinary tract, including the kidneys, ureters, bladder, urethra, and the male and female genitals.

Nephrectomy—Surgical removal of a kidney.

Neurogenic bladder—Bladder dysfunction caused by neurological diseases that alter the brain's messages to the bladder.

Prostatectomy—Prostate cancer surgery that includes partial or complete removal of the prostate.

ulcerative colitis; penile dysfunction; and infections of the genitourinary tract.

Urologic surgery has been revolutionized by striking advances in urodynamic diagnostic systems. Changes in these areas have been particularly beneficial for urologic surgery: **laparoscopy**, endoscopic examination for colon cancer, implantation procedures, and imaging techniques. These procedural and imaging advances have brought the field of urology to a highly active and innovative stage, with new surgical options created each year.

Demographics

According to the National Kidney Foundation, kidney and urologic diseases affect at least 5% of the American population, and cause over 260,000 deaths. As the population ages, these conditions are expected to increase, especially among ethnic minorities who have a disproportionate share of urologic diseases. Major urologic surgery includes radical and partial resections for malignant and benign conditions; and implantation and diversion surgeries.

Cancer

Prostate cancer is the most common cancer affecting males in the United States. One in six men will have the disease at some time in his life. It is, however, treated successfully with surgery.

According to the Urological Foundation, more than 63,200 new cases of bladder cancer are detected each year. In the United States, bladder cancer is the fourth most common cancer in men and the eighth most common for women.

Kidney cancer occurs in 51,190 new patients per year, with almost 13,000 deaths. It is the eighth most common cancer in men and the tenth most common cancer in women. Renal cell carcinoma makes up 85% of all kidney tumors. In adults ages 50–70 years, kidney cancer occurs twice as often in men as women. At the time of diagnosis, metastasis is present in 25–30% of patients with renal cell carcinoma.

Other conditions

Enlarged prostate (benign prostate hyperplasia, BPH) is very common, and often treated with surgery. Interstitial cystitis (bladder infection of unknown origin) often affects women with severe pain and incontinence. The condition, like other forms of severe incontinence, requires surgery.

Incontinence is increasingly diagnosed as a problem among the aging population in the United States, and is gaining recognition for its highly debilitating effects both in its fecal and urinary forms. According to the National Institute of Diabetes & Digestive & Kidney Diseases (NIDDK), more than 6.5 million Americans have fecal incontinence. Fecal incontinence affects people of all ages; many cases are never reported. Women are five times more likely than men to have fecal incontinence. This is primarily due to obstetric injury, especially with forceps delivery and anal sphincter laceration.

Urinary incontinence affects an estimated 38% of women aged 60 or older, and an estimated 17% of men aged 60 or older. According to one study published in the *American Journal of Gastroenterology*, only 34% of incontinent patients have ever mentioned their problem to a physician, even though 23% wear absorbent pads, 12% take medications, and 11% lead lives restricted by their incontinence.

Many surgical procedures are now available to correct both fecal and urinary incontinence. They include retropubic slings for urinary incontinence, artificial sphincter implants for urinary and fecal incontinence, and bladder and colon diversion surgeries for restoration of voiding and waste function with an outside appliance called an ostomy. Kidney surgery and transplantation account for a large segment of urologic surgery. Benign conditions include sexual dysfunction, kidney stones, and fertility issues.

Description

Until the late twentieth century, urological operations usually involved open abdominal surgery with full incision, lengthy hospital stays, and long recovery periods. Today, surgery is less traumatic, with shortened hospitalizations. Minimally invasive surgeries are the norm in many cases, with new laparoscopic procedures developed each year. Laparoscopic surgery is effective for many kidney tumors and kidney removal (**nephrectomy**), lymph node excision, prostate and ureteral cancers, as well as incontinence, urological reconstruction, kidney stones, and some cases of bladder dysfunction.

Diagnosis/Preparation

Testing is often required to determine if a patient is better suited for open or laparoscopic surgery. Blood tests for some cancers, as well as function tests for the affected organs, will be required. Radiographic or **ultrasound** techniques are helpful in providing images of abnormalities.

Cystoscopy is often used with bladder and urethra surgery. In this procedure, a thin telescope-like instrument is inserted directly into the bladder. Disorders of the colon may be studied with endoscopes, imaging instruments inserted directly into the colon. Urodynamic studies of the bladder and sphincter determine how the bladder fills and empties. Digital rectal exams diagnose prostatic disorders. In this procedure, the physician feels the prostate with a gloved, lubricated finger inserted into the rectum.

Aftercare

Hospital stays range from one day to one week, depending upon the level of organ involvement and type of urologic surgery (open versus laparoscopic). Major urologic surgeries may require stents (temporary diversion of urine or feces) and catheters that are removed after surgery. Some surgeries are staged in two parts to accommodate the removal of diseased tissue, and the augmentation or reconstruction to replace function. Laparoscopic surgery patients benefit from shorter hospital stays, more rapid recovery, and possibly lower morbidity rates than open surgery procedures. This is increasingly true for prostate cancer surgeries.

Risks

The risks of urologic surgery vary with the type of surgical procedure (open or laparoscopic), and the extent of organ involvement. According to one study of 2,407 urologic surgeries in four centers, the overall complication rate was 4.4%, with a mortality rate of 0.08%.

Open surgery poses the standard surgery and anesthetic risks associated with strain on the heart and lungs. Risks of infection at the wound site accompany all surgeries, open and laparoscopic. The risk of injury to adjacent organs is higher in laparoscopic surgery. Kidney removal and transplantation have many risks because of the extent of the surgery, as do surgeries of the colon, bladder, and prostate.

Significant gains have been made in prostate surgery. Urinary control issues following prostate surgery, especially radical prostatectomy, have improved. However, postoperative urinary incontinence remains a significant risk, with 27% of patients in one study reporting the need for some kind of leakage protection. In the same study, only 14.2% of previously potent men reported the ability to achieve and maintain a postoperative erection that is sufficient for sexual intercourse. Urologic surgeons are well versed in the risks and benefits of the surgeries they perform, and they expect to be asked questions related to these issues.

WHO PERFORMS THE PROCEDURE AND WHERE IS IT PERFORMED?

Urologic surgery is performed by surgeons who specialize in the treatment of urologic conditions. Surgery is performed in a general hospital, regional center, or clinic, depending upon the type of procedure.

Normal results

The expected surgery result is a topic that the urologic surgeon and patient should address prior to surgery. It is important that the patient understands the issues of recovery, rehabilitation, training or retraining, and the limitations surgery may offer for basic daily functions and enjoyment. Results of urologic surgery are individual, and depend upon the health of the patient and his or her motivation to deal with postoperative recovery issues and changes to organ function brought about by the surgery.

Alternatives

Many urological diseases can be dealt with through diet, weight loss, and lifestyle changes. These modifications are especially significant in preventing and treating conditions of the urinary tract. Obesity and nutrition play a significant role in urologic diseases, and impact many urologic cancers, inflammatory and ulcerative conditions, incontinence, and sexual dysfunction.

QUESTIONS TO ASK THE DOCTOR

- How many procedures does this physician and hospital perform compared to other facilities?
- What are the urination and sexual intercourse risks of this surgery?
- Does this condition offer alternatives to surgery without risks of exacerbating the condition?
- How often are patients dissatisfied with their outcomes?

Medical interventions are another form of treatment, particularly for infectious and inflammatory urologic conditions. They are particularly useful along with special adjunctive surgical procedures for the treatment of incontinence and painful bladder and kidney conditions. While many cancers must be treated surgically, prostate cancer is often treated with a "wait and see" approach due to its slow rate of growth. There is an increasing trend for men with slow-growing prostate cancers to have regular check-ups instead of immediate treatment.

Resources

BOOKS

Khatri, V. P., and J. A. Asensio. *Operative Surgery Manual*, 1st ed. Philadelphia: Saunders, 2003.

Townsend, C. M., et al. *Sabiston Textbook of Surgery*, 17th ed. Philadelphia: Saunders, 2004.

Wein, A. J., et al. *Campbell-Walsh Urology*, 9th ed. Philadelphia: Saunders, 2007.

ORGANIZATIONS

American Society of Nephrology. 1725 Eye Street, NW Suite 510, Washington, DC 20006. (202) 659-0599. Fax: (202) 659-0709.

American Society of Transplantation. 236 Route 38 West, Suite 100, Moorestown, NJ 08057. (856) 608-1104. Fax: (856) 608-1103. http://www.a-s-t.org (accessed April 15, 2008).

National Institute of Diabetes and Digestive and Kidney Diseases. National Institutes of Health, Information Office. 31 Center Drive, MSC 2560, Building 31, Room 9A-04, Bethesda, MD 20892-2560. (800) 860-8747, (800) 891-5389, (800) 891-5390, (301) 496-3583. Fax: (301) 496-7422. http://www.niddk.nih.gov/ (accessed April 15, 2008).

National Kidney Foundation. Director of Communications, 30 East 33rd Street, New York, NY 10016. (800) 622-9010, (212) 889-2210. Fax: (212) 689-9261. http://www.kidney.org (accessed April 15, 2008).

OTHER

"Resource Guide: Prostate Cancer." American Foundation for Urologic Diseases. http://www.auafoundation.org (accessed April 15, 2008).

Nancy McKenzie, PhD

Uterine fibroid removal *see* **Myomectomy**

Uterine stimulants

Definition

Uterine stimulants (uterotonics) are medications given to cause a woman's uterus to contract, or to increase the frequency and intensity of the contractions. These drugs are used to: induce (start) or augment (speed) labor; facilitate uterine contractions following a miscarriage; induce abortion; or reduce hemorrhage following childbirth or abortion. The three uterotonics used most frequently are the oxytocins, prostaglandins, and ergot alkaloids. Uterotonics may be given intravenously (IV), intramuscularly (IM), as a vaginal gel or suppository, or by mouth.

Purpose

Uterine stimulants are used to induce labor in certain circumstances when the mother's labor has not started naturally. These circumstances may include the mother's being past her due date; that is, the pregnancy has lasted longer than 40 weeks. Labor is especially likely to be induced if tests indicate a decrease in the volume of amniotic fluid. Uterotonics may also be used in cases of premature rupture of the membranes; preeclampsia (elevated blood pressure in the later stages of pregnancy); diabetes; and intrauterine growth retardation (IUGR), if these conditions require delivery before labor has begun. These medications may be recommended if the expectant mother lives a great distance from the healthcare facility and there is concern for either her or her baby's safety if she were unable to reach the facility once labor begins.

Uterine stimulants are also used in the augmentation of existing contractions, to increase their strength and frequency when labor does not move along well.

According to the American College of Obstetrics and Gynecology (ACOG), there continues to be an increase in the rate of induced labor. The ACOG reported that the increase in the rate of Caesarian sections is not due to the induction process but to other factors, such as the condition of the mother's cervix at the time of induction and whether the pregnancy was the woman's first.

Precautions

It is important to establish a clear baseline of **vital signs** before a woman is given any uterine stimulant. Consistent reevaluation and documentation of vital signs permit faster recognition of an abnormal change in a woman's condition. Documentation includes the time and dosage of any medications given, as well as a record of any side effects. A faster pulse and a drop in blood pressure signal a potential hemorrhage. When oxytocin is given intravenously, it must be diluted in IV fluid and never given as a straight IV. PGs should not be administered if there is any question about the condition of the fetus—for example, an abnormal fetal heart rate tracing. Methergine should never be given intravenously, and never to a woman with hypertension (high blood pressure).

Description

Oxytocin

Oxytocin is a naturally occurring hormone used to induce labor. The production and secretion of natural oxytocin is stimulated by the pituitary gland. It is also available in synthetic form under the trade names of Pitocin and Syntocinon.

Oxytocin is used in a contraction **stress test** (CST). A CST is done prior to the onset of labor to evaluate the fetus's ability to withstand the contractions of the uterus. To avoid the possibility of exogenous (introduced) oxytocin putting the woman into labor, she may instead be asked to stimulate her nipples to release her natural oxytocin. A negative, or normal, CST result is three contractions within a 10-minute period with no abnormal slowing of the fetal heart rate (FHR). The CST occasionally produces false positives, however.

Oxytocin may be used in the treatment of a miscarriage to assure that all the products of conception (POC) are expelled from the uterus. If the fetus died but was not expelled, a prostaglandin (PGE_2) may be given to ripen the cervix to facilitate a dilatation and evacuation, or to encourage uterine contractions. The prostaglandin may be administered either in gel form or as a vaginal suppository.

In a routine delivery, oxytocin may be given to the mother after the placenta has been delivered in order to help the uterus contract and minimize bleeding. It is also used to treat uterine hemorrhage. While hemorrhage occurs in about 4% of vaginal deliveries and 6% of Caesarian deliveries, it accounts for about 35% of maternal deaths due to bleeding during pregnancy. If the bleeding started at the placental detachment site, contractions of the uterus help to close off the blood vessels and thereby stop excessive bleeding. Additional medications may be used, including $PGF2_{alpha}$ (Hemabate), misoprostol (Cytotec), or the ergot alkaloid methylergonovine (Methergine).

Prostaglandins

Prostaglandins (PGs) play a major role in stimulating the uterine contractions at the beginning of labor. Research indicates that PGs are also involved in the

KEY TERMS

Alkaloid—Any of a group of bitter-tasting alkaline compounds that contain nitrogen and are commonly found in plants. Alkaloids derived from ergot can be used as uterine stimulants.

Antidiuretic—A medication or other compound that suppresses the production of urine.

Caesarian section—An incision made through the wall of a pregnant woman's abdomen and uterus in order to deliver the fetus. It is commonly abbreviated as C-section.

Cyanosis—A bluish discoloration of the skin and mucous membranes caused by low levels of oxygen in the blood.

Ergot alkaloids—Compounds derived from a fungus, *Claviceps purpurea,* which grows on rye plants and forms a hard blackish body. Ergot itself is toxic.

Hemorrhage—The loss of an excessive amount of blood in a short period of time. After childbirth, a loss of more than 500 mL over a 24-hour period is considered a postpartum hemorrhage.

Induce—To begin or start.

Miscarriage—The loss of a fetus before it is viable, usually between the third and seventh months of pregnancy. A miscarriage is sometimes called a spontaneous abortion.

Postpartum—After childbirth or after delivery.

Prostaglandins—A group of unsaturated fatty acids involved in the contraction of smooth muscle, control of body temperature, and other body functions.

Vital signs—Measurements of a patient's essential body functions, usually defined as pulse rate, breathing rate, and body temperature.

transition from the early phase of labor to the later stages. In addition, PGs may be used to ripen the cervix prior to induction. Administration of prostaglandins is sometimes sufficient to stimulate labor, and the woman needs no further medication for labor to progress. There are many PGs used in medicine, but the most significant are PGE_1, PGE_2, and $PGF2_{alpha}$. Researchers are investigating which prostaglandins are the most effective for specific purposes. For example, PGE_2 in the form of dinoprostone (Cervidil and Prepidil) has proved to be superior to the PGF series for cervical ripening. Misoprostol (Cytotec), a synthetic form of PGE_1, is also effective in cervical ripening and labor induction, while the $PGF2_{alpha}$ analogue, carboprost (Prostin 15-M or Hemabate), is the preferred prostaglandin for stimulating the uterus.

Ergot alkaloids

Ergot alkaloids are derived from a fungus, *Claviceps purpurea*, which grows primarily on rye grain. The fungus forms a hard blackish body known as a sclerotium, which contains alkaloid compounds that can be used to treat migraine headache. Ergot by itself, however, is toxic to the central nervous system of humans and animals, producing irritability, spasms, cramps, and convulsions. Because of its potentially harmful side effects, one ergot-based drug (Ergonovine or Ergotrate) was taken off the American market in 1993. Methylergonovine maleate (Methergine) is now the only ergot derivative in use in the United States. It is given only as a uterine stimulant to control PPH. Because of the risk of complications, and because the use of Methergine is contraindicated in many women, it has largely been replaced by the PGs as a second-line uterotonic.

Preparation

A healthcare professional should review information about a medication or procedure with the pregnant woman before administering it to make sure that she understands what will happen during the procedure or the potential side effects of the medication. The patient should inform the doctor or nurse about any allergies to medications, as well as any side effects she may have experienced previously.

If the patient is anxious about induction of labor or augmentation of contractions, the nurse or doctor should discuss these concerns and relieve the patient's anxiety.

Aftercare

The expectant mother should be monitored closely during induction of labor or cervical ripening. The FHR and uterine contractions are usually monitored for an hour after induction. Frequent checks of the patient's vital signs alert the nurse to any potential complications.

Risks

Oxytocin

Oxytocin takes effect rapidly when it is given intravenously. Individual responses to oxytocin vary considerably; for this reason, the drug dosage is usually increased slowly and incrementally. Oxytocin can cause hyperstimulation of the uterus, which in turn can place the fetus at risk for asphyxia. Hyperstimulation is defined as more than five contractions in 10 minutes, contractions lasting longer than 60 seconds, and increased uterine tonus either with or without significant decrease in FHR. Uterine rupture has also been linked to oxytocin administration, particularly when the drug is given for four hours or longer.

Oxytocin has a mild antidiuretic effect that is usually dose related; it can lead to water intoxication (hyponatremia). Onset occurs gradually and may go unnoticed. Signs of water intoxication may include reduced urine output, confusion, nausea, convulsions, and coma. Expectant mothers receiving oxytocin should have their blood pressure monitored closely, as both hypotension and hypertension can occur.

Although the subject remains controversial, some evidence suggests oxytocin increases the incidence of neonatal jaundice. Although oxytocin may increase the risk of uterine rupture in women who were delivered by Caesarian section in a previous pregnancy, contraindications to the use of the drug are virtually the same as contraindications for labor. Other side effects of oxytocin include nausea, vomiting, cardiac arrhythmias, and fetal bradycardia (slowing of the heartbeat). When used judiciously, oxytocin is a very effective medication for the progression of labor.

Prostaglandins

PGs have significant systemic side effects. These include headache, nausea, diarrhea, tachycardia (rapid heartbeat), vomiting, chills, fever, sweating, hypertension, and hypotension (low blood pressure). There is also an increased risk of uterine hyperstimulation and uterine rupture. $PGF2_{alpha}$ (carboprost—Prostin 15-M or Hemabate) can cause hypotension, pulmonary edema, and intense bronchospasms in women with asthma. Because carboprost stimulates the production of steroids, it may be contraindicated in women with disorders of the adrenal gland. When used for abortion, it may result in sufficient blood loss to cause anemia, which may make a **transfusion** necessary. Medical problems (or a history) of diabetes, epilepsy, heart or blood vessel disease, jaundice, kidney disease, or liver disease should be brought to the attention of the health care practitioner before the patient is given carboprost. The use of this PG has been reported to increase the fluid pressure in the eyes in women with glaucoma; however, this side effect is fortunately rare.

Ergot alkaloids

Ergot alkaloids have an alpha-adrenergic action with a vasoconstrictive effect, which means that they cause the blood vessels to become narrower. These drugs can cause hypertension, cardiovascular changes, cyanosis, muscle pain, tingling, other symptoms associated with decreased blood circulation, and severe uterine cramping. The healthcare professional should be informed of other medications taken by the patient. The presence or history of such medical problems as angina, hypertension, stroke, infection, kidney and liver disease, and Raynaud's phenomenon may be contraindications to the use of ergot alkaloids.

Normal results

The normal results of uterine stimulants, when administered in appropriate circumstances and correct dosages, are preparation of the cervix for childbirth; induction or stimulation of uterine contractions to produce a safe delivery of a newborn; encouragement of a complete spontaneous or **induced abortion**; elimination of blood clots or other tissue debris from the uterus; and the slowing or cessation of hemorrhage following childbirth or abortion.

Normal results would include the achievement of these outcomes without significant side effects for the mother or fetus.

Resources

BOOKS

Gabbe, S. G., et al. *Obstetrics: Normal and Problem Pregnancies*, 5th ed. London: Churchill Livingstone, 2007.

Katz, V. L., et al. *Comprehensive Gynecology*, 5th ed. St. Louis: Mosby, 2007.

Marx, John A., et al. *Rosen's Emergency Medicine*, 6th ed. St. Louis, MO: Mosby, Inc., 2006.

Roberts, J. R., et al. *Clinical Procedures in Emergency Medicine*, 6th ed. Philadelphia: Saunders, Inc., 2004.

PERIODICALS

Ovelese, Y. "Postpartum hemorrhage." *Obstetrics and Gynecology Clinics of North America* 34 (September 2007): 421–441.

Sanchez-Ramos, L. "Induction of labor." *Obstetrics and Gynecology Clinics of North America* 32 (June 2005): 181–200.

ORGANIZATIONS

American College of Obstetricians and Gynecologists (ACOG). 409 12th St. SW, PO Box 96920, Washington, DC 20090-6920. http://www.acog.com (accessed April 15, 2008).

United States Food and Drug Administration (FDA). 5600 Fishers Lane, Rockville, MD 20857-0001. (888) INFO-FDA. http://www.fda.gov (accessed April 15, 2008).

Esther Csapo Rastegari, RN, BSN, EdM
Sam Uretsky, PharmD

Uterus removal *see* **Hysterectomy**

Uvulopalatoplasty *see* **Snoring surgery**

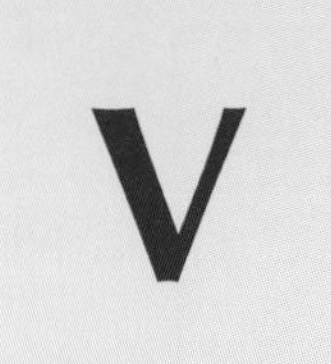

Vagal nerve stimulation

Definition

Vagal nerve stimulation is a treatment for epilepsy in which an electrode is implanted in the neck to deliver electrical impulses to the vagus nerve.

Purpose

Vagal nerve stimulation is an alternative to medication or surgical removal of brain tissue in controlling epileptic seizures. The seizures of epilepsy are caused by uncontrolled electrical discharges spreading through the brain. Antiseizure drugs interrupt this process by reducing the sensitivity of individual brain cells to stimulation. Brain surgery for epilepsy either removes the portion of the brain where seizures originate, or cuts nerve fibers to prevent the nerve impulses that occur during a seizure from spreading to other parts of the brain. Vagal nerve stimulation uses a different approach: It provides intermittent electrical stimulation to a nerve outside the brain—the vagus, or tenth cranial nerve, which influences certain patterns of brain activity.

The vagus nerve is a major connection between the brain and the rest of the body. It carries sensory information from the body to the brain, and motor commands from the brain to the body. The vagus is involved in complex control loops between these destinations; its precise pathways and mechanisms are still not fully understood. It is also not known how stimulation of the vagus nerve works to reduce seizure activity—it may stimulate inhibitory pathways that prevent the brain's electrical activity from getting out of control, interrupt some feedback loops that worsen seizures, or act in some other fashion.

Vagal nerve stimulation has been effective in reducing seizure frequency in patients whose seizures are not controlled by drugs, and who are either not candidates for other types of brain surgery or who have chosen not to undergo these procedures.

Demographics

About 2.7 million people in the United States have been diagnosed with epilepsy. Ten percent of patients who are newly diagnosed with epilepsy do not respond well to medications, however, and so may be candidates for surgical treatment. Vagus nerve stimulation was first performed in the United States in 1988 and received final approval by the United States Food and Drug Administration (FDA) in July 1997. As of 2007, approximately 32,000 people worldwide are being treated with vagus nerve stimulation. One registry of patients who are being treated with vagus nerve stimulation shows that 60% were performed for patients with partial seizures, 15% were performed for patients with Lennox-Gastaut syndrome (also known as mixed seizures), and 25% were performed for patients with generalized seizures.

Description

The vagal nerve stimulator (VNS) has two parts: an electrode that wraps around the left vagus nerve in the neck, and a pulse generator, which is implanted under the skin below the collarbone. The two parts are connected by a wire. Stimulation is performed only on the left vagal nerve, as the right vagal nerve helps control the heartbeat.

Surgery to implant a VNS device takes about two hours. A neurosurgeon implants the electrode and generator while the patient is under **general anesthesia**. A vertical incision is made in the left side of the neck, and the helical electrode is attached to the nerve itself. A second incision is made on the left side of the chest below the collarbone, and the pulse generator (a disc about 2 in [5 cm] in diameter) is implanted under the skin. The connecting wire is threaded around the muscles and bones to join the electrode and generator.

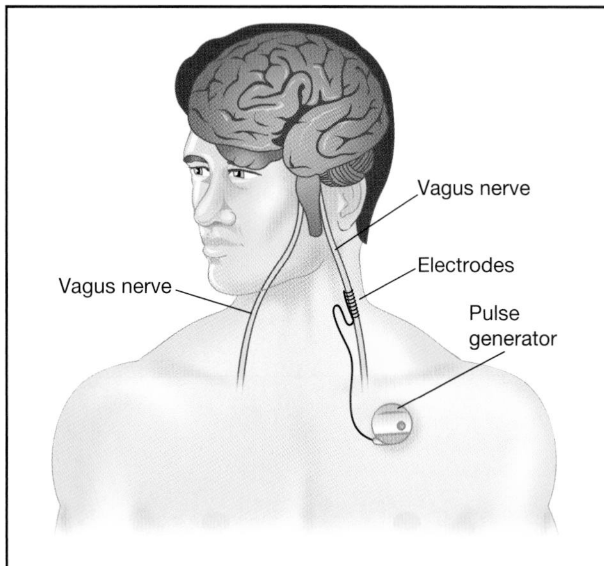

(Illustration by Electronic Illustrators Group.)

KEY TERMS

Epilepsy—The name for a group of syndromes characterized by periodic temporary disturbances of brain function. The symptoms of an epileptic seizure may include loss of consciousness, abnormal movements, falling, emotional reactions, and disturbances of sight or hearing.

Helical—Having a spiral shape.

Neurologist—A physician who specializes in diagnosing and treating disorders of the nervous system.

Seizure—A single episode of epilepsy. Seizures are also called convulsions or fits.

Vagus nerve—The tenth cranial nerve, running from the head through the neck and chest into the abdomen. Intermittent electrical stimulation of the vagus nerve can help to control epileptic seizures.

The generator makes a small bulge under the skin, but is hidden by clothing after the operation.

Before the neurosurgeon closes the incisions, he or she tests the VNS device to make sure it is working, and programs it to deliver the lowest amount of stimulation. The device is usually timed to stimulate the vagus nerve for 30 seconds every five minutes.

Diagnosis/Preparation

A candidate for vagal nerve stimulation will have had many tests already to determine the focal point of seizure activity. Preoperative tests include neuroimaging, as well as psychological tests to determine the patient's cognitive (thinking) strengths and weaknesses.

The patient must be fully informed about VNS—how it works, its advantages and disadvantages, what will happen during surgery—before the operation is scheduled. A video as well as written material about VNS is available to view and discuss with the doctor.

Aftercare

Implantation of the stimulator in an adult may be performed as either an outpatient or inpatient procedure. In the latter case, the patient will remain in the hospital overnight for monitoring of heart function and other **vital signs**. Children who are receiving a VNS are usually scheduled for an overnight stay. Pain medication is given as needed.

The stimulation parameters are adjustable, and the neurologist may require several visits to find the right settings. Settings are adjusted with a magnetic wand that delivers commands to the stimulator's computer chip. The patient will be taught how to use a magnet to temporarily increase stimulation, to prevent a seizure, or to abort it once it begins.

The VNS generator is powered by a battery that lasts several years. It is replaced during an outpatient procedure under **local anesthesia**.

Risks

The most common adverse effects from vagal nerve stimulation are a hoarse voice, cough, headache, and ear pain. These side effects can be reduced by adjusting the stimulation settings, and may subside on their own over time. Infection and device malfunction are possible, though rare.

Patients who have had a VNS implanted must avoid strong magnets, which may affect the stimulator settings. Areas with warning signs posted regarding **pacemakers** should be avoided. The patient should consult with the neurologist and the neurosurgeon about other hazards.

Normal results

Approximately half of all patients who have received vagal nerve stimulation experience about a 50% reduction in seizures. Another 9% of patients obtain complete relief from seizures. Most patients who continue to take antiseizure medications can

WHO PERFORMS THE PROCEDURE AND WHERE IS IT PERFORMED?

The implanting of a VNS device is performed by a neurosurgeon in a hospital, in consultation with a neurologist.

QUESTIONS TO ASK THE DOCTOR

- What will the procedure cost? Will my insurance cover the cost?
- How often will I need to return to have the stimulator adjusted?
- Will my medication dosages be reduced after this procedure?
- How long will the procedure take?
- How many VNS devices have you implanted? What is your success rate?

reduce their dosage, however, which offers some relief from the side effects of these drugs.

Morbidity and mortality rates

Vagal nerve stimulation is a relatively safe procedure. Pilot studies of 300 patients that were done prior to FDA approval of VNS reported the following complication rates: hoarseness, 37% of patients; coughing, 14%; voice alteration, 13%; chest pain, 12%; and nausea, 2%.

Alternatives

Some candidates for vagal nerve stimulation are also likely to be candidates for a **corpus callosotomy**, temporal lobectomy, or other surgical procedures.

Resources

BOOKS

Goetz, C. G. *Goetz's Textbook of Clinical Neurology*, 3rd ed. Philadelphia: Saunders, 2007.

PERIODICALS

DeGiorgio, C. "Vagus nerve stimulation for intractable seizures in children." *Pediatric Neurology* 35 (November 2006): 323–326.

Rielo, Diego, MD, and Selim R. Benbadis, MD. "Vagus Nerve Stimulation." *eMedicine*, April 12, 2002 [June 10, 2003]. http://www.emedicine.com/neuro/topic559.htm (accessed April 16, 2008).

Saneto, R. P. "Vagus nerve stimulation for epilepsy: randomized comparison of three stimulation paradigms." *Neurology* 65 (July 2005): 317–319.

ORGANIZATIONS

American Association of Neurological Surgeons (AANS). 5550 Meadowbrook Drive, Rolling Meadows, IL 60008. (847) 378-0500. http://www.neurosurgery.org (accessed April 16, 2008).

Epilepsy Foundation. 4351 Garden City Drive, Landover, MD 20785-7223. (800) 332-1000. http://www.epilepsyfoundation.org (accessed April 16, 2008).

Richard Robinson

Vaginal wall repair *see* **Colporrhaphy**

Vaginotomy *see* **Colpotomy**

Vagotomy

Definition

Vagotomy is the surgical cutting of the vagus nerve to reduce acid secretion in the stomach.

Purpose

The vagus nerve trunk splits into branches that go to different parts of the stomach. Stimulation from these branches causes the stomach to produce acid. Too much stomach acid leads to ulcers that may eventually bleed and create an emergency situation.

A vagotomy is performed when acid production in the stomach can not be reduced by other means. The purpose of the procedure is to disable the acid-producing capacity of the stomach. It is used when ulcers in the stomach and duodenum do not respond to medication and changes in diet. It is an appropriate surgery when there are ulcer complications, such as obstruction of digestive flow, bleeding, or perforation. The frequency with which elective vagotomy is performed has decreased in the past 20 years as it has become clear that the primary cause of ulcers is an infection by a bacterium called *Helicobacter pylori*. Drugs have become increasingly effective in treating ulcers. However, the number of vagotomies performed in emergency situations has remained about the same.

A vagotomy procedure is often performed in conjunction with another gastrointestinal surgery, such as partial removal of the stomach (**antrectomy** or subtotal **gastrectomy**).

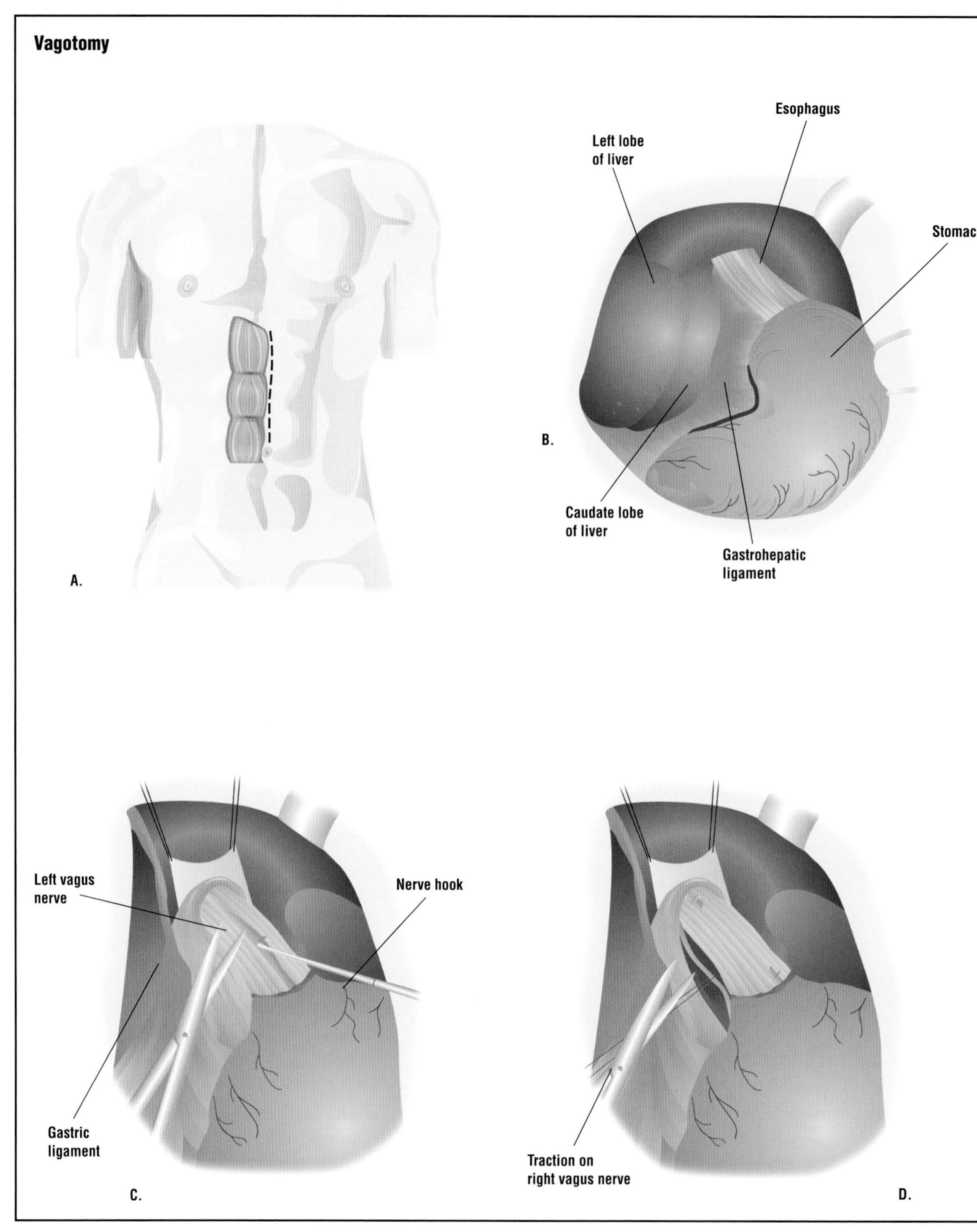

To perform a vagotomy, the surgeon makes an incision in the patient's abdomen (A). The stomach is located (B), and the vagus nerves are cut in turn (C and D). *(Illustration by GGS Information Services. Cengage Learning, Gale.)*

KEY TERMS

Duodenum—The section of the small intestine closest to the stomach.

Gastric glands—Branched tubular glands located in the stomach.

Gastric ulcer—An ulcer of the stomach, duodenum, or other part of the gastrointestinal system. Also called a peptic ulcer.

Latarjet's nerve—Terminal branch of the anterior vagal trunk, which runs along the lesser curvature of the stomach.

Parietal cells—Cells of the gastric glands that secrete hydrochloric acid and intrinsic factor.

Peristalsis—The rhythmic contractions that move material through the bowel.

Pyloroplasty—Widening of the pyloric canal and any adjacent duodenal structure by means of a longitudinal incision.

Demographics

Gastric (peptic) ulcers are included under the general heading of gastrointestinal (GI) diseases. GI disorders affect an estimated 25–30% of the world's population. In the United States, 60 million adults experience gastrointestinal reflux at least once a month, and 25 million adults suffer daily from heartburn. Left untreated, these conditions often evolve into ulcers. Four million people have active peptic ulcers; about 350,000 new cases are diagnosed each year. Four times as many duodenal ulcers as gastric ulcers are diagnosed. The first-degree relatives of patients with duodenal ulcer have a two to three times greater risk of developing duodenal ulcer. Relatives of gastric ulcer patients have a similarly increased risk of developing a gastric ulcer.

Description

A vagotomy can be performed using closed (laparoscopic) or open surgical technique. The indications for a laparoscopic vagotomy are the same as open vagotomy.

There are four basic types of vagotomy procedures:

- Truncal or total abdominal vagotomy. The main vagal trunks are divided, and surgery is accompanied by a drainage procedure, such as pyloroplasty.
- Selective (total gastric) vagotomy. The main vagal trunks are dissected to the point where the branch leading to the biliary tree divides, and there is a cut at the section of vagus close to the hepatic branch. This procedure is rarely indicated or performed.
- Highly selective vagotomy (HSV). HSV selectively deprives the parietal cells of vagal nerves, and reduces their sensitivity to stimulation and the release of acid. It does not require a drainage procedure. The branches of Latarjet's nerve are divided from the esophagogastric junction to the crow's foot along the lesser curvature of the stomach.
- Thoracoscopic vagotomy. Performed through the third, sixth, and seventh left intercostal spaces, the posterior vagus trunk is isolated, clipped, and a segment excised.

A vagotomy is performed under **general anesthesia**. The surgeon makes an incision in the abdomen and locates the vagus nerve. Either the trunk or the branches leading to the stomach are cut. The abdominal muscles are sewn back together, and the skin is closed with sutures.

Often, other gastrointestinal surgery is performed (e.g., part of the stomach may be removed) at the same time. Vagotomy causes a decrease in peristalsis, and a change in the emptying patterns of the stomach. To ease this, a **pyloroplasty** is often performed to widen the outlet from the stomach to the small intestine.

Diagnosis/Preparation

A gastroscopy and x rays of the gastrointestinal system determine the position and condition of the ulcer. Standard preoperative blood and urine tests are done. The patient discusses with the anesthesiologist any medications or conditions that might affect the administration of anesthesia.

Aftercare

Patients who have had a vagotomy stay in the hospital for about seven days. Nasogastric suctioning is required for the first three or four days. A tube is inserted through the nose and into the stomach. The stomach contents are then suctioned out. Patients eat a clear liquid diet until the gastrointestinal tract regains function. When patients return to a regular diet, spicy and acidic foods should be avoided.

It takes about six weeks to fully recover from the surgery. The sutures that close the skin can be removed in seven to 10 days. Patients are encouraged to move around soon after the operation to prevent the formation of deep vein blood clots. Pain medication, stool softeners, and **antibiotics** may be prescribed following the operation.

WHO PERFORMS THE PROCEDURE AND WHERE IS IT PERFORMED?

Patients who receive vagotomies are most often seen in emergency situations where bleeding and perforated ulcers require immediate intervention. A vagotomy is usually performed by a board-certified surgeon, either a general surgeon who specializes in gastrointestinal surgery or a gastrointestinal endoscopic surgeon. The procedure is performed in a hospital setting.

QUESTIONS TO ASK THE DOCTOR

- What are the possible complications involved in vagotomy surgery?
- What surgical preparation is needed?
- What type of anesthesia will be used?
- How is the surgery performed?
- How long is the hospitalization?
- How many vagotomies does the surgeon perform in a year?

Risks

Standard surgical risks, such as excessive bleeding and infection, are potential complications. In addition, the emptying patterns of the stomach are changed. This can lead to dumping syndrome and diarrhea. Dumping syndrome is a condition in which the patient experiences palpitations, sweating, nausea, cramps, vomiting, and diarrhea shortly after eating.

The following complications are also associated with vagotomy surgery:

- Gastric or esophageal perforation. May occur from an electrocautery injury or by clipping the branch of the nerve of Latarjet.
- Delayed gastric emptying. Most common after truncal and selective vagotomy, particularly if a drainage procedure is not performed.

People who use alcohol excessively, smoke, are obese, and are very young or very old are at higher risk for complications.

Normal results

Normal recovery is expected for most patients. Ulcers recur in about 10% of those who have vagotomy without stomach removal. Recurrent ulcers are also found in 2–3% of patients who have some portion of their stomach removed.

Morbidity and mortality rates

In the United States, approximately 3,000 deaths per year are due to duodenal ulcer and 3,000 to gastric ulcer. There has been a marked decrease in reported hospitalization and mortality rates for gastric ulcer.

Alternatives

The preferred short-term treatment for gastric ulcers is drug therapy. A recent review surveying medical articles published from 1977 to 1994 concluded that drugs such as cimetidine, ranitidine, famotidine, H2 blockers, and sucralfate were efficient, with omeprazole considered the "gold standard" for active gastric ulcer treatment. Surgical intervention, however, is recommended for people who do not respond to medical therapy.

Resources

BOOKS

Ansolon, K. B. *Developmental Technology of Gastrectomy & Vagotomy*. Rockville, MD: Kabel Publishers, 1995.

Kral, J. *Vagal Nerve Function*. New York: Elsevier Science Ltd., 1984.

"Stomach and Duodenum." In *Current Surgical Diagnosis and Treatment*, 10th ed. Edited by Lawrence W. Day. Stamford: Appleton & Lange, 1994.

PERIODICALS

Chang, T. M., D.C. Chan, Y.C. Liu, S.S. Tsou, and T. H. Chen. "Long-term Results of Duodenectomy with Highly Selective Vagotomy in the Treatment of Complicated Duodenal Ulcers." *American Journal of Surgery* 181 (April 2001): 372-6.

Gilliam, A. D., W.J. Speake, and D. N. Lobo. "Current Practice of Emergency Vagotomy and Helicobacter Pylori Eradication for Complicated Peptic Ulcer in the United Kingdom." *British Journal of Surgery* 90 (January 2003): 88-90.

Saindon, C. S., F. Blecha, T.I. Musch, D.A. Morgan, R.J. Fels, and M. J. Kenney. "Effect of Cervical Vagotomy on Sympathetic Nerve Responses to Peripheral Interleukin-1beta." *Autonomic Neuroscience* 87 (March 2001): 243-8.

ORGANIZATIONS

American College of Surgeons. 633 N. Saint Clair St., Chicago, IL 60611. (312) 202-5000. www.faacs.org.

Society of American Gastrointestinal Endoscopic Surgeons. 2716 Ocean Park Boulevard, Suite 3000, Santa Monica, CA 90405. (310) 314-2404. www.sages.org.

OTHER

"Laparoscopic Vagotomy." *SAGES web center*.www.sages.org/primarycare/chapter19.html.

Tish Davidson, A.M.
Monique Laberge, Ph.D.

Valvuloplasty, balloon *see* **Balloon valvuloplasty**

Varicose vein sclerotherapy *see* **Sclerotherapy for varicose veins**

Vascular study *see* **Angiography**

Vascular surgery

Definition

Vascular surgery is the treatment of surgery on diagnosed patients with diseases of the arterial, venous, and lymphatic systems (excluding the intracranial and coronary arteries).

Purpose

Vascular surgery is indicated when a patient has vascular disease that cannot be treated by less invasive, non-surgical treatments. The purpose of vascular surgery is to treat vascular diseases, which are diseases of the arteries and veins. Arterial disease is a condition in which blood clots, arteriosclerosis, and other vascular conditions occur in the arteries. Venous disease involves problems that occur in the veins. Some vascular conditions occur only in arteries, others occur only in the veins, and some affect both veins and arteries.

Demographics

As people age, vascular diseases are very common. Since they rarely cause symptoms in the early stages, many people do not realize that they suffer from these diseases. A large percentage of the 10 million people in the United States who may have peripheral vascular disease (PVD) are males. In the majority of cases, the blockage is caused by one or more blood clots that travel to the lungs from another part of the body. Factors that increase the chances of vascular disease include:

- increasing age (which results in a loss of elasticity in the veins and their valves)
- a family history of heart or vascular disease
- illness or injury
- pregnancy
- prolonged periods of inactivity sitting, standing, or bed rest
- smoking
- obesity
- hypertension, diabetes, high cholesterol, or other conditions that affect the health of the cardiovascular system
- lack of exercise

Description

Vascular surgery involves techniques relating to endovascular surgeries, including balloon **angioplasty** and/or stenting, aortic and peripheral vascular endovascular stent/graft placement, thrombolysis, and other adjuncts for vascular reconstruction.

The vascular system is the network of blood vessels that circulate blood to and from the heart and lungs. The circulatory system (made up of the heart, arteries, veins, capillaries, and the circulating blood) provides nourishment to the body's cells and removes their waste. The arteries carry oxygenated blood from the heart to the cells. The veins return the blood from the cells back to the lungs for reoxygenation and recirculation by the heart. The aorta is the largest artery leaving the heart; it then subdivides into smaller arteries going to every part of the body. The arteries, as they narrow, are connected to smaller vessels called capillaries. In these capillaries, oxygen and nutrients are released from the blood into the cells, and cellular wastes are collected for the return trip. The capillaries then connect to veins, which return the blood back to the heart.

The aorta stems from the heart, arches upward, and then continues down through the chest (thorax) and the abdomen. The iliac arteries, which branch out from the aorta, provide blood to the pelvis and legs. The thoracic section of the aorta supplies blood to the upper body, as it continues through the chest. The abdominal section of the aorta, which supplies blood to the lower body, continues through the abdomen.

Vascular diseases are usually caused by conditions that clog or weaken blood vessels, or damage valves that control the flow of blood in and out of the veins, thus robbing them of vital blood nutrients and oxygen.

KEY TERMS

Ankle-brachial index (ABI) test—A means of checking the blood pressure in the arms and ankles using a regular blood pressure cuff and a special ultrasound stethoscope (Doppler). The pressure in the ankle is compared to the pressure in the arm.

Aorta—A large, elastic artery beginning at the upper part of the left ventricle of the heart that becomes the main trunk of the arterial system.

Aortic aneurysms—Occurs when an area in the aorta (the main artery of the heart) is weakened and bulges like a balloon.

Arteriogram—A test to check the blood pressure at several points in the leg by using a blood pressure cuff and a Doppler. The patient is then asked to walk on a treadmill, after which the ankle pressure is taken again to determine if the pressure decreased after walking.

Abdominal aortic aneurysm—Occurs when an area in the aorta (the main artery of the heart) is weakened and bulges like a balloon. The abdominal section of the aorta supplies blood to the lower body.

Aneurysm—A weakening of the artery wall, due to atherosclerosis, causing a bulge that can rupture, and lead to thrombosis or embolism.

Angiography or angiogram—An x-ray exam of the arteries and veins (blood vessels) to diagnose blockages and other blood vessel problems.

Atherosclerosis— A form of arteriosclerosis affecting the innermost area of the artery; a series of calcified deposits that can close down the vessel.

Arteriogram—An x-ray picture of an artery achieved by injecting an opaque dye with a needle or tube into the affected artery.

Artery—A blood vessel conveying blood in a direction away from the heart.

Bruit—A roaring sound created by a partially blocked artery.

Capillary—Smallest extremity of the arterial vessel, where oxygen and nutrients are released from the blood into the cells, and cellular waste is collected.

Carotid artery—Major artery leading to the brain, blockages of which can cause temporary or permanent strokes.

Carotid artery disease—A condition in which the arteries in the neck that supply blood to the brain become clogged, causing the danger of a stroke.

Carotid endarterectomy—A surgical technique for removing intra-arterial obstructions of the internal carotid artery.

Cerebral aneurysm—The dilation, bulging, or ballooning out of part of the wall of a vein or artery in the brain.

Cholesterol—An abundant fatty substance in animal tissues. High levels in the diet are a factor in the cause of atherosclerosis.

Claudication—Attacks of lameness or pain chiefly in the calf muscles, brought on by walking because of a lack of oxygen reaching the muscle.

Computed tomography (CT) scan—A special type of x ray that can produce detailed pictures of structures inside the body.

A few common diseases affecting the arteries are peripheral vascular disease (PVD), carotid artery disease, and aortic aneurysms.

Surgery is used to treat specific diseased arteries, such as atherosclerosis, to help prevent strokes or heart attacks, improve or relieve angina or hypertension, remove aneurysms, improve claudication, and save legs that would otherwise have to be amputated. The choices involve repairing the artery, bypassing it, or replacing it.

As people age, atherosclerosis, commonly called hardening of the arteries, occurs with the constant passage of blood through the arteries. It can take on a number of forms, of which atherosclerosis (hardening of the innermost portion) is the most common. This occurs when fatty material containing cholesterol or calcium (plaque) is deposited on the innermost layer of the artery. This causes a narrowing of the inside diameter of the blood vessel. Eventually, the artery becomes so narrow that a blood clot (thrombus) forms, and blocks blood flow to an entire portion of the body. This condition is called PVD, or peripheral arterial disease. In another form of atherosclerosis, a rough area or ulcer forms in the diseased interior of the artery. Blood clots then tend to develop on this ulcer, break off, and travel further along, forming a blockage where the arteries get narrower. A blockage resulting from a clot formed elsewhere in the body is called an embolism.

Collaterals—Alternate pathways for arterial blood.

Coronary—Of or relating to the heart.

Embolism—Obstruction or closure of a vessel by a transported clot of foreign matter.

Endovascular grafting—A procedure that involves the insertion of a delivery catheter through a groin artery into the abdominal aorta under fluoroscopic guidance.

Intracranial—Existing or occurring within the cranium; affecting or involving intracranial structures.

Lower extremity amputation—To cut a limb from the body.

Lymphangiography—Injection of dye into lymphatic vessels followed by x rays of the area. It is a difficult procedure, as it requires surgical isolation of the lymph vessels to be injected.

Lymphoscintigraphy—A technique in which a radioactive substance that concentrates in the lymphatic vessels is injected into the affected tissue and mapped using a gamma camera, which images the location of the radioactive tracer.

Magnetic resonance imaging (MRI)—A noninvasive diagnostic technique that produces computerized images of internal body tissues and is based on nuclear magnetic resonance of atoms within the body induced by the application of radio waves.

Plethysmography—A test in which a patient sits inside a booth called a plethysmograph and breathes through a mouthpiece, while pressure and air flow measurements are collected to measure the total lung volume.

Pulmonary embolism—A blocked artery in the lung.

Renal artery aneurysm—An aneurysm relating to, involving, or located in the region of the kidneys.

Thoracic aortic aneurysm—Occurs when an area in the thoracic section of the aorta (the chest) is weakened and bulges like a balloon. The thoracic section supplies blood to the upper body.

Thrombus—A blood clot that may form in a blood vessel or in one of the cavities of the heart.

Thrombosis—The formation or presence of a blood clot within a blood vessel.

Thrombolysis—A treatment that opens up blood flow and may prevent permanent damage to the blood vessels.

Ulcer—A lesion or rough spot formed on the surface of an artery.

Vascular—Relating to the blood vessels.

Ultrasound scan—The scan produces images of arteries on a screen and is used to evaluate the blood flow, locate blockages, and measure the size of the artery.

Vasculogenic erectile dysfunction—The inability to attain or sustain an erection satisfactory for coitus, due to atherosclerotic disease of penile arteries, inadequate impedance of venous outflow (venous leaks), or a combination of both.

Venous stasis disease—A condition in which there is pooling of blood in the lower leg veins that may cause swelling and tissue damage, and lead to painful sores or ulcers.

Varicose veins —Twisted, enlarged veins near the surface of the skin, which develop most commonly in the legs and ankles.

People who have few areas affected by PVD may be treated with angioplasty by opening up the blood vessel with a balloon placed on the end of a catheter. A stent is often used with angioplasty to help keep the artery open. The type of surgery used to treat PVD is based upon the size and location of the damaged artery. The surgery techniques used for severe PVD include:

- Bypass surgery is preferred for people who have many areas of blockage or a long, continuous blockage.
- Aortobifemoral bypass is used for PVD affecting the major abdominal artery (aorta) and the large arteries that branch off of it.
- In a technique called thromboendarterectomy, the inner diseased layers of the artery are removed, leaving the relatively normal outer coats of the artery.
- Resection involves a technique to remove a diseased artery following an aneurysm; a bypass is created with a synthetic graft.
- In a bypass graft, a vein graft from another part of the body or a graft made from artificial material is used to create a detour around a blocked artery.
- Tibioperoneal bypass is used for PVD affecting the arteries in the lower leg or foot.
- Femoropopliteal (fem-pop) bypass surgery is used for PVD affecting the arteries above and below the knee.

- Embolectomy is a technique in which an embolic clot on the wall of the artery is removed, using an inflatable balloon catheter.
- Thrombectomy is a technique in which a balloon catheter is inserted into the affected artery beyond a blood clot. The balloon is then inflated and pulled back, bringing the clot with it.

An aneurysm occurs when weakened blood vessels bulge like balloons as blood flows through them. Once they have grown to a certain size, there is a risk of rupture and life-threatening bleeding. There are two types of aortic aneurysms: abdominal aortic aneurysm (AAA) and thoracic aortic aneurysm. This classification is based on where the aneurysm occurs along the aorta. Aneurysms are more common in the abdominal section of the aorta than the thoracic section.

Most blood clots originate in the legs, but they can also form in the veins of arms, the right side of the heart, or even at the tip of a catheter placed in a vein. Venous disease conditions that usually occur in the veins of the legs include:

- varicose veins
- phlebitis
- venous stasis disease
- deep vein thrombosis (DVT)
- claudication
- blood clots

Carotid artery disease is a condition in which the arteries in the neck that supply blood to the brain become clogged; this condition can cause a stroke.

Lymphatic obstruction involves blockage of the lymph vessels, which drain fluid from tissues throughout the body and allow immune cells to travel where they are needed. Some of the causes of lymphatic obstruction (also known as swelling of the lymph passages), include infections such as chronic cellulitis, or parasitic infections such as filariasis, trauma, tumors, certain surgeries including **mastectomy**, and radiation therapy. There are rare forms of congenital lymphedema that probably result from abnormalities in the development of the lymphatic vessels. Most patients with lymphedema will not need surgery, as the symptoms are usually managed by other techniques. Surgical therapy for lymphedema includes removal of tissue containing abnormal lymphatics, and less commonly, transplant of tissue from areas with normal lymphatic tissues to areas with abnormal lymphatic drainage. In rare cases, bypass of abnormal lymphatic tissue is attempted, sometimes using vein grafts.

Other examples of vascular surgery include:

- cerebral aneurysm
- acute arterial and graft occlusion
- carotid endarterectomy
- endovascular grafting
- vasculogenic erectile dysfunction
- renal artery aneurysm
- surgery on varicose veins
- lower extremity amputation

Diagnosis/Preparation

In order for a patient to be diagnosed with a vascular disease, he or she must be clinically evaluated by a vascular surgeon, which includes a history and **physical examination**. A vascular surgeon also treats vascular disorders by non-operative means, including drug therapy and risk factor management.

The symptoms produced by atherosclerosis, thrombosis, embolisms, or aneurysms depend on the particular artery affected. These conditions can sometimes cause pain, but often there are no symptoms at all.

A physician has many ways of feeling, hearing, measuring, and even seeing arterial blockages. Many arteries in the body can be felt or palpated. A doctor can feel for a pulse in an area he or she believes afflicted. Usually, the more advanced the arteriosclerosis, the less pulse in a given area.

As the artery becomes blocked, it can cause a noise very much like water roaring over rocky rapids. The physician can listen to this noise (bruit) directly, or can use special amplification systems to hear the noise.

There are other tests that can be done to determine if arterial blood flow is normal, including:

- ankle-brachial index (ABI) test
- arteriogram
- segmental pressure test
- ultrasound scan
- magnetic resonance imaging (MRI)
- computed tomography (CT) scan
- angiography
- lymphangiography
- lymphoscintigraphy
- plethysmography
- duplex ultrasound scanning

There may be no symptoms of vascular disease caused by blood clots until the clot grows large enough to block the flow of blood through the vein. Symptoms that may come on suddenly include:

- pain
- sudden swelling in the affected limb

- reddish blue discoloration
- enlargement of the superficial veins
- skin that is warm to the touch

The physician will probably do an evaluation of all organ systems, including the heart, lungs, circulatory system, kidneys, and the gastrointestinal system. The decision whether to have surgery or not is based on the outcome of these evaluations.

For high-risk patients undergoing vascular surgery, research has shown that taking oral beta-blockers one to two weeks before surgery and continuing for at least two weeks after the operation can significantly reduce the chance of **dying** or having a heart attack. Scientists suspect that the drug improves oxygen balance in the wall of the heart and stabilizes plaques in the arteries.

WHO PERFORMS THE PROCEDURE AND WHERE IS IT PREFORMED?

A vascular surgeon performs the procedure in a hospital operating room. Applicants for residency training in vascular surgery must have successfully completed a general surgery residency and be eligible for the board examination in general surgery. An individual must meet the standards set by the Vascular Surgery Board of the American Board of Surgery for cognitive knowledge and hypothetical case management. At the completion of a vascular surgery residency, both a written and oral examination must be completed before certification. A vascular surgeon is required to undergo periodic written reexamination.

Aftercare

The length of time in intensive care and hospitalization will vary with each surgery, as will the recovery time, depending on numerous factors. Because surgery for an AAA is more serious, the patient can expect to be in intensive care for 24 hours, and in the hospital for five to 10 days, providing the patient was healthy and had a smooth operative and postoperative course. The hospital stay will likely increase if there are complications. It may take as long as six months to fully recover from surgery for an AAA.

Living a heart-healthy lifestyle is the best way of preventing and controlling vascular disease: quit smoking; eat nutritious foods low in fat; **exercise**; maintain a healthy weight; and control risk factors such as high blood pressure, high cholesterol, diabetes, hypertension, and other factors that contribute to vascular disease.

Medications that may be used to treat PVD include:

- aspirin and other antiplatelet medications to treat leg pain
- statins to lower cholesterol levels
- medications to control high blood pressure
- medications to control diabetes
- anticoagulants (these are rarely, but not generally, used to treat PVD unless the person is at an increased risk for forming blood clots)

Risks

All surgeries carry some risks. There is a risk of infection whenever incisions are required. Operations in the chest or those that involve major blood vessels carry a higher risk of complications. Patients that have high blood pressure, chronic lung or kidney disease, or other illnesses are at greater risk of complications during and after surgery. Other risks of vascular surgery include:

- bleeding
- failed or blocked grafts
- heart attack or stroke
- smoking
- leg swelling if a leg vein is used
- people over 65 years are at greater risk for brain impairment after major surgery
- the more damaged the circulatory system is before surgery, the higher susceptibility to mental decline after vascular surgery
- impotence

The patient should discuss risks with the surgeon after careful review of the patient's medical history and a physical examination.

Normal results

The success rate for vascular surgery varies depending on a number of factors that may influence the decision on whether to have surgery or not, as well as the results.

The chance that an aneurysm will rupture generally increases with the size of the aneurysm; AAAs smaller than 1.6 in (4 cm) in diameter have up to a 2% risk of rupture, while ones larger than 2 in (5 cm) in diameter have a 22% risk of rupture within two years.

Arterial bypass surgery and peripheral bypass surgery have very good success rates. Most of those who

QUESTIONS TO ASK THE DOCTOR

- Can my vascular disease be controlled with lifestyle changes?
- If a procedure is required, am I a candidate for a less invasive, interventional radiology treatment?
- What are the risks and benefits of this operation?
- What are the normal results of this operation?
- What happens if this operation does not go as planned?
- What is the expected recovery time?

undergo AAA surgery recover well, except in the case of a rupture. Most patients who have a ruptured aortic aneurysm die due to excessive, rapid blood loss.

Surgical therapy for lymphedema has met with limited success, and requires significant experience and technical expertise.

Morbidity and mortality rates

Peripheral vascular disease affects 10 million people in the United States, including 5% of those over 50. Only a quarter of PVD sufferers are receiving treatment. More than two million people in the United States develop DVT each year. More than 650,000 Americans experience a pulmonary embolism every year. Of those, approximately 200,000 people die from the condition.

Alternatives

There a few alternatives to treating vascular disease, although extensive research has not been done. Acupuncture is used to aid in hypertension and chelation therapy is thought to stabilize the effects of vascular disease. The focus should be on maintaining a proper diet and being aware of a family history of vascular disease so as to catch it as early as possible.

Resources

BOOKS

Khatri, V. P., and J. A. Asensio. *Operative Surgery Manual*, 1st ed. Philadelphia: Saunders, 2003.

Libby, P., et al. *Braunwald's Heart Disease*, 8th ed. Philadelphia: Saunders, 2007.

Mason, R. J., et al. *Murray & Nadel's Textbook of Respiratory Medicine*, 4th ed. Philadelphia: Saunders, 2007.

Townsend, C. M., et al. *Sabiston Textbook of Surgery*, 17th ed. Philadelphia: Saunders, 2004.

PERIODICALS

Abir, Farshad, Iannis Kakisis, and Bauer Sumpio. "Do Vascular Surgery Patients Need a Cardiology Work-up? A Review of Preoperative Cardiac Clearance Guidelines in Vascular Surgery." *European Journal of Vascular and Endovascular Surgery* 25, no. 2 (2003): 110–117.

Moore, Wesley S., M.D., G. Patrick Clagett, M.D., Frank J. Veith, M.D., Gregory L. Moneta, M.D., Marshall W. Webster, M.D. et al. "Guidelines for Hospital Privileges in Vascular Surgery: An Update by an Ad Hoc Committee of the American Association for Vascular Surgery and the Society for Vascular Surgery." *Journal of Vascular Surgery* 36, no. 6 (2002): 1276–1282.

ORGANIZATIONS

American Board of Vascular Surgery (ABVS). 900 Cummings Center, #221-U, Beverly, MA 01915. http://abvs.org (accessed April 16, 2008).

The National Heart, Lung and Blood Institute. 6701 Rockledge Drive, P.O. Box 30105, Bethesda, MD 20824-0105. (301) 592-8573. E-mail: nhlbiinfo@rover.nhlbi.nih.gov. http://www.nhlhi.nih.gov (accessed April 16, 2008).

National Institutes of Health (NIH), Department of Health and Human Services. 9000 Rockville Pike, Bethesda, MD 20892.

The Society for Vascular Surgery. 900 Cummings Center, #221-U, Beverly, MA 01915. http://www.vascularweb.org (accessed April 16, 2008).

Society of Interventional Radiology. 10201 Lee Highway, Suite 500. Fairfax, VA. 22030. (800) 488-7284. E-mail: info@sirweb.org. http://www.sirweb.org/index.shtml (accessed April 16, 2008).

The U.S. Department of Health and Human Services. 200 Independence Avenue, S.W., Washington, DC 20201. (877) 696-6775.

Valley Baptist Heart and Vascular Institute. 2101 Pease Street, P.O. Drawer 2588, Harlingen, TX 78550. (956) 389-4848.

Crystal H. Kaczkowski, MSc
Rosalyn Carson-DeWitt, MD

Vasectomy

Definition

A vasectomy is a surgical procedure performed on adult males in which the vasa deferentia (tubes that carry sperm from the testicles to the seminal

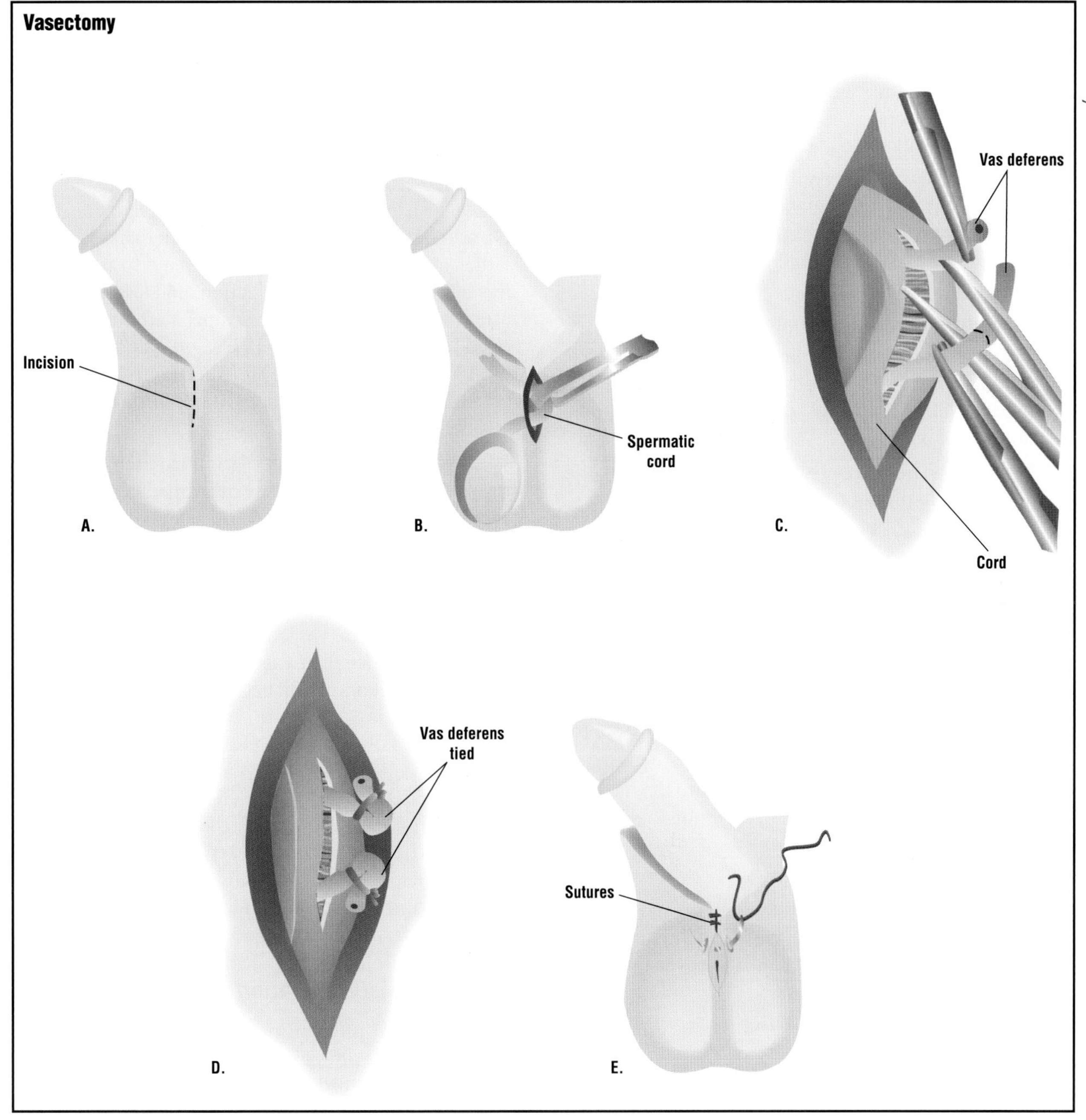

In a vasectomy, an incision is made in the man's scrotum. The spermatic cord is pulled out (B) and incised to expose the vas deferens, which is then severed (C). The ends may be cauterized or tied off (D). After the procedure is repeated on the opposite cord, the scrotal incision is closed (E). *(Illustration by GGS Information Services. Cengage Learning, Gale.)*

vesicles) are cut, tied, cauterized (burned or seared), or otherwise interrupted. The semen no longer contains sperm after the tubes are cut, so conception cannot occur. The testicles continue to produce sperm, but the sperm die and are absorbed by the body.

Purpose

The purpose of the vasectomy is to provide reliable contraception. Research indicates that the level of effectiveness is 99.6%. Vasectomy is the most reliable method of contraception and has fewer complications

KEY TERMS

Ejaculation—The act of expelling the sperm through the penis during orgasm. The fluid that is released is called the ejaculate.

Epididymitis—Inflammation of the small tube that rests on top of the testicle and is part of the system that carries sperm from the testicle to the penis. The condition can be successfully treated with antibiotics, if necessary.

Scrotum—The sac that contains the testicles.

Sperm granuloma—A collection of fluid that leaks from an improperly sealed or tied vas deferens. The fluid usually disappears on its own, but can be drained, if necessary.

Testicles—The two egg-shaped organs found in the scrotum that produce sperm.

Tubal ligation—A female sterilization surgical procedure in which the fallopian tubes are tied in two places and cut between. This prevents eggs from moving from the ovary to the uterus.

Vas deferens (plural, vasa deferentia)—The Latin name for the duct that carries sperm from the testicle to the epididymis. In a vasectomy, a portion of each vas deferens is removed to prevent the sperm from entering the seminal fluid.

Vasovasostomy—A surgical procedure that is done to reverse a vasectomy by reconnecting the ends of the severed vasa deferentia.

and a faster recovery time than female sterilization methods. Some insurance plans will cover the cost of the procedure.

Demographics

Approximately 500,000 vasectomies are performed annually in the United States. About one out of every six men over the age of 35 has had a vasectomy. Higher vasectomy rates are associated with higher levels of education and income.

Description

Vasectomies are usually performed in the doctor's office or an outpatient clinic using **local anesthesia**. The area around the patient's scrotum (the sac containing the testicles that produce sperm) is shaved and cleaned with an antiseptic solution to reduce the chance of infection. A small incision is made in the scrotum. Each vas deferens (one from each testicle) is tied in two places with nonabsorbent (permanent) sutures and the tube is severed between the ties. The ends may be cauterized (burned or seared) to decrease the chance that they will leak or grow back together.

"No-scalpel" vasectomies are gaining in popularity. Instead of an incision, a small puncture is made into the scrotum. The vasa deferentia are cut and sealed in a manner similar to that described above. No **stitches** are necessary and the patient has less pain. Other advantages include less damage to the tissues, less bleeding, less risk of infection, and less discomfort after the procedure. The no-scalpel method was developed in China in the mid-1970s and has been used in the United States since 1988. About one-third of vasectomies in the United States are performed with this technique.

The patient is not sterile immediately following the procedure. Men must use other methods of contraception until two consecutive semen analyses confirm that there are no sperm present in the ejaculate. It takes about four to six weeks, or 15–20 ejaculations, to clear all of the sperm from the tubes.

In some cases, vasectomies may be reversed by a procedure known as a **vasovasostomy**. In this procedure, the surgeon reconnects the ends of the severed vasa deferentia. A vasectomy should be considered permanent, however, as there is no guarantee of successful reversal. Vasovasostomies are successful in approximately 40–50% of men, although the success rate varies considerably with the individual surgeon. In the mid 2000s between 6% and 12% of American men were requesting reversals of their vasectomies. The cost of the procedure in the United States can be considerable, ranging from $5,000–20,000.

Diagnosis/Preparation

No special physical preparation is required for a vasectomy. The physician will first assess the patient's general health in order to identify any potential problems that could occur. The doctor will then explain the possible risks and side effects of the procedure. The patient is asked to sign a consent form that indicates that he understands the information he has received, and gives the doctor permission to perform the operation.

Aftercare

Following the surgery, ice packs are often applied to the scrotum to decrease pain and swelling. A dressing (or athletic supporter) that supports the scrotum can also reduce pain. Mild over-the-counter (OTC) pain medication such as **aspirin** or **acetaminophen**

WHO PERFORMS THE PROCEDURE AND WHERE IS IT PERFORMED?

Vasectomy is a minor procedure that can be performed in a clinic or doctor's office on an outpatient basis. The procedure is generally performed by a urologist, who is a medical doctor that has completed specialized training in the diagnosis and treatment of diseases of the urinary tract and genital organs.

QUESTIONS TO ASK THE DOCTOR

- How often do you perform vasectomies?
- What is your rate of complications?
- How long will the procedure take?
- What will the procedure cost?
- Will my insurance cover the cost?
- Do you perform vasectomy reversal? If so, what is your success rate?

(Tylenol) should be able to control any discomfort. Activities may be restricted for one or two days, and no sexual intercourse for three or four days.

Risks

There are very few risks associated with vasectomy other than infection, bruising, epididymitis (inflammation of the tube that carries the sperm from the testicle to the penis), and sperm granulomas (collections of fluid that leaks from a poorly sealed or tied vas deferens). These complications are easily treated if they do occur. Patients do not experience difficulty achieving an erection, maintaining an erection, or ejaculating. There is no decrease in the production of the male hormone (testosterone), and the patient's sex drive and sexual performance are not altered. Vasectomy is safer and less expensive than **tubal ligation** (sterilization of a female by cutting the fallopian tubes to prevent conception).

According to both the World Health Organization (WHO) and the National Institutes of Health (NIH), there is no evidence that a vasectomy will increase a man's long-term risk of testicular cancer, prostate cancer, or heart disease.

Normal results

Vasectomies are more than 99% successful in preventing conception. As such, male sterilization is one of the most effective methods of contraception available.

Morbidity and mortality rates

Complications occur in approximately 5% of vasectomies. The rates of incidence of some of the more common complications include:

- mild bleeding into the scrotum: one in 400
- major bleeding into the scrotum: one in 1,000
- infection: one in 100
- epididymitis: one in 100
- sperm granuloma: one in 500
- persistent pain: one in 1,000

Fournier gangrene is a very rare but possible complication of vasectomy in which the lining of tissue underneath the skin of the scrotum becomes infected (a condition called fasciitis). Fournier gangrene progresses very rapidly and is treated with aggressive antibiotic therapy and surgery to remove necrotic (dead) tissue. Despite treatment, a mortality rate of 45% has been reported for this condition.

Alternatives

There are numerous options available to couples who are interested in preventing pregnancy. The most common methods are female sterilization, oral contraceptives, and the male condom. Female sterilization has a success rate of 99.5%; oral contraceptives, 95–99.5%; and the male condom, 86–97%.

Resources

ORGANIZATIONS

Alan Guttmacher Institute. 1302 Connecticut Ave., NW, Suite 700, Washington, DC 20036. (202) 296-4012 or toll free (877) 823-0262. http://www.guttmacher.org (accessed April 16, 2008).

Planned Parenthood Federation of America. 434 West 33rd Street, New York, NY 10001. 212-541-7800. http://www.plannedparenthood.org (accessed April 16, 2008).

OTHER

"Facts About Vasectomy Safety." *National Institute of Child Health and Human Development*, August 17, 2006 [cited January 5, 2008]. http://www.nichd.nih.gov/publications/pubs/vasectomy_safety.cfm (accessed April 16, 2008).

"Vasectomy." *Planned Parenthood Federation of America*, [cited January 5, 2008]. http://www.plannedparen

thood.org/midsouthmi/vasectomy.htm (accessed April 16, 2008).

VasectomyMedical.com. April 4, 2007 [cited January 5, 2008]. http://www.vasectomymedical.com (accessed April 16, 2008).

Donald G. Barstow, RN
Stephanie Dionne Sherk
Tish Davidson, AM

Vasectomy reversal *see* **Vasovasostomy**

Vasovasostomy

Definition

A vasovasostomy is a surgical procedure in which the effects of a **vasectomy** (male sterilization) are reversed. During a vasectomy, the vasa deferentia, which are ducts that carry sperm from the testicles to the seminal vesicles, are cut, tied, cauterized (burned or seared), or otherwise interrupted. A vasovasostomy creates an opening between the separated ends of each vas deferens so that the sperm may enter the semen before ejaculation.

Purpose

The purpose of a vasovasostomy is to restore a man's fertility, whereas a vasectomy, or male sterilization, is performed to provide reliable contraception (birth control). Research indicates that the level of effectiveness in preventing pregnancy is 99.6%. Vasectomy is the most reliable method of contraception and has less risk of complications and a faster recovery time than female sterilization methods.

In many cases, a vasectomy can be reversed. Vasectomy reversal does not, however, guarantee a successful pregnancy. The longer the time elapsed since a man has had a vasectomy, the more difficult the

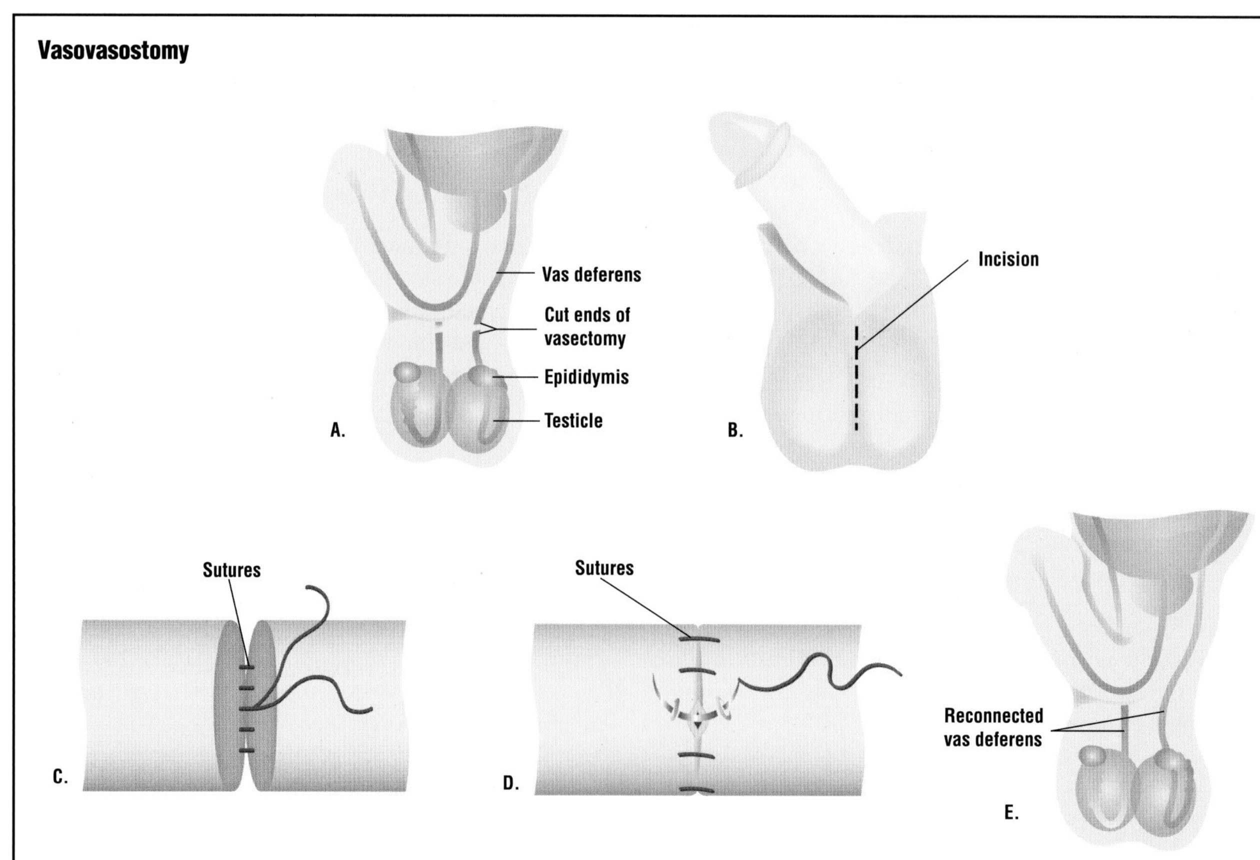

In a vasovasostomy, the surgeon makes an incision in scrotum at the site of the vasectomy scar (B). The spermatic cords are located, and the two vas deferens are reconnected with two layers of suture (C and D). *(Illustration by GGS Information Services. Cengage Learning, Gale.)*

KEY TERMS

Atrophy—Withering away.

Congenital—Present at birth.

Epididymis—A coiled cordlike structure at the upper border of the testis, in which sperm mature and are stored.

Hematoma—A localized collection of blood in an organ or tissue due to broken blood vessels.

Intracytoplasmic sperm injection (ICSI)—A process in which a single sperm is injected into a female egg.

In vitro fertilization (IVF)—A process in which sperm are incubated with a female egg under carefully controlled conditions, then transferred to the female uterus once fertilization has occurred.

Scrotum—The sac that contains the testicles.

Vas deferens (plural, vasa deferentia)—The Latin name for the duct that carries sperm from the testicle to the epididymis. In a vasectomy, a portion of each vas deferens is removed to prevent the sperm from entering the seminal fluid.

Vasoepididymostomy—A type of vasectomy reversal in which the vas deferens is attached to the epididymis, the structure where sperm matures and is stored.

reversal and the lower the success rate. The rate of sperm return if a vasovasostomy is performed within three years of a vasectomy is 97%; this number decreases to 88% by three to eight years after vasectomy, 79% at nine to 14 years, and 71% after 15 years. In addition, other factors affect the success rate of vasectomy reversal, including the age of the female partner, her fertility potential, the method of reversal used, and the experience of the surgeon performing the procedure.

Vasovasostomies are also performed in men who are sterile because of genital tract obstructions rather than prior vasectomies. A vasovasostomy may also be performed on occasion to relieve pain associated with postvasectomy pain syndrome.

Demographics

An estimated 5% of men who have had a vasectomy later decide that they would like to have children. Some reasons for wanting a vasectomy reversal include **death** of a child, death of a spouse, divorce, or experiencing a change in circumstances so that having more children is possible. One study found that divorce was the most commonly reported reason for a vasovasostomy and that the average age of men requesting a vasovasostomy is approximately 40 years.

About 7.4% of infertile men have primary genital tract obstructions caused by trauma, gonorrhea or other venereal infections, or congenital malformations of the vasa deferentia. Many of these men are good candidates for surgical treatment of their infertility.

Description

Most surgeons prefer to have the patient given either a continuous anesthetic block or **general anesthesia** because of the length of time required for the operation. A vasovasostomy generally takes two to three hours to perform, depending on the complexity of the surgery and the experience of the operating physician. More complex surgeries may take as long as five hours. The advantage of general anesthesia is that the patient remains unconscious for the duration of the surgery, which ensures that he remains comfortable. Regional anesthesia, such as a spinal block, allows the patient to remain awake during the procedure while blocking pain in the area of the surgery.

After an adequate level of anesthesia has been reached, the surgeon will make an incision from the top of one side of the scrotum, sometimes moving upward as far as several inches into the abdominal area. A similar incision will then be made on the other side of the scrotum. The vasa deferentia will be identified and isolated from surrounding tissue. Fluid will be removed from the testicular end of each vas deferens and analyzed for presence of sperm. If sperm are found, then a simpler procedure to connect the cut ends of the vasa deferentia will be performed. If no sperm are found, a more complex procedure called a vasoepididymostomy or epididymovasostomy (in which the vas deferens is attached to the epididymis, a structure in which the sperm mature and are stored) may be more successful in restoring sperm flow.

There are two techniques that may be used to reconnect the cut ends of the vasa deferentia. A single-layer closure involves stitching the outer layer of each cut end of the tube together with a very fine suture thread. This procedure takes less time but is often less successful in restoring sperm flow. A double-layer closure, however, involves stitching the inner layer of each cut end of the tube first, and then stitching the outer layer. After reconnection is established, the vasa deferentia are returned to their anatomical place and the scrotal incisions closed.

Diagnosis/Preparation

Before a vasovasostomy is performed, the patient will undergo a preoperative assessment, including a **physical examination** of the scrotum. This evaluation will allow the surgeon to determine what sort of vasectomy reversal should be performed and how extensive the surgery might be. A medical history will be taken. The physician will review the patient's medical records in order to determine how the patient's vasectomy was performed; if large portions of the vasa deferentia were removed during surgery, the vasectomy reversal will be more complicated and may have a lower chance of success. The patient's partner should also undergo a fertility assessment, including a gynecologic exam, to assess her reproductive health.

Some surgeons prefer to give the patient a broad-spectrum antibiotic about half an hour before surgery as well as a mild sedative.

Aftercare

After the procedure the patient will be transferred to a **recovery room** where he will remain for approximately three hours. The patient will be asked to void urine before discharge. Pain medication is prescribed and usually required for one to three days after the procedure. **Antibiotics** may be given after the procedure as well as beforehand to prevent infection. Ice packs applied to the scrotum will help to decrease swelling and discomfort. Heavy lifting, **exercise**, and sexual activity should be avoided for up to four weeks while the vasovasostomy heals.

Patients are usually allowed to return to work within three days. They may shower within two days after surgery, but should avoid soaking the incision (by taking a tub bath or going swimming) for about two weeks. The surgeon will schedule the patient for an incision check about a week after surgery and a semen analysis three months later.

Risks

The complications that most commonly occur after vasovasostomy include swelling, bruising, and symptoms associated with anesthesia (nausea, headache, etc.). There is a risk of low sperm count if the operation is done inadequately or if scarring partially blocks the channel inside the vasa deferentia. Less common complications are infection or severe hematoma (collection of blood under the skin). The most serious potential complication of a vasovasostomy is testicular atrophy (wasting away), which may result from damage to the spermatic artery during the procedure.

WHO PERFORMS THE PROCEDURE AND WHERE IS IT PERFORMED?

A vasovasostomy can be performed in a hospital, clinic, or doctor's office on an outpatient basis. The procedure is generally performed by a urologist, a medical doctor who has completed specialized training in the diagnosis and treatment of diseases of the urinary tract and genital organs.

Normal results

If a successful vasectomy reversal has been performed, the average time to achieving pregnancy after the procedure is one year, with most pregnancies occurring within the first two years. A good sperm count usually returns within three to six months.

Morbidity and mortality rates

The chance that the vasa deferentia will become obstructed after a successful reversal is approximately 10%. Some doctors recommend that patients bank their sperm as a precautionary measure. Scrotal hematoma occurs in 1–2% of patients after vasovasostomy, and infection in less than 1%.

Alternatives

A vasoepididymostomy may be performed if the physician determines that a vasovasostomy will be insufficient in restoring sperm flow. The determining factor is usually the absence of sperm or fluid in the testicular end of the cut vas deferens (which is found during surgery), although a swollen or blocked epididymis found during a preoperative scrotal examination may also indicate a vasoepididymostomy will be necessary.

There are some options available to men and their partners who are seeking to conceive after a vasectomy but wish to avoid vasectomy reversal. As sperm are no longer present in the man's ejaculate, they may be retrieved from the testicle or epididymis by extraction (removal of tissue) or aspiration (removed by a needle). The sperm may then be incubated with a female egg under carefully controlled conditions, then transferred to the female uterus once fertilization has

QUESTIONS TO ASK THE DOCTOR

- How often do you perform vasectomy reversals?
- What is your success rate?
- What is your rate of complications?
- What technique do you recommend for reestablishing sperm flow?
- How long will the procedure take?
- What will vasectomy reversal cost me? Will my insurance cover the cost?

occurred; this process is called in vitro fertilization (IVF). A process called intracytoplasmic sperm injection (ICSI) may be used to improve the success rate of IVF; in this procedure, a single sperm is injected into the female egg.

Resources

BOOKS

"Family Planning: Sterilization." Section 18, Chapter 246 in *The Merck Manual of Diagnosis and Therapy*, edited by Mark H. Beers, MD, and Robert Berkow, MD. Whitehouse Station, NJ: Merck Research Laboratories, 1999.

PERIODICALS

Sabanegh, Edmund, MD. "Vasovasostomy and Vasoepididymostomy." *eMedicine*, February 13, 2002 [June 5, 2003]. www.emedicine.com/med/topic3090.htm.

Schroeder-Printzen, I., T. Diemer, and W. Weidner. "Vasovasostomy." *Urologia Internationalis* 70, no. 2 (2003): 101-107.

ORGANIZATIONS

American Board of Urology (ABU). 2216 Ivy Road, Suite 210, Charlottesville, VA 22903. (434) 979-0059. www.abu.org.

Center for Male Reproductive Medicine. 2080 Century Park East, Suite 907, Los Angeles, CA 90067. (310) 277-2873. www.malereproduction.com.

OTHER

"Alternatives to Vasectomy Reversal." *VasectomyMedical.com*. December 3, 2002 [cited March 22, 2003]. www.vasectomymedical.com/vasectomy-reversal-alternatives.html.

Fisch, Harry. *The Patient's Guide to Vasectomy Reversal.* [cited March 22, 2003]. www.cpmcnet.columbia.edu/dept/urology/infertility.html.

Silber, Sherman J. *Microscopic Vasectomy Reversal.* 2002 [cited March 22, 2003]. www.infertile.com/treatmnt/treats/mvr/mvr.htm.

"Vasectomy Reversal." *Center for Male Reproductive Medicine.* [cited March 22, 2003]. www.malereproduction.com/08_vasectomyrev.html.

Stephanie Dionne Sherk

Vein ligation and stripping

Definition

Vein ligation and stripping is a surgical approach to the treatment of varicose veins. It is also sometimes called phlebectomy. Ligation refers to the surgical tying-off of a large vein in the leg called the greater saphenous vein, while stripping refers to the removal of this vein through incisions in the groin area or behind the knee. If some of the valves in the saphenous vein are healthy, the weak portion of the vein can be closed off by ligation. If the entire vein is weak, it is closed off and pulled downward and out through an incision made below it. Tying and removal of the greater saphenous vein are done to reduce the pressure of blood flowing backward through this large vein into the smaller veins that feed into it.

Phlebectomy is one of the oldest forms of treatment for varicose veins; the earliest description of it was written by Aulus Cornelius Celsus, a Roman historian of medicine, in 45 A.D. The first description of a phlebectomy hook comes from a textbook on surgery published in 1545. The modern technique of ambulatory (outpatient) phlebectomy was developed around 1956 by a Swiss dermatologist named Robert Muller. As of 2008, surgical ligation and stripping of the saphenous vein are performed less frequently because of the introduction of less invasive forms of treatment.

Purpose

The purpose of vein ligation and stripping is to reduce the number and size of varicose veins that cannot be treated or closed by other measures. The reasons for **vascular surgery** in general include:

- Improvement of the appearance of the legs; large varicose veins are considered disfiguring by many people.
- Relief from pain, leg cramps, and fatigue that may be associated with varicose veins.
- Treatment of skin problems that may develop as complications of varicose veins; these include chronic

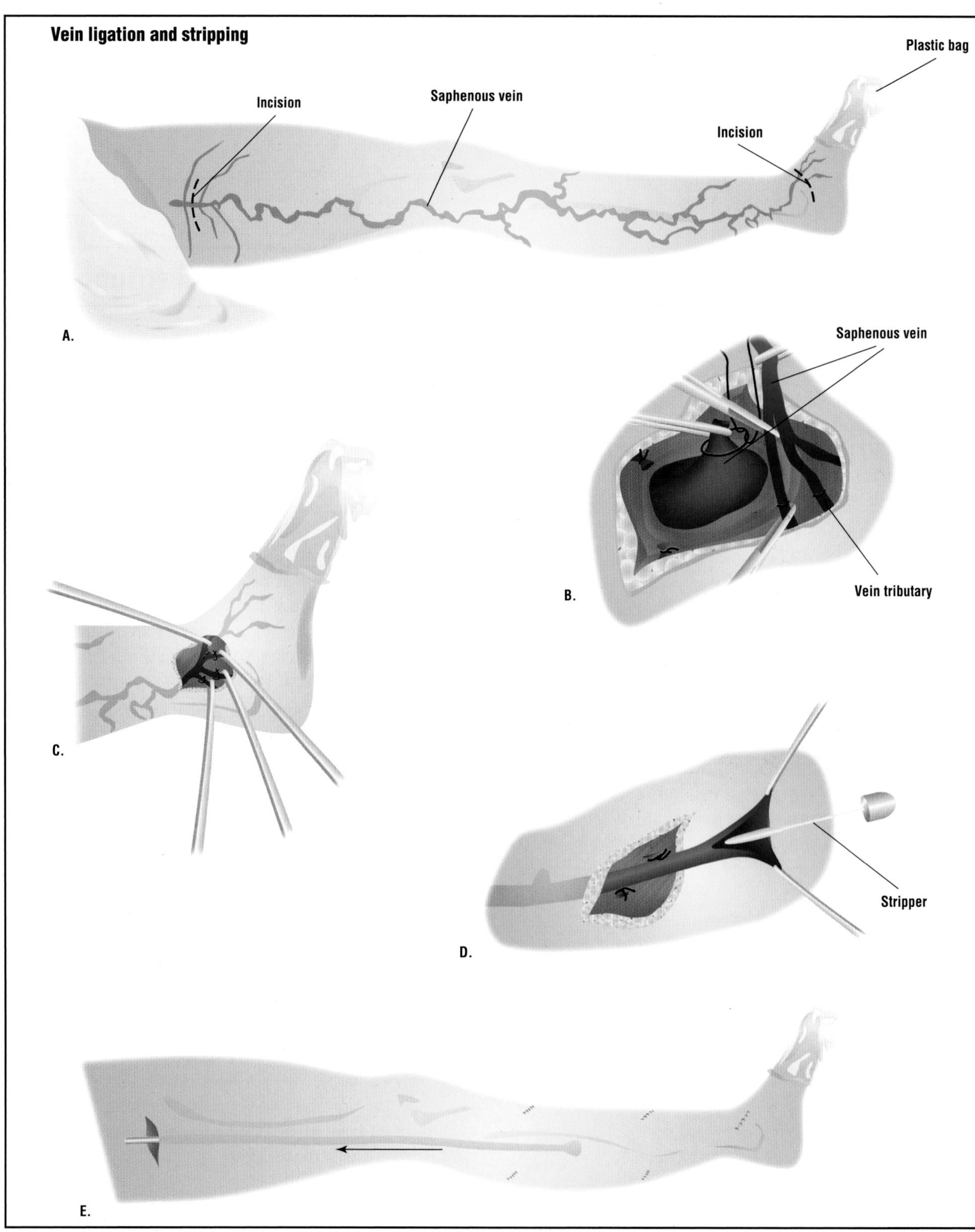

To treat varicose veins in the leg, the saphenous vein may be removed by ligation and stripping (A). First an incision is made in the upper thigh, and the saphenous vein is separated from its tributaries (B). Another incision is made above the foot (C). The lower portion of the vein is cut, and a stripper is inserted into the vein (D). The stripper is pulled through the vein and out the incision in the upper thigh (E). *(Illustration by GGS Information Services. Cengage Learning, Gale.)*

KEY TERMS

Ablation—The destruction or removal of a body part. Saphenous ablation refers to several techniques for closing and destroying the greater saphenous vein without cutting or stripping.

Edema—The presence of abnormally large amounts of fluid in the soft tissues of the body.

Endovascular—Inside a blood vessel. Endovascular treatments of varicose veins are those that are performed inside the veins.

Incompetent—In a medical context, insufficient. An incompetent vein is one that is not performing its function of carrying blood back to the heart.

Ligation—The act of tying off a blood vessel.

Lumen—The channel or cavity inside a tube or hollow organ of the body.

Palpation—Examining by touch as part of the process of physical diagnosis.

Percussion—Thumping or tapping a part of the body with the fingers for diagnostic purposes.

Phlebectomy—Surgical removal of a vein or part of a vein.

Phlebology—The study of veins, their disorders, and their treatments. A phlebologist is a doctor who specializes in treating spider veins, varicose veins, and associated disorders.

Saphenous veins—Two large superficial veins in the leg that may be treated by ligation and stripping as therapy for varicose veins. The greater saphenous vein runs from the foot to the groin area, while the short saphenous vein runs from the ankle to the knee.

Sclerose—To harden or undergo hardening. Sclerosing agents are chemicals that are used in sclerotherapy to cause swollen veins to fill with fibrous tissue and close down.

Seroma—A collection of blood serum or lymphatic fluid in body tissues. It is an occasional complication of vascular surgery.

Telangiectasia—The medical term for the visible discolorations produced by permanently swollen capillaries and smaller veins.

Thrombophlebitis—The inflammation of a vein associated with the formation of blood clots.

Trendelenburg's test—A test that measures the speed at which the lower leg fills with blood after the leg has first been raised above the level of the heart. It is named for Friedrich Trendelenburg (1844–1924), a German surgeon.

Tumescent anesthesia—A type of local anesthesia originally developed for liposuction in which a large volume of diluted anesthetic is injected into the tissues around the vein until they become tumescent (firm and swollen).

Varicose—Abnormally enlarged and distended.

Varix (plural, varices)—The medical term for an enlarged blood vessel.

eczema, skin ulceration, external bleeding, and abnormal pigmentation of the skin.

- Prevention of such disorders as thrombophlebitis and pulmonary blood clots.

Demographics

The World Health Organization (WHO) estimates that about 25% of adults around the world have some type of venous disorder in the legs. The proportion of the general population with varicose veins is higher, however, in the developed countries. The American College of Phlebology (ACP), which is a group of dermatologists, plastic surgeons, gynecologists, and general surgeons with special training in the treatment of venous disorders, states that more than 80 million people in the United States suffer from varicose veins. In the past, the female-to-male ratio has been close to four to one, but this figure is changing due to the rapid rise in obesity among adult males in the past two decades.

Varicose veins are more common in middle-aged and elderly adults than in children or young adults. Although varicose veins tend to run in families, they do not appear to be associated with specific racial or ethnic groups.

Description

Causes of varicose veins

The venous part of the circulatory system returns blood to the heart to be pumped to the lungs for oxygenation, in contrast to the arterial system, which carries oxygenated blood away from the heart to be distributed throughout the body. Veins are more likely than arteries to expand or dilate if blood volume or pressure increases, because they consist of only one layer of tissue; this is in contrast to arteries, in which there are three layers.

There are three major categories of veins: superficial veins, deep veins, and perforating veins. All varicose veins are superficial veins; they lie between the skin and a layer of fibrous connective tissue called fascia, which cover and support the muscles and the internal organs. The deep veins of the body lie within the muscle fascia. This distinction helps to explain why a superficial vein can be removed or closed without damage to the deep circulation in the legs. Perforating veins are veins that connect the superficial and deep veins.

Veins contain one-way valves that push blood inward and upward toward the heart against the force of gravity when they are functioning normally. The blood pressure in the superficial veins is usually low, but if it rises and remains at a higher level over a period of time, the valves in the veins begin to fail. The blood flows backward and collects in the lower veins, and the veins dilate, or expand. Veins that are not functioning properly are said to be incompetent. As the veins expand, they become more noticeable under the surface of the skin. Small veins, or capillaries, often appear as spider-shaped or tree-like networks of reddish or purplish lines under the skin. The medical term for these is telangiectasias, but they are commonly known as spider veins or thread veins. Larger veins that form flat, blue-green networks often found behind the knee are called reticular varicosities. True varicose veins are formed when the largest superficial veins become distorted and twisted by a long-term rise in blood pressure in the legs.

The most important veins in the lower leg are the two saphenous veins: the greater saphenous vein, which runs from the foot to the groin area, and the short saphenous vein, which runs from the ankle to the knee. It is thought that varicose veins develop when the valves at the top of the greater saphenous vein fail, allowing more blood to flow backward down the leg and increase the pressure on the valves in the smaller veins in turn. The practice of ligation and stripping of the greater saphenous vein is based on this hypothesis.

Some people are at increased risk for developing varicose veins. These risk factors include:

- Sex. Females in any age group are more likely than males to develop varicose veins. It is thought that female sex hormones contribute to the development of varicose veins by making the veins dilate more easily. Many women experience increased discomfort from varicose veins during their menstrual periods.
- Genetic factors. Some people have veins with abnormally weak walls or valves. They may develop varicose veins even without a rise in blood pressure in the superficial veins. This characteristic tends to run in families.
- Pregnancy. A woman's total blood volume increases during pregnancy, which increases the blood pressure in the venous system. In addition, the hormonal changes of pregnancy cause the walls and valves in the veins to soften.
- Using birth control pills.
- Obesity. Excess body weight increases the pressure on the veins.
- Occupational factors. People who have jobs that require standing or sitting for long periods of time—without the opportunity to walk or move around—are more likely to develop varicose veins.

Ambulatory phlebectomy

Ambulatory phlebectomy is the most common surgical procedure for treating medium-sized varicose veins, as of early 2008. It is also known as stab avulsion or micro-extraction phlebectomy. An ambulatory phlebectomy is performed under **local anesthesia**. After the patient's leg has been anesthetized, the surgeon makes a series of very small vertical incisions 0.39–1.18 in (1–3 mm) in length along the length of the affected vein. These incisions do not require **stitches** or tape closure afterward. Beginning with the more heavily involved areas of the leg, the surgeon inserts a phlebectomy hook through each micro-incision. The vein segment is drawn through the incision, held with a mosquito clamp, and pulled out through the incision. This technique requires the surgeon to be especially careful when removing varicose veins in the ankle, foot, or back of the knee. The procedure takes about 45–50 minutes.

After all the vein segments have been removed, the surgeon washes the patient's leg with hydrogen peroxide and covers the area with a foam wrap, several layers of cotton wrap, and an adhesive bandage. A compression stocking is then drawn up over the wrapping. The **bandages** are removed three to seven days after surgery, but the compression stocking must be worn for another two to four weeks to minimize bruising and swelling. The patient is encouraged to walk around for 10 or so minutes before leaving the office; this mild activity helps to minimize the risk of a blood clot forming in the deep veins of the leg.

Transilluminated powered phlebectomy

Transilluminated powered phlebectomy (TIPP) is a newer technique that avoids the drawbacks of stab avulsion phlebectomy, which include long operating times, the risk of scar formation, and a relatively high risk of infection developing in the micro-incisions. Transilluminated powered phlebectomy is performed with an illuminator and a motorized resector. After the patient has been anesthetized with light **general anesthesia**, the surgeon makes only two small incisions: one for the illuminating device and the other for the resector. After making the first incision and introducing the illuminator, the surgeon uses a technique called tumescent anesthesia to plump up the tissues around the veins and make the veins easier to remove. Tumescent anesthesia was originally developed for **liposuction**. It involves the injection of large quantities of a dilute anesthetic into the tissues surrounding the veins until they become firm and swollen.

After the tumescent anesthesia has been completed, the surgeon makes a second incision to insert the resector, which draws the vein by suction toward an inner blade. The suction then removes the tiny pieces of venous tissue left by the blade. After all the clusters of varicose veins have been treated, the surgeon closes the two small incisions with a single stitch or Steri-Strips. The incisions are covered with a gauze dressing and the leg is wrapped in a sterile compression dressing.

Diagnosis/Preparation

Diagnosis

Vein ligation and stripping and ambulatory phlebectomies are considered elective cosmetic procedures; they are not performed on an emergency basis. For this reason, patients should check with their insurance provider to see whether these procedures are covered. Costs vary but generally run between $600 and $2,000 per leg for the surgeon's fee; anesthesia and hospitalization are extra.

The process of diagnosis may begin with the patient's complaints about the appearance of the legs or of pain and cramps, as well as with the physician's observations. It is important to note that there is no correlation between the size or number of a patient's varicose veins and the amount of pain that is experienced. Some people experience considerable discomfort from fairly small varices, while others may have no symptoms from clusters of extremely swollen varicose veins. If the patient mentions pain, burning sensations, or other physical symptoms, the doctor will need to rule out other possible causes, such as nerve root irritation, osteoarthritis, diabetic neuropathy, or problems in the arterial circulation. Relief of pain when the leg is elevated is the most significant diagnostic sign of varicose veins.

After taking the patient's medical history and a family history of venous disorders, the doctor examines the patient from the waist down to note the location of varicose veins and to palpate (touch with gentle pressure) for signs of other venous disorders. Palpation helps the doctor locate both normal and abnormal veins; further, some varicose veins can be detected by touch even though they cannot be seen through the skin. Ideally, the examiner will have a small raised platform for the patient to stand on during the **physical examination**. The doctor will ask the patient to turn slowly while standing, and will be looking for scars or other signs of trauma, bulges, and areas of discoloration in the skin, or other indications of chronic venous insufficiency. While palpating the legs, the doctor will note areas of unusual warmth or soreness, cysts, and edema (swelling of the soft tissues due to fluid retention). Next, the doctor will percuss (tap on) certain parts of the legs where the larger veins lie closer to the surface. By gently tapping or thumping on the skin over these areas, the doctor can feel if there are any fluid waves in the veins and determine whether further testing for venous insufficiency is required.

The next stage of the diagnostic examination is an evaluation of the valves in the patient's greater saphenous vein. The doctor places a tourniquet around the patient's upper thigh while the patient is lying on the examination table with the leg raised. The patient is then asked to stand on the floor. If the valves in this vein are working properly, the lower superficial veins should not fill up rapidly as long as the tourniquet remains tied. This test is known as Trendelenburg's test. It has, however, been largely replaced by the use of duplex Doppler **ultrasound**, which maps the location of the varicose veins in the patient's leg and provides information about the condition of the valves in the veins. Most insurance companies now also require a Doppler test before authorizing surgical treatment. The doctor's findings will determine whether the greater saphenous vein will require ligation and stripping or endovenous ablation before smaller varicose veins can be treated.

Some disorders or conditions are contraindications for vascular surgery, including:

- cellulitis and other infectious diseases of the skin
- severe edema associated with heart or kidney disease (these disorders should be brought under control before a phlebectomy is performed)
- uncontrolled diabetes
- disorders that affect the immune system, including HIV infection
- severe heart or lung disorders

Preparation

Patients preparing for vascular surgery are asked to discontinue **aspirin** or aspirin-related products for a week before the procedure. They should not eat or drink after midnight on the day of surgery. They should not apply any moisturizers, creams, tanning lotions, or sun block to the legs on the day of the procedure.

A patient scheduled for an ambulatory phlebectomy should arrive at the surgical center about an hour and a half before the procedure. All clothing must be removed before changing into a hospital gown. The patient is asked to walk up and down in the room or hallway for about 20 minutes to make the veins stand out. The surgeon marks the outlines of the veins with an indelible ink marker on the patient's legs while he or she is standing up. An ultrasound may be done at this point to verify the location and condition of the veins. The patient is then taken into the **operating room** for surgery.

Although patients are encouraged to walk around for a few minutes after an ambulatory phlebectomy, they should make arrangements for a friend or relative to drive them home from the surgical facility.

Aftercare

Surgical ligation and stripping of the greater saphenous vein usually requires an overnight stay in the hospital and two to eight weeks of **recovery at home** afterward.

Aftercare following surgical treatment of varicose veins includes wearing medical compression stockings that apply either 20–30 mmHg or 30–40 mmHg of pressure for two to six weeks after the procedure. Wearing compression stockings minimizes the risk of edema, discoloration, and pain. Fashion support stockings are a less acceptable alternative because they do not apply enough pressure to the legs.

The elastic surgical dressing applied at the end of an ambulatory phlebectomy should be left in place after returning home. Mild pain-killing medications may be taken for discomfort.

The patient is advised to watch for redness, swelling, pus, fever, and other signs of infection.

Patients are encouraged to walk, ride a bicycle, or participate in other low-impact forms of **exercise** (such as yoga and tai chi) to prevent the formation of blood clots in the deep veins of the legs. They should lie down with the legs elevated above heart level for 15 minutes at least twice a day, and use a foot stool when sitting to keep the legs raised.

Risks

Vein ligation and stripping carries the same risks as other surgical procedures under general anesthesia, such as bleeding, infection of the incision, and an adverse reaction to the anesthetic. Patients with leg ulcers or fungal infections of the foot are at increased risk of developing infections in the incisions following surgical treatment of varicose veins.

Specific risks associated with vascular surgery include:

- Deep venous thrombosis.
- Bruising. Bruising is the most common complication of phlebectomies, but heals itself in a few days or weeks.
- Scar formation. Phlebectomy has been found to produce permanent leg scars more frequently than sclerotherapy.
- Injury to the saphenous nerve. This complication results in numbness, tingling, or burning sensations in the area around the ankle. It usually goes away without further treatment within six to 12 months.
- Seromas. A seroma is a collection of uninfected blood serum or lymphatic fluid in the tissues. Seromas usually resolve without further treatment, but can be drained by the surgeon, if necessary.
- Injury to the arteries in the thigh and groin area. This complication is extremely rare, but it can have serious consequences. One example is amputation of the leg.
- Leg swelling. This complication is caused by disruption of the lymphatic system during surgery. This lasts about two to three weeks and can be managed by wearing compression stockings.
- Recurrence of smaller varicose veins.

Normal results

Normal results of vein ligation and stripping, or ambulatory phlebectomy, include reduction in the size and number of varicose veins in the leg. About 95% of patients also experience significant relief of pain.

Morbidity and mortality rates

The mortality rate following vein ligation and stripping has been reported to be one in 30,000. The incidence of deep venous thrombosis (DVT) following vascular surgery is estimated to be 0.6%.

Alternatives

Conservative treatments

Patients who are experiencing discomfort from varicose veins may be helped by any or several of the following approaches:

- Exercise. Walking or other forms of exercise that activate the muscles in the lower legs can relieve aching and cramping because these muscles keep the blood moving through the leg veins. One specific exercise that is often recommended is repeated flexing of the ankle joint. Flexing the ankles five to 10 times every few minutes and walking around for one to two minutes every half hour throughout the day helps to prevent the venous congestion that results from sitting or standing in one position for hours at a time.
- Avoiding high-heeled shoes. Shoes with high heels do not allow the ankle to flex fully when the patient is walking. This limitation of the range of motion of the ankle joint makes it more difficult for the leg muscles to contract and force venous blood upwards toward the heart.
- Elevating the legs for 15–30 minutes once or twice a day. This change of position is frequently recommended for reducing edema of the feet and ankles.
- Wearing compression hosiery. Compression benefits the leg veins by reducing inflammation as well as improving venous outflow. Most manufacturers of medical compression stockings now sell some relatively sheer hosiery that looks attractive in addition to providing support.
- Medications. Drugs that have been used to treat the discomfort associated with varicose veins include nonsteroidal anti-inflammatory drugs (NSAIDs) and preparations of vitamins C and E. One prescription medication that is sometimes given to treat circulatory problems in the legs and feet is pentoxifylline, which improves blood flow in the smaller capillaries. Pentoxifylline is sold under the brand name Trendar.

If appearance is the patient's primary concern, varicose veins can be partially covered with specially formulated cosmetics that come in a wide variety of skin tones. Some of these preparations are available in waterproof formulations for use during swimming and other athletic activities.

Endovenous ablation

Endovenous ablation refers to two newer and less invasive methods for treating incompetent saphenous veins. In the Closure® method, which was approved by the Food and Drug Administration (FDA) in 1999, the surgeon passes a catheter into the lumen of the saphenous vein. The catheter is connected to a radiofrequency generator and delivers heat energy to the vein through an electrode in its tip. As the tissues in the wall of the vein are heated, they shrink and coagulate, which closes and seals the vein. The temperature inside the wall of the vein is limited to 185°F (85°C) to prevent heat damage to surrounding tissues. Radiofrequency ablation of the saphenous vein has been demonstrated to be safe and at least as effective as surgical stripping of the vein; in addition, patients can return to work the next day. About 95% of patients are satisfied with the procedure and would recommend it to others. The procedure produces good cosmetic results that last at least 5 years; the longer-term effectiveness of radiofrequency ablation, however, is not known, as of 2008. Its chief risk is loss of feeling in a patch of skin about the size of a quarter above the knee. This numbness usually resolves in about six months. One limitation of radiofrequency ablation is that present catheters cannot be used with extremely twisted or crooked veins. The most frequent complication reported with this procedure is deep vein thrombosis.

Endovenous laser treatment, or EVLT, uses a laser instead of a catheter with an electrode to heat the tissues in the wall of an incompetent vein in order to close the vein. Although EVLT appears to be as safe and effective as radiofrequency ablation, patients experience more discomfort and bruising afterward;

WHO PERFORMS THE PROCEDURE AND WHERE IS IT PERFORMED?

Surgical treatment of varicose veins is usually performed by general surgeons or by vascular surgeons, who are trained in the diagnosis and medical management of venous disorders as well as surgical treatment of them. Most vascular surgeons have completed five years of residency training in surgery after medical school, followed by one to two years of specialized fellowship training.

Phlebectomies and endovenous ablation treatments are performed in ambulatory surgery centers as outpatient procedures. Ligation and stripping of the greater saphenous vein, however, is more commonly performed in a hospital as an inpatient operation.

QUESTIONS TO ASK THE DOCTOR

- Can my varicose veins be treated without ligation and stripping?
- Am I a candidate for treatment with EVLT or radiofrequency ablation?
- What specific technique(s) do you perform most frequently?
- Which treatment technique(s) do you recommend and why?
- What are the risks of these techniques?
- Are other patients satisfied with the results?

most require two to three days of recovery at home after laser treatment. EVLT is reported to give as good results as surgery or laser ablation, with a low rate (less than 7%) of varicose vein recurrence after two years. As with radiofrequency ablation, EVLT cannot be used in extremely crooked veins. EVLT is not yet widely used; fewer than 10,000 cases worldwide have been reported, as of 2007. The major side effect that has been described is skin burns.

Sclerotherapy

Sclerotherapy is a treatment method in which irritating chemicals in liquid or foam form are injected into spider veins or smaller reticular varicosities to close them off. The chemicals cause the vein to become inflamed, and lead to the formation of fibrous tissue and closing of the lumen, or central channel of the vein. Sclerotherapy is sometimes used in combination with other techniques to treat larger varicose veins.

Complementary and alternative (CAM) treatments

According to Dr. Kenneth Pelletier, former director of the program in complementary and alternative treatments at Stanford University School of Medicine, horse chestnut extract works as well as compression stockings when used as a conservative treatment for varicose veins. Horse chestnut (*Aesculus hippocastanum*) preparations have been used in Europe for some years to treat circulatory problems in the legs; most recent research has been carried out in Great Britain and Germany. The usual dosage is 75 mg twice a day, at meals. The most common side effect of oral preparations of horse chestnut is occasional indigestion in some patients.

Resources

BOOKS

Bergan, John, ed. *The Vein Book*. Boston: Elsevier Academic Press, 2007.

Pelletier, Kenneth R., MD. *The Best Alternative Medicine*, Part II, "CAM Therapies for Specific Conditions: Varicose Veins." New York: Simon & Schuster, 2002.

Weiss, Robert, Craig Feied, and Margaret Weiss, eds. *Vein Diagnosis and Treatment: A Comprehensive Approach*. New York: McGraw-Hill, Health Professions Division, 2001.

PERIODICALS

Beale, R. J., and M. J. Gough. "Treatment Options for Primary Varicose Veins—A Review." *European Journal of Vascular and Endovascular Surgery* 30 (July 2005): 83–95.

Bergan, J. J., N. H. Kumins, E. L. Owens, and S. R. Sparks. "Surgical and Endovascular Treatment of Lower Extremity Venous Insufficiency." *Journal of Vascular and Interventional Radiology* 13 (June 2002): 563–568.

De Roos, K. P., F. H. Nieman, and H. A. Neumann. "Ambulatory Phlebectomy Versus Compression Sclerotherapy: Results of a Randomized Controlled Trial." *Dermatologic Surgery* 29 (March 2003): 221–226.

Hingorani, A. P., E. Ascher, N. Marcevich, et al. "Deep Venous Thrombosis after Radiofrequency Ablation of Greater Saphenous Vein: A Word of Caution." *Journal of Vascular Surgery* 40 (March 2004): 500–504.

Johnson, C. M., and R. B. McLafferty. "Endovenous Laser Ablation of Varicose Veins: Review of Current Technologies and Clinical Outcome." *Vascular* 15 (September–October 2007): 250–254.

Ramelet, A. A. "Phlebectomy. Technique, Indications and Complications." *International Angiology* 21 (June 2002): 46–51.

Sadick, N. S. "Advances in the Treatment of Varicose Veins: Ambulatory Phlebectomy, Foam Sclerotherapy, Endovascular Laser, and Radiofrequency Closure." *Dermatologic Clinics* 23 (July 2005): 443–455.

Vardanian, A. J., H. L. Cao, and P. F. Lawrence. "Light-Assisted Stab Phlebectomy: Early Postoperative Experience." *American Surgeon* 73 (October 2007): 1067–1070.

Zotto, Lisa M., RN. "Treating Varicose Veins with Transilluminated Powered Phlebectomy." *AORN Journal* 76 (December 2002): 981–990.

ORGANIZATIONS

American Academy of Dermatology. 930 East Woodfield Rd., PO Box 4014, Schaumburg, IL 60168. (847) 330-0230 or (866) 503-SKIN. http://www.aad.org (accessed April 17, 2008).

American College of Phlebology. 100 Webster Street, Suite 101, Oakland, CA 94607-3724. (510) 834-6500. http://www.phlebology.org (ACCESSED April 17, 2008).

Peripheral Vascular Surgery Society (PVSS). 824 Munras Avenue, Suite C, Monterey, CA 93940. (831) 373-0508. http://www.pvss.org (accessed April 17, 2008).

Society for Vascular Surgery. 633 N. St, 24th floor, Chicago, IL 60611. http://www.vascularweb.org (accessed April 17, 2008).

OTHER

Bergan, John J., MD. *Surgery of Varicose Veins*, [cited April 13, 2003]. http://www.phlebology.org/surgery.html (accessed April 17, 2008).

Feied, Craig, MD. "Varicose Veins Treated with Radiofrequency Ablation Therapy." *eMedicine*, September 29, 2005 [cited January 12, 2008]. http://www.emedicine.com/derm/topic751.htm (accessed April 17, 2008).

Feied, Craig, MD. *Venous Anatomy and Physiology*, [cited April 10, 2003]. http://www.phlebology.org/ (accessed April 17, 2008).

Feied, Craig, MD, Robert Min, MD, and Steven E. Zimmet, MD. "Varicose Vein Treatment with Endovenous Laser Therapy." *eMedicine*, February 15, 2007 [cited January 12, 2008]. http://www.emedicine.com/derm/topic750.htm (accessed April 17, 2008).

Feied, Craig, MD, Robert Weiss, MD, and Robert B. Hashemiyoon, MD. "Varicose Veins and Spider Veins." *eMedicine*, September 29, 2005 [cited January 12, 2008]. http://www.emedicine.com/derm/topic475.htm (accessed April 17, 2008).

Fronek, Helane S., MD. *Conservative Therapy for Venous Disease*, [cited April 10, 2003]. http://www.phlebology.org/ (accessed April 17, 2008).

Fronek, Helane S., MD. *Functional Testing for Venous Disease*, [cited April 10, 2003]. http://www.phlebology.org/ (accessed April 17, 2008).

Marley, Wayne, MD. *Physical Examination of the Phlebology Patient*, [cited April 10, 2003]. www.phlebology.org/ (accessed April 17, 2008).

Olivencia, José A., MD. *Ambulatory Phlebectomy*, [cited April 13, 2003]. http://www.phlebology.org/ (accessed April 17, 2008).

Weiss, Robert, MD. *Radiofrequency Endovenous Occlusion (Closure(R) Technique)*, [cited April 13, 2003]. http://www.phlebology.org/ (accessed April 17, 2008).

Rebecca Frey, PhD

Venography *see* **Phlebography**

Venous thrombosis prevention

Definition

Venous thrombosis prevention refers to the use of medications, other devices, or behavioral changes to prevent blood clots from forming in veins within the body.

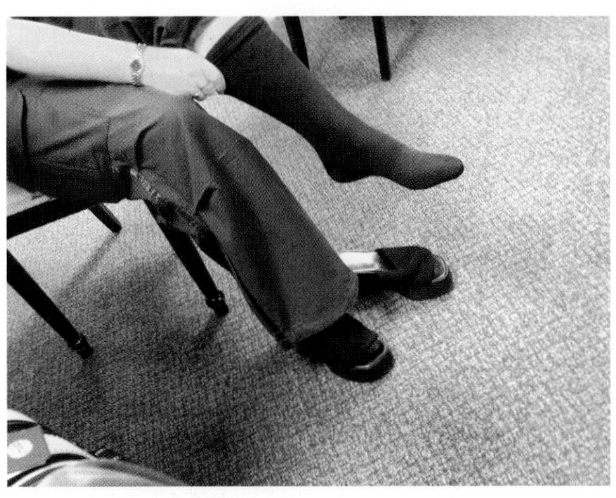

Putting on flight socks before a long flight can help prevent venous thrombosis. *(Slick Stock Images / Alamy)*

Purpose

Different preventative methods can also maintain normal blood flow and therefore enable oxygen and nutrients to reach the cells of the body. Blood clots can be painful and can cause serious damage to tissues and organs. Sometimes, they can cause rapid **death**. Blood clot prevention can enhance blood flow and save lives.

Description

Blood clots can form in any vein within the body. Deep vein thrombosis (DVT) can be quite serious. DVT occurs when a blood clot (thrombus) forms in the legs or pelvis; in a few cases, DVT occurs in the arms. If the thrombus is large enough, it can block the blood flow within the vein, cutting off oxygen to the tissues. An embolus (a clot that breaks away from the wall of the blood vessel) can travel into the lung, the heart, or the brain where it can disrupt the normal functioning of these organs and become life threatening. Some blood clots distend the walls of the blood vessel, creating a sac called an aneurysm. Sometimes the aneurysm bursts, causing blood to leak out. If this occurs within the brain, the heart, or the lungs, it can be fatal.

Venous thrombosis can occur for a number of reasons. There are three large categories of factors that influence the likelihood of DVT: changes in the rate of blood flow; injuries to the tissue lining the inner walls of the veins; and changes in the thickness of the blood or its ability to coagulate. These three categories are known as Virchow's triad, named for Rudolf Virchow (1821–1902), a German physician and pathologist.

Patients with DVT may have disease within the blood vessels such as an inflammation of the walls of the vein (phlebitis) or hereditary blood clotting disorders. The patient may also develop blood clots because of other medical conditions such as heart disease, heart failure, stroke, or cancer. Some drugs used in cancer chemotherapy increase the risk of DVT. Clots can also occur after surgery or prolonged bed rest or inactivity. People who smoke and take oral contraceptives may be more susceptible to blood clots. Pregnancy and childbirth also increase the risk of DVT, as do Crohn's disease and ulcerative colitis. Such autoimmune disorders as systemic lupus erythematosus (SLE) increase the risk of DVT; about 9% of lupus patients develop spontaneous DVT. Last, people who have had surgery to remove or close varicose veins have an increased risk of DVT.

The classical symptoms of DVT include pain, swelling, and redness of the affected leg, and dilation of the surface veins. The doctor can examine the leg for possible DVT by measuring the circumference of both legs at the same point to see whether one is swollen, or palpate (touch with light pressure) the veins in the affected leg to see whether the area is sore or tender. The absence of these signs and symptoms, however, does not mean that the patient does not have DVT. As of 2008, there is no laboratory blood test that can definitely confirm or exclude a diagnosis of DVT.

Pulmonary embolism (PE) is one of the most common, but highly fatal, types of blood clots that patients experience. Sometimes there is little or no warning, causing sudden death. On the other hand, some doctors think that cases of DVT and PE are underdiagnosed; one researcher estimates that one of every 9 persons in the United States develops recognized DVT before the age of 80. Studies of autopsies indicate that approximately 80% of all cases of DVT and PE remain undiagnosed even when they are the immediate cause of death. About 90% of pulmonary embolisms are the result of DVT in the legs or the pelvis; the clot moves into the lung and blocks the pulmonary artery. Most often, the DVT occurs in the recovery period after surgery, though there is an alarming trend of DVT events that are the result of airline travel. In 1999, nearly 2,000 Americans, many of them young and fit, died from travel-related DVT strokes. In 2003, NBC reporter David Bloom, who was embedded with the United States Army as he covered the war in Iraq, died of a pulmonary embolism due to his riding in a cramped position for long hours over several days.

KEY TERMS

Aneurysm—A sac created by the distention of the walls of a blood vessel.

Embolus—A clot that breaks away from the wall of the blood vessel and travels throughout the body.

Phlebitis—An inflammation of the walls of a vein.

Prophylaxis—A measure designed to preserve health and/or prevent the spread of disease.

Thrombus—A clot that forms within a blood vessel and remains attached to its place of origin.

Venous thrombosis—The formation or presence of a blood clot in a vein.

Virchow's triad—Three categories of factors that affect a patient's risk of venous thrombosis: alterations in the rate of blood flow; injuries to the tissue lining the walls of the veins; and alterations in the blood's ability to coagulate.

Prevention methods

There are several methods physicians use to prevent blood clots. Some use medications, others use mechanical means, and still others require behavioral changes, or a combination of all of these.

Heparin and other blood thinners

Anticoagulants (blood thinners) such as heparin are often prescribed as prophylactics for venous thrombosis. These drugs decrease the clotting ability of the blood. A study published in 2008 indicates that anticoagulant prophylaxis prevents about 48% of cases of DVT. There has been very good success combining heparin and pneumatic compression stockings, especially for colorectal and cardiac surgery patients.

There are some precautions, however, for using this drug. People who have had an unusual reaction to the drug should not take it, as well as those with allergies to beef and pork. Women who are pregnant and nursing should only use anticoagulants with caution. In addition, certain medications should not be used with heparin. They include **aspirin**, hyperthyroid medication, and drugs for pain or inflammation.

Mechanical leg pumps (pneumatic compression stockings)

Mechanical stimulation of the calf muscles of the leg can help stimulate blood flow. Many hospitals require all surgery patients, especially those who have abdominal or cardiac surgery, to wear pneumatic compression stockings. These devices wrap around the lower leg from ankle to the knee, and some reach as high as the thigh. When plugged in and turned on, a pneumatic device pumps air into chambers within the stocking, which gently tighten around the legs for a few seconds and then are released. This pulsing massage keeps the blood flowing and discourages venous thrombosis.

Compression stockings

Often physicians recommend compression stockings for patients to prevent DVT and edema, and to treat varicose veins and phlebitis. Graduated compression stockings apply more pressure at the ankle and less up the leg and closer to the knee. This pressure prevents backflow of blood and clot formation. A controlled trial to measure the effectiveness of compression stockings in preventing DVT is underway in Canada, as of the summer of 2007.

Exercise

Sitting for long periods or being confined to bed after surgery or during a long illness can slow blood flow, allowing clots to form. As soon as possible after surgery, the patient should move the legs, stand, and begin taking short walks. Travelers or people who work sitting at a desk or computer for several hours at a time should take a break every hour to get up and move around. People can also do such specific exercises as ankle circles or leg lifts while sitting in the confines of an airplane or lying in bed.

Fluids

It is important not to restrict fluids when recovering from surgery, traveling, or working for long periods in a seated position. Not only will the body be kept hydrated, but drinking fluids will help prevent venous thrombosis. Drinking fluids keeps the blood liquid and moving, discouraging clot formation. Travelers should drink something every hour. This may be difficult since some air carriers may not have frequent beverage service.

Preparation

The most important preparation that the patient can do is discuss his or her own personal risk of developing blood clots with a physician. If medication is given, the patient should be instructed how to take it and what side effects to look for. Special exercises should be explained to the patient, and a daily walk should be encouraged.

Normal results

Any of these prevention methods can help a patient avoid having a blood clot after surgery or during long periods of inactivity such as bed rest or while traveling. Travelers and sedentary workers may find moving around and drinking fluids are the best methods for them to prevent blood clots. For patients recovering from surgery, however, a combination of methods is usually necessary. Pneumatic compression pumps with or without a round of heparin may be the best option for surgery patients.

Resources

BOOKS

Bergan, John, ed. *The Vein Book*. Boston: Elsevier Academic Press, 2007.

Weiss, Robert, Craig Feied, and Margaret Weiss, eds. *Vein Diagnosis and Treatment: A Comprehensive Approach.* New York: McGraw-Hill, Health Professions Division, 2001.

PERIODICALS

Agnelli, G., and C. Becattini. "Treatment of DVT: How Long Is Enough and How Do You Predict Recurrence?" *Journal of Thrombosis and Thrombolysis* 25 (February 2008): 37–44.

Ball, Kay. "Deep Vein Thrombosis and Airline Travel—The Deadly Duo." *AORN Journal* 77 (February 2003): 346–354.

Dalen, James E. "Pulmonary Embolism: What Have We Learned Since Virchow? Treatment and Prevention." *Chest* 122 (November 2002): 1801–1818.

Kahn, S. R., H. Shbaklo, S. Shapiro, et al. "Effectiveness of Compression Stockings to Prevent the Post-Thrombotic Syndrome (the SOX Trial and Bio-SOX Biomarker Substudy): A Randomized Controlled Trial." *BMC Cardiovascular Disorders* 7 (July 24, 2007): 21.

Sherman, D. G. "Prevention of Venous Thromboembolism, Recurrent Stroke, and Other Vascular Events after Acute Ischemic Stroke: The Role of Low-Molecular-Weight Heparin and Antiplatelet Therapy." *Journal of Stroke and Cerebrovascular Diseases* 15 (November–December 2006): 250–259.

Själander, A., J. H. Jansson, D. Bergqvist, et al. "Efficacy and Safety of Antocoagulant Prophylaxis to Prevent Venous Thromboembolism in Acutely Ill Medical Inpatients: A Meta-Analysis." *Journal of Internal Medicine* 263 (January 2008): 52–60.

ORGANIZATIONS

American College of Phlebology. 100 Webster Street, Suite 101, Oakland, CA 94607-3724. (510) 834-6500. http://www.phlebology.org (accessed April 17, 2008).

American Heart Association. 7272 Greenville Avenue, Dallas, TX 75231. (800) 242-8721. http://www.americanheart.org (accessed April 17, 2008).

Society for Clinical Vascular Surgery (SCVS). 900 Cummings Center, #221-U, Beverly, MA 01915. (978) 927-8330. http://scvs.vascularweb.org/index.html (accessed April 17, 2008).

OTHER

Feied, Craig. "Deep Venous Thrombosis." *eMedicine*, March 20, 2005 [cited January 13, 2008]. http://www.emedicine.com/med/topic2785.htm (accessed April 17, 2008).

Wille-Jørgensen, P., M. S. Rasmussen, B. R. Andersen, and L. Borly. "Heparins and Mechanical Methods for Thromboprophylaxis in Colorectal Surgery." *The Cochrane Library*. Update Software, 2003.

Janie Franz
Rebecca Frey, PhD

Ventilation *see* **Mechanical ventilation**

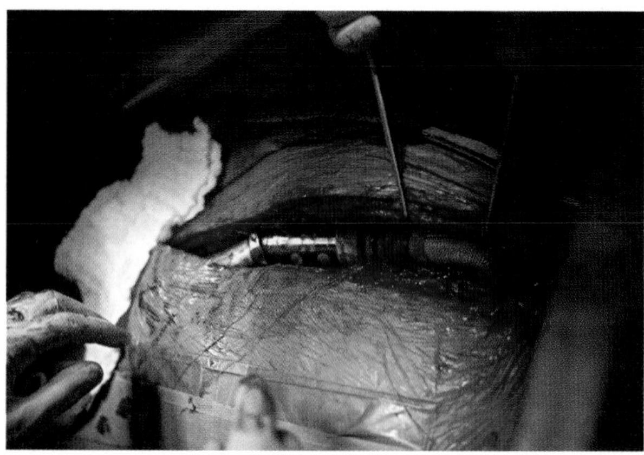

A ventricular assist device being removed. *(Michelle Del Guercio / Photo Researchers, Inc.)*

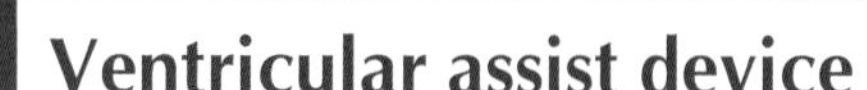

Ventricular assist device

Definition

A ventricular assist device (VAD) is a battery-operated mechanical system consisting of a blood pump and a control unit used for temporary support of blood circulation. The VAD decreases the workload of the heart while maintaining adequate blood flow and blood pressure.

Purpose

A VAD is a temporary life-sustaining device. VADs can replace the left ventricle (LVAD), the right ventricle (RVAD), or both ventricles (BIVAD). They are used when the heart muscle is damaged and needs to rest in order to heal, or when blood flow from the heart is inadequate. In November 2002, the Food and Drug Administration (FDA) approved the use of one type of LVAD as a form of permanent treatment for patients who are ineligible for a heart transplant. VADs can also be used as a bridge in patients awaiting **heart transplantation** or in patients whose bodies have rejected a transplanted heart.

Examples of patients who might be candidates for a VAD are those who:

- have suffered a massive heart attack
- cannot be weaned from heart-lung bypass after treatment with intravenous fluids, medications, and insertion of a balloon pump in the aorta
- have an infection in the heart wall that does not respond to conventional treatment
- are awaiting a heart transplant and are unresponsive to drug therapy and intravenous fluids
- are undergoing high-risk procedures to clear blockages in a coronary artery

Although one in five people suffer left-side ventricular failure, only a minority are candidates for VADs. To be considered for a VAD, patients must meet specific criteria with regard to blood flow, blood pressure, and general health.

Demographics

About 40,000 people in the United States need a heart from a compatible donor, but only 2,200 donor hearts become available each year; hence there is a great need for mechanical devices that can keep patients alive during the wait for transplantation.

VADs are available to all patients in cardiovascular crisis, but their use is contraindicated in patients with:

- irreversible renal failure
- severe peripheral vascular disease
- irreversible brain damage
- cancer that has spread (metastasized)
- severe liver disease
- blood clotting disorders
- severe lung disease
- infections that do not respond to antibiotics
- advanced age

Description

A VAD is selected based on specific patient criteria, including the patient's size; the length of time that support will be needed; the amount of support (total or partial) required; and the type of flow desired (pulsatile or continuous). Different heart problems require different types of flow.

KEY TERMS

Anticoagulant—A type of medication given to prevent the formation of blood clots in the circulatory system.

Aorta—The main artery in humans and other mammals, arising from the left ventricle of the heart.

Artery—A blood vessel that carries blood from the heart to other parts of the body.

Coronary blood vessels—The arteries and veins that supply blood to the heart muscle.

Pulmonary artery—The major artery that carries blood from the right ventricle of the heart to the lungs.

Ventricles—The two thickly walled lower chambers of the heart that receive blood from the upper chambers and send it into the major arteries.

A VAD is implanted under **general anesthesia** in a hospital **operating room**. After the patient has been anesthetized, the surgeon makes an incision in the chest. He or she then inserts a catheter into the jugular vein in the neck. The catheter is threaded through the pulmonary artery, which carries blood from the right ventricle of the heart to the lungs. The catheter is used to measure the oxygen levels in the blood and to administer medications. A urinary catheter is also inserted and used to measure the output of urine. The surgeon sutures the catheters in place, then attaches tubing to connect the catheters to the VAD's pump. Once the pump is turned on, blood flows out of the diseased ventricle and into the pump. The blood is then returned to the proper artery; an LVAD is connected to the aorta, which leaves the heart from the left ventricle, whereas an RVAD is connected to the pulmonary artery. After the VAD has been implanted, the surgeon closes the incisions in the heart and the chest wall. The complete operation may take several hours.

Preparation

VADs are used in patients who have not benefited from other forms of treatment for heart disease. In order to evaluate a patient's eligibility for a VAD, the doctor will use **cardiac catheterization** to demonstrate poor cardiac function and make pressure measurements of the chambers in the patient's heart. Blood samples are drawn in order to measure the levels of blood cells and electrolytes in the patient's circulation. Monitoring of the heart includes an **electrocardiogram** (EKG) as well as measurements of arterial and venous blood pressures.

Aftercare

After a VAD implant, the patient is monitored in an **intensive care unit** (ICU) with follow-up laboratory studies. He or she will remain in the hospital for at least five to seven days. A breathing tube may be left in place until the patient is awake and able to breathe comfortably. Anticoagulant (blood thinning) medications are given to prevent the formation of blood clots, and **antibiotics** are given to prevent infections.

Patients are slowly and gradually weaned from the VAD, except for those patients awaiting a heart transplant or approved for long-term use of the VAD. As the patient improves, he or she will begin a regular **exercise** program. Some VADs require drive lines connected to the control console that penetrate the chest or abdominal cavity. These connections must be cleansed and bandaged to prevent infection of the device. With appropriate training, the patient can continue treatment at home, returning to the hospital only when necessary.

Fully implanted VADs do not require the patient to remain connected to a bedside control console and power unit. He or she will need to carry battery packs in a waistband or shoulder harness, however. In addition, some fully implanted VADs require the patient to plug a cord attached to their body into an electrical outlet at night.

Risks

VAD insertion carries risks of severe complications. Bleeding from the surgery is common; it occurs in as many as 30–50% of patients. Other complications include the development of blood clots; partial paralysis of the diaphragm; respiratory failure; kidney failure; failure of the VAD; damage to the coronary blood vessels; stroke; and infection.

An additional risk is physical dependency on the device. If VADs are inserted in both ventricles, the heart may become so dependent that the patient cannot be weaned from ventricular support.

In addition to physical complications, many patients find that their emotions and cognitive functions are affected by the implantation procedure. Depression, mood swings, and memory loss are not unusual in patients with VADs.

WHO PERFORMS THIS PROCEDURE AND WHERE IS IT PERFORMED?

A VAD is implanted by a cardiothoracic surgeon. A cardiothoracic surgeon is a physician who has completed medical school followed by an internship and residency program for specialized training in cardiac and thoracic surgery.

VADs are implanted in hospitals that are equipped to handle cardiopulmonary bypass procedures, with surgeons that have been trained in the specific techniques required by a given type of VAD. The cost of supplies and the special training required limit the type and number of devices that can be implanted in a specific hospital. Patients are transported to specialized transplant centers for continued support and treatment if their heart function is not expected to return to normal.

Normal results

Because VADs are used in the treatment of critically ill patients, outcomes vary widely according to the state of the patient's health before treatment. The signs of a successful implant include normal cardiac output with normal blood pressure and systemic and pulmonary vascular resistance.

If the patient is a candidate for a heart transplant, a successful VAD transplant may allow him or her to continue treatment at home. The goal of this extended support is to survive the wait for a donor organ. As many as 5% of patients with implanted VADs may recover an adequate level of heart muscle function, however, and avoid the need for a heart transplant.

Resources

BOOKS

Hensley, Frederick A., et al., eds. *A Practical Approach to Cardiac Anesthesia*, 3rd ed. Philadelphia, PA: Lippincott Williams & Wilkins, 2003.

"Ventricular Assist Device." In *The Patient's Guide to Medical Tests*, ed. Barry L. Zaret et al. Boston, MA: Houghton Mifflin, 1997.

PERIODICALS

Rose, Eric A., Annetine C. Gelijns, Alan J. Moskowitz, et al. "Long-Term Use of a Left-Ventricular Assist Device for End-Stage Heart Failure." *New England Journal of Medicine* 345 (November 15, 2001): 1435-1443.

QUESTIONS TO ASK THE DOCTOR

- What types of VAD are available for implant at your institution?
- Which of these devices have you been trained to implant?
- What is the success rate for VAD patients at your hospital?
- What institutions are available for transport for patients waiting for a heart transplant?

ORGANIZATIONS

American Association for Thoracic Surgery (AATS). 900 Cummings Center, Suite 221-U, Beverly, MA 01915. (978) 927-8330. www.aats.org.

American Heart Association (AHA), National Center. 7272 Greenville Avenue, Dallas, TX 75231. (800) 242-8721. www.americanheart.org.

United States Food and Drug Administration (FDA). 5600 Fishers Lane, Rockville, MD 20857-0001. (888) INFO-FDA. www.fda.gov.

OTHER

Department of Biological and Agricultural Engineering, New York State University. *Ventricular Assist Devices*. www.bae.ncsu.edu

Tish Davidson, A.M.
Allison J. Spiwak, MSBME

Ventricular shunt

Definition

A ventricular shunt is a tube that is surgically placed in one of the fluid-filled chambers inside the brain (ventricles). The fluid around the brain and the spinal column is called cerebrospinal fluid (CSF). When infection or disease causes an excess of CSF in the ventricles, the shunt is placed to drain it and thereby relieve excess pressure.

Purpose

A ventricular shunt relieves hydrocephalus, a condition in which there is an increased volume of CSF within the ventricles. In hydrocephalus, pressure from the CSF usually increases. It may be caused by a tumor of the brain or of the membranes covering the brain (meninges), infection of or bleeding into the CSF, or

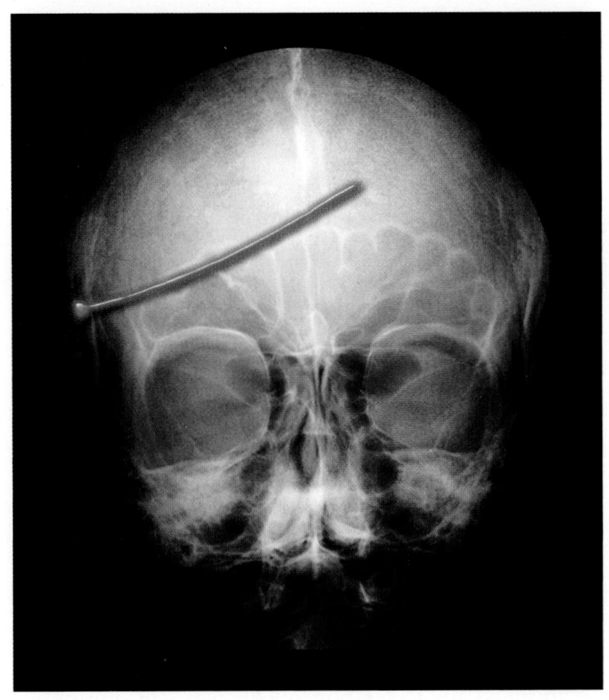

An x ray of a skull with a ventricular shunt. *(Living Art Enterprises, LLC / Photo Researchers, Inc.)*

inborn malformations of the brain. Symptoms of hydrocephalus may include headache, personality disturbances and loss of intellectual abilities (dementia), problems in walking, irritability, vomiting, abnormal eye movements, or a low level of consciousness.

Normal pressure hydrocephalus (a condition in which the volume of CSF increases without an increase in pressure) is associated with progressive dementia, problems walking, and loss of bladder control (urinary incontinence). Even though CSF is not thought to be under increased pressure in this condition, it may also be treated by ventricular shunting.

Demographics

The congenital form of hydrocephalus is believed to occur at an incidence of approximately one to four out of every 1,000 births. The incidence of acquired hydrocephalus is not exactly known. The peak ages for the development of hydrocephalus are in infancy, between four and eight years, and in early adulthood. Normal pressure hydrocephalus generally occurs in patients over the age of 60.

Description

The ventricular shunt tube is placed to drain fluid from the ventricular system in the brain to the cavity of the abdomen or to the large vein in the neck (jugular vein). Therefore, surgical procedures must be done both in the brain and at the drainage site. The tubing contains valves to ensure that fluid can only flow out of the brain and not back into it. The valve can be set at a desired pressure to allow CSF to escape whenever the pressure level is exceeded.

A small reservoir may be attached to the tubing and placed under the scalp. This reservoir allows samples of CSF to be removed with a syringe to check the pressure. Fluid from the reservoir can also be examined for bacteria, cancer cells, blood, or protein, depending on the cause of hydrocephalus. The reservoir may also be used to inject **antibiotics** for CSF infection or chemotherapy medication for meningeal tumors.

KEY TERMS

Cerebrospinal fluid—Fluid bathing the brain and spinal cord.

Computed tomography (CT) scan—An imaging technique in which cross-sectional x rays of the body are compiled to create a three-dimensional image of the body's internal structures.

Dementia—Progressive loss of mental abilities.

Magnetic resonance imaging (MRI)—An imaging technique that uses a large circular magnet and radio waves to generate signals from atoms in the body. These signals are used to construct images of internal structures.

Diagnosis/Preparation

The diagnosis of hydrocephalus should be confirmed by diagnostic imaging techniques, such as computed tomography scan (CT scan) or **magnetic resonance imaging** (MRI), before the shunting procedure is performed. These techniques will also show any associated brain abnormalities. CSF should be examined if infection or tumor of the meninges is suspected. Patients with dementia or mental retardation should undergo neuropsychological testing to establish a baseline psychological profile before the shunting procedure.

As with any surgical procedure, the surgeon must know about any medications or health problems that may increase the patient's risk. Because infections are both common and serious, antibiotics are often given before and after surgery.

WHO PERFORMS THE PROCEDURE AND WHERE IS IT PERFORMED?

Ventricular shunting is performed in a hospital operating room by a neurosurgeon, a surgeon who specializes in the treatment of diseases of the brain, spinal cord, and nerves.

Aftercare

To avoid infections at the shunt site, the area should be kept clean. CSF should be checked periodically by the doctor to be sure there is no infection or bleeding into the shunt. CSF pressure should be checked to be sure the shunt is operating properly. The eyes should be examined regularly because shunt failure may damage the nerve to the eyes (optic nerve). If not treated promptly, damage to the optic nerve causes irreversible loss of vision.

Risks

Serious and long-term complications of ventricular shunting are bleeding under the outermost covering of the brain (subdural hematoma), infection, stroke, and shunt failure. When a shunt drains to the abdomen (ventriculoperitoneal shunt), fluid may accumulate in the abdomen or abdominal organs may be injured. If CSF pressure is lowered too much, patients may have severe headaches, often with nausea and vomiting, whenever they sit up or stand.

Normal results

After shunting, the ventricles get smaller within three or four days. This shrinkage occurs even when hydrocephalus has been present for a year or more. Clinically detectable signs of improvement occur within a few weeks. The cause of hydrocephalus, duration of hydrocephalus before shunting, and associated brain abnormalities affect the outcome.

Of patients with normal pressure hydrocephalus who are treated with shunting, 25–80% experience long-term improvement. Normal pressure hydrocephalus is more likely to improve when it is caused by infection of or bleeding into the CSF than when it occurs without an underlying cause.

Morbidity and mortality rates

Complications of shunting occur in 30% of cases, but only 5% are serious. Infections occur in 5–10% of patients, and as many as 80% of shunts develop a mechanical problem at some point and need to be replaced.

QUESTIONS TO ASK THE DOCTOR

- Why is a ventricular shunt recommended in my case?
- What is the cause of the hydrocephalus?
- What diagnostic tests will be performed prior to the shunt being placed?
- Where will the shunt be placed?
- Are there any alternatives to a ventricular shunt?

Alternatives

In some cases of hydrocephalus, certain drugs may be administered to temporarily decrease the amount of CSF until surgery can be performed. In patients with hydrocephalus caused by a tumor, removal of the tumor often cures the buildup of CSF. Approximately 25% of patients respond to therapies other than shunt placement.

Patients with normal pressure hydrocephalus may experience a temporary improvement in walking and mental abilities upon the temporary drainage of a moderate amount of CSF. This improvement may be an indication that shunting will improve their condition.

Resources

BOOKS

Aldrich, E. Francois, Lawrence S. Chin, Arthur J. DiPatri, and Howard M. Eisenberg. "Hydrocephalus." In *Sabiston Textbook of Surgery*, edited by Courtney M. Townsend Jr. 16th ed. Philadelphia: W. B. Saunders Company, 2001.

Golden, Jeffery A., and Carsten G. Bonnemann. "Hydrocephalus." In *Textbook of Clinical Neurology*, edited by Christopher G. Goetz and Eric J. Pappert. Philadelphia: W. B. Saunders Company, 1999.

PERIODICALS

Hamid, Rukaiya K. A., and Philippa Newfield. "Pediatric Neuroanesthesia: Hydrocephalus." *Anesthesiology Clinics of North America* 19, no. 2 (June 1, 2001): 207–18.

ORGANIZATIONS

American Academy of Neurology. 1080 Montreal Ave., St. Paul, MN 55116. (800) 879-1960. http://www.aan.com.

OTHER

Dalvi, Arif. "Normal Pressure Hydrocephalus." *eMedicine*, January 14, 2002 [cited May 21, 2003]. http://www.emedicine.com/neuro/topic277.htm.

Hord, Eugenia-Daniela. "Hydrocephalus." *eMedicine*, January 14, 2002 [cited May 21, 2003]. http://www.emedicine.com/neuro/topic161.htm.

Sgouros, Spyros. "Management of Spina Bifida, Hydrocephalus, and Shunts." *eMedicine*, May 14, 2003. [cited May 21, 2003]. http://www.emedicine.com/ped/topic2976.htm.

Laurie Barclay, MD
Stephanie Dionne Sherk

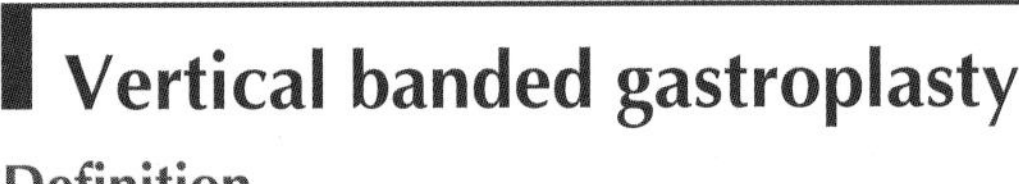

Vertical banded gastroplasty

Definition

Vertical banded gastroplasty, or VBG, is an elective surgical procedure in which the stomach is partitioned with **staples** and fitted with a plastic band to limit the amount of food that the stomach can hold at one time. Gastroplasty is a term that comes from two Greek words, *gaster*, or "stomach," and *plassein*, "to form or shape." Stomach stapling, also known as VBG, is part of a relatively new surgical subspecialty called bariatric surgery. The word "bariatric" is also derived from two Greek words, *barys*, which means "heavy," and *iatros*, which means "healer." A restrictive bariatric procedure, VBG controls the amount of food that the stomach can hold—in contrast to malabsorptive surgeries, in which the food is rerouted within the digestive tract to prevent complete absorption of the nutrients in the food.

Purpose

The purpose of VBG is the treatment of morbid (unhealthy) obesity. It is one of the first successful procedures in bariatric surgery. VBG was developed in its present form in 1982 by Dr. Edward E. Mason, a professor of surgery at the University of Iowa.

Bariatric surgery in general is important in the management of severe obesity because it is the only method, as of 2008, that has demonstrated long-term success in the majority of patients. Weight reduction diets, **exercise** programs, and appetite suppressant medications have had a very low long-term success rate in managing morbid obesity. Most people who try to lose weight on reduced-calorie diets regain two-thirds of the weight lost within one year; within five

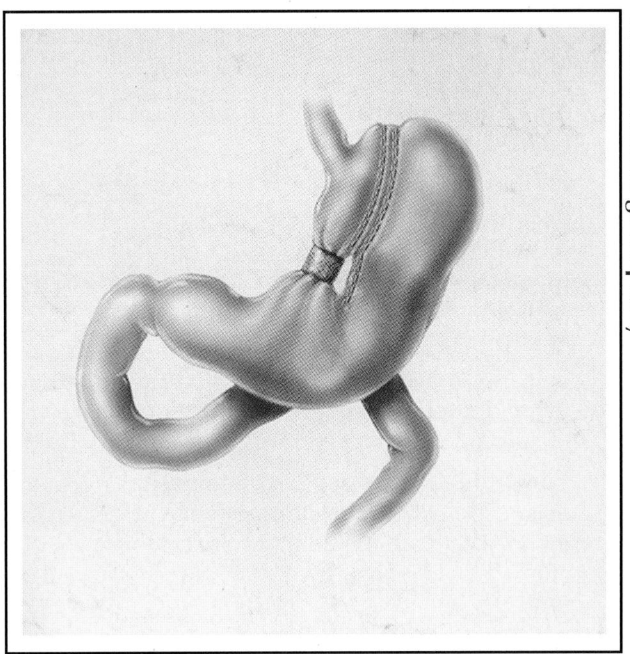

Vertical banded gastroplasty. *(PHOTOTAKE Inc. / Alamy)*

years, they have gained more weight in addition to all the weight they had lost previously. Appetite suppressants often have undesirable or harmful side effects, as well as having a low rate of long-term effectiveness; in 1997, the Food and Drug Administration (FDA) banned the sale of fenfluramine and phentermine ("fen-phen") when these substances were discovered to cause damage to heart valves.

Obesity is a major health problem not only because it is widespread in the American population—as of 2008, 35% of adults in the United States meet the National Institutes of Health (NIH) criteria for obesity—but because it greatly increases a person's risk of developing potentially life-threatening disorders. Obesity is associated with type 2 (non-insulin-dependent) diabetes, hypertension, abnormal blood cholesterol levels, liver disease, coronary artery disease, sleep apnea syndrome, and certain types of cancer. In addition to these disorders, obesity is a factor in what has been called lifestyle-limiting conditions. These conditions are not life-threatening, but they can have an enormous impact on people's day-to-day lives, particularly in their relationships and in the working world. Lifestyle-limiting conditions related to obesity include osteoarthritis and gout; urinary stress incontinence; heartburn; skin disorders caused by heavy perspiration accumulating in folds of skin; leg swelling and varicose veins; gallstones; and abdominal hernias. Obese women frequently suffer from irregular menstrual

KEY TERMS

Appetite suppressant—A medication given to reduce the desire to eat.

Bariatrics—The branch of medicine that deals with the prevention and treatment of obesity and related disorders.

Body mass index (BMI)—A measurement that has replaced weight as the preferred determinant of obesity. The BMI can be calculated (in American units) as 703.1 times a person's weight in pounds divided by the square of the person's height in inches.

Comorbid—A term applied to a disease or disorder that occurs at the same time as another disease condition. There are a number of health problems that are comorbid with obesity.

Dehiscence—A separation or splitting apart. In a vertical banded gastroplasty, dehiscence refers to the coming apart of the line of staples used to form the stomach pouch.

Gastric pacing—An experimental form of obesity surgery in which electrodes are implanted in the muscle of the stomach wall. Electrical stimulation paces the timing of stomach contractions so that the patient feels full on less food.

Hernia—The protrusion of a loop or piece of tissue through an incision or abnormal opening in other tissues. Incisional hernias sometimes occur after open VBGs.

Laparoscope—An instrument that allows a doctor to look inside the abdominal cavity. A less invasive form of VBG can be performed with the help of a laparoscope.

Malabsorptive—A type of bariatric surgery in which a part of the stomach is partitioned off and connected to a lower portion of the small intestine in order to reduce the amount of nutrients that the body absorbs from the food.

Morbid—Unwholesome or bad for health. Morbid obesity is a condition in which the patient's weight is a very high risk to his or her health. The NIH (National Institutes of Health) prefers the term "severely obese" to "morbidly obese."

Obesity—Excessive weight gain due to accumulation of fat in the body, sometimes defined as a BMI (body mass index) of 30 or higher, or body weight greater than 30% above one's desirable weight on standard height-weight tables.

Prevalence—The number of cases of a disease or disorder that are present in a given population at a specific time.

Restrictive—A type of bariatric surgery that works by limiting the amount of food that the stomach can hold. Vertical banded gastroplasty is a restrictive procedure.

Sleep apnea syndrome—A disorder in which the patient's breathing temporarily stops at intervals during the night due to obstruction of the upper airway. People with sleep apnea syndrome do not get enough oxygen in their blood and often develop heart problems.

Stricture—An abnormal narrowing of a body canal or opening. Sometimes strictures form near the plastic band in a VBG. A stricture may also be called a stenosis.

periods and infertility. Finally, societal prejudice against obese people is widespread and frequently mentioned as a source of acute psychological distress. Surgical treatment of obesity has been demonstrated to relieve emotional pain as well as to reduce risks to the patient's physical health.

Demographics

Like other procedures in bariatric surgery, VBG is performed only on patients who are severely or morbidly obese by NIH standards. Severe obesity is presently defined as a body mass index (BMI) of 35 or higher. Nonetheless, it is the epidemic with the greatest prevalence in the United States, as of 2003. One out of every 20 adults, or 15 million people in the United States, has a BMI greater than 35. In addition to the increase in the sheer number of people defined as obese between 1986 and 2000, the increase in those defined as morbidly obese (BMI > 40) or super-obese (BMI > 50) has risen even faster. According to the American Society for Bariatric Surgery (ASBR), while the prevalence of obesity in the United States doubled between 1986 and 2000, the prevalence of morbid obesity quadrupled and the prevalence of super-obesity increased fivefold.

At present, few figures are available regarding the number of VBGs performed in the United States each year compared with other types of obesity surgery, although there is evidence that the number of VBGs has steadily declined each year since 1991. The International Bariatric Surgery Registry (IBSR) at the University of Iowa is presently compiling a database to monitor the outcomes of different procedures and to analyze statistical data about patients undergoing obesity surgery. In 2000, the IBSR analyzed data on a group of 14,641 people who had had obesity surgery as of 1998. The patients weighed an average of 280 lb (127 kg) at the time of surgery and had an average BMI of 46. Slightly less than 20% of the patients had BMIs between 35 and 39.9; 76.1% had BMIs of 40 or higher.

Description

There are two major types of VBG—open, which is the older of the two procedures; and the laparoscopic VBG, which is performed through very small incisions with the help of special instruments.

Open vertical banded gastroplasty

The open VBG is done under **general anesthesia**. In most cases, it takes one to two hours to perform. The surgeon makes an incision several inches long in the patient's upper abdomen. After cutting through the layers of tissue over the stomach, the surgeon cuts a hole, or "window," into the upper part of the stomach a few inches below the esophagus. The second step involves placing a line of surgical staples from the window in the direction of the esophagus, which creates a small pouch at the upper end of the stomach. The surgeon must measure the size of this pouch very carefully; when completed, it is about 10% of the size of a normal stomach and will hold about a tablespoon of solid food.

After forming the pouch and checking its size, the surgeon takes a band made out of polypropylene plastic and fits it through the window around the outlet of the stomach pouch. The vertical band is then stitched into place. Because the polypropylene does not stretch, it holds food in the stomach longer, which allows the patient to feel full on only a small amount of food.

Following the placement of the band, the surgeon will check to make sure that there is no leakage around the window and the line of surgical staples. The area of surgery will then be washed out with a sterile saline solution and the incision closed.

Laparoscopic vertical banded gastroplasty

A laparoscopic vertical banded gastroplasty, or LVBG, is performed with the help of a bariatric laparoscope. A laparoscope is a small tube, 0.39 in (10 mm) in diameter, that holds a fiberoptic cable that allows the surgeon to view the inside of the abdominal cavity on a high-resolution video screen and record the operation on a video recorder. In a laparoscopic VBG, the surgeon makes three small incisions on the left side of the abdomen for inserting the laparoscope, and a fourth incision about 2.5 in (14 cm) long on the right side. The formation of the stomach pouch and insertion of the plastic band are done through these small incisions. Because it is more difficult for the surgeon to maneuver the instruments through the small openings, an LVBG takes longer than an open VBG, about two to four hours.

A laparoscopic VBG requires that the surgeon spend more training and practice than with an open VBG. In the event of complications developing during a laparoscopic VBG, the surgeon usually completes the operation using the open procedure.

Diagnosis/Preparation

Diagnosis

DETERMINATION OF OBESITY. The diagnosis of a patient for bariatric surgery begins with measuring the degree of the patient's obesity. This measurement is crucial because the NIH and almost all health insurers have established specific limits for approval of bariatric procedures.

The obesity guidelines that are cited most often were drawn up by Milliman and Robertson, a nationally recognized company that establishes medical need for a wide variety of procedures for health insurers. The Milliman and Robertson criteria for a patient to qualify for weight loss surgery include:

- Be least 100 lb (45 kg) over ideal weight, as defined by life insurance tables; have a BMI of 40 or higher; or have a BMI over 35 with a coexisting serious medical condition (for example: severe diabetes or coronary artery disease).
- Demonstrate failure to lose or regain of weight despite having tried a multidisciplinary weight control program.
- Have another cause of obesity, such as an endocrine disorder.
- Have attained full adult height.

The patient must be treated not only by a doctor with special training in obesity surgery, but in a comprehensive program that includes preoperative psychological screening and medical examination; nutritional counseling; exercise counseling; and participation in support groups.

There are several ways to measure obesity. Some are based on the relationship between a person's height and weight. The older measurements of this correlation are the so-called height-weight tables that listed desirable weights for a given height. The limitation of height-weight tables is that they do not distinguish between weight of human fatty tissue and weight of lean muscle tissue—many professional athletes and bodybuilders are overweight by the standards of these tables. A more accurate measurement of obesity is body mass index, or BMI. The BMI is an indirect measurement of the amount of body fat. The BMI is calculated in American measurements by multiplying a person's weight in pounds by 703.1, then dividing that number by the person's height in inches squared. A BMI between 19 and 24 is considered normal; 25–29 is overweight; 30–34 is moderately obese; 35–39 is severely obese; 40 or higher is defined as morbidly obese; and 50 or higher is super-obese.

More direct methods of measuring body fat include measuring the thickness of the skinfold at the back of the upper arm, and bioelectrical impedance analysis (BIA). Bioelectrical impedance measures the total amount of water in the body, using a special instrument that calculates the different degrees of resistance to a mild electrical current in different types of body tissue. Fatty tissue has a higher resistance to the current than body tissues containing larger amounts of water. A higher percentage of body water indicates a greater amount of lean tissue.

PSYCHOLOGICAL EVALUATION. Psychiatric and psychological screening before a VBG is done to evaluate the patient's emotional stability and to ensure the expectations of the results of weight loss are not unrealistic. Because of social prejudice against obesity, some obese people who have felt isolated from others or suffered job discrimination come to think of weight loss surgery as a magical or quick solution to all the problems in their lives. In addition, the surgeon will want to make sure that the patient understands the long-term lifestyle adjustments that are necessary after surgery, and that the patient is committed to making those changes. A third reason for a psychological assessment before a VBG is to determine whether the patient's eating habits are compulsive; these would be characterized by the persistent and irresistible impulse to eat from unknown or unconscious purposes. Compulsive eating is not a reason for not having weight loss surgery, but it does mean that the psychological factors contributing to the patient's obesity will also require treatment.

OTHER TESTS AND EXAMINATIONS. Patients must have a complete **physical examination** and blood tests before being considered for a VBG. Some bariatric surgeons will not accept patients with histories of major psychiatric illness; alcohol or drug abuse; previous abdominal surgery; or collagen vascular diseases, which include systemic lupus erythematosus (SLE) and rheumatoid arthritis. Many will not accept patients younger than 16 or older than 55, although some surgeons report successful VBGs in patients over 70. In any event, the patient will need to provide documentation of physical condition, particularly comorbid diseases or disorders, to their insurance company.

Preparation

Preparation for bariatric surgery requires more attention to certain matters than most other forms of surgery requiring hospitalization.

HEALTH INSURANCE ISSUES. Both bariatric surgeons and people who have had weight loss surgery report that obtaining preauthorization for a VBG from insurance companies is a lengthy, complicated, and frequently frustrating process. Insurance companies tend to reflect the prejudices against obese people that exist in the wider society. In addition, bariatric surgery is expensive—between $20,000 and $35,000 per procedure, according to the National Institutes of Health. Although this situation is slowly changing because of increasingly widespread recognition of the high costs of obesity-related diseases, people considering a VBG should start early to secure approval for their operation.

LIFESTYLE CHANGES. A VBG requires a period of **recovery at home** after **discharge from the hospital**. Since the patient's physical mobility will be limited, the following should be done before the operation:

- Arrange for leave from work, assistance at home, help with driving, and similar tasks and commitments.
- Obtain a handicapped parking permit.
- Check the house or apartment thoroughly for needed adjustments to furniture, appliances, lighting, and personal conveniences; specific recommendations include the purchase of a shower chair and toilet seat lift. People recovering from bariatric surgery must minimize bending, stooping, and any risk of falling.
- Stock up on prescription medications, nonperishable groceries, cleaning supplies, and similar items to minimize shopping. Food items should include plenty of clear liquids (juices, broth, soups) and soft foods (oatmeal and other cooked cereals, gelatin dessert mixes).

- Have a supply of easy-care clothing with elastic waistbands and simple fasteners. Shoes should be slip-ons or fastened with Velcro.
- Take "before" photographs prior to the operation, and make a written record of body measurements. These should include measurements of the neck, waist, wrist, widest part of hips, bust or chest, knees, and ankles, as well as shoe size. The pre-operation photographs and measurements help to document the rate and amount of weight lost. Patients who have had weight loss surgery also point out that these records serve to boost morale by allowing the patient to measure progress in losing weight after the surgery.

PRE-OPERATION CLASSES AND SUPPORT GROUPS. In line with the Milliman and Robertson guidelines, most bariatric surgeons now have "preop" classes and ongoing support groups for patients scheduled for VBG and other types of bariatric surgery. Facilitators of these classes can answer questions regarding preparation for the operation and what to expect during recovery, particularly about changes in eating patterns. In addition, they provide opportunities for patients to share concerns and experiences. Patients who have attended group meetings for weight loss surgery often report that simply sharing accounts of the effects of severe obesity on their lives strengthened their resolve to have the operation. In addition, clinical studies indicate that patients who have attended preop classes are less anxious before surgery and generally recover more rapidly.

MEDICAL PREPARATION. Patients scheduled for a gastroplasty are advised to eat lightly the day before surgery. The surgeon will provide specific instructions about taking medications prescribed for other health conditions. The patient will be given pre-operation medications that usually include a laxative to clear the lower digestive tract, an anti-nausea drug, and an antibiotic to lower the risk of infection. Some surgeons ask patients to shower on the morning of their surgery with a special antiseptic skin cleanser.

Aftercare

Aftercare following a gastroplasty has long-term as well as short-term aspects.

Short-term aftercare

Patients who have had an open VBG usually remain in the hospital for four to five days after surgery; those who have had a laparoscopic VBG may return home after two to three days. Aftercare in the hospital typically includes:

- Pain medication. After returning from surgery, patients are given a patient-controlled anesthesia, or PCA device. The PCA is a small pump that delivers a dose of medication into the IV when the patient pushes a button.
- Clear fluids. Inpatient food is limited to a liquid diet following a VBG.
- Oxygen treatment and breathing exercises to get the patient's lungs back into shape. Patients are encouraged to get out of bed and walk around as soon as possible to prevent pneumonia.
- Regular change of surgical dressings. Patients may be given additional dressings for use at home, if needed.

Long-term aftercare

Long-term aftercare includes several adjustments to the patient's lifestyle:

- Slow progression from consuming foods and liquids to eating a normal diet. For the first two weeks after surgery, the patient is limited to liquids and foods that have been pureed in a blender. The reintroduction of solid foods takes place gradually over several months. In addition, patients sometimes have unpredictable reactions to specific foods; most of these resolve over time.
- Lifelong changes in eating habits. Patients who have had a VBG must learn to chew food thoroughly and to eat slowly to reduce the risk of nausea and vomiting. They must also be careful to avoid eating too many soft foods or sweets, to reduce the risk of regaining weight.
- A minimum of five years of follow-up visits to the surgeon to monitor weight maintenance and other health concerns. Patients considering bariatric surgery should choose a surgeon with whom they feel comfortable, as they are making a long-term commitment to aftercare with this professional.
- Ongoing support group meetings to deal with the physical and psychological aftereffects of surgery and weight loss.
- Beginning and maintaining an appropriate exercise program.

Risks

Patients who undergo a VBG are at risk for some of the same complications that may follow any major operation, including **death**, pulmonary embolism, the formation of blood clots in the deep veins of the leg, and infection of the surgical incision. These risks are increased for severely obese patients; for example, the risk of infection is about 10% for obese patients compared to 2% for patients of normal weight. With specific regard to VBGs, recent studies indicate that the risks of complications after surgery are about the same for open and laparoscopic VBGs. The ASBR reported in 2005 that about 5% of VBGs result in complications; the mortality rate is 0.1%.

Specific risks of VBGs

Specific risks associated with vertical banded gastroplasty include:

- Incisional hernia. An incisional hernia is the protrusion of a loop or piece of tissue through a reopened incision. It results from the stress placed on the stitches holding the incision closed in extremely obese patients. Most can be repaired by resuturing the incision. Incisional hernias are more likely to occur with open VBGs than with laparoscopic procedures.
- Dehiscence. Dehiscence is the medical term for splitting open; it can occur in a VBG if the staples forming the pouch at the upper end of the stomach come loose.
- Nausea and vomiting. Nausea and vomiting usually result from eating more food than the stomach pouch can hold, or eating the food too quickly. In most cases, the vomiting disappears as the patient learns different eating habits.
- Formation of a stricture at the site of the plastic band. A stricture is an abnormal narrowing of a body canal or opening. It is also called a stenosis.
- Lodging of a food particle, pill, or capsule within the band or ring. If the object does not move further down the digestive tract within 24 hours, it must be removed by an endoscope.
- Damage to the spleen. The spleen lies very close to the stomach and can be injured in the process of bariatric surgery. In most cases, it can be repaired during the operation.

Long-term risks

The long-term risks of vertical banded gastroplasty include:

- Regaining weight. Patients who have had a VBG are more likely to regain lost weight than those who have had gastric bypass surgery. This is partly because the patient's digestive tract continues to absorb nutrients in food in normal fashion. Because the stomach pouch in a VBG is small, many patients are tempted to eat ice cream and high-calorie liquids that pass quickly through the pouch. A 10-year follow-up study of 70 patients who had had a VBG found that only 20% of the patients had lost and kept off the loss of 50% of their excess body weight.
- Ongoing vomiting and heartburn. About 20% of patients with VBGs report long-term digestive difficulties.
- Psychological problems. Some people have difficulty adjusting to the changes in their outward appearance and to others' changed reactions to them. Others experience feelings of depression, which are thought to be related to biochemical changes resulting from the weight loss.

Normal results

The most rapid weight loss following a VBG takes place in the first six months. It usually takes between 18 and 24 months after the operation for patients to lose 50% of their excess body weight, which is the measurement used to define success in bariatric surgery. At this point, most patients feel much better physically and psychologically; diabetes, high blood pressure, urinary stress incontinence, and other complications associated with severe obesity have either improved or completely resolved.

The primary drawback of VBG is its relatively high rate of failure in maintaining the patient's weight loss over a five-year period. The most common form of revision surgery for a failed VBG is the Roux-en-Y **gastric bypass**. For this reason, some bariatric surgeons recommend VBGs for patients at the lower end of the severe obesity spectrum—those with BMIs between 35 and 40. The chief advantage of VBGs over malabsorptive types of weight loss surgery is that there is little risk of malnutrition or vitamin deficiencies.

Although bariatric surgeons advise patients to wait for two years after a VBG to have **plastic surgery** procedures, it is not unusual for patients to require operations to remove excess skin from the upper arms, abdomen, and other parts of the body that had large accumulations of fatty tissue.

Morbidity and mortality rates

According to the American Society of Bariatric Surgery, the rates of postsurgical complications are about 2% for leaks leading to infection and a need to reoperate; 1.5% for dehiscence; 1% for injury to the spleen; and 1% for pulmonary embolisms.

Alternatives

Established surgical alternatives

The primary restrictive alternative to a VBG is implanting a Lap-Band, which is an adjustable band

WHO PERFORMS THE PROCEDURE AND WHERE IS IT PERFORMED?

A VBG is performed in a hospital whether the operation is an open or a laparoscopic gastroplasty. It is done by a bariatric surgeon, who is a medical doctor (MD) or doctor of osteopathy (DO) who has completed at least three years' training in general surgery after medical school and internship. Most bariatric surgeons have had additional training in gastrointestinal or biliary surgery before completing a fellowship in bariatric surgery with an experienced practitioner in this subspecialty.

In addition to demonstrating the technical skills necessary to perform a VBG, bariatric surgeons seeking hospital privileges must show that they are competent to provide the psychological and nutritional assessments and counseling included in weight loss surgery programs.

QUESTIONS TO ASK THE DOCTOR

- Do I meet the eligibility criteria for bariatric surgery?
- Would you recommend a vertical banded gastroplasty (VBG) for me, a gastric bypass operation, IGS, or staged surgery?
- Am I a candidate for a laparoscopic VBG?
- How long have you been practicing bariatric surgery?
- How many VBGs do you perform each year?

that the surgeon positions around the upper end of the stomach to form the small pouch instead of using staples. The Lap-Band was approved by the Food and Drug Administration (FDA) for use in the United States in 2001. It can be implanted with the laparoscopic technique. When the band is in place, it is inflated with saline solution. It can be tightened or loosened after the operation through a portal under the skin. Although the Lap-Band eliminates the risk of dehiscence, it produces such side effects as vomiting, heartburn, abdominal cramps, or enlargement of the stomach pouch due to the band slipping out of place. In one American study, 25% of patients eventually had the band removed.

The other major type of obesity surgery combines restriction of the size of the stomach with a malabsorptive approach. The combination surgery that is considered the safest and performed most frequently in the United States is the Roux-en-Y gastric bypass. In this procedure, the surgeon forms a stomach pouch and then divides the small intestine, connecting one part of it to the new pouch and reconnecting the other portion to the intestines at some distance from the stomach. The food bypasses the section of the stomach and the small intestine, where most nutrients are absorbed. The procedure takes its name from Cesar Roux, a Swiss surgeon who first performed it, and the "Y" shape formed by the reconnected intestines.

Experimental procedures

A newer technique in obesity surgery is known as gastric pacing or implantable gastric stimulation (IGS). In IGS, the surgeon implants electrodes in the muscle of the stomach wall that deliver a mild electrical current. These electrical impulses regulate the pace of stomach contractions so that the patient feels full on smaller amounts of food. Preliminary results from a team of Italian researchers on patients followed since 1995 indicate that gastric pacing is both safe and effective. As of 2005, published reports of two ongoing clinical trials of IGS in the United States involving over 130 patients showed that IGS is a safe and effective procedure in selected patients.

Another experimental surgical alternative in obesity surgery is staged surgery. This approach involves a first-stage less invasive procedure—usually a Lap-Band—that helps the patient reduce his or her weight to a safer level. Once the patient has lost some weight, the more complex Roux-en-Y gastric bypass is performed.

Resources

BOOKS

Cantor Goldberg, Merle, William Y. Marcus, and George Cowan, Jr. *Weight-Loss Surgery: Is It Right for You?* Garden City, NY: Square One Publishers, 2006.

Flancbaum, Louis, MD, with Erica Manfred and Deborah Biskin. *The Doctor's Guide to Weight Loss Surgery*. West Hurley, NY: Fredonia Communications, 2001.

Hochstrasser, April. *The Patient's Guide to Weight Loss Surgery: Everything You Need to Know about Gastric Bypass and Bariatric Surgery*. Long Island City, NY: Hatherleigh Press, 2004.

Thompson, Barbara. *Weight Loss Surgery: Finding the Thin Person Hiding Inside You*, 4th ed. Tarentum, PA: Word Association Publishers, 2008.

PERIODICALS

Buchwald, H. "Consensus Conference Statement. Bariatric Surgery for Morbid Obesity: Health Implications for Patients, Health Professionals, and Third-Party Payers." *Surgery for Obesity and Related Diseases* 1 (2005): 371–381.

Cigaina, V. "Gastric Pacing as Therapy for Morbid Obesity: Preliminary Results." *Obesity Surgery* 12 (April 2002), Supplement 1: 12S–16S.

Cummings, S., E. S. Parham, and G. W. Strain. "Position of the American Dietetic Association: Weight Management." *Journal of the American Dietetic Association* 102 (August 2002): 1145–1155.

Guisado, J. A., F. J. Vaz, J. Alarcon, et al. "Psychopathological Status and Interpersonal Functioning Following Weight Loss in Morbidly Obese Patients Undergoing Bariatric Surgery." *Obesity Surgery* 12 (December 2002): 835–840.

Gumbs, A. A., A. Pomp, and M. Gagner. "Revisional Bariatric Surgery for Inadequate Weight Loss." *Obesity Surgery* 17 (September 2007): 1137–1145.

Magnusson, M., J. Freedman, E. Jonas, et al. "Five-Year Results of Laparoscopic Vertical Banded Gastroplasty in the Treatment of Massive Obesity." *Obesity Surgery* 12 (December 2002): 826–830.

Regan, J. P., et al. "Early Experience with Two-Stage Laparoscopic Roux-en-Y Gastric Bypass as an Alternative in the Super-Super Obese Patient." *Obesity Surgery* 13 (December 2003): 861–864.

Shai, I., Y. Henkin, S. Weitzman, and I. Levi. "Long-Term Dietary Changes After Vertical Banded Gastroplasty: Is the Trade-Off Favorable?" *Obesity Surgery* 12 (December 2002): 805–811.

Shikora, S. A. "'What Are the Yanks Doing?' The U.S. Experience with Implantable Gastric Stimulation (IGS) for the Treatment of Obesity—Update on the Ongoing Clinical Trials." *Obesity Surgery* 14 (September 2004): S40–S48.

Shikora, S. A., J. J. Kim, and M. E. Tarnoff. "Nutrition and Gastrointestinal Complications of Bariatric Surgery." *Nutrition in Clinical Practice* 22 (February 2007): 29–40.

Sugerman, H. J., E. L. Sugerman, E. J. DeMaria, et al. "Bariatric Surgery for Severely Obese Adolescents." *Journal of Gastrointestinal Surgery* 7 (January 2003): 102–108.

van Hout, G. C., J. J. Jakimowicz, F. A. Fortuin, et al. "Weight Loss and Eating Behavior following Vertical Banded Gastroplasty." *Obesity Surgery* 17 (September 2007): 1226–1234.

ORGANIZATIONS

American Society of Bariatric Physicians (ASBP). 5453 East Evans Place, Denver, CO 80222-5234. (303) 770-2526. http://www.asbp.org (accessed April 18, 2008).

American Society for Metabolic and Bariatric Surgery. 100 SW 75th Street, Suite 201, Gainesville, FL 32607. (352) 331-4900. http://www.asbs.org (accessed April 18, 2008).

International Bariatric Surgery Registry (IBSR). University of Iowa Hospitals and Clinics, 200 Hawkins Drive, Iowa City, IA 52242. (319) 384-7359. http://www.healthcare.uiowa.edu/surgery/ibsr/ (accessed April 18, 2008).

Obesity Society (formerly the American Obesity Association). 8630 Fenton Street, Suite 814, Silver Spring, MD 20910. (301) 563-6526. http://www.obesity.org (accessed April 18, 2008).

Weight-control Information Network (WIN). 1 WIN Way, Bethesda, MD 20892-3665. (202) 828-1025 or (877) 946-4627.

OTHER

FDA Talk Paper. *FDA Approves Implanted Stomach Band to Treat Severe Obesity*, T01-26, June 5, 2001 [cited March 18, 2003]. http://www.fda.gov/bbs/topics/ANSWERS/2001/ANS01087.html (accessed April 18, 2008).

LeMont, Diane, Melodie Moorehead, Michael Parish, et al. *Suggestions for the Pre-Surgical Psychological Assessment of Bariatric Surgery Candidates*, Gainesville, FL: ASBR, 2004.

MacGregor, Alex, MD. *The Story of Surgery for Obesity*. Updated May 2005 [cited January 14, 2008]. http://www.asbs.org/Newsite07/patients/resources/asbs_story.htm (accessed April 18, 2008).

Weight-control Information Network. *Gastrointestinal Surgery for Severe Obesity*, Bethesda, MD: National Institutes of Health (NIH), 2004. NIH Publication No. 04-4006. http://win.niddk.nih.gov/publications/gastric.htm (accessed April 18, 2008).

Rebecca Frey, PhD

Vital signs

Definition

Vital signs, or signs of life, include the following objective measures for a person: temperature, respiratory rate, heart beat (pulse), and blood pressure. When these values are not zero, they indicate that a person is alive. All of these vital signs can be observed, measured, and monitored. This will enable the assessment of the level at which an individual is functioning. Normal ranges of measurements of vital signs change with age and medical condition.

Purpose

The purpose of recording vital signs is to establish a baseline on admission to a hospital, clinic, professional office, or other encounter with a health care provider. Vital signs may be recorded by a nurse, physician, physician's assistant, or other health care professional. The health care professional has the responsibility of interpreting data and identifying

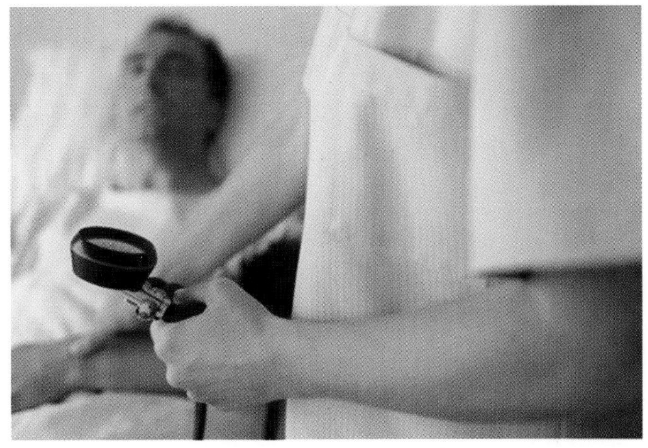

A nurse taking a patient's vital signs. *(moodboard / Alamy)*

any abnormalities from a person's normal state, and of establishing if current treatment or medications are having the desired effect.

Abnormalities of the heart are diagnosed by analyzing the heartbeat (or pulse) and blood pressure. The rate, rhythm and regularity of the beat are assessed, as well as the strength and tension of the beat, against the arterial wall.

Vital signs are usually recorded from once hourly to four times hourly, as required by a person's condition.

The vital signs are recorded and compared with normal ranges for a person's age and medical condition. Based on these results, a decision is made regarding further actions to be taken.

All persons should be made comfortable and reassured that recording vital signs is normal part of health checks, and that it is necessary to ensure that the state of their health is being monitored correctly. Any abnormalities in vital signs should be reported to the health care professional in charge of care.

Description

Temperature

Temperature is recorded to check for fever (pyrexia or a febrile condition), or to monitor the degree of hypothermia.

Manufacturer guidelines should be followed when recording a temperature with an electronic **thermometer**. The result displayed on the liquid crystal display (LCD) screen should be read, then recorded in a person's medical record. Electronic temperature monitors do not have to be cleaned after use. They have protective guards that are discarded after each use. This practice ensures that infections are not spread.

KEY TERMS

Auscultation—The process of listening to sounds that are produced in the body. Direct auscultation uses the ear alone, such as when listening to the grating of a moving joint. Indirect auscultation involves the use of a stethoscope to amplify sounds from within the body, such as those coming from the heart or intestines.

Blood pressure—The pressure exerted by arterial blood on the walls of arteries. This depends on the strength of the heart beat, elasticity of the arterial walls, and volume and viscosity (resistance to flow) of blood. The pressure of blood in the arteries measured in millimeters of mercury by a sphygmomanometer or by an electronic device.

Hypothermia —An abnormally low body temperture.

Pyrexia—Fever or a febrile condition.

Respiration—The exchange of gases between red blood cells and the atmosphere.

Stethoscope—A Y-shaped instrument that amplifies body sounds such as heartbeat, breathing, and air in the intestine. Used in auscultation.

An alcohol or mercury thermometer can be used to monitor a temperature by three methods:

- Axillary, under the armpit. This method provides the least accurate results.
- Orally, under the tongue. This method is never used with infants or very young children because they may accidentally bite or break the thermometer. They also have difficulty holding oral thermometers under their tongues long enough for their temperatures to be accurately measured.
- Rectally, inserted into the rectum. This method provides the most accurate recording of recording the temperature. It is most often used for infants. A recent study reported that rectal thermometers were more accurate than ear thermometers in detecting high fevers. With the ability to detect low-grade fevers, rectal thermometers can be useful in discovering serious illnesses, such as meningitis or pneumonia. The tip of a rectal thermometer is usually blue, which distinguishes it from the silver tip of an oral, or axillary thermometer.

To record the temperature using an alcohol or mercury thermometer, one should shake down the thermometer by holding it firmly at the clear end and flicking it quickly a few times, with the silver end pointing downward. The health care provider who is taking the temperature should confirm that the alcohol or mercury is below a normal **body temperature**.

To record an axillary temperature, the silver tip of the thermometer should be placed under the right armpit. The arm clamps the thermometer into place, against the chest. The thermometer should stay in place for three to four minutes. After the appropriate time has elapsed, the thermometer should be removed and held at eye level. During this waiting period, the body temperature will be measured The alcohol or mercury will have risen to a mark that indicates the temperature of a person.

To record an oral temperature, the axillary procedure should be followed, except that the silver tip of the thermometer should be placed beneath the tongue for three to four minutes, then read as described previously.

In both cases, the thermometer should be wiped clean with an antiseptic and stored in an appropriate container to prevent breakage.

To record a rectal temperature, a rectal thermometer should be shaken down, as described previously. A small amount of water-based lubricant should be placed on the colored tip of the thermometer. Infants must be placed on their stomachs and held securely in place. The tip of the thermometer is inserted into the rectum no more than 0.5 in (1.3 cm) and held there for two to three minutes. The thermometer is removed, read as before, and wiped with an antibacterial wipe. It is then stored in an appropriate container to prevent breakage, because ingestion of mercury can be fatal.

Respiratory rate

An examiner's fingers should be placed on the person's wrist, while the number of breaths or respirations in one minute is recorded. Every effort should be made to prevent people from becoming aware that their breathing is being checked. Respiration results should be noted in the medical chart.

Heartbeat (pulse)

The pulse can be recorded anywhere that a surface artery runs over a bone. The radial artery in the wrist is the point most commonly used to measure a pulse. To measure a pulse, one should place the index, middle, and ring fingers over the radial artery. It is located above the wrist, on the anterior or front surface of the thumb side of the arm. Gentle pressure should be applied, taking care to avoid obstructing blood flow. The rate, rhythm, strength, and tension of the pulse should be noted. If there are no abnormalities detected, the pulsations can be counted for half a minute, and the result doubled. However, any irregularities discerned indicate that the pulse should be recorded for one minute. This will eliminate the possibility of error. Pulse results should be noted in the health chart.

Blood pressure

To record blood pressure, a person should be seated with one arm bent slightly, and the arm bare or with the sleeve loosely rolled up. With an aneroid or automatic unit, the cuff is placed level with the heart and wrapped around the upper arm, one inch above the elbow. Following the manufacturer's guidelines, the cuff is inflated and then deflated while an attendant records the reading.

If the blood pressure is monitored manually, a cuff is placed level with the heart and wrapped firmly but not tightly around the arm one inch above the elbow over the brachial artery. Wrinkles in the cuff should be smoothed out. Positioning a **stethoscope** over the brachial artery in front of the elbow with one hand and listening through the earpieces, the cuff is inflated well above normal levels (to about 200 mmHg), or until no sound is heard. Alternatively, the cuff should be inflated 10 mm Hg above the last sound heard. The valve in the pump is slowly opened. Air is allowed to escape no faster than 5 mmHg per second to deflate the pressure in the cuff to the point where a clicking sound is heard over the brachial artery. The reading of the gauge at this point is recorded as the systolic pressure.

The sounds continue as the pressure in the cuff is released and the flow of blood through the artery is no longer blocked. At this point, the noises are no longer heard. The reading of the gauge at this point is noted as the diastolic pressure. "Lub-dub" is the sound produced by the normal heart as it beats. Every time this sound is detected, it means that the heart is contracting once. The noises are created when the heart valves click to close. When one hears "lub," the atrioventricular valves are closing. The "dub" sound is produced by the pulmonic and aortic valves.

With children, the clicking noise does not disappear but changes to a soft muffled sound. Because sounds continue to be heard as the cuff deflates to zero, the reading of the gauge at the point where the sounds change is recorded as the diastolic pressure.

Blood pressure readings are recorded with the systolic pressure first, then the diastolic pressure (e.g., 120/70).

Blood pressure should be measured using a cuff that is correctly sized for the person being evaluated. Cuffs that are too small are likely to yield readings that can be 10 to 50 millimeters (mm) Hg too high. Hypertension (high blood pressure) may be incorrectly diagnosed.

Preparation

As there may be no recorded knowledge of a person's previous vital signs for comparison, it is important that a health care professional be aware that there is a wide range of normal values that can apply to persons of different ages. The health care professional should obtain as detailed a medical history from the person as soon as possible. Any known medical or surgical history, prior measurements of vital signs, and details of current medications should be recorded, as well. Physical exertion prior to measurement of vital signs, such as climbing stairs, may affect the measurements. This should be avoided immediately before the measurement of one's blood pressure. Tobacco, caffeinated drinks, and alcohol should be avoided for 30 minutes prior to recording.

A person should be sitting down or lying comfortably to ensure that the readings are taken in a similar position each time. There should be little excitement, which can affect the results. The equipment required include a watch with a second hand, an electronic or other form of thermometer, an electronic or manual **sphygmomanometer** with an appropriate sized cuff, and a stethoscope.

Normal results

A normal body temperature taken orally is 98.6°F (37°C), with a range of 97.8–99.1°F (36.5–37.2°C). A fever is a temperature of 101°F (38.3°C) or higher in an infant younger than three months or above 102°F (38.9°C) for older children and adults. Hypothermia is recognized as a temperature below 96°F (35.5°C).

Respirations are quiet, slow, and shallow when the adult is asleep, and rapid, deeper, and noisier during and after activity.

Average respiration rates at rest are:

- Infants: 34–40 per minute.
- Children five years of age: 25 per minute.
- Older children and adults: 16–20 per minute.

Tachypnea is rapid respiration above 20 per minute.

The strength of a heart beat is raised during conditions such as fever and lowered by conditions such as shock or elevated intracranial pressure. The average heart rate for older children (aged 12 and older) and adults is approximately 72 beats per minute (bpm). Tachycardia is a pulse rate over 100 bpm, while bradycardia is a pulse rate of under 60 bpm.

Blood pressure is recorded for older children and adults. A normal adult blood pressure reading is 120/80.

Resources

BOOKS

Bickley, L. S., P. G. Szilagyi, J. G. Stackhouse. *Bates' Guide to Physical Examination & History Taking, 8th edition.* Philadelphia: Lippincott Williams & Wilkins, 2002.

Chan, P. D., and P. J. Winkle. *History and Physical Examination in Medicine, 10th ed.* New York: Current Clinical Strategies, 2002.

Seidel, Henry M. *Mosby's Physical Examination Handbook, 4th ed.*St. Louis: Mosby-Year Book, 2003.

Swartz, Mark A., and William Schmitt. *Textbook of Physical Diagnosis: History and Examination, 4th edition.* Philadelphia: Saunders, 2001.

PERIODICALS

Ahmed A. M. "Deficiences of physical examination among medical students." *Saudi Medical Journal* 24, no. 1 (2003): 108-111.

ORGANIZATIONS

American Academy of Family Physicians, 11400 Tomahawk Creek Parkway, Leawood, KS 66211-2672. (913) 906-6000. E-mail: fp@aafp.org. http://www.aafp.org.

American Academy of Pediatrics, 141 Northwest Point Boulevard, Elk Grove Village, IL 60007-1098. 847) 434-4000. Fax: (847) 434-8000. E-mail: kidsdoc@aap.org. http://www.aap.org/default.htm,

American College of Physicians. 190 N. Independence Mall West, Philadelphia, PA 19106-1572. (800) 523-1546, x2600 or (215) 351-2600. http://www.acponline.org

OTHER

Karolinska Institute. [cited March 1, 2003] <http://isp.his.ki.se/text/physical.htm>.

Loyola University Chicago Stritch School of Medicine. [cited March 1, 2003] http://www.meddean.luc.edu/lumen/MedEd/MEDICINE/PULMONAR/PD/Pdmenu.htm.

National Library of Medicine. [cited March 1, 2003] http://www.nlm.nih.gov/medlineplus/ency/article/002274.htm.

Review of Systems School of Medical Transcription. [cited March 1, 2003] http://www.mtmonthly.com/student corner/cpe.htm.

L. Fleming Fallon, Jr., M.D., DrPH

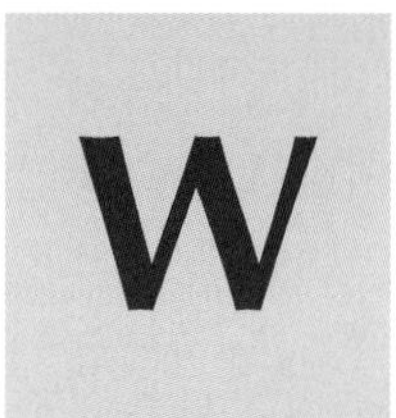

Water pills *see* **Diuretics**

Webbed finger or toe repair

Definition

Webbed finger or toe repair refers to corrective or **reconstructive surgery** performed to repair webbed fingers or toes, also called syndactyly. The long and ring fingers or the second and third toes are most often affected. Generally, syndactyly repairs are done between the ages of six months and two years.

Purpose

Webbing, or syndactyly, is a condition characterized by the incomplete separation or union of two or more fingers or toes, and usually only involves a skin connection between the two (simple syndactyly), but may—rarely— also include fusion of bones, nerves, blood vessels, and tendons in the affected digits (complex syndactyly). Webbing may extend partially up between the digits, frequently just to the first joint, or may extend the entire length of the digits. Polysyndactyly describes both webbing and the presence of an extra number of fingers or toes. The condition usually develops within six weeks after birth. Syndactyly can also occur in victims of fires, as the intense heat can melt the skin and fuse the epidermis and dermis of the phalanges, fingers, or toes. Burn victim syndactyly is always less invasive because bone fusion is not present in these cases. The purpose of repair surgery is to improve the appearance of the hand or foot and to prevent progressive deformity from developing as the child grows.

Demographics

In the United States, approximately one infant in every 2,000 births is born with webbed fingers or toes. Both hands are involved in 50% of cases; the middle finger and ring finger in 41%; the ring finger and little finger in 27%; the index finger and middle finger in 23%; and the thumb and index finger in 9%.

Description

Polydactyly can be corrected by surgical removal of the extra digit or partial digit. Syndactyly can also be corrected surgically. This is usually accomplished with the addition of a skin graft from the groin.

There are several ways to perform this type of surgery; the design of the operation depends both on the features of the hand or foot and the surgeon's experience. The surgery is usually performed with zigzag cuts that cross back and forth across the fingers or toes so that the scars do not interfere with growth of the digits.

The procedure is performed under **general anesthesia**. The skin areas to be repaired are marked and the surgeon then proceeds to incise the skin, lifting small flaps at the sides of the fingers or toes and in the web. These flaps are sutured into position, leaving absent areas of skin. These areas may be filled in with full thickness skin grafts, usually taken from the skin in the groin area. The hand or foot is then immobilized with bulky **dressings**, or a cast. Webbed or toe repair surgery usually takes two to four hours.

Diagnosis/Preparation

Syndactyly may be diagnosed during an examination of an infant or child, with the aid of x rays. In its most common form, it is seen as webbing between the second and third toes. This form is often inherited. Syndactyly can also occur as part of a pattern of other congenital defects involving the skull, face, and bones.

An infant with webbed fingers or toes may have other symptoms that, when observed together, define a specific syndrome or medical condition. For example, syndactyly is a characteristic of Apert syndrome,

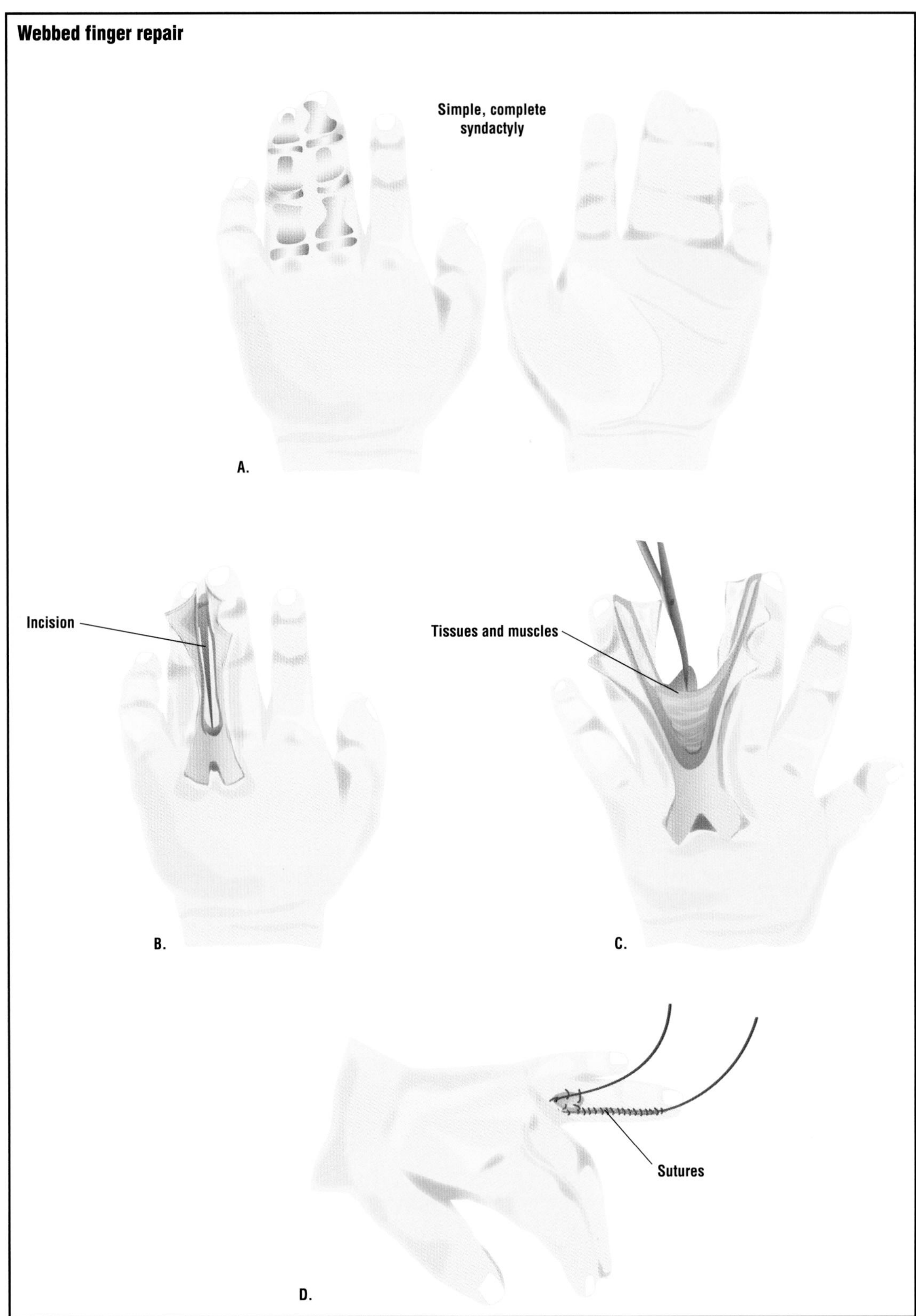

This webbed finger shows a simple, complete syndactyly, meaning the bones for two fingers are complete, and only the soft tissues form the webbed section (A). To repair this, an incision is made in the skin of the webbing (B). Tissues and muscles are severed (C), and the two separated fingers are stitched (D). *(Illustration by GGS Information Services. Cengage Learning, Gale.)*

KEY TERMS

Congenital—Condition or disorder present at birth.

Graft—The implantation of a portion of living flesh or skin in a lesion to form an organic union.

Polysyndactyly—Condition involving both webbing and the presence of an extra number of fingers or toes.

Syndactyly—Union or webbing of two or more fingers or toes, which usually only involves a skin connection between the two.

Syndrome—A set of signs or a series of events occurring together that often point to a single disease or condition as the cause.

Poland syndrome, Jarcho-Levin syndrome, oral-facial-digital syndrome, Pfeiffer syndrome, and Edwards syndrome. Diagnosis of a syndrome is made on family history, medical history, and thorough physical evaluation. The medical history questions documenting the condition in detail usually include:

- Which fingers (toes) are involved?
- Are any other family members affected by the same condition?
- What other symptoms or abnormalities are also present?

To prepare for surgery, seven to 10 days before surgery, the child visits the family physician or pediatrician for a general **physical examination** and blood tests. The child cannot have solid food after midnight before surgery. Breast milk, formula, or milk (no pablum or other cereal may be added) up to six hours before the scheduled start of surgery is allowed, and then only clear fluids up to three hours before surgery. Thereafter, the child may not have anything else to eat or drink.

Aftercare

Hospital stays of one or two days are common for webbed finger or toe repair surgery. There is usually some swelling and bruising. Pain medications are given to alleviate any discomfort. The **bandages** must be kept clean and dry and must remain for two to three weeks for proper healing and protection. Skin grafts and the hand or foot may become very dry, so it is encouraged to dampen them with a good moisturizer such as Lubriderm or Nivea. Small children with hand syndactylies may have a cast put on that extends above the flexed elbow. Sometimes, the cast extends beyond the fingers or toes. This protects the repaired areas from trauma.

The treating physician should be informed of any post-operative swelling, severe pain, fever, or fingers that tingle, are numb, or have a bluish discoloration.

WHO PERFORMS THE PROCEDURE AND WHERE IS IT PERFORMED?

Webbed finger or toe repair surgery is usually performed in a children's hospital by a pediatric surgeon or orthopedic surgeon specializing in syndactyly surgery.

If prenatal screening indicates syndactyly in the fetus, arrangements are usually made so that the baby is delivered at a hospital with a pediatric surgeon on staff.

Risks

Webbed finger or toe repair surgery carries the risks associated with any anesthesia, such as adverse reactions to medications, breathing problems, and sore throat from intubation. Risks associated with any surgery are excessive bleeding and infection.

Specific risks associated with the repair surgery include possible loss of skin graft and circulation damage from the cast or bandages.

Normal results

The results of webbed finger or toe repair depend on the degree of fusion of the digits and the repair is usually successful. When joined fingers share a single fingernail, the creation of two normal-looking nails is rarely possible. One nail will look more normal than the other. Some children may require a second surgery, depending on the type of syndactyly. If polydactyly or syndactyly are just cosmetic and not symptomatic of a condition or disorder, the outcome of surgery is usually very good. If it is symptomatic, the outcome will rely heavily on the management of the disorder.

Alternatives

Syndactyly does not generally pose any health risk, so that it is not mandatory that the repair be performed. However, if the thumb is joined, or if the fingers are joined out toward their tips, they will grow in a progressively worsening bend over time.

QUESTIONS TO ASK THE DOCTOR

- What will happen during the surgery?
- Does my baby have any other birth defect?
- How long will it take to recover from surgery?
- Will my baby have normal fingers/toes?
- How many webbed finger/toe repair surgeries do you perform each year?
- Will the syndactyly return?

Resources

BOOKS

Jones, Kenneth Lyons. *Smith's Recognizable Patterns of Human Malformation,* 5th ed. Philadelphia: W.B. Saunders, 1997.

Moore, K. L., and T. V. N. Persaud. *Before We Are Born: Essentials of Embryology and Birth Defects.* New York: Elsevier Science, 2003.

PERIODICALS

Ad-El, D. D., A. Neuman, and A. Eldad. "Syndactyly repair in Kindler syndrome." *Plastic and Reconstructive Surgery* 111 (January 2003): 504-505.

Benatar, N. "The open finger technique for release of syndactyly." *The Journal of Hand Surgery: Journal of the British Society for Surgery of the Hand* 26 (October 2001): 500-501.

Deunk, J., J. P. Nicolai, and S. M. Hamburg. "Long-term results of syndactyly correction: Full-thickness versus split-thickness skin grafts." *The Journal of Hand Surgery: Journal of the British Society for Surgery of the Hand* 28 (April 2003): 125-130.

Greuse, M., and B. C. Coessens. "Congenital syndactyly: defatting facilitates closure without skin graft." *Journal of Hand Surgery (American)* 26 (July 2001): 589-594.

Takagi, S., K. Hosokawa, U. Haramoto, and T. Kubo. "A new technique for the treatment of syndactyly with osseous fusion of the distal phalanges." *Annals of Plastic Surgery* 44 (June 2000): 660-663.

ORGANIZATIONS

The American Academy of Orthopaedic Surgeons. 6300 North River Road, Rosemont, IL 60018-4262. (847) 823-7186; (800) 346-AAOS. www.aaos.org.

The American Society for Surgery of the Hand. 6300 North River Road, Suite 600, Rosemont, IL 60018-4256. (847) 384-8300. www.assh.org.

Office of Rare Diseases (NIH). 6100 Executive Boulevard, Room 3A07, MSC 7518 Bethesda, MD 20892-7518. (301) 402-4336. <rarediseases.info.nih.gov/info-diseases.html>.

OTHER

"Before and after webbed finger repair." *Medline Plus*.www.nlm.nih.gov/medlineplus/ency/imagepages/10034.htm.

"Repair of webbed fingers or toes." *PennHealth*.www.pennhealth.com/ency/article/002969.htm

Monique Laberge, Ph.D.

Weight management

Definitions

Weight management refers to a set of practices and behaviors that are necessary to keep one's weight at a healthful level. It is preferred to the term "dieting," because it involves more than regulation of food intake or treatment of overweight people. People diagnosed with eating disorders that are not obese or overweight still need to practice weight management. Some healthcare professionals use the term "nutritional disorders" to cover all disorders related to weight.

The term "weight management" also reflects a change in thinking about treatment of obesity and overweight during the past 20 years. Before 1980, treatment of overweight people focused on weight loss, with the goal of helping the patient reach an ideal weight as defined by standard life insurance height-weight charts. In recent years, however, researchers have discovered that most of the negative health consequences of obesity are improved or controlled by a relatively modest weight loss, perhaps as little as 10% of the patient's body weight. It is not necessary for the person to reach the ideal weight to benefit from weight management. Some nutritionists refer to this treatment goal as the "10% solution." Second, the fact that most obese people who lose large amounts of weight from reduced-calorie diets regain it within five years has led nutrition experts to emphasize weight management rather than weight loss as an appropriate outcome of treatment.

Overweight and obese

Overweight and obese are not the same thing. People who are overweight weigh more than they should compared with set standards for their height. The excess weight may come from muscle tissue, body water, or bone, as well as from fat. A person who is obese has too much fat in comparison to other types of body tissue; hence, it is possible to be overweight without being obese.

KEY TERMS

Anorexia nervosa—An eating disorder marked by refusal to eat, intense fear of obesity, and distortions of body image.

Appetite suppressant—A medication given to reduce the desire to eat.

Bariatrics—The branch of medicine that deals with the prevention and treatment of obesity and related disorders.

Binge—A time-limited bout of excessive indulgence in eating; consuming a larger amount of food within a limited period of time than most people would eat in similar circumstances.

Binge eating disorder—An eating disorder in which the person binges but does not try to get rid of the food afterward by vomiting, using laxatives, or exercising.

Body mass index (BMI)—A measurement that has replaced weight as the preferred determinant of obesity. The BMI can be calculated (in American units) as 703.1 times a person's weight in pounds divided by the square of the person's height in inches.

Bulimia nervosa—An eating disorder marked by episodes of binge eating followed by purging, over-exercising, or other behaviors intended to prevent weight gain.

Ephedra—A herb used in traditional Chinese medicine to treat asthma and hay fever. It should never be used for weight management.

Hoodia—A succulent African plant resembling a cactus said to contain a natural appetite suppressant.

Obesity—Excessive weight gain due to accumulation of fat in the body, sometimes defined as a BMI of 30 or higher, or body weight greater than 30% above one's desirable weight on standard height-weight tables.

Prevalence—The number of cases of a disease or disorder that are present in a given population at a specific time.

Sedentary—Characterized by inactivity and lack of exercise. A sedentary lifestyle is a major risk factor for becoming overweight or obese.

There are several ways to determine whether someone is obese. Some measures are based on the relationship between the person's height and weight. The older measurements of this correlation are the so-called height-weight tables that list desirable weights for a given height. A more accurate measurement of obesity is body mass index, or BMI. The BMI is an indirect measurement of the amount of body fat. The BMI is calculated in American measurements by multiplying a person's weight in pounds by 703.1, and dividing that number by the person's height in inches squared. A BMI between 19 and 24 is considered normal; 25–29 is overweight; 30–34 is moderately obese; 35–39 is severely obese; and 40 or higher is defined as morbidly obese. More direct methods of measuring body fat include measuring the thickness of the skin fold at the back of the upper arm, and bioelectrical impedance analysis (BIA). Bioelectrical impedance analysis measures the total amount of water in the body using a special instrument that calculates the different degrees of resistance to an electrical current in different types of body tissue. Fatty tissue has a higher resistance to the current than body tissues containing larger amounts of water. A higher percentage of body water indicates a greater amount of lean tissue.

Eating disorders

Eating disorders are a group of psychiatric disturbances defined by unhealthy eating or weight management practices. Anorexia nervosa is an eating disorder in which people restrict their food intake severely, refuse to maintain a normal body weight, and express intense fear of becoming obese. Bulimia nervosa is a disorder marked by episodes of binge eating followed by attempts to avoid weight gain from the food by abusing **laxatives**, forcing vomiting, or over-exercising. A third type, binge eating disorder, is found in some obese people, as well as in people of normal weight. In binge eating disorder, the person has an eating binge but does not try to get rid of the food after eating it. Although most patients diagnosed with anorexia or bulimia are women, 40% of patients with binge eating disorder are men.

Purpose

The purpose of weight management is to help each patient achieve and stay at the best weight possible in the context of their overall health, occupation, and living situation. A second purpose is the prevention and treatment of diseases and disorders associated with obesity or with eating disorders. These disorders include depression and other psychiatric disturbances, in addition to the physical problems associated with nutritional disorders.

Demographics and statistics

Obesity has become a major public health concern in the United States in the last decade. As of 2007, obesity ranks second only to smoking as a major cause of preventable deaths. It is estimated that 300,000 people die in the United States each year from weight-related causes. The proportion of overweight adults in the general population has continued to rise since the 1960s. According to the National Health and Nutrition Examination Survey (NHANES) of 2004, almost two-thirds of American adults are overweight, and almost a third is obese. In addition, there has been a 42% increase in the rate of childhood obesity since 1980.

The prevalence of obesity in the United States varies somewhat according to sex, age, race, and socioeconomic status. Among adults, 35% of women are considered obese, compared to 31% of men. The rate of obesity increases as people get older; those aged 55 or older are more than twice as likely to be obese as those in their 20s. African American men have the same rate of obesity as Caucasian men; however, African American women are almost twice as likely as Caucasian women to be obese by the time they reach middle age. The same ratio holds true for socioeconomic status; people in the lowest third of the income and educational level distribution are twice as likely to be obese as those with more education and higher income.

From the economic standpoint, obesity costs the United States more than $117 billion each year. This amount includes the direct costs of hospital care and medical services, which come to $61 billion annually, or 7% of all healthcare costs. Another $56 billion represents the indirect costs of obesity, such as disabilities related to overweight or work days lost to obesity-related illnesses.

Obesity is considered responsible for:

- 88–97% of cases of type 2 diabetes
- 57–70% of cases of coronary heart disease
- 70% of gallstone attacks
- 35% of cases of hypertension
- 11% of breast cancers
- 10% of colon cancers

In addition, obesity intensifies the pain of osteoarthritis and gout; increases the risk of complications in pregnancy and childbirth; contributes to depression and other mental disorders; and makes a person a poor candidate for surgery. Many surgeons refuse to operate on patients who weigh more than 300 lb (136 kg).

Although fewer people suffer from eating disorders than from obesity, the National Institutes of Mental Health (NIMH) reports that 10 million adults in the United States meet the diagnostic criteria for anorexia or bulimia. Although eating disorders are stereotyped as affecting only adolescent or college-aged women, as of 2007 at least 10% of people with eating disorders are males—and the proportion of males to females is rising. Moreover, the number of women over 45 years of age who are diagnosed with eating disorders is also rising; many doctors attribute this startling new trend to fear of aging, as well as fear of obesity.

The long-term health consequences of eating disorders include gum disease and loss of teeth, irregular heart rhythm, disturbances in the chemical balance of the blood, and damage to the digestive tract. At least 50,000 people die each year in the United States as the direct result of an eating disorder; anorexia is the leading cause of **death** in women between the ages of 17 and 25.

Description

To understand the goals and structure of nutritionally sound weight management programs, it is helpful to look first as the causes of being overweight, obesity, and eating disorders.

Causes of nutrition-related disorders

GENETIC/BIOLOGIC. Studies of twins separated at birth and research with genetically altered mice have shown that there is a genetic component to obesity. Some researchers think that there are also genetic factors involved in eating disorders.

LIFESTYLE-RELATED. The ready availability of relatively inexpensive, but high-caloric snacks and "junk food" is considered to contribute to the high rates of obesity in developed countries. In addition, the fast pace of modern life encourages people to select quick-cooking processed foods that are high in calories, rather than making meals that are more healthful but take longer to prepare. Lastly, changes in technology and transportation patterns mean that people today do not do as much walking or hard physical labor as earlier generations did. This sedentary or inactive lifestyle makes it easier for people to gain weight.

SOCIOCULTURAL. In recent years, many researchers have examined the role of advertising and the mass media in encouraging unhealthy eating patterns. On the one hand, advertisements for such items as fast food, soft drinks, and ice cream often convey the message that food can be used to relieve stress, reward, or comfort oneself, or substitute for a fulfilling human relationship. On the other hand, the media also portray unrealistic images of human physical perfection. Their emphasis on slenderness as essential to beauty, particularly in women, is often cited as a major factor in the increase of eating disorders over the past three decades.

Another sociocultural factor that contributes to obesity among some Hispanic and Asian groups is the belief that children are not healthy unless they look plump. Overfeeding in infancy and early childhood, unfortunately, makes weight management in adolescence and adult life much more difficult.

MEDICATIONS. Recent research has found that a number of prescription medications can contribute to weight gain. These drugs include steroid hormones, antidepressants, benzodiazepine tranquilizers, lithium, and antipsychotic medications.

Aspects of weight management

Since the late 1980s, nutritionists and healthcare professionals had come to recognize that successful weight management programs have three characteristics, including:

- They present weight management as a lifetime commitment to healthful patterns of eating and exercise, rather than emphasize strict dieting alternating with carelessness about eating habits.
- They are tailored to each person's age, general health, living situation, and other individual characteristics.
- They recognize that the emotional, psychological, and spiritual dimensions of human life are as important to maintaining a healthy lifestyle as the medical and nutritional facets.

NUTRITION. The nutritional aspect of weight management programs includes education about healthful eating, as well as modifying the person's food intake.

DIETARY REGULATION. Most weight-management programs are based on a diet that supplies enough vitamins and minerals; 50–63 grams of protein each day; an adequate intake of carbohydrates (100 g) and dietary fiber (20–30 g); and no more than 30% of each day's calories from fat. Good weight-management diets are intended to teach people how to make wise food choices and to encourage gradual weight loss. Some diets are based on fixed menus, while others are based on food exchanges. In a food-exchange diet, a person can choose among several items within a particular food group when following a menu plan. For example, if a person's menu plan allows for two items from the vegetable group at lunch, they can have one raw and one cooked vegetable, or one serving of vegetable juice along with another vegetable.

NUTRITIONAL EDUCATION. Nutritional counseling is important to successful weight management because many people, particularly those with eating disorders, do not understand how the body uses food. They may also be trying to manage their weight in unhealthy ways. One recent study of adolescents found that 32% of the females and 17% of the males were using such potentially dangerous methods of weight control as smoking, fasting, over-the-counter (OTC) diet pills, or laxatives.

Exercise

Regular physical **exercise** is a major part of weight management because it increases the number of calories used by the body and because it helps the body to replace fat with lean muscle tissue. Exercise also serves to lower emotional stress levels and to promote a general sense of well-being. People should consult a doctor before beginning an exercise program, however, to make sure that the activity that interests them is safe relative to any other health problems they may have. For example, people with osteoarthritis should avoid high-impact sports that are hard on the knee and ankle joints. Good choices for most people include swimming, walking, cycling, and yoga or other stretching exercises.

Psychological/psychiatric

Both obesity and eating disorders are associated with a variety of psychiatric disorders, most commonly major depression and substance abuse. Almost all obese people feel harshly judged and criticized by others, and fear of obesity is a major factor in the development of both anorexia and bulimia. Many people find medications and/or psychotherapy to be a helpful part of a weight management program.

MEDICATIONS. In recent years, doctors have been cautious about prescribing appetite suppressants, which are drugs given to reduce the desire for food. In 1997, the Food and Drug Administration (FDA) banned the sale of two drugs: fenfluramine and phentermine (known as "fen-phen") when they were discovered to cause damage to heart valves. A newer appetite suppressant, known as sibutramine (Meridia), was approved as safe in 1997. The drug is being monitored by the FDA as of 2007, however, because of reports linking it to heart failure, kidney failure, and stomach problems. Another new drug that is sometimes prescribed for weight management is called orlistat (Xenical). It works by lowering the amount of dietary fat that is absorbed by the body. However, it can cause significant diarrhea or intestinal gas.

People with eating disorders are sometimes given antidepressant medications, most often fluoxetine (Prozac) or venlafaxine, to relieve the symptoms of depression or anxiety that often accompany eating disorders.

COGNITIVE-BEHAVIORAL THERAPY. Cognitive-behavioral therapy (CBT) is a form of psychotherapy that has been shown to be effective in reinforcing the changes in food selection and eating patterns that are necessary to successful weight management. In this form of therapy, usually offered in specialized clinics, patients learn to modify their eating habits by keeping diaries and records of what they eat, what events or feelings trigger overeating, and any other patterns that they notice about their choice of foods or eating habits. They also examine their attitudes toward food and weight management, and work to change any attitudes that are self-defeating or interfere with a healthy lifestyle. Most CBT programs also include nutritional education and counseling. As of 2007, however, some researchers maintain that more work needs to be done on the use of CBT in real-world settings, not just university-related specialized clinics.

WEIGHT-MANAGEMENT GROUPS. Many doctors and nutritional counselors suggest that patients attend a weight-management group for social support. Social support is essential in weight management, because many who suffer from obesity or an eating disorder struggle with intense feelings of shame. Many isolate themselves from others because they are afraid of being teased or criticized for their appearance. Such groups as Overeaters Anonymous (OA) or Take Off Pounds Sensibly (TOPS) help members in several ways: They help to reduce the levels of shame and anxiety that most members feel; they teach strategies for coping with setbacks in weight management; they provide settings for making new friends; and they help people learn to handle problems in their workplace or in relationships with family members.

ANTI-DISCRIMINATION GROUPS. Another approach to weight-related psychological issues is tackling public discrimination against overweight people, including educational and employment discrimination as well as verbal harassment and teasing. The two major groups in the United States are the Council on Size and Weight Discrimination (CSWD) and the National Association to Advance Fat Acceptance (NAAFA). The CWSD describes itself as "a not-for-profit group which works to change people's attitudes about weight. We act as consumer advocates for larger people, especially in the areas of medical treatment, job discrimination, and media images." NAAFA states its goals as "eliminat[ing] discrimination based on body size and provid[ing] fat people with the tools for self-empowerment through public education, advocacy, and member support."

Surgical

As of 2007, bariatric surgery is the most successful approach to weight management for people who are morbidly obese (BMI of 40 or greater), or severely obese with additional health complications. Surgical treatment of obesity usually results in a large weight loss that is successfully maintained for longer than five years. The most common surgical procedures for weight management are **vertical banded gastroplasty** (VBG), sometimes referred to as "stomach stapling," and **gastric bypass**. Vertical banded gastroplasty works by limiting the amount of food the stomach can hold, while gastric bypass works by preventing normal absorption of the nutrients in the food.

Complementary and alternative medicine (CAM) approaches

Some forms of complementary and alternative medicine are beneficial additions to weight management programs.

MOVEMENT THERAPIES. Movement therapies include a number of forms of exercise, such as tai chi, yoga, dance therapy, Trager work, and the Feldenkrais method. Many of these approaches help people improve their posture and move their bodies more easily as well as keeping active. Tai chi and yoga, for example, are good for people who must avoid high-impact physical workouts. Yoga can also be adapted to a person's individual needs or limitations with the help of a qualified teacher following a doctor's recommendations. Books and videos on yoga and weight management are available through most bookstores or the American Yoga Association.

SPIRITUAL AND RELIGIOUS PRACTICE. Prayer, meditation, and regular religious worship have been linked to reduced emotional stress in people struggling with weight issues. In addition, many people find that spiritual practice helps them to keep a healthy perspective on weight management, so that it does not crowd out other important interests and concerns in their lives.

HERBAL PREPARATIONS. The one type of alternative treatment that people should be extremely cautious about making part of a weight management program is over-the-counter herbal preparations advertised as "fat burners," muscle builders, or appetite suppressants. Within a two-week period in early 2003, the national media carried accounts of death or serious illness from taking these substances. One is ephedra, an herb used in traditional Chinese medicine that can cause strokes, heart attacks, seizures, and psychotic episodes. The other is usnic acid, a compound derived from lichens that can cause liver damage.

Another herbal preparation that has received considerable media attention since 2004 is hoodia (*Hoodia gordonii*), a succulent plant similar to a cactus that is native to South Africa and Namibia. Used for generations by the native inhabitants of these parts of Africa to treat indigestion, hoodia was studied by several pharmaceutical companies in the early 2000s as a natural appetite suppressant. In 2002, one such company stopped its research into hoodia on the grounds that it has potentially severe side effects on the liver. Nonetheless, hoodia has been featured on such popular television shows as *60 Minutes*, and is marketed as of 2007 in tablets, shakes, teas, and other diet products. As of 2007, however, there is no scientific evidence that hoodia is effective in curbing appetite, and is not recommended by any professional medical or nutrition society.

Normal results

As of 2007, much more research needs to be done to improve the success of weight management programs. A position paper published by the American Dietetic Association in the summer of 2002 summarizes the present situation: "Although our knowledge base has greatly expanded regarding the complex causation of increased body fat, little progress has been made in long-term maintenance interventions, with the exception of surgery." A study published in the *Journal of the American Medical Association* in 2003 showed that neither subjects randomly assigned to a commercial weight loss program nor those assigned to a self-help weight loss program lost more than a modest amount of weight and succeeded in keeping it off over a two-year period. Most adults in weight maintenance programs find it difficult to change eating patterns learned over a lifetime. Furthermore, their efforts are all too often undermined by friends or relatives, as well as by media messages that encourage overeating or the use of food as a mood-enhancing drug. More effective weight maintenance programs may well depend on broad-based changes in society.

Resources

BOOKS

American Psychiatric Association. "Eating Disorders." In *Diagnostic and Statistical Manual of Mental Disorders*, 4th ed., text revision. Washington, DC: American Psychiatric Association, 2000.

Brownell, Kelly, ed. *Weight Bias: Nature, Consequences, and Remedies*. New York: Guilford Press, 2005.

Fairburn, Christopher, and Kelly Brownell. *Eating Disorders and Obesity: A Comprehensive Handbook*, 2nd ed. New York: Guilford Press, 2002.

Hornbacher, Marya. *Wasted: A Memoir of Anorexia and Bulimia*. New York: Harper Perennial Editions, 1999.

Murphy, Wendy. *Weight and Health*. Minneapolis, MN: Twenty First Century Books, 2008.

Pelletier, Kenneth R., M.D. "CAM Therapies for Specific Conditions: Obesity." In *The Best Alternative Medicine*, Part II. New York: Simon & Schuster, 2002.

Schauer, Philip. *Bariatric Surgery and Weight Management*. Cleveland, OH: Cleveland Clinic Press, 2008.

PERIODICALS

Bellafante, Ginia. "When Midlife Seems Just an Empty Plate." *New York Times* March 9, 2003 [cited March 12, 2003]. http://query.nytimes.com/gst/fullpage.html?res=950DEED6103FF93AA35750C0A9659C8B63&scp=1&sq=When+Midlife+Seems+Just+an+Empty+Plate&st=nyt (accessed April 18, 2008).

Bindra, Jasjit S. "A Popular Pill's Hidden Dangers." *New York Times*, April 26, 2005 [cited December 31, 2007]. http://query.nytimes.com/gst/fullpage.html?res=9505E3D71231F935A15757C0A9639C8B63 (accessed April 18, 2008).

Chass, Murray. "Pitcher's Autopsy Points to Ephedra As One Factor." *New York Times* March 14, 2003 [cited March 14, 2003]. http://www.nytimes.com/2003/03/14/sports/baseball/14BASE.html (accessed April 18, 2008).

Cummings, S., E. S. Parham, and G. W. Strain. "Position of the American Dietetic Association: Weight Management." *Journal of the American Dietetic Association* 102 (August 2002): 1145–1155.

Drohan, S. H. "Managing Early Childhood Obesity in the Primary Care Setting: A Behavior Modification Approach." *Pediatric Nursing* 28 (November–December 2002): 599–610.

Foster, Gary D., Angela P. Makris, and Brooke A. Bailer. "Behavioral Treatment of Obesity." *American Journal of Clinical Nutrition* 82 (July 2005): 2305–2355.

Heshka, Stanley, James W. Anderson, Richard L. Atkinson, et al. "Weight Loss with Self-help Compared with a Structured Commercial Program." *Journal of the American Medical Association* 289 (April 9, 2003): 1792–1798.

Holt, Richard I. G. "Obesity—An Epidemic of the Twenty-First Century: An Update for Psychiatrists." *Journal of Psychopharmacology* 19, no. 6 (2005): 6–15.

"Hoodia: Lose Weight without Feeling Hungry?" *Consumer Reports* 71 (March 2006): 49.

James, W. Philip T. "The SCOUT Study: Risk-Benefit Profile of Sibutramine in Overweight High-Risk Cardiovascular Patients." *European Heart Journal* 7 (2005, Supplement 7): L44–L48.

Lowry, R., D. A. Galuska, J. E. Fulton, et al. "Weight Management Goals and Practices Among U. S. High School Students: Associations with Physical Activity, Diet, and Smoking." *Journal of Adolescent Health* 31 (August 2002): 133–144.

ORGANIZATIONS

American Dietetic Association. (800) 877-1600. http://www.eatright.org (accessed April 18, 2008).

American Society for Metabolic and Bariatric Surgery. 100 SW 75th Street, Suite 201, Gainesville, FL 32607. (352) 331-4900. http://www.asbs.org (accessed April 18, 2008).

American Yoga Association. http://www.americanyoga association.org (accessed April 18, 2008).

Council on Size and Weight Discrimination (CSWD). P. O. Box 305, Mt. Marion, NY 12456. (845) 679-1209. http://www.cswd.org/index.html (accessed April 18, 2008).

National Association to Advance Fat Acceptance (NAAFA). P.O. Box 22510, Oakland, CA 94609. (916) 558-6880. http://www.naafa.org/ (accessed April 18, 2008).

Obesity Society (formerly the American Obesity Association). 8630 Fenton Street, Suite 814, Silver Spring, MD 20910. (301) 563-6526. http://www.obesity.org (accessed April 18, 2008).

Overeaters Anonymous (OA). World Service Office, P. O. Box 44020, Rio Rancho, NM 87174-4020. (505) 891-2664. http://www.oa.org(accessed April 18, 2008).

Shape Up America! c/o WebFront Solutions Corporation, 15757 Crabbs Branch Way, Rockville, MD 20855. (301) 258-0540. http://www.shapeup.org(accessed April 18, 2008).

Weight-control Information Network (WIN). 1 WIN Way, Bethesda, MD 20892-3665. (202) 828-1025 or (877) 946-4627.

OTHER

National Institutes of Health, National Institute of Diabetes & Digestive & Kidney Diseases (NIDDK). *Choosing a Safe and Successful Weight-Loss Program*. Bethesda, MD: NIDDK, 2006. NIH Publication No. 03-3700.

National Institutes of Health, National Institute of Diabetes & Digestive & Kidney Diseases (NIDDK). *Do You Know the Health Risks of Being Overweight?* Bethesda, MD: NIDDK, 2004. NIH Publication No. 04-4098.

National Institutes of Health, National Institute of Diabetes & Digestive & Kidney Diseases (NIDDK). *Weight Loss for Life*. Bethesda, MD: NIDDK, 2006. NIH Publication No. 94-3700.

Rebecca Frey, PhD

Whipple procedure

Definition

A Whipple procedure, or pancreaticoduodenectomy, is a surgical procedure which is most often performed to treat pancreatic cancer. The operation may also be performed for cancer of the duodenum, cholangiocarcinoma (cancer of the bile duct), cancer of the ampulla (the area where the bile and pancreatic ducts enter the small intestine), and for chronic pancreatitis and benign (noncancerous) tumors involving the pancreatic head.

During the course of a Whipple procedure, the surgeon removes the head of the pancreas, the majority of the first part of the small intestine (the duodenum), part of the bile duct, and in some cases part of the stomach. Variations on the operation may include removal of the body of the pancreas and/or the entire gall bladder.

Purpose

The Whipple procedure is the most common operation performed for treatment of cancer of the pancreas. The pancreas is an organ located near the liver on the right side of the body. It produces both digestive juices and hormones that are involved in regulation of blood sugar. Pancreatic cancer most often affects what is called the exocrine pancreas, which is the portion of the pancreas involved in producing digestive juices.

Because it initially causes only vague symptoms, pancreatic cancer is often not diagnosed until later stages of the disease. Additionally, it spreads very quickly, so when the disease is often quite widespread by the time it is finally diagnosed. Symptoms of pancreatic cancer can include pain in the upper abdomen, often radiating to the back; jaundice (yellow eyes and skin); decreased appetite; weight loss; and depression.

Demographics

The American Cancer Society estimates that approximately 37,680 people will be diagnosed with pancreatic cancer in the United States in 2008. About 34,290 people will die of pancreatic cancer in 2008, making pancreatic cancer the fourth leading cause of cancer death in the United States. Most people who are diagnosed with pancreatic cancer are over age 60. Men and women are about equally at risk. Risk factors for the development of pancreatic cancer include smoking, history of diabetes, family history, and a personal history of chronic pancreatitis. Researchers

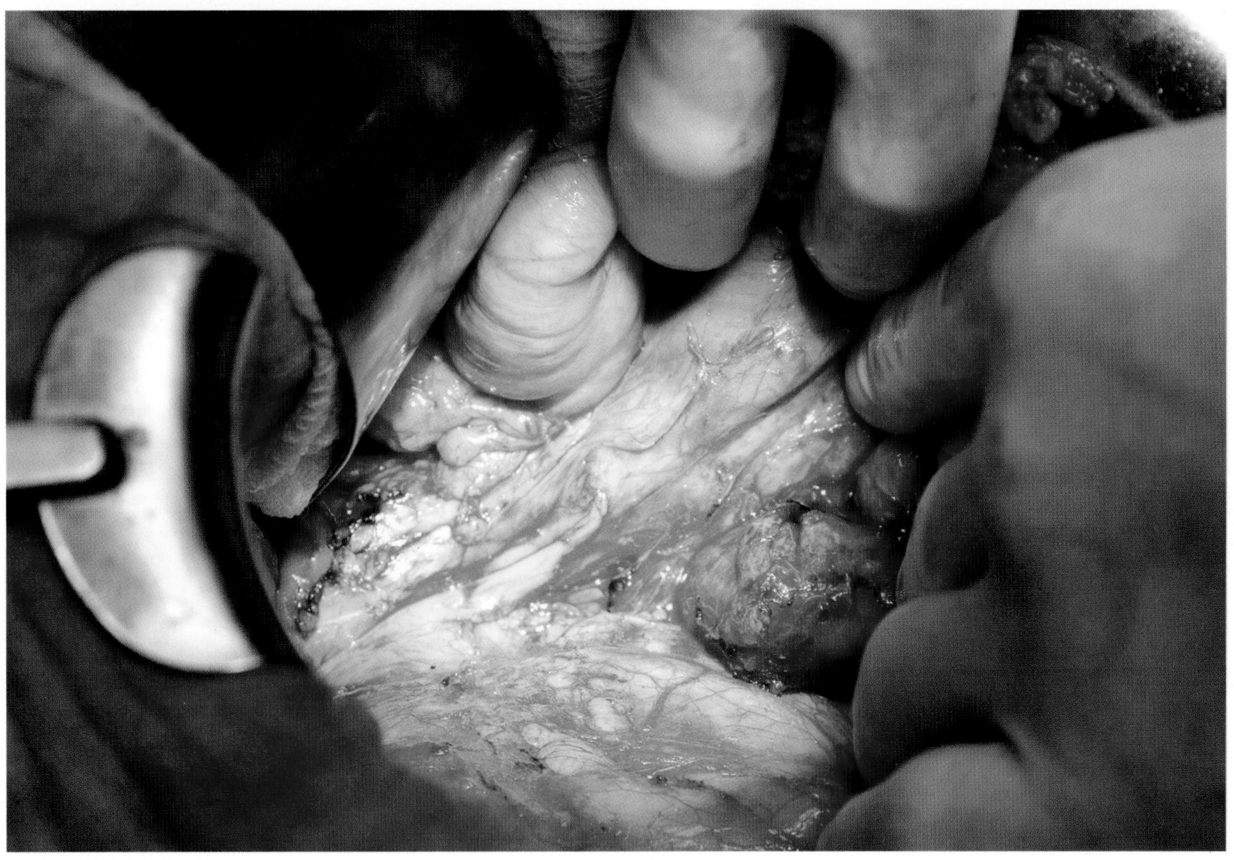

Whipple procedure. *(Barry Slaven, MD, PhD / Phototake. Reproduced by permission.)*

are still examining the possibility that other factors, such as certain workplace exposures or a high fat diet, may also increase an individual's risk of pancreatic cancer.

Description

A Whipple procedure is a lengthy operation, taking about four to six hours. **General anesthesia** is required. A classic operation requires a large abdominal incision through which the operation occurs. There are some centers that offer **laparoscopic** Whipple procedure performed with or without **robotic assistance**. This minimally invasive method of surgery is performed through four small incisions with the use of a fiberoptic scope and miniaturized surgical instruments.

After the head of the pancreas has been removed during the operation, three important connections (anastamoses) must be performed. The intestine must be connected to the remains of the pancreas, to the bile duct, and to the stomach. These anastamoses must be very carefully achieved, since any leak may allow pancreatic juices to enter the abdomen, risking severe complications.

Diagnosis/Preparation

The patient meets with the operating physician prior to surgery to discuss the details of the surgery and receive instructions on **preoperative** and **postoperative care**. Blood tests to evaluate bleeding time and an EKG to evaluate cardiac function may be performed several days prior to the operation. Directly preceding surgery, an intravenous (IV) line is placed to administer fluid and medications, and the patient is given a **bowel prep** to cleanse the bowel and prepare it for surgery.

Aftercare

Recuperation from Whipple procedure may be slow and difficult. Depending on the type of surgery (traditional open incision or minimally invasive), inpatient stay will range from five to 14 days. Because of the high likeilhood of gastroparesis (slow gastric emptying), patients will remain on intravenous feeding

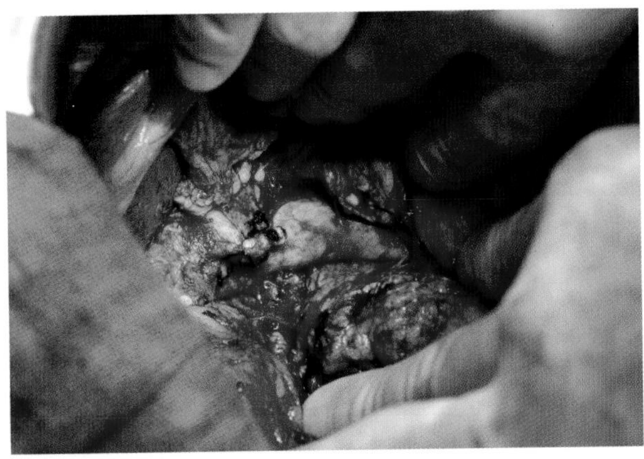

Surgeons performing a Whipple procedure, the removal of the pancreatic head. *(Barry Slaven, MD, PhD/Phototake. Reproduced by permission.)*

for five or six days following the operation. A nasogastric tube may be required to remove excess stomach acid and juices that accumulate. Advancement of diet through clear liquids, full liquids, soft foods, to regular diet will be slow and the timeframe will depend on the patient's tolerance of each new step. Some patients take as long as 4-6 weeks to have normal stomach emptying return. A feeding tube that delivers a nutritional formula directly into the jejunum may be used if recovery is overly slow.

Risks

Risks associated with the Whipple procedure include excessive bleeding, infection, and complications due to general anesthesia. Delayed gastric emptying after eating affects about 19% of patients. Leakage of pancreatic juices into the abdomen is a serious problem, since these digestive juices are strong enough to actually begin to digest the internal organs themselves. This can result in perforations (holes) in the intestine, stomach, or other nearby organs; abnormal communication between organs (fistulas); or necrosis (cell death) within an affected organ. Some patients may develop diabetes following Whipple procedure. Weight loss of 5-10% of original body weight is common after the operation, as is the need to take oral enzyme supplements to aid digestion.

Normal results

Although the recuperative time may be long, most patients return to their usual level of functioning and their usual quality of life after a Whipple procedure. However, the risk for further advancement of pancreatic cancer is very high. Many patients receive chemotherapy and radiation for further treatment of the cancer.

KEY TERMS

Anastomosis—A surgically created joining or opening between two organs or body spaces.

Fistula—An abnormal connection between two organs, or between an organ and the outside of the body.

Jaundice—A yellowish cast to the whites of the eyes and/or the skin, caused by excess bilirubin circulating in the bloodstreatm.

Morbidity and mortality rates

The Whipple procedure has a high morbidity and mortality rate. It requires the expertise of a surgeon who has performed a large number of these types of procedures. Even when highly skilled surgeons in cancer centers operate, 2-5% of patients die due to surgical complications. When less skilled surgeons perform this procedure, or when it is undertaken at smaller hospitals rather than major medial centers, the death rate from surgical complications may be as high as 15%. The complication rate is very high as well, between 30-50%. Possible complications include leakage from the anastomoses (connections) between organs, infection, bleeding, and slow gastric (stomach) emptying following meals. Risk of death from advancement of the original pancreatic cancer also is quite high, with only about 20% of all Whipple procedure patients surviving for five years after their initial diagnosis. Patients with no lymph node involvement at the time of surgery may have a higher five-year survival rate (about 40%). However, patients who receive chemotherapy but no surgery have only a 5% survival rate at five years.

Resources

BOOKS

Abeloff, M. D., et al. *Clinical Oncology*. 3rd ed. Philadelphia: Elsevier, 2004.

Feldman, M., et al. *Sleisenger & Fordtran's Gastrointestinal and Liver Disease*. 8th ed. St. Louis: Mosby, 2005.

Khatri, V. P., and J. A. Asensio. *Operative Surgery Manual*. 1st ed. Philadelphia: Saunders, 2003.

Townsend, C. M., et al. *Sabiston Textbook of Surgery*. 17th ed. Philadelphia: Saunders, 2004.

Rosalyn Carson-DeWitt, MD

WHO PERFORMS THE PROCEDURE AND WHERE IS IT PERFORMED?

A Whipple procedure is performed in a hospital operating room. It is considered one of the most technically difficult operations, and should be performed by a very experienced, skilled surgeon who has successfully performed many of these same procedures. Some of the doctors who perform these operations include general surgeons, surgical gastroenterologists, and surgical oncologists.

QUESTIONS TO ASK THE DOCTOR

- Why is a Whipple procedure being recommended?
- What type of Whipple procedure would work best for me?
- What are the risks and complications associated with the recommended procedure?
- Are any nonsurgical treatment alternatives available?
- How soon after surgery may I resume my normal diet and activities?
- If the Whipple procedure is being done to treat pancreatic cancer, will I require any other treatment?

White blood cell count and differential

Definition

A white blood cell (WBC) count determines the concentration of white blood cells in the patient's blood. A differential determines the percentage of each of the five types of mature white blood cells.

Purpose

A WBC count is included in general health examinations and to help investigate a variety of illnesses. An elevated WBC count occurs in infection, allergy, systemic illness, inflammation, tissue injury, and leukemia. A low WBC count may occur in some viral infections, immunodeficiency states, and bone marrow failure. The WBC count provides clues about certain illnesses, and helps physicians monitor a patient's recovery from others. Abnormal counts that return to normal indicate that the condition is improving, while counts that become more abnormal indicate that the condition is worsening. The differential will reveal which WBC types are affected most. For example, an elevated WBC count with an absolute increase in lymphocytes having an atypical appearance is most often caused by infectious mononucleosis. The differential will also identify early WBCs, which may be reactive (e.g., a response to acute infection) or the result of a leukemia.

Precautions

Many medications affect the WBC count. Both prescription and non-prescription drugs, including herbal supplements, should be noted. Normal values for both the WBC count and differential are age-related.

Sources of error in manual WBC counting are due largely to variance in the dilution of the sample and the distribution of cells in the chamber, as well as the small number of WBCs that are counted. For electronic WBC counts and differentials, interference may be caused by small fibrin clots, nucleated red blood cells (RBCs), platelet clumping, and unlysed RBCs. Immature WBCs and nucleated RBCs may cause interference with the automated differential count. Automated cell counters may not be acceptable for counting WBCs in other body fluids, especially when the number of WBCs is less than 1,000/μL or when other nucleated cell types are present.

Description

White cell counts are usually performed using an automated instrument, but may be done manually using a microscope and a counting chamber, especially when counts are very low, or if the patient has a condition known to interfere with an automated WBC count.

An automated differential may be performed by an electronic cell counter or by an image analysis instrument. When the electronic WBC count is abnormal or a cell population is flagged, meaning that one or more of the results is atypical, a manual differential is performed. The WBC differential is performed manually by microscopic examination of a blood sample that is spread in a thin film on a glass slide. White blood cells are identified by their size, shape, and texture.

Causes for abnormalities in the white blood cell (WBC) differential count

Type of WBC and normal differential count	Elevated	Decreased
Neutrophils 55–70%	Neutrophilia Physical or emotional stress Acute suppurative infection Myelocytic leukemia Trauma Cushing's syndrome Inflammatory disorders Metabolic disorders	Neutropenia Aplastic anemia Dietary deficiency Overwhelming bacterial infection Viral infections Radiation therapy Addison's disease Drug therapy: myelotoxic drugs (as in chemotherapy)
Lymphocytes 20–40%	Lymphocytosis Chronic bacterial infection Viral infection Lymphocytic leukemia Multiple myeloma Infectious mononucleosis Radiation Infectious hepatitis	Lymphocytopenia Leukemia Sepsis Immunodeficiency diseases Lupus erythematosus Later stages of HIV infection Drug therapy: adrenocorticosteroids, antineoplastics Radiation therapy
Monocytes 2–8%	Monocytosis Chronic inflammatory disorders Viral infections Tuberculosis Chronic ulcerative colitis Parasites	Monocytopenia Drug therapy: prednisone
Eosinophils 1–4%	Eosinophilia Parasitic infections Allergic reactions Eczema Leukemia Autoimmune diseases	Eosinopenia Increased adrenosteroid production
Basophils 0.5–1.0%	Basophilia Myeloproliferative disease (e.g., myelofibrosis, polycythemia rubra vera) Leukemia	Basopenia Acute allergic reactions Hyperthyroidism Stress reactions

SOURCE: Pagana, K.D. and T.J. Pagana. *Mosby's Diagnostic and Laboratory Test Reference*. 3rd ed. St. Louis: Mosby, 1997.

(*Cengage Learning, Gale.*)

The manual WBC differential involves a thorough evaluation of a stained blood film. In addition to determining the percentage of each mature white blood cell, the following tests are preformed as part of the differential:

- Evaluation of RBC morphology. This includes grading of the variation in RBC size (anisocytosis) and shape (poikilocytosis); reporting the type and number of any abnormal or immature RBCs; and counting the number of nucleated RBCs per 100 WBCs.
- An estimate of the WBC count is made and compared with the automated or chamber WBC count. An estimate of the platelet count is made and compared with the automated or chamber platelet count. Abnormal platelets, such as clumped platelets or excessively large platelets, are noted on the report.
- Any immature WBCs are included in the differential count of 100 cells, and any inclusions or abnormalities of the WBCs are reported.

Preparation

This test requires a 3.5 mL sample of blood. Vein puncture with a needle is usually performed by a nurse or phlebotomist, a person trained to draw blood. There is no restriction on diet or physical activity.

Aftercare

Discomfort or bruising may occur at the puncture site. Pressure to the puncture site until the bleeding stops reduces bruising; warm packs relieve discomfort. Some people feel dizzy or faint after blood has been drawn and should be allowed to lie down and relax until they are stable.

KEY TERMS

Band cell—An immature neutrophil at the stage just preceding a mature cell. The nucleus of a band cell is unsegmented.

Basophil—Segmented white blood cell with large dark blue-black granules that releases histamine in allergic reactions.

Cytoplasm—The part of a cell outside of the nucleus.

Differential—Blood test that determines the percentage of each type of white blood cell in a person's blood.

Eosinophil—Segmented white blood cell with large orange-red granules that increases in response to parasitic infections and allergic reactions.

Lymphocyte—Mononuclear white blood cell that is responsible for humoral (antibody mediated) and cell mediated immunity.

Monocyte—Mononuclear phagocytic white blood cell that removes debris and microorganisms by phagocytosis and processes antigens for recognition by immune lymphocytes.

Nucleus—The part of a cell that contains the DNA.

Neutrophil—Segmented white blood cell normally comprising 50–70% of the total. The cytoplasm contains both primary and secondary granules that take up both acidic and basic dyes of the Wright stain. Neutrophils remove and kill bacteria by phagocytosis.

Phagocytosis—A process by which a white blood cell envelopes and digests debris and microorganisms to remove them from the blood.

Risks

Other than potential bruising at the puncture site, and/or dizziness, there are no complications associated with this test.

Normal results

Normal values vary with age. White blood cell counts are highest in children under one year of age, and then decrease somewhat until adulthood. The increase is largely in the lymphocyte population. Adult normal values include:

- WBC count: 4,500–11,000/μL
- polymorphonuclear neutrophils: 1800–7800/μL; (50–70%)

- band neutrophils: 0–700/μL; (0–10%)
- lymphocytes: 1,000–4,800/μL; (15–45%)
- monocytes: 0–800/μL; (0–10%)
- eosinophils: 0–450/μL; (0–6%)
- basophils: 0–200/μL; (0–2%)

Resources

BOOKS

Cohen, J., et al. *Infectious Diseases*, 2nd ed. St. Louis: Mosby, 2004.

Gershon, A. A., et al. *Infectious Diseases of Children*, 11th ed. St. Louis: Mosby, 2004.

Hoffman, R., et al. *Hematology: Basic Principles and Practice*, 4th ed. Philadelphia: Elsevier, 2005.

Long, S. S., et al. *Principles and Practice of Pediatric Infectious Diseases*, 2nd ed. London: Churchill Livingstone, 2003.

Mandell, G. L., et al. *Principles and Practice of Infectious Diseases*, 6th ed. London: Churchill Livingstone, 2005.

McPherson, R. A., et al. *Henry's Clinical Diagnosis and Management By Laboratory Methods*, 21st ed. Philadelphia: Saunders, 2007.

OTHER

National Institutes of Health, [cited April 5, 2003]. http://www.nlm.nih.gov/medlineplus/encyclopedia.html (accessed April 18, 2008).

Victoria E. DeMoranville
Mark A. Best
Rosalyn Carson-DeWitt, MD

Wound care

Definition

A wound is a disruption in the continuity of cells—anything that causes cells that would normally be connected to become separated. Wound healing is the restoration of that continuity. Several effects may result from the occurrence of a wound: immediate loss of all or part of organ functioning, sympathetic stress response, hemorrhage and blood clotting, bacterial contamination, and **death** of cells. The most important factor in minimizing these effects and promoting successful care is careful prevention of infection, which can be accomplished using sterile techniques when treating a wound.

Description

Wound healing is a biological process that begins with trauma and ends with scar formation. There are two types of tissue injury: full and partial thickness. Partial thickness injury is limited to the outermost layers of skin, with no damage to the dermal blood vessels. Healing occurs by regeneration of the outer layers of tissue. Full thickness injury involves loss of the dermis, extends to deeper tissue layers, and disrupts blood vessels. Wound healing involves the synthesis of several types of tissue and scar formation.

The three phases of repair are lag, proliferative, and remodeling. Shortly after an injury, blood flow ceases when a clot is formed. The initial clot acts like a magnet for the migration of more platelets and protein strands, called fibrin, which seal the wound from the inside. Within the first four hours of injury, certain white blood cells called neutrophils begin to appear. These inflammatory cells kill microbes, and prevent infection of the wound. Next, white blood cells called leukocytes also arrive and act to kill microbes and break down wound debris. The inflammatory response is dependent on the depth and volume of tissue loss from the injury. Leukocytes also secrete cytokines that initiate the proliferative phase of repair.

During the proliferative phase, synthetic cells, or fibroblasts, proliferate and synthesize new connective tissue, replacing the fibrin matrix. At this time, an efficient nutrient supply develops through the arborization (terminal branching) of adjacent blood vessels. This in-growth of new blood vessels is called angiogenesis. This new and very vascular connective tissue is referred to as granulation tissue. In this process, acute inflammation releases cytokines, promoting fibroblast infiltration of the wound site, and then creating a high density of cells. Collagen is the major connective tissue protein produced and released by fibroblasts. The connective tissue physically supports the new blood vessels that form, and endothelial cells promote ingrowth of new vessels. These new blood vessels are necessary to meet the nutritional needs of the wound healing process. The mark of wound closure is when a new epidermal cover seals the defect. The process of wound healing continues beneath the new surface. This is the remodeling or maturation phase and is the third phase of healing.

The first principle of wound care is the removal of nonviable tissue, including dead tissue, slough, foreign debris, and residual material from **dressings**. Removal of nonviable tissue is referred to as **debridement**; removal of foreign matter is referred to as cleansing. Chronic wounds are colonized with bacteria, but not necessarily infected. A wound is colonized when a limited number of bacteria are present in the wound and are of no consequence in the healing process. A wound is infected when the bacterial burden

KEY TERMS

Allograft—Skin donated from another person to treat burns.

Asepsis—Freedom from infection or infectious material; also, the absence of viable pathogenic organisms. Asepsis can be accomplished using aseptic techniques, which are the use of surgical practices that restrict microorganisms in the environment and prevent contamination of the surgical wound; they include sterilization of instruments and the wearing of sterile caps, gloves, and masks.

Cadaver skin—Skin donated from another person to treat burns.

Cytokine—A protein that regulates the duration and intensity of the body's immune response.

Dermis—The thick layer of skin below the epidermis.

Epidermis—The outermost layer of the skin.

Exudate—Fluid, cells, or other substances that are slowly discharged by tissue, especially due to injury or inflammation.

Fibroblast—An undifferentiated connective tissue cell that is capable of forming collagen fibers.

Hemostasis—Slowing down or stopping bleeding.

Langerhans' cells—Cells in the epidermis that help protect the body against infection.

Melanocytes—Cells within the epidermis that give skin its color

Neutrophil—A type of white blood cell.

Scar tissue—Scar tissue is the fibrous tissue that replaces normal tissue destroyed by injury or disease.

overwhelms the immune response of the host and bacteria grow unchecked. Clinical signs of infection are redness of the skin around the wound, purulent (pus-containing) drainage, foul odor, and edema.

The second principle of wound care is to provide a moist environment. This has been shown to promote re-epithelialization and healing. Exposing wounds to air dries the surface and may impede the healing process. Gauze dressings provide a moist environment provided they are kept moist in the wound. These are referred to as wet-to-dry dressings. Generally, a saline-soaked gauze dressing is loosely placed into the wound and covered with a dry gauze dressing to prevent drying and contamination. It also supports autolytic debridement (the body's own capacity to dissolve dead tissue), absorbs exudate (thick layer of discharge), and traps bacteria in the gauze, which are removed when the dressing is changed.

Preventing further injury is the third principle of wound care. This involves elimination or reduction of the condition that allowed the wound to develop. Factors that contribute to the development of chronic wounds include losses in mobility, mental status changes, deficits of sensation, and circulatory deficits. Patients must be properly positioned to eliminate continued pressure to the chronic wound. Pressure-reducing devices, such as mattresses, cushions, supportive boots, foam wedges, and fitted shoes can be used to keep pressure off wounds.

Providing nutrition, specifically protein for healing, is the fourth principle of healing. Protein is essential for wound repair and regeneration. Without essential amino acids, angiogenesis, fibroblast proliferation, collagen synthesis, and scar remodeling will not occur. Amino acids also support the immune response. Adequate amounts of carbohydrates and fats are needed to prevent the amino acids from being oxidized for caloric needs. Glucose is also needed to meet the energy requirements of the cells involved in wound repair.

Diagnosis/Preparation

Effective wound care begins with an assessment of the entire patient. This includes obtaining a complete **health history** and a physical assessment. Assessing the patient assists in identifying causes and contributing factors of the wound. When examining the wound, it is important to document its size, location, appearance, and the surrounding skin. The healthcare professional also examines the wound for exudate, dead tissue, signs of infection, and drainage, and documents how long the patient has had the wound. It is also important to know what treatment, if any, the patient has previously received for the wound.

Actual components of wound care include cleaning, dressing, determining frequency of dressing changes, and reevaluation. Dead tissue and debris can impede healing: the goal of cleaning the wound is its removal. When cleaning the wound, protective goggles should be worn and sterile saline solution should be used. Providone iodine, sodium hypochlorite, and hydrogen peroxide should never be used, as they are toxic to cells.

Gentle pressure should be used to clean the wound if there is no dead tissue. This can be accomplished by utilizing a syringe to apply the cleaning solution. If the wound has dead tissue, more pressure may be needed.

Whirlpools can also be used for wounds having a thick layer of discharge, known as exudate. At times, chemical or surgical debridement may be needed to remove debris.

Dressings are applied to wounds to provide the proper environment for healing, to absorb drainage, to immobilize the wound, to protect the wound and new tissue growth from mechanical injury and bacterial contamination, to prevent bleeding, and to provide mental and physical patient comfort. There are several types of dressings and most are designed to maintain a moist wound bed, including:

- Alginate. Made of non-woven fibers derived from seaweed, alginate forms a gel as it absorbs exudate. It is used for wounds with moderate-to-heavy exudate or drainage, and is changed every 12 hours to three days, depending on when the exudate penetrates the secondary dressing.
- Composite dressings. Combining physically distinct components into a single dressing, composite dressings provide bacterial protection, absorption, and adhesion. The frequency of dressing changes vary.
- Foam. Made from polyurethane, foam comes in various thicknesses having different absorption rates. It is used for wounds with moderate-to-heavy exudate or drainage. Dressing change is every three to seven days.
- Gauze. Available in a number of forms, including sponges, pads, ropes, strips, and rolls, gauze can be impregnated with petroleum jelly, antimicrobials, and saline. Frequent changes are needed because gauze has limited moisture retention properties, and there is little protection from contamination. With removal of a dried dressing, there is a risk of wound damage to the healing skin surrounding the wound. Gauze dressings are changed two to three times a day.
- Hydrocolloid. Made of gelatin or pectin, hydrocolloid is available as a wafer, paste, or powder. While absorbing exudate, the dressing forms a gel. Hydrocolloid dressings are used for light-to-moderate exudate or drainage. This type of dressing is not used for wounds with exposed tendon or bone, third-degree burns, or in the presence of bacterial, fungal, or viral infection or active cellulitis or vasculitis because it is almost totally occlusive. Dressings are changed every three to seven days.
- Hydrogel. Composed primarily of water, hydrogel dressings are used for wounds with minimal exudate. Some are impregnated in gauze or non-woven sponge. Dressings are changed one or two times a day.
- Transparent film. An adhesive, waterproof membrane that keeps contaminants out while allowing oxygen and water vapor to cross through, it is used primarily for wounds with minimal exudate. It is also used as a secondary material to secure non-adhesive gauzes. Dressings are changed every three to five days if the film is used as a primary dressing.

In cases where a wound is particularly severe, large, or, if it is a third-degree burn, cellular wound healing products may be used to close the wound and speed recovery. In some cases (i.e., a third-degree burn), a skin graft will often be used. Although most surgeons prefer to use skin donated from another person (known as cadaver skin, or human allograft), skin donations are not always available. Then surgeons must rely on other available products such as cellular wound dressings for the treatment of burns. For **skin grafting** of full-thickness burn wounds, surgeons use healthy skin from another part of the person's own body (autografting) as a permanent treatment. Surgeons may use cellular wound dressings as a temporary covering when the skin damage is so extensive that there is not enough healthy skin available to graft initially. This helps prevent infection and fluid loss until autografting can be performed.

The survival rate for burn patients has increased considerably through the process of quickly removing dead tissue and immediately covering the wound. Burns covering half the body were routinely fatal 20 years ago, but today even people with extensive and severe burns have a good chance of survival, according to the American Burn Association.

Cellular wound dressings

In recent years, the technology of burn and wound care using cellular wound dressings and grafts has helped to transform the treatment of burns and chronic wounds by decreasing the risk of infection, protecting against fluid loss, requiring fewer skin grafts, and promoting and speeding the healing process. These dressings provide a cover that keeps fluids from evaporating and prevents blood from oozing out once the dead skin has been removed. Some of these products grow in place and expand natural skin when it heals.

Cellular wound dressings may look and feel like skin, but they do not function exactly the same as skin because they are missing hair follicles, sweat glands, melanocytes, and Langerhans' cells. Some cellular wound dressings have a synthetic top layer structured like an epidermis. It peels away over time, or is replaced with healthy skin through skin grafting.

How these products are involved in wound repair is a subject of great scientific interest; it is known that they promote a higher rate of healing than does standard wound care.

People with severe wounds, chronic wounds, burns, and ulcers can benefit from cellular wound dressings. Several artificial skin products for non-healing wounds or burns include:

- Apligraf is a two-layer wound dressing that contains live human skin cells combined with cow collagen. It delivers live cells from a different donor (circumcised infant foreskin). Thousands of pieces of Apligraf are produced in the laboratory from one small patch of cells from a single donor.
- Dermagraft is made from human cells placed on a dissolvable mesh material. The mesh material is gradually absorbed and the human cells grow and replace the damaged skin after being placed on the wound or ulcer.
- Biobrane is used as a temporary dressing for a variety of wounds, including ulcers, lacerations, and full-thickness burns. It may also be used on wounds that develop on areas from which healthy skin is transplanted to cover damaged skin. It consists of an ultrathin silicone film and nylon fabric. As the wound heals, or until autografting becomes possible, the Biobrane is trimmed away.
- TransCyte is used as a temporary covering over full-thickness and some partial-thickness burns until autografting is possible, as well as a temporary covering for some burn wounds that heal without autografting. It consists of human cells from circumcised infant foreskin, and is grown on nylon mesh, combined with a synthetic epidermal layer. TransCyte starts with living cells, but these cells die when it is shipped in a frozen state to burn treatment facilities. The product is then thawed and stretched over a burn site. In one to two weeks, the TransCyte starts peeling off, and the surgeon trims it away as it peels.
- Integra Dermal Regeneration Template is used to treat full-thickness and some partial-thickness burns. Integra consists of two layers. The bottom layer, made of shark cartilage and collagen from cow tendons, acts as a matrix onto which a person's own cells migrate over two to three weeks. A new dermis is created as the cells gradually absorb the cartilage and collagen. The top layer is a protective silicone sheet that is peeled off after several weeks, while the bottom layer is a permanent cover. A very thin layer of the person's own skin is then grafted onto the neo-dermis.
- OrCel is also made from circumcised infant foreskin, grown on a cow collagen matrix, and used to treat donor sites in burn patients. It is also used to help treat epidermolysis bullosa, a rare skin condition in children.

Risks

Various risks from wounds include:

- Hematoma. Dressings should be inspected for hemorrhage at intervals during the first 24 hours after surgery. A large amount of bleeding should be reported to a healthcare professional immediately. Concealed bleeding sometimes occurs in the wound, beneath the skin. If the clot formed is small, it will be absorbed by the body, but if large, the wound bulges and the clot must be removed for healing to continue.
- Infection. The second most frequent nosocomial (hospital-acquired) infection in hospitals is surgical wound infections with *Staphylococcus aureus*, *Escherichia coli*, and *Pseudomonas aeruginosa*. Prevention is accomplished with meticulous wound management. Cellulitis is a bacterial infection that spreads into tissue planes; systemic antibiotics are usually prescribed to treat it. If the infection is in an arm or leg, elevation of the limb reduces dependent edema and heat application promotes blood circulation. Abscess is a bacterial infection that is localized and characterized by pus. Treatment consists of surgical drainage or excision with the concurrent administration of antibiotics.
- Dehiscence (disruption of the surgical wound) and evisceration (protrusion of wound contents). This condition results from sutures giving way, from infection, distention, and coughs. Dehiscence results in pain; the surgeon should be called immediately. Prophylactically, an abdominal binder may be utilized.
- Keloid, which refers to excessive growth of scar tissue. Careful wound closure, hemostasis, and pressure support are used to ward off this complication.

Normal results

The goals of wound care include reducing risks that inhibit wound healing, enhancing the healing process, and lowering the incidence of wound infections.

Resources

BOOKS

Baranoski, Sharon and Elizabeth A. Ayello. *Wound Care Essentials: Practice Principles*, 2nd ed. Philadelphia: Lippincott Williams & Wilkins., 2008.

Dipietro, Luisa A. and Aime L. Burns, eds. *Wound Healing: Methods and Protocols (Methods in Molecular Medicine Ser)*. Totowa, NJ: Humana Press, 2003.

Hess, Cathy Thomas. *Clinical Guide to Wound Care*, 4th ed. Philadelphia, PA: Lippincott Williams & Wilkins, 2002.

Sheffield, Paul J., Adrianne P.S. Smith and Caroline E. Fife, eds. *Wound Care Practice*, 2nd ed. Flagstaff, AZ: Best Pub Co., 2007.

PERIODICALS

Collins, Nancy. "Obesity and Wound Healing." *Advances in Wound Care* 16, no 1. (January/February 2003): 45.

Collins, Nancy. "Vegetarian Diets and Wound Healing." *Advances in Wound Care* 16, no. 2 (March/April 2003): 65.

McGuckin, Maryanne, Robert Goldman, Laura Bolton, and Richard Salcido. "The Clinical Relevance of Microbiology in Acute and Chronic Wounds." *Advances in Wound Care* 16, no 1. (January/February 2003): 12.

Trent, Jennifer T. and Robert S. Kirsner. "Wounds and Malignancy." *Advances in Wound Care* 16, no 1. (January/February 2003): 31.

ORGANIZATIONS

American Diabetes Association. 1701 North Beauregard Street, Alexandria, VA 22311. (800) 342-2383. E-mail: AskADA@diabetes.org. http://www.diabetes.org (accessed April 18, 2008).

American Professional Wound Care Association (APWCA). 853 Second Street Pike, Suite #A-1, Richboro, PA 18954. (215) 364-4100. Fax: (215) 364-1146. E-mail: wounds@apwca.org. http://www.apwca.org (accessed April 18, 2008).

National Institutes of Health. 9000 Rockville Pike, Bethesda, MD 20892. (301) 496-4000. Email: NIHInfo @OD.NIH.GOV. http://www.nih.gov (accessed April 18, 2008).

OTHER

Lippincott Williams & Wilkins. *Advances in Skin & Wound Care*, 2007, [cited December 29, 2007]. http:// www.aswcjournal.com/ (accessed April 18, 2008).

René A. Jackson, RN
Crystal H. Kaczkowski, MSc
Robert Bockstiegel

Wound culture

Definition

A wound culture is a diagnostic laboratory test in which microorganisms—such as bacteria or fungi from an infected wound, are grown in the laboratory on nutrient-enriched substance called media—then identified. Wound cultures always include aerobic (with oxygen) culture, but direct smear evaluation by Gram stain and anaerobic (without oxygen) culture are not performed on every wound. These tests are performed when indicated or requested by the physician.

Purpose

The purpose of a wound culture is to isolate and identify bacteria or fungi causing an infection of the wound. Only then can **antibiotics** that will be effective in destroying the organism be identified.

Preparation

A biopsy sample is usually preferred by clinicians, but this is a moderately invasive procedure and may not always be feasible. The health-care professional prepares the patient by cleansing the affected area with a sterile solution, such as saline. **Antiseptics** such as ethyl alcohol are not recommended, because they kill bacteria and cause the culture results to be negative. The patient is given a local anesthetic and the tissue is removed by the practitioner, who uses a cutting sheath. Afterwards, pressure is applied to the wound to control bleeding.

Needle aspiration is less invasive and is a good technique to use in wounds where there is little loss of skin, such as in the case of puncture wounds. The skin around the wound is cleaned with an antiseptic to kill bacteria on the skin's surface, and a small needle is inserted. To obtain a sample of the fluid to be biopsied, the clinician pulls back on the plunger, then changes the angle of the needle two or three times to remove fluid from different areas of the wound. This procedure may be painful for the patient, so many initial cultures are done with the swab technique.

For a sample to be collected using the swab technique some of the wound must be exposed. A small sterile swab is inserted into the wound, or rubbed on top of the wound, rotated, and moved back and forth to collect as much fluid as possible from the wound. This is usually the least painful of the collection techniques, although it cannot be used with every type of wound. After completion of any of the three procedures, the wound should be cleaned thoroughly and bandaged.

Description

Wounds are injuries to body tissues caused by physical trauma or disease processes that may include surgery, diabetes, burns, punctures, gunshots, lacerations, bites, bed sores, and broken bones. Types of wounds may include:

KEY TERMS

Aerobe—Bacteria that require oxygen to live.

Agar—A gelatinous material extracted from red algae that is not digested by bacteria. It is used as a support for growth in plates.

Anaerobe—Bacteria that live only where there is no oxygen.

Antibiotic—A medicine that can be used topically or taken orally, intramuscularly, or intravenously to limit the growth of bacteria.

Antimicrobial—A compound that prevents the growth of microbes which may include bacteria, fungi, and viruses.

Antimycotic—A medicine that can be used to kill yeast and fungus.

Antiseptic—A compound that kills all bacteria, also known as a bactericide.

Broth—A growth mixture for bacteria. Different compounds, such as sugars or amino acids, may be added to increase the growth of certain organisms. Also known as media.

Exudate—Any fluid that has been released by tissue or its capillaries due to injury or inflammation.

Normal flora—The mixture of bacteria normally found at specific body sites.

Purulent—Containing, consisting of or forming pus.

Pus—A fluid that is the product of inflammation and infection containing white blood cells and debris of dead cells and tissue.

- Abraded or abrasion: Caused by scraping, such as falling on concrete.
- Contused or contusion: A bruise or bleeding into the tissue.
- Incised or incision: A wound formed by a clean cut, as by a sharp instrument like a knife.
- Lacerated or laceration: A wound caused by heavy pressure, causing tearing of the skin or other tissues.
- Nonpenetrating: An injury caused without disruption of the surface of the body. These wounds are usually in the thorax or abdomen and can also be termed blunt trauma wounds.
- Open: A wound in which tissues are exposed to the air.
- Penetrating: Disruption of the body surface and extension into the underlying tissue.
- Perforating: A wound with an exit and an entry, such as a gunshot wound.
- Puncture: A wound formed when something goes through the skin and into the body tissues. This wound has a very small opening, but can be very deep.

The chance of a wound becoming infected depends on the nature, size, and depth of the wound, its proximity to and involvement of nonsterile areas, such as the skin and gastrointestinal (GI) tract, the opportunity for organisms from the environment to enter the wound, and the immunologic, nutritional, and general health status of the person. In general, acute (sudden onset) wounds are more prone to infection than chronic (long-lasting) wounds. Wounds with a large loss of body surface, such as abrasions, are also easily infected. Puncture wounds can permit the growth of microorganisms because there is a break in the skin with minimal bleeding; they are also difficult to clean. Deep wounds, closed off from oxygen, are an ideal breeding environment for anaerobic infections. Foul-smelling odors, gas, or dead tissue at the infection site are signs of an infection caused by anaerobic bacteria. Surgical wounds can also cause infection by introducing bacteria from one body compartment into another.

Diagnosing infection in a wound may be difficult. One of the chief signs the clinician looks for is slow healing. Within hours of injury, most wounds display a release of fluid, called exudate. This fluid contains compounds that aid in healing, and is normal. It should not be present 48–72 hours after injury. Exudate indicative of infection may be thicker than the initial exudate and may also be purulent (containing pus) and foul smelling. Clinicians will look at color, consistency, and the amount of exudate to monitor early infection. In addition, infected wounds may display skin discoloration, swelling, warmth to touch, and an increase in pain.

Wound infection prevents healing, and the bacteria or yeast can spread from wounds to other body parts, including the blood. Infection in the blood is termed septicemia and can be fatal. Symptoms of a systemic infection include a fever and rise in white blood cells (WBCs), along with confusion and mental status changes in the elderly. It is important to treat the infected wound early with a regimen of antibiotics to prevent further complications.

Wound infections often contain multiple organisms, including both aerobic and anaerobic gram-positive cocci and Gram-negative bacilli and yeast. The most common pathogens isolated from wounds are *Streptococcus* group A, *Staphylococcus aureus*, *Escherichia coli*, *Proteus*, *Klebsiella*, *Pseudomonas*, *Enterobacter*, Enterococci, *Bacteroides*, *Clostridium*, *Candida*, *Peptostreptococcus*, *Fusobacterium*, and *Aeromonas*.

The tissue used for the tests is obtained by three different methods: tissue biopsy, needle aspiration, or the swab technique. The biopsy method involves the removal of tissue from the wound using a cutting sheath. The swab technique is most commonly used, but contains the least amount of specimen.

Wound specimens are cultured on both nonselective enriched and selective media. Cultures are examined each day for growth and any colonies are Gram stained and subcultured (i.e., transferred) to appropriate media. The subcultured isolates are tested via appropriate biochemical identification panels to identify the species present. In some cases sensitivity testing will also be done. Sensitivity testing exposes the grown colonies to one or more antibiotics and monitors the response. This helps determine which antibiotics will be effective at treating the infection. The selection of antibiotics for testing depends on the organism isolated.

Normal results

The initial Gram-stain result is available the same day, or in less than an hour, if requested by the doctor. An early report, known as a preliminary report, is usually available after one day. After that, preliminary reports will be posted whenever an organism is identified. Cultures showing no growth are signed out after two to three days unless a slow-growing mycobacterium or fungus is found. These organisms take several weeks to grow and are held for four to six weeks. The final report includes complete identification, an estimate of the quantity of the microorganisms, and a list of the antibiotics to which each organism is sensitive and resistant.

Risks

The physician may choose to start the person on an antibiotic before the specimen is collected for culture. This may alter results, since antibiotics in the person's system may prevent microorganisms present in the wound from growing in culture. In some cases, the patient may begin antibiotic treatment after the specimen is collected. The antibiotic chosen may or may not be appropriate for one or more organisms recovered by culture.

Clinicians must be very careful when finishing a wound culture collection to make ensure that the wound has been cleaned thoroughly and is bandaged properly. It is important to watch for bleeding and further infection from the procedure. In addition, patients may be in pain from the manipulation, so giving pain-killing drugs, such as **acetaminophen**, may be advised.

Resources

BOOKS

Dealey, Carol and Janice Cameron. *Wound Management.* Malden, MA: Blackwell, 2008.

Krasner, Diane L., George T. Rodeheaver and R. Gary Sibbald, eds. *Chronic Wound Care: a Clinical Source Book for Healthcare Professionals*, 4th Ed. Malvern, PA: HMP Communications, 2007.

Myers, Betsy A. *Wound Management: Principles and Practice*, 2nd Ed. Upper Saddle River, NJ: Pearson/Prentice Hall, 2008.

PERIODICALS

Baer, Daniel M. "Extent of Wound-Culture Work-Up." *Medical Laboratory Observer* 38.10 (Oct 2006): 39-40.

Sardina, Donna. "Is a Swab Culture Still an Acceptable Method to Culture a Wound?" *McKnight's Long-Term Care News* (Feb 2006): 8-9.

ORGANIZATIONS

The Wound Healing Society. 13355 Tenth Ave., Suite 108, Minneapolis, MN 55441-5554. [cited April 4, 2003] http://www.woundheal.org/.

Jane E. Phillips, Ph.D.
Mark A. Best, M.D.
Robert Bockstiegel

Wrist replacement

Definition

Wrist replacement surgery is performed to replace a wrist injured or damaged beyond repair. An artificial wrist joint replacement is implanted.

Purpose

Traumatic injuries or severe degenerative diseases affecting the wrist (such as osteoarthritis and rheumatoid arthritis with bony destruction) may require replacement of the painful wrist joint with an artificial wrist joint. The purpose of wrist replacement surgery is to restore wrist motion for activities of daily living and non-contact sports. A wrist replacement recovers lost strength by restoring length to the muscles and tendons of the fingers and wrist, and maintains a useful arc of motion and provides the stability required for an active life.

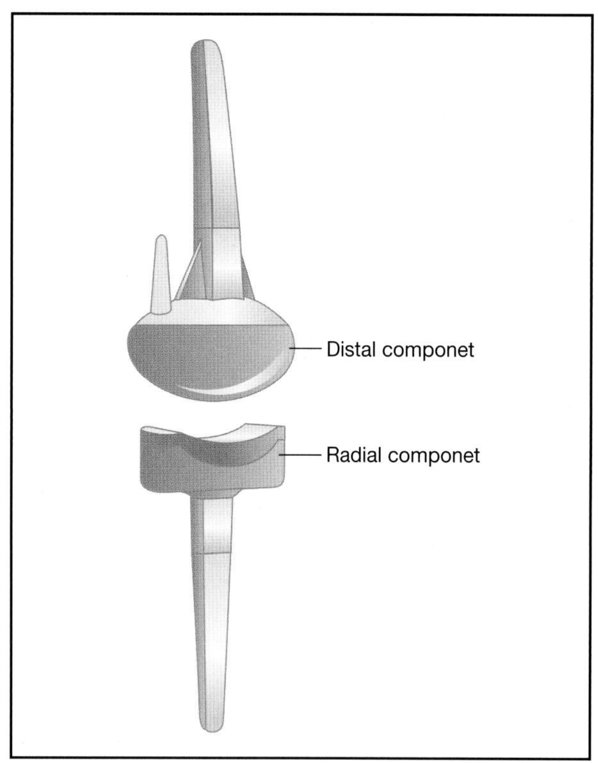

Two pieces of an artificial wrist joint. *(Illustration by Electronic Illustrators Group.)*

Description

Surgery to replace a wrist starts with an incision through the skin on the back of the wrist. The surgeon then moves the tendons extending over the back of the wrist out of the way to access the joint capsule on the back of the wrist joint, which is then opened to expose the wrist joint area. A portion of the carpal bones and the end of the radius and ulna are then removed from the wrist to allow room for the new artificial wrist joint. The bones of the hand and the radius bone of the forearm are prepared with the use of special instruments to form holes in the bones; the stems of the artificial joint components can then fit in. Next, the components are inserted into the holes. After obtaining a proper fit, the surgeon verifies the range of motion of the joint to ensure that it moves correctly. Finally, the surgeon cements the two sides of the joint and replaces the tendons back into their proper position before closing the wound.

A total wrist replacement implant consists of the following components:

- An ellipsoid head that simulates the curvature of the natural wrist joint and allows for a functional range of motion. This ensures that the patient may flex and extend the wrist and move it side-to-side.
- An offset radial stem that anchors the implant in the forearm. The special shape of this component is designed to assist the function of the tendons used to extend the wrist and to ensure the stability of the implant.
- An elongated radial tray surface with a molded bearing usually made of polyethylene. This component is required to distribute forces over the entire surface of the artificial joint.
- A fixation stem that is secured to the patient's bone to add stability and eliminate rotation of the artificial joint within the bone.
- A curved metacarpal stem that secures the artificial wrist within the hand.

KEY TERMS

Arthritis— An inflammatory condition that affects joints.

Carpal bones—Eight wrist bones arranged in two rows that articulate proximally with the radius and indirectly with the ulna, and distally with the five metacarpal bones.

Metacarpal bones—Five cylindrical bones extending from the wrist to the fingers.

Osteoarthritis—Non-inflammatory degenerative joint disease occurring mostly in older persons accompanied by pain and stiffness, especially after prolonged activity.

Radius—One of the two forearm bones. The largest portion of the radius is at the wrist joint where it articulates with the carpal bones of the hand. Above, the radius articulates with the humerus at the elbow joint.

Rheumatoid arthritis—Chronic inflammatory disease in which there is destruction of joints.

Tendon—A fibrous, strong, connective tissue that connects muscle to bone.

Ulna—One of the two bones of the forearm. The largest section articulates with the humerus at the elbow joint and the smallest portion of the ulna articulates with the carpal bones in the wrist.

Diagnosis/Preparation

The orthopedic surgeon who will perform the surgery will usually require a complete **physical examination** of the patient by the primary care physician to ensure that the patient will be in the best possible condition to undergo the surgery. The patient

WHO PERFORMS THE PROCEDURE AND WHERE IS IT PERFORMED?

Wrist replacement surgery is performed by an orthopedic surgeon in an orthopedic hospital or in a specialized clinic.

QUESTIONS TO ASK THE DOCTOR

- Will the surgery restore my wrist flexibility?
- How long will rehabilitation require?
- What are the chances of infection?
- Is alternative treatment available?
- How much wrist replacement surgery do you perform each year?
- What appearance will my wrist have after surgery?

may also need to see the physical therapist responsible for managing rehabilitation after wrist replacement. The therapist prepares the patient before surgery to ensure readiness for rehabilitation post-surgery. The purpose of the preoperative examination is also for the physician to prerecord a baseline of information that will include measurements of the patient's current pain levels, functional wrist capacity, and the range of motion and strength of each hand.

Before surgery, patients are advised to take all of their normal medications, with the exception of blood thinners such as **aspirin**, ibuprofen, and other anti-inflammatory drugs that may cause greater blood loss during surgery. Patients may eat as they please the night before surgery, including solid food, until midnight. After midnight, patients should not eat or drink anything unless told otherwise by their doctor.

Aftercare

Following surgery, the patient's wrist, hand, and lower arm are placed into a bulky bandage and a splint. A small plastic tube may be inserted to drain any blood that gathers under the incision to prevent excessive swelling (hematoma). The tube is usually removed within 24 hours. Sutures may be removed 10–14 days after surgery.

Risks

Some of the most common risks associated with wrist replacement surgery are:

- Infection. Infection can be a very serious complication following wrist replacement surgery. Infection following wrist replacement occurs in approximately 1–2% of cases. Some infections may appear before the patient leaves the hospital, while others may not become apparent for months, or even years, after surgery.
- Loosening. There is also a risk that the artificial joints may eventually fail, due to a loosening process where the metal or cement meets the bone. There have been great advances in extending how long an artificial joint will last, but most will eventually loosen and require revision surgery. The risk of loosening is much greater in younger, more active people. A loose artificial wrist is a problem because of the resulting pain. Once the pain becomes unbearable, another operation is usually required to either revise the wrist replacement or perform a wrist fusion.
- Nerve injury. All of the nerves and blood vessels that go to the hand travel across the wrist joint. Wrist replacement surgery is performed very close to these structures, introducing a risk of injury either to the nerves or the blood vessels.

Normal results

Wrist replacement surgery often succeeds at restoring wrist function. On average, a wrist replacement is expected to last for 10–15 years.

Alternatives

An alternative to wrist replacement is wrist fusion (arthrodesis). Wrist fusion surgery eliminates pain by allowing the bones that make up the joint to grow together, or fuse, into one solid bone. The surgery reduces pain, but also reduces the patient's ability to move the wrist. Wrist fusions were very common before the invention of artificial joints, and they are still performed often.

Resources

BOOKS

Browner, B. D., et al. *Skeletal Trauma: Basic Science, Management, and Reconstruction*, 3rd ed. Philadelphia: Elsevier, 2003.

Canale, S. T., ed. *Campbell's Operative Orthopaedics*, 10th ed. St. Louis: Mosby, 2003.

DeLee, J. C., and D. Drez. *DeLee and Drez's Orthopaedic Sports Medicine*, 2nd ed. Philadelphia: Saunders, 2005.

ORGANIZATIONS

The American Academy of Orthopaedic Surgeons (AAOS). 6300 North River Road, Rosemont, Illinois 60018-4262. (847) 823-7186; (800) 346-AAOS. http://www.aaos.org (accessed April 18, 2008).

OTHER

"Wrist Replacement." *University of Maryland Information Page*. http://www.wristreplacement.com/ (accessed April 18, 2008).

"Wrist Joint Replacement (Arthroplasty)." AAOS. http://orthoinfo.aaos.org/topic.cfm?topic=A00019 (accessed April 18, 2008).

Monique Laberge, PhD

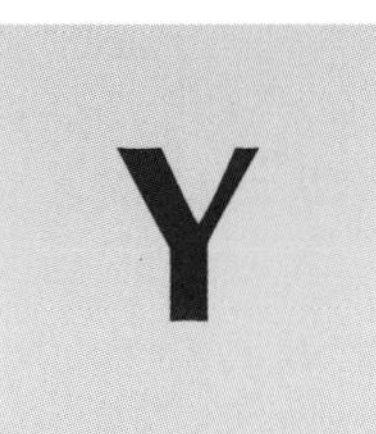

YAG laser capsulotomy *see* **Laser posterior capsulotomy**

ORGANIZATIONS

A

AARP. 601 E Street NW, Washington, DC 20049. (888) 687-2277. http://www.aarp.org.

Academic Orthopaedic Society (AOS). 6300 N. River Rd., Suite 505, Rosemont, IL 60018. (847) 318-7330. http://www.a-o-s.org/.

Academy of General Dentistry, 211 East Chicago Avenue, Chicago, IL 60611. (312) 440-4300. http://www.agd.org.

Accreditation Association for Ambulatory Health Care (AAAHC). 3201 Old Glenview Road, Suite 300, Wilmette, IL 60091-2992. (847) 853-6060. http://www.aahc.org.

Action on Smoking and Health. 2013 H Street, NW, Washington, DC 20006. (202) 659-4310. http://ash.org.

Agency for Health Care Policy and Research (AHCPR), Publications Clearinghouse. P.O. Box 8547, Silver Spring, MD, 20907. (800) 358-9295. http://www/ahcpr.gov.

Agency for Healthcare Research and Quality (AHRQ). 540 Gaither Road, Rockville, MD 20850. (301) 427-1364. http://www.ahrq.gov/.

Alan Guttmacher Institute. 1302 Connecticut Ave., NW, Suite 700, Washington, DC 20036. (202) 296-4012 or toll free (877) 823-0262. http://www.guttmacher.org.

Alden March Bioethics Institute. 47 New Scotland Avenue, MC 153, Albany, NY 12208-3478. (518) 262-6082. http://bioethics.org.

Alexander Graham Bell Association for the Deaf. 3417 Volta Place NW, Washington, DC 20007. (202) 337-5220. http://www.agbell.org.

ALS Association. 27001 Agoura Road, Suite 150 Calabasas Hills, CA 91301-5104. (800) 782-4747. http://www.alsa.org.

Alzheimer's Association. 225 N. Michigan Ave., Fl. 17, Chicago, IL 60601-7633. (312) 335-8700, (800) 272-3900. Fax: (866) 699-1246. Email: info@alz.org. http://www.alz.org.

America's Blood Centers. 725 15th St., NW, Suite 700, Washington, DC 20005. (202) 393-5725. http://www.americasblood.org.

America's Health Insurance Plans, 601 Pennsylvania Avenue, NW, South Building, Suite 500, Washington, DC 20004, Phone: (202) 778-3200. Fax: (202) 331-7487. http://www.ahip.org/.

American Academy for Thoracic Surgery. 900 Cummings Center, Suite 221-U, Beverly, Massachusetts 01915. (978)927-8330. Fax: (978)524-8890. http://www.aats.org.

American Academy of Allergy, Asthma and Immunology. 611 East Wells Street, Milwaukee, WI 53202. Telephone: (414) 272–6071. Web site:. http://www.aaaai.org.

American Academy of Anesthesiologist Assistants. 2209 Dickens Road, Richmond, VA 23230-2005. (804) 565-6353, (866) 328-5858. Fax: (804) 822-0090. http://www.anesthetist.org.

American Academy of Audiology. 11730 Plaza America Drive, Suite 300, Reston, VA 20190. (703) 790-8466. http://www.audiology.org.

American Academy of Cosmetic Surgery. 737 N. Michigan Ave., Suite 820, Chicago, IL 60611. (312) 981-6760. http://www.cosmeticsurgery.org.

American Academy of Cosmetic Surgery. 737 North Michigan Avenue, Suite 820, Chicago, IL 60611-5405. (312) 981-6760. http://www.cosmeticsurgery.org.

American Academy of Dermatology Association. 1350 I Street NW, Suite 880, Washington, DC 20005. (202) 842-3555. http://www.aadassociation.org/.

American Academy of Dermatology. 930 East Woodfield Rd., PO Box 4014, Schaumburg, IL 60168. (847) 330-0230 or (866) 503-SKIN. http://www.aad.org.

American Academy of Emergency Medicine (AAEM). 611 East Wells Street, Milwaukee, WI 53202. (800) 884-2236. http://www.aaem.org.

American Academy of Facial Plastic and Reconstructive Surgery (AAFPRS). 310 South Henry Street, Alexandria, VA 22314. (703) 299-9291. http://www.facemd.org.

American Academy of Family Physicians. 11400 Tomahawk Creek Parkway, Leawood, KS 66211-2672. (913) 906-6000. Email: fp@aafp.org. http://www.aafp.org.

American Academy of Hospice and Palliative Medicine (AAHPM). 4700 West Lake Avenue, Glenview, IL 60025-1485. (847) 375-4712. http://www.aahpm.org.

American Academy of Implant Dentistry. 211 E. Chicago Avenue, Suite 750, Chicago, IL 60611. (312) 335-1550. Fax: (312) 335-9090. http://www.aaid-implant.org.

American Academy of Medical Acupuncture (AAMA). 4929 Wilshire Boulevard, Suite 428, Los Angeles, CA 90010. (323) 937-5514. http://www.medicalacupuncture.org.

American Academy of Neurological and Orthopaedic Surgeons (AANOS). 2300 South Rancho Drive, Suite 202, Las Vegas, NV 89102. (702) 388-7390. http://www.aanos.org.

American Academy of Neurology. 1080 Montreal Avenue, St. Paul, Minnesota 55116. (651) 695-1940. Fax: (651) 695-2791. Email: info@aan.org. http://www.aan.com/.

American Academy of Ophthalmology. 655 Beach Street, P.O. Box 7424, San Francisco, CA 94120-7424. http://www.aao.org.

American Academy of Orthopaedic Surgeons (AAOS). 6300 North River Road, Rosemont, IL 60018. (847) 823-7186 or (800) 346-AAOS. http://www.aaos.org.

American Academy of Otolaryngology—Head and Neck Surgery. One Prince Street, Alexandria, VA 22314. (703) 806-4444. www.entnet.org.

American Academy of Pediatric Dentistry. 211 East Chicago Avenue, Ste. 700, Chicago, IL 60611-2616. (312) 337- 2169. Fax: (312) 337-6329. http://www.aapd.org.

American Academy of Pediatric Ophthalmology and Strabismus (AAPOS). P.O. Box 193832, San Francisco, CA 94119-3832. (415) 561-8505. Fax: (415) 561-8531. http://www.aapos.org/ [accessed May 16, 2008].

American Academy of Pediatrics (AAP), 141 Northwest Point Boulevard, Elk Grove Village, IL 60007-1098. (847) 434-4000. Fax: (847) 434-8000. Email: kidsdoc @aap.org. http://www.aap.org/default.htm.

American Academy of Sleep Medicine. One Westbrook Corporate Center, Suite 920, Westchester, IL 60154. (708) 492-0930. http://www.aasmnet.org.

American Academy of Wound Management. 1255 23rd St., NW, Washington, DC 20037. (202) 521-0368. http://www.aawm.org.

American Association for Accreditation of Ambulatory Surgery Facilities (AAAASF). 1202 Allanson Road, Mundelein, IL 60060. (888) 545-5222.

American Association for Cardiovascular and Pulmonary Rehabilitation (AACVPR). 7600 Terrace Avenue, Suite 203, Middleton, Wisconsin 53562. (608) 831-6989. Email: aacvpr@tmahq.com. http://www.aacvpr.org.

American Association for Clinical Chemistry. 1850 K Street, NW, Suite 625, Washington, DC 20006. (800) 892-1400. http://www.aacc.org.

American Association for Hand Surgery. 20 North Michigan Avenue, Suite 700, Chicago, IL 60602. (321) 236-3307; Fax: (312) 782-0553. Email: contact @handssurgery.org. http://www.handsurgery.org.

American Association for Respiratory Care (AARC). 11030 Ables Lane, Dallas, TX 75229. (972) 243-2272. Email: info@aarc.org. http://www.aarc.org.

American Association for the Surgery of Trauma. 633 N Saint Clair St, Suite 2400, Chicago, Illinois 60611. (312)202-5252, (800)789-4006. Fax: (312)202-5013. http://www.aast.org/index.aspx.

American Association for Thoracic Surgery (AATS). 900 Cummings Center, Suite 221-U, Beverly, MA 01915. (978) 927-8330. Fax: (978) 524-8890. Email: aats@prri.com. www.aats.org.

American Association for Vascular Surgery (AAVS). 900 Cummings Center, #221-U, Beverly, MA 01915. www.aavs.vascularweb.org.

American Association of Ambulatory Surgical Centers (AAASC). P. O. Box 23220, San Diego, CA 92193. (800) 237-3768. http://www.aaasc.org.

American Association of Blood Banks (AABB). 8101 Glenbrook Road, Bethesda, MD 20814-2749. (301) 907-6977 Fax: (301) 907-6895. http://www.aabb.org.

American Association of Clinical Endocrinologists (AACE). 1000 Riverside Ave., Suite 205, Jacksonville, FL 32204. (904) 353-7878. http://www.aace.com/.

American Association of Critical Care Nurses (ACCN). 101 Columbia, Aliso Viejo, CA 92656-4109. (800) 889-AACN [(800) 889-2226] or (949) 362-2000. http://www.aacn.org.

American Association of Endocrine Surgeons (AAES). MetroHealth Medical Center, H920, 2500 MetroHealth Drive, Cleveland, OH 44109-1908. (216) 778-4753. http://www.endocrinesurgeons.org.

American Association of Endodontists, 211 E. Chicago Ave., Suite 1100, Chicago, IL 60611-2691. (800) 872-3636 or (312) 266-7255. Fax: (866) 451-9020 or (312) 266-9867. Email: info@aae.org. http://www.aae.org.

American Association of Gynecologic Laparoscopists. 6757 Katella Avenue. Cypress, CA, 90630-5105. (800) 554-AAGL, (800) 554-2245, (714) 503-6200. http://www.aagl.org/.

American Association of Hip and Knee Surgeons (AAHKS). 704 Florence Drive, Park Ridge, IL 60068-2104. (847) 698-1200. hhtp://. www.aahks.org.

The American Association of Immunologists (AAI). 9650 Rockville Pike, Bethesda, MD 20814. (301) 634-7178. www.12.17.12.70/aai/default/asp..

American Association of Kidney Patients. 3505 E. Frontage Rd., Suite 315, Tampa, FL 33607. (800) 749-2257. Fax: 813-636-8122. Email: info@aakp.org. http://www.aakp.org.

American Association of Managed Care Nurses. 4435 Waterfront Drive, Suite 101, Glen Allen, VA 23060. (804) 747-9698. http://www.aamcn.org/.

American Association of Neurological Surgeons. 5550 Meadowbrook Drive, Rolling Meadows, IL 60008. (888) 566-AANS (2267). Fax: (847) 378-0600. Email: info@aans.org. http://www.neurosurgery.org/aans/index.asp.

American Association of Neuromuscular and Electrodiagnostic Medicine (AANEM). 421 First Avenue SW, Suite 300 East, Rochester, MN 55902. (507) 288–0100. Fax: (507) 288–1225. Email: aanem@aanem.org. http://www.aanem.org/index.cfm.

American Association of Nurse Anesthetists (AANA). 222 South Prospect Avenue, Park Ridge, IL 60068-4001.

(847) 692-7050; Fax: (847) 692-6968. Email: info@aana.com. http://www.aana.com.
American Association of Oral and Maxillofacial Surgeons. 9700 West Bryn Mawr Avenue, Rosemont, IL 60018-5701. (847) 678-6200. http://www.aaoms.org.
American Association of Orthopaedic Surgeons. http://www.aaos.org/.
American Association of Retired Persons (AARP). 601 E. Street NW, Washington, DC 20049. (800) 424-3410,. http://www.aarp.org/.
American Association of Retired Persons. 601 E. Street NW, Washington, DC 20049. (888) 687-2277. http://www.aarp.org.
American Association of Tissue Banks. 1320 Old Chain Bridge Road, Suite 450, McLean, VA 22101. (703) 827-9582. Fax: (703) 356-2198. Email: aatb@aatb.org. http://www.aatb.org.
American Bar Association. 321 N Clark St., Chicago, IL 60610. 800-285-2221. http://www.abanet.org/home.html.
American Board of Anesthesiology. 4101 Lake Boone Trail, Suite 510, Raleigh, NC 27607-7506. (919) 881-2570. Fax: (919) 881-2575. http://www.theaba.org.
American Board of Medical Specialties (ABMS). 1007 Church St., Suite 404, Evanston, IL 60201. (866) ASK-ABMS. (847) 491-9091. http://www.abms.org.
American Board of Neurological Surgery. 6550 Fannin Street, Suite 2139 Houston, TX 77030. (713) 441-6015. http://www.abns.org.
The American Board of Obstetrics and Gynecology. 2915 Vine Street, Suite 300, Dallas, TX 75204. (214) 871-1619; Fax: (214) 871-1943. Email: info@abog.org. http://www.abog.org.
American Board of Ophthalmology. 111 Presidential Boulevard, Suite 241, Bala Cynwyd, PA 19004-1075. (610) 664-1175. info@abop.org. http://www.abop.org.
American Board of Oral and Maxillofacial Surgery. 625 North Michigan Avenue, Suite 1820, Chicago, IL 60611. (312) 642-0070; FAX: (312) 642-8584. www.aboms.org.
American Board of Plastic Surgery. 7 Penn Center, Suite 400, 1635 Market St., Philadelphia, PA 19103-2204. (215) 587-9322. http://www.abplsurg.org(accessed March 11, 2008).
American Board of Surgery. 1617 John F. Kennedy Boulevard, Suite 860, Philadelphia, PA 19103. (215) 568-4000. Fax: (215) 563-5718. http://www.absurgery.org.
American Board of Surgery. 1617 John F. Kennedy Blvd., Suite 860, Philadelphia, PA 19103-1847. (215) 568-4000. Fax: (215) 563-5718. http://www.absurgery.org.
American Board of Urology (ABU). 2216 Ivy Road, Suite 210, Charlottesville, VA 22903. (434) 979-0059. http://www.abu.org.
American Board of Vascular Surgery (ABVS). 900 Cummings Center. #221-U Beverly, MA 01915. http://abvs.org.
American Burn Association. 625 North Michigan Avenue, Suite 1530, Chicago, IL 60611. (312) 642-9260. www.ameriburn.org.
American Cancer Society. 1875 Connecticut Avenue, NW, Suite 730, Washington, DC 20009. (800) ACS-2345. http://www.cancer.org.
American Chiropractic Association. 1701 Clarendon Blvd., Arlington, VA 22209. (800) 986-4636. http://www.amerchiro.org.
American Chronic Pain Association (ACPA). P.O. Box 850, Rocklin, CA 95677-0850. (800) 533-3231. http://www.theacpa.org/index.asp.
American Cleft Palate-Craniofacial Association. 104 South Estes Drive, Suite 204, Chapel Hill, NC 27514. (919) 933-9044. www.cleftline.org.
American College of Cardiology. Heart House, 2400 N Street, NW, Washington, DC 20037. (202) 375-6000. http://www.acc.org.
American College of Chest Physicians. 3300 Dundee Road, Northbrook, IL 60062-2348. (847) 498-1400. http://www.chestnet.org.
American College of Clinical Pharmacology. 3 Ellinwood Court, New Hartford, NY 13413-1105. (315) 768-6117. Fax: (315) 768-6119. http://www.accp1.org.
American College of Clinical Pharmacy. 13000 W. 87th St. Parkway, Lenexa KS 66215-4530. (913) 492-3311. Fax: (913) 492-0088. Email: accp@accp.com. http://www.accp.com.
American College of Emergency Physicians (ACEP). 1125 Executive Circle, Irving, TX 75038-2522. (800) 798-1822 or (972) 550-0911. http://www.acep.org/.
American College of Eye Surgeons. 2665 Oak Ridge Court, Suite A, Fort Myers, FL 33901. (239) 275-8881. http://www.aces-abes.org/.
American College of Foot and Ankle Surgeons. 8725 West Higgins Road, Suite 555, Chicago, IL 60631-2724. (773) 693-9300, (800) 421-2237. Email: info@acfas.org. http://www.acfas.org.
American College of Gastroenterology. P.O. Box 342260, Bethesda, MD 20827-2260. (301) 263-9000. http://www.acg.gi.org.
American College of Healthcare Executives. One North Franklin, Suite 1700, Chicago, IL 60606-4425. (312) 424-2800. Fax: 312-424-0023. http://www.ache.org/.
American College of Nurse Practitioners. 503 Capitol Ct. NE #300, Washington, DC 20002. (202) 546-4825. acnp@nurse.org.
American College of Nurse-Midwives. 8403 Colesville Road, Suite 1550, Silver Spring, MD 20910. (240) 485-1800. http://www.midwife.org.
American College of Obstetricians and Gynecologists. 409 12th St., SW, P.O. Box 96920, Washington, DC 20090-6920. (202) 638-5577. http://www.acog.org.
American College of Phlebology. 100 Webster Street, Suite 101, Oakland, CA 94607-3724. (510) 834-6500. http://www.phlebology.org.
American College of Physicians—American Society of Internal Medicine. Washington Office: 2011 Pennsylvania Avenue NW, Suite 800, Washington, DC 20006-1837. (202) 261-4500 or (800) 338-2746. http://www.acponline.org.

American College of Physicians. 190 N. Independence Mall West, Philadelphia, PA 19106-1572. (800) 523-1546, x2600 or (215) 351-2600. http://www.acponline.org.

American College of Physicians. 190 N. Independence Mall West, Philadelphia, PA 19106-1572. (215) 351-2400, (800) 523-1546. http://www.acponline.org.

American College of Radiology. 1891 Preston White Drive, Reston, VA 20191-4397. (800) 227-5463. (703) 648-8900. http://www.acr.org.

American College of Sports Medicine. 401 West Michigan Street, Indianapolis, IN 46202-3233 (Mailing Address: P.O. Box 1440, Indianapolis, IN 46206-1440). (317) 637-9200. Fax: (317) 634-7817. http://www.acsm.org.

American College of Surgeons. 633 N. Saint Clair Street, Chicago, IL 60611-3231. (312) 202-5000. Fax: (312) 202-5001. Email: postmaster@facs.org. http://www.facs.org.

American Council on Exercise (ACE). 4851 Paramount Drive, San Diego, CA 92123. (888) 825-3636. http://www.acefitness.org/default.aspx.

American CPR Training. 444 Sante Fe Drive #127, Encinitas, CA 92024-5134. (760) 944-1048. http://www.cpr-training-classes.com.

American Dental Association. 211 E. Chicago Avenue, Chicago, IL 60611. (312) 440-2500. Fax: (312) 440-7494. http://www.ada.org.

American Diabetes Association. National Call Center. 1701 North Beauregard Street, Alexandria, VA 22311. (800) 342-2383. Email: AskADA@diabetes.org. http://www.diabetes.org.

American Dietetic Association. Headquarters: 120 South Riverside Plaza, Suite 2000. Chicago, IL 60606-6995. (800) 877-1600. Washington, D.C., Office: 1120 Connecticut Avenue NW, Suite 480. Washington, D.C. 20036. (800) 877-0877. http://www.eatright.org.

American Epilepsy Society. 342 North Main Street, West Hartford, CT 06117-2507. (860) 586-7505. http://www.aesnet.org/.

The American Fertility Association. 305 Madison Avenue Suite 449, New York, NY 10165. (888) 917-3777. http://www.afafamilymatters.com/.

American Gastroenterological Association (AGA). 4930 Del Ray Avenue, Bethesda, MD 20814. (301) 654-2055. Fax: (301) 654-5920. http://www.gastro.org.

American Health Lawyers Association. Suite 600, 1025 Connecticut Avenue NW, Washington, DC 20036-5405. (202) 833-1100. http://www.healthlawyers.org.

American Hearing Research Foundation. 8 S. Michigan Avenue, Suite 814, Chicago, IL 60603. (312) 726-9670. http://www.american-hearing.org.

American Heart Association (AHA). 7272 Greenville Ave. Dallas, TX 75231. (800) 242-8721 or (214) 373-6300. http://www.americanheart.org.

American Herbal Products Association. 8484 Georgia Avenue, Suite 370, Silver Spring, MD 20910. (301) 588-1171. http://www.ahpa.org.

American Hospital Association (AHA). One North Franklin, Chicago, IL 60606-3421. (312) 422-3000 fax: (312) 422-4796. http://www.aha.org.

American Institute of Ultrasound in Medicine. 14750 Sweitzer Lane, Suite 100, Laurel, MD 20707-5906. (301) 498-4100 or (800) 638-5352. http://www.aium.org.

American Kidney Fund (AKF). 6110 Executive Boulevard, Suite 1010. Rockville, MD 20852. (800) 638-8299, (301) 881-3052. Email: helpline@akfinc.org. http://www.akfinc.org.

American Lithotripsy Society. 305 Second Avenue, Suite 200, Waltham, MA 02451.

American Liver Foundation. 75 Maiden Lane, Suite 603, New York, NY. 10038. (800) 465-4837 or (888) 443-7872. Fax: (212) 483.8179. Email: info@liverfoundation.org. http://www.liverfoundation.org.

American Lung Association and American Thoracic Society. 1740 Broadway, New York, NY 10019-4374. (800) 586-4872 or (212) 315-8700. http://www.lungusa.org and. http://www.thoracic.org.

American Medical Association. 515 N. State Street, Chicago, IL 60610. (312) 464-5000. http://www.ama-assn.org.

American Medical Informatics Association. 4915 St. Elmo Avenue, Suite 401, Bethesda, MD 20814. (301) 657-1291. Fax: (301) 657-1296. http://www.amia.org.

American Medical Technologists. 710 Higgins Road, Park Ridge, IL 60068-5765. (847) 823-5169. www.amt1.com.

American Nurses Association. 8515 Georgia Avenue, Suite 400, Silver Spring, MD 20910. (800) 274-4ANA (4262). http://www.nursingworld.org.

American Obesity Association. 1250 24th Street, NW, Suite 300, Washington, DC 20037. (202) 776-7711. http://www.obesity.org.

American Optometric Association. 243 North Lindbergh Blvd., St. Louis, MO 63141. (314) 991-4100. http://www.aoanet.org.

American Orthopaedic Foot & Ankle Society. 2517 Eastlake Avenue East, Seattle, WA 98102. http://www.aofas.org.

American Osteopathic Association (AOA). 142 East Ontario Street, Chicago, IL 60611. (800) 621-1773 or (312) 202-8000. http://www.aoa-net.org.

American Osteopathic College of Otolaryngology—Head and Neck Surgery. 405 W. Grand Avenue, Dayton, OH 45405. (937) 222-8820 or (800) 455-9404. Fax: (937) 222-8840. Email: info@aocoohns.org.

American Osteopathic College of Radiology. 119 East Second St., Milan, MO 63556. (660) 265-4011. www.aocr.org.

American Pain Society. 4700 West Lake Ave., Glenview, IL 60025. (847) 375-4715. http://www.ampainsoc.org.

American Pediatric Surgical Association (APSA). 60 Revere Drive, Suite 500, Northbrook, Il 60062. (847) 480-9576. Fax: (847) 480-9282 Email: eapsa@eapsa.org.

The American Physical Therapy Association (APTA). 1111 North Fairfax Street, Alexandria, VA 22314. (703) 684-APTA or (800) 999-2782. http://www.apta.org.

American Podiatric Medical Association. 9312 Old Georgetown Road, Bethesda, MD 20814-1621. (301) 581-9200. http://www.apma.org.

American Podiatric Medical Association. 9312 Old Georgetown Road, Bethesda, MD 20814. (301) 581-9200. http://www.apma.org.

American Professional Wound Care Association (APWCA). 853 Second Street Pike, Suite #A-1, Richboro, PA 18954. (215) 364-4100. Fax: (215) 364-1146. Email: wounds@apwca.org. http://www.apwca.org.

American Prostate Society. P. O. Box 870, Hanover, MD 21076. (800) 308-1106. http://www.ameripros.org.

American Psychiatric Association. 1000 Wilson Boulevard, Suite 1825, Arlington, VA 22209-3901. (703) 907-7300. Email: apa@psych.org. http://www.psych.org.

American Psychological Association. 750 First Street, NE, Washington, DC 20002-4242. (202) 336-5500, (800) 374-2721. http://www.apa.org.

American Red Cross National Headquarters. 2025 E Street, NW. Washington, DC 20006. (703) 206-6000. http://www.redcross.org.

American Registry of Diagnostic Medical Sonographers (ARDMS). 51 Monroe Street, Plaza East One, Rockville, MD 20850-2400. (800) 541-9754, (301) 738-8401. Fax: (301) 738-0312. http://www.ardms.org.

American Shoulder and Elbow Surgeons. 6300 N. River Road, Suite 727, Rosemont, IL 60018. (847) 698-1629. http://www.ases-assn.org.

American Sleep Apnea Association. 1424 K Street NW, Suite 302, Washington, DC 20005. (202) 293-3650. http://www.sleepapnea.org.

American Society for Aesthetic Plastic Surgery. 11081 Winners Circle, Los Alamitos, CA 90720. (800) 364-2147 or (562) 799-2356. http://www.surgery.org.

American Society for Bariatric Surgery. 7328 West University Avenue, Suite F, Gainesville, FL 32607. (352) 331-4900. http://www.asbs.org.

American Society for Blood and Marrow Transplantation (ASBMT). 85 W. Algonquin Road, Suite 550 Arlington Heights, IL 60005. (847) 427-0224. mail@asbmt.org.

American Society for Bone and Mineral Research. 2025 M Street, NW, Suite 800, Washington, DC 20036-3309. (202) 367-1161. http://www.asbmr.org/.

American Society for Clinical Laboratory Science. 6701 Democracy Boulevard, Suite 300. Bethesda, MD 20817. (301) 657-2768. Fax: (301) 657-2909. Email: ascls@ascls.org. http://www.ascls.org.

The American Society for Clinical Pathology. 1225 New York Ave., NW, Suite 250, Washington, DC 20005. (202) 347-4450. http://www.ascp.org.

American Society for Colposcopy and Cervical Pathology. 152 West Washington Street, Hagerstown, MD 21740. (301) 733-3640, (800) 787-7227. http://www.asccp.org.

American Society for Dermatologic Surgery (ASDS). 5550 Meadowbrook Dr., Suite 120, Rolling Meadows, IL 60008. (847) 956-0900. Fax: 8470-956-0999. http://www.asds-net.org.

American Society for Gastrointestinal Endoscopy (ASGE). 1520 Kensington Rd., Suite 202, Oak Brook, IL 60523. (630) 573-0600, (866) 353-ASGE (2743). Fax: (630) 573-0691. Email: info@asge.org. http://www.asge.org.

American Society for Laser Medicine and Surgery. 2404 Stewart Square, Wausau, WI 54401.(715) 845-9283. http://www.aslms.org.

American Society for Metabolic and Bariatric Surgery. 100 SW 75th Street, Suite 201, Gainesville, FL 32607. (352) 331-4900. http://www.asbs.org.

American Society for Microbiology. 1752 N Street, NW, Washington, DC 20036. (202) 737-3600. http://www.asm.org.

American Society for Mohs Surgery. Private Mail Box 391, 5901 Warner Avenue, Huntington Beach, CA 92649-4659. (714) 840-3065. (800) 616-ASMS (2767). www.mohssurgery.org.

American Society for Reconstructive Microsurgery. 20 North Michigan Ave., Suite 700, Chicago, IL 60602. (312) 456-9579. http://www.microsurg.org.

American Society for Reproductive Medicine. 1209 Montgomery Highway, Birmingham, AL 35216-2809. (205) 978-5000. http://www.asrm.com.

American Society for Surgery of the Hand. 6300 North River Road, Suite 600, Rosemont, IL 60018-4256. (847) 384-8300. www.assh.org.

The American Society of Anesthesiologists (ASA). 520 North Northwest Highway, Park Ridge, IL 60068-2573. (847) 825-5586. Fax: (847) 825-1692. Email: mail@asahq.org. http://www.asahq.org.

American Society of Bariatric Physicians (ASBP). 5453 East Evans Place, Denver, CO 80222-5234. (303) 770-2526. http://www.asbp.org.

American Society of Cataract and Refractive Surgery (ASCRS). 4000 Legato Road, Suite 700, Fairfax, VA 22033. (703) 591-2220. Fax: (703) 591-0614. http://www.ascrs.org.

American Society of Clinical Oncology (ASCO). 1900 Duke Street, Suite 200, Alexandria, VA 22314. (703) 299-0150. www.asco.org.

American Society of Clinical Pathologists. Corporate Headquarters: 33 West Monroe Street, Suite 1600. Chicago, IL 60603. (312) 541-4999. Fax: (312) 541-4998. Board of Registry (Certification Maintenance, Exam Application and Eligibility, International Certification): (800) 267-2727, option 2, 2. Fax: (312) 541-4845. Email: bor@ascp.org. Indianapolis (Check-Path, Cytology, GYN, Non-GYN, Proficiency Testing): 8900 Keystone Crossing, Suite 620. Indianapolis, IN 46240. (317) 569-9470. Fax: (317) 569-0221. Washington (Advocacy, ePolicy, Government Relations): 1225 New York Avenue, NW, Suite 250. Washington, DC 20005. (202) 347-4450. Fax: (202) 347-4453. http://www.ascp.org.

American Society of Colon and Rectal Surgeons. 85 W. Algonquin Rd., Suite 550. Arlington Heights, IL 60005. (847) 290-9184. Fax: (847) 290-9203. Email: ascrs@fascrs.org. http://www.fascrs.org.

American Society of Echocardiography. 1500 Sunday Drive, Suite 102, Raleigh, NC 27607. (919) 861-5574. http://www.asecho.org.

American Society of Electroneurodiagnostic Technologists Inc, 204 W. 7th Carroll, IA 51401. (712) 792–2978. http://www.aset.org/.

American Society of Health-System Pharmacists (ASHP). 7272 Wisconsin Avenue, Bethesda, MD 20814. (301) 657-3000; toll free: (866) 279-0681 (United States and Canada only); International: 001-301-664-8700. www.ashp.org.

American Society of Nephrology. 1725 I Street, NW, Suite 510. Washington, DC 20006. (202) 659-0599. Fax: (202) 659-0709. Email: email@asn-online.org. http://www.asn-online.org.

The American Society of Perianesthesia Nurses (ASPAN). 10 Melrose Avenue, Suite 110, Cherry Hill, NJ 08003-3696. (877) 737-9696 or (856) 616-9600. Fax: (856) 616-9601. Email: aspan@aspan.org. http://www.aspan.org.

American Society of Plastic and Reconstructive Surgeons. 444 E. Algonquin Road, Arlington Heights, IL 60005. (847) 228-9900. http://www.plasticsurgery.org.

American Society of Plastic Surgeons, Plastic Surgery Educational Foundation. 444 E. Algonquin Rd., Arlington Heights, IL 60005. Public Relations: (847) 228-9900. Email: media@plasticsurgery.org. http://www.plasticsurgery.org.

American Society of Radiologic Technologists. 15000 Central Ave. SE. Albuquerque, NM 87123-3909. (800) 444-2778, (505) 298-4500. Fax: (505) 298-5063. Email: customerinfo@asrt.org. http://www.asrt.org.

American Society of Transplant Surgeons (ASTS). 2461 South Clark St., Suite 640, Arlington, VA 22202. (703) 414-7870. http://www.asts.org.

American Society of Transplantation (AST). 15000 Commerce Parkway, Suite C. Mt.Laurel, NJ,08054. (856) 439-9986. Fax: (856) 439-9982. Email: ast@ahint.com. http://www.a-s-t.org.

American Society Parenteral and Enteral Nutrition. 8630 Fenton St., Suite 412, Silver Springs, Maryland 20910. (301) 587-6315. Fax: (301) 587-2365. www.clinnutr.org.

American Speech-Language-Hearing Association. 2200 Research Boulevard, Rockville, MD 20850-3289. (800) 638-8255. http://www.asha.org.

American Urological Association Foundation. 1000 Corporate Boulevard, Linthicum, MD 21090. 1-866-RING AUA (1-866-746-4282). (410) 689-3700. Fax: (410) 689-3800. Email: auafoundation@auafoundation.org. http://www.auafoundation.org.http://www.urologyhealth.org.

American Yoga Association. P.O. Box 19986. Sarasota, FL 34276. Email: info@americanyogaassociation.org. http://www.americanyogaassociation.org.

Anesthesia Patient Safety Foundation (APSF). Building One, Suite Two, 8007 South Meridian Street, Indianapolis, IN 46217-2922. www.apsf.org.

Applied Biometrics. 501 East Highway Thirteen, Suite 108, Burnsville, MN 55337. (952) 890-1123

Arthritis Foundation. P.O. Box 7669, Atlanta, GA 30357-0669. (800) 283-7800. http://www.arthritis.org.

Associated Jehovah's Witnesses for Reform on Blood (AJWRB). P. O. Box 190089, Boise, ID 83719-0089. http://www.ajwrb/org.

Association for Applied Psychotherapy and Biofeedback. 10200 W. 44th Avenue, Suite 304, Wheat Ridge, CO 80033. (303) 422-8436. http://www.aapb.org..

Association for Research in Otolaryngology. 19 Mantua Rd., Mt. Royal, NJ 08061. (856) 423-0041. (301) 733-3640. http://www.aro.org/index.html.

Association of periOperative Registered Nurses (AORN). 2170 South Parker Road, Suite 300. Denver, CO 80231. (800) 755-2676. (303) 755-6304. Fax: (303) 750-3212. Email: custsvc@aorn.org. http://www.aorn.org.

Association of Surgical Technologists. 6 West Dry Creek Circle, Suite 200, Littleton, CO 80120-8031. (303) 694-9130. Fax: (303) 694-9169. http://www.ast.org.

Association of Thyroid Surgeons. 717 Buena Vista St., Ventura, CA 93001. Fax: (509) 479-8678. Email: info@thyroidsurgery.org. www.thyroidsurgery.org.

Association of Women's Health, Obstetric, and Neonatal Nurses. 2000 L St., NW, Suite 740, Washington, DC 20036. (202) 261-2400, (800) 673-8499. http://www.awhonn.org.

Asthma and Allergy Foundation of America. 1125 15th Street NW, Suite 502, Washington, DC 20005. Telephone: (800) 727–8462. Web site:. http://www.aafa.org.

B

Better Hearing Institute. 515 King Street, Suite 420, Alexandria, VA 22314. (703) 684-3391.

Biofeedback Certification Institute of America. 10200 W. 44th Avenue, Suite 310, Wheat Ridge, CO 80033. (303) 420-2902. http://www.bcia.org..

BMT Infonet (Blood and Marrow Transplant Information Network). 2900 Skokie Valley Road, Suite B, Highland Park, IL 60035. (847) 433-3313, (888) 597-7674. help@bmtinfonet.org. http://www.bmtinfonet.org.

Brain Injury Association. 1608 Spring Hill Road, Suite 110, Vienna, VA 22182. (703) 761-0750. http://www.biausa.org.

Breast Cancer Network of Strength Headquarters (formerly known as Y-ME National Breast Cancer Organization). 212 W. Van Buren, Suite 1000, Chicago, IL 60607-3903. (312) 986-8338. Fax: (312) 294-8597. http://www.networkofstrength.org.

British Association of Oral and Maxillofacial Surgeons, Royal College of Surgeons. 35–43 Lincoln's Inn Fields, London, UK WC2A 3PN. www.baoms.org.uk.

C

California Association for Adult Day Services. 921 11th Street Suite 1101, Sacramento, CA 95814. (916) 552-7400. Fax: (916) 552-7404. Email: caads@caads.org. http://www.caads.org.

Canadian Association of Gastroenterology (CAG). 2902 South Sheridan Way, Oakville, ON L6J 7L6 (888) 780-0007 or (905) 829-2504. www.cag-acg.org.

Canadian Institute for Health Information/Institut canadien d' information sur la santé (CIHI). 377 Dalhousie Street, Suite 200, Ottawa, ON K1N 9N8. (613) 241-7860. http://secure.cihi.ca/cihiweb.

Canadian Ophthalmological Society (COS). 610-1525 Carling Avenue, Ottawa ON K1Z 8R9 Canada. http://www.eyesite.ca.

Canadian Prostate Cancer Network. P. O. Box 1253, Lakefield, ON K0L 2H0 Canada. (705) 652-9200. http://www.cpcn.org.

Cancer Information Service. National Cancer Institute, Public Inquiries Office. 6116 Executive Boulevard, Room 3036A. Bethesda, MD 20892-8322. (800) 4-CANCER (800-422-6237). TTY: (800) 332-8615. http://www.cancer.gov.

Cancer Research Institute. 681 Fifth Avenue, New York, NY 10022. (800) 992-2623. http://www.cancerresearch.org.

Cancercare. Health Resources and Services Administration. 5600 Fishers Lane, Rm. 14-45, Rockville, MD 20857. (301) 443-3376. (800) 813-HOPE (4673). http://www.cancercare.org.

Cardiac Arrhythmia Research and Education Foundation (C.A.R.E.). 2082 Michelson Dr. #301, Irvine, CA 92612. (800) 404–9500. www.longqt.com/.

Cardiac Electrophysiology Society. http://www.cardiaceps.org/.

Center for Biologics Evaluation and Research (CBER), U.S. Food and Drug Administration (FDA). 1401 Rockville Pike, Rockville, MD 20852-1448. (800) 835-4700 or (301) 827-1800. http://www.fda.gov/cber.

Center for Devices and Radiological Health. United States Food and Drug Administration. 1901 Chapman Ave., Rockville, MD 20857. (301) 443-4109. http://www.fda.gov/cdrh.

Center for Emergency Medicine of Western Pennsylvania. 230 McKee Place, Suite 500, Pittsburgh, PA 15213. (412) 647-5300. http://www.centerem.org.

Center for Fetal Diagnosis and Treatment, Children's Hospital of Philadelphia. 34th Street and Civic Center Boulevard, Philadelphia, PA 19104-4399. (800) IN-UTERO. http://fetalsurgery.chop.edu.

Center for Hip and Knee Replacement, Columbia University. Department of Orthopaedic Surgery, Columbia Presbyterian Medical Center, 622 West 168th Street, PH11-Center, New York, NY 10032. (212) 305-5974. www.hipnknee.org.

Center for Male Reproductive Medicine. 2080 Century Park East, Suite 907, Los Angeles, CA 90067. (310) 277-2873. www.malereproduction.com.

Center for Medicare Advocacy, P.O. Box 350, Willimantic, CT 06226. (860) 456-7790 or (202) 216-0028. http://www.medicareadvocacy.org.

Center for Uterine Fibroids, Brigham and Women's Hospital. 623 Thorn Building, 20 Shattuck Street, Boston, MA 02115. (800) 722-5520. http://www.fibroids.net.

Centers for Disease Control and Prevention (CDC). 1600 Clifton Rd, Atlanta, GA 30333. (404) 498-1515, (800) 311-3435. http://www.cdc.gov.

Centers for Disease Control and Prevention (CDC). Cancer Prevention and Control Program. 4770 Buford Highway, NE, MS K64, Atlanta, GA 30341. (888) 842-6355. http://www.cdc.gov/cancer/comments.htm.

Centers for Disease Control and Prevention (CDC). Division of Diabetes Translation, National Center for Chronic Disease Prevention and Health Promotion. TISB Mail Stop K-13, 4770 Buford Highway NE, Atlanta, GA 30341-3724. (770) 488-5080. http://www.cdc.gov/diabetes.

Centers for Disease Control and Prevention, Division of Reproductive Health. 4770 Buford Highway, NE, Mail Stop K-20, Atlanta, GA 30341-3717. (770) 488-5200. http://www.cdc.gov/reproductivehealth.

Centers for Medicare & Medicaid Services. 7500 Security Boulevard, Baltimore MD 21244-1850. (800) MEDICARE (800-633-4227). TTY: (877) 486-2048. http://www.cms.hhs.gov/.

Centre for Minimal Access Surgery (CMAS). 50 Charlton Avenue E., Hamilton, Ontario L8N 4A6 Canada. (905) 522-1155 x 5144. http://www.cmas.ca/.

Charles P. Felton National Tuberculosis Center, 2238 Fifth Avenue, First Floor, New York, NY 10037. (212)939-8254. http://www.harlemtbcenter.org/.

Children's Health Information Network. 1561 Clark Drive, Yardley, PA 19067. (215) 493-3068. http://www.tchin.org.

Children's Hospice International (CHI). 1101 King Street, Suite 360, Alexandria, VA 22314. (703) 684-0330 or (800) 2-4-CHILD. http://www.chionline.org.

Children's Organ Transplant Association, Inc. 2501 West COTA Drive, Bloomington, IN 47403. (800) 366-2682. http://www.cota.org.

The Cleveland Clinic Heart and Vascular Institute, The Cleveland Clinic Foundation. 9500 Euclid Avenue, F25, Cleveland, Ohio, 44195. (216) 445-9288. http://www.clevelandclinic.org/heartcenter.

The Cleveland Clinic Heart Center, The Cleveland Clinic Foundation. 9500 Euclid Avenue, F25, Cleveland, OH 44195. (800) 223-2273 ext. 46697 or (216) 444-6697. http://www.clevelandclinic.org/heartcenter.

The Coalition on Donation. 700 North 4th Street, Richmond, VA 23219. (804)782-4920. http://www.organtransplants.org/donor/coalition/.

College of American Pathologists. 325 Waukegan Rd., Northfield, IL 60093-2750. (800) 323-4040. http://www.cap.org/apps/cap.portal.

Colorectal Cancer Network (CCNetwork). P.O. Box 182, Kensington, MD 20895-0182. (301) 879-1500. http://clickonium.com/colorectal-cancer.net/html.

Congenital Heart Anomalies Support, Education & Resources, Inc. 2112 North Wilkins Road, Swanton, OH 43558. (419) 825-5575. http://www.csun.edu/~hfmth006/chaser.

Council for Refractive Surgery Quality Assurance. 8543 Everglade Drive, Sacramento, CA 95826-0769.

(916) 381-0769. Email: info@usaeyes.org. www.usaeyes.org.

Council on Size and Weight Discrimination (CSWD). P. O. Box 305, Mt. Marion, NY 12456. (845) 679-1209. http://www.cswd.org/index.html.

Crohn's and Colitis Foundation of America. 386 Park Ave. S., 17th Floor, New York, NY 10016. (800) 932-2423. www.ccfa.org.

D

DES Action USA. 158 S. Stanwood Rd., Columbus, OH 43209. (800) 337-9288. http://www.desaction.org.

Diabetic Retinopathy Foundation. 350 North LaSalle, Suite 800, Chicago, IL 60610. www.retinopathy.org.

Division of Blood Diseases and Resources. The National Heart, Lung and Blood Institute (NHLBI). Two Rockledge Center, Suite 10138, 6701 Rockledge Drive, MSC 7950, Bethesda, MD 20892-7950. http://www.nhlbi.nih.gov/about/dbdr.

Division of Transplantation, Health Resources and Services Administration (HRSA). 5600 Fishers Lane, Rm. 14-45, Rockville, MD 20857. 301-443-3376. http://www.organdonor.gov/.

E

e-Healthcare Solutions, Inc., 953 Route 202 North, Branchburg, N.J. 08876. (908) 203-1350. Fax: (908) 203-1307. info@e-healthcaresolutions.com. http://www.digitalhealthcare.com/.

EA/TEF Child and Family Support Connection. 111 West Jackson Blvd., Suite 1145, Chicago, IL 60604. (312) 987-9085. www.eatef.org.

Emphysema Anonymous, Inc. P.O. Box 3224, Seminole FL 34642. (813) 391–9977.

Endometriosis Association. 8585 North 76th Place, Milwaukee, WI 53223. (414) 355-2200. http://www.endometriosisassn.org.

Epilepsy Foundation of America. 8301 Professional Place, Landover MD 20785. (800) 332-1000. http://www.epilepsyfoundation.org.

The European Institute of TeleSurgery (EITS). Hôpitaux Universitaires 1, place de l'Hôpital 67091 Strasbourg Cedex, France. +33 (0)3 88 11 90 00. http://www.eits.fr/homepage.php.

Extracorporeal Life Support Organization (ELSO). 1327 Jones Dr., Ste. 101, Ann Arbor, MI 48105. (734) 998-6600. http://www.elso.med.umich.edu/.

Eye Bank Association of America. 1015 Eighteenth Street NW, Suite 1010, Washington, D.C. 20036. (202) 775-4999. http://www.restoresight.org.

F

FACES: The National Craniofacial Association. P. O. Box 11082, Chattanooga, TN 37401. (800) 332-2373. http://www.faces-cranio.org.

Federal Bureau of Investigation (FBI), Laboratory Division. J. Edgar Hoover Building, 935 Pennsylvania Avenue, NW, Washington, DC 20535-0001. www.fbi.gov/hq/lab/labhome.htm.

Federal Drug Administration (FDA), 5600 Fishers Ln., Rockville, MD 20857. (800) 532-4440. http://www.fda.gov.

Federated Ambulatory Surgery Association (FASA). 700 North Fairfax Street, #306, Alexandria, VA 22314. (703) 836-8808. http://www.fasa.org.

Federation of State Medical Boards. P.O. Box 619850, Dallas, TX 75261-9850. (817) 868-4000. Fax: (817) 868-4099. http://www.fsmb.org.

Fetal Treatment Center, University of California San Francisco. 513 Parnassus Ave., HSW 1601, San Francisco, CA 94143-0570. (800) RX-FETUS or (415) 353-8489. http://www.fetus.ucsf.edu.

Franklin Institute Science Museum. 222 North 20th Street, Philadelphia, PA, 19103. (215) 448-1200. http://sln2.fi.edu/biosci/heart.html.

G

The Glaucoma Foundation. 116 John Street, Suite 1605, New York, NY 10038. (212) 285-0080 or (800) 452-8266. Email: info@glaucomafoundation.org. http://www.glaucoma-foundation.org.

The Glaucoma Research Foundation. 490 Post Street, Suite 1427, San Francisco, CA 94102. (415) 986-3162 or (800) 826-6693. http://www.glaucoma.org.

Gynecologic Surgery Society. 2440 M Street, NW, Suite 801, Washington, DC 20037. (202) 293-2046. http://www.gynecologicsurgerysociety.org.

H

Harry Benjamin International Gender Dysphoria Association, Inc. (HBIGDA). 1300 South Second Street, Suite 180, Minneapolis, MN 55454. (612) 625-1500. http://www.hbigda.org.

Health Canada/Santé Canada. A.L. 0900C2, Ottawa, Canada K1A 0K9. (613) 957-2991. http://www.hc-sc.gc.ca.

Health Insurance Association of America. 601 Pennsylvania Avenue, NW, South Building, Washington, DC 20004-1204. (202) 778-3200. http://www.hiaa.org.

Hearing Loss Link. 2600 W. Peterson Ave., Ste. 202, Chicago, IL 60659. (312) 743-1032, (312) 743-1007 (TDD).

Hepatitis Foundation International (HFI). 504 Blick Drive, Silver Spring, MD. 20904-2901. (800) 891-0707 or (301) 622-4200. Fax: (301) 622-4702. Email: hfi@comcast.net. http://www.hepfi.org

Hospice Foundation of America. 2001 S. Street NW, Suite 300, Washington, DC 20009. (800) 854-3402. (202) 638-54191. Fax: (202) 638-5312. Email: jon@hospicefoundation.org. http://www.hospicefoundation.org.

I

ICU-USA. 29 Summerhill, Suite 100, St. Louis, MO 63017. (866) 377-4442. Email: charlie.owen@icu-usa.com. http://www.icu-usa.com.

Immune Tolerance Network (ITN). 5743 South Drexel Avenue, Suite 200, Chicago, IL 60637. (773) 834-5341. Http://www.immunetolerance.org.

Infusion Nurses Society. 315 Norwood Park South, Norwood, MA 02062. (781) 440.9408. http://www.ins1.org.

Institute for Bone and Joint Disorders. 2222 East Highland Avenue, Phoenix, AZ 85016; 602-553-3113. http://www.ibjd.com.

Institute of Medicine (IOM). The National Academies. 500 Fifth Street, NW, Washington, DC 20001. www.iom.edu.

Inter-Institutional Collaborating Network on End-of-Life Care (IICN). (415) 863-3045. http://www.growthhouse.org.

International Association for the Study of Pain (IASP). 111 Queen Anne Avenue North, Suite 501, Seattle, WA 98109-4955. (206) 283-0311. http://www.iasp-pain.org//AM/Template.cfm?Section = Home.

International Association of Laryngectomees (IAL). http://www.larynxlink.com/.

International Bariatric Surgery Registry (IBSR). University of Iowa Hospitals and Clinics, 200 Hawkins Drive, Iowa City, IA 52242. (319) 384-7359. http://www.healthcare.uiowa.edu/surgery/ibsr/.

International Bone Marrow Transplant Registry/Autologous Blood and Marrow Transplant Registry N. America. Health Policy Institute, Medical College of Wisconsin, 8701 Watertown Plank Road, P.O. Box 26509, Milwaukee, WI 53226. (414) 456-8325. ibmtr@mcw.edu.

International Cesarean Awareness Network. 1304 Kingsdale Ave., Redondo Beach, CA 90278. (310) 542-6400. http://www.ican-online.org.

International Council on Infertility Information Dissemination, Inc. P.O. Box 6836, Arlington, VA 22206. (703) 379-9178. http://www.inciid.org.

International Craniofacial Institute, Cleft Lip & Palate Treatment Center. Medical City Dallas. 7777 Forest Lane, Suite C-717, Dallas, TX 75230. (972) 566-6555, (800) 344-4068. Fax: (972) 566-6017. Email: info@craniofacial.net. http://www.craniofacial.net.

International EECP Therapists Association. P.O. Box 650005, Vero Beach, FL 32965-0005. (800) 376-3321, ext. 140. http://www.ietaonline.com.

International Foundation for Functional Gastrointestinal Disorders (IFFGD). P.O. Box 170864, Milwaukee, WI 53217-8076. (888) 964-2001 or (414) 964-1799. fax: (414) 964-7176. http://www.iffgd.org.

International Pancreas Transplant Registry (IPTR). University of Minnesota Department of Surgery, Mayo Mail Code 280, 420 Delaware Street SE, Minneapolis, MN 55455-0392. http://www.iptr.umn.edu/.

International Radiosurgery Support Association (IRSA). 3005 Hoffman Street, Harrisburg, PA 17110. (717) 260-9808. www.irsa.org.

Interstitial Cystitis Association. 51 Monroe Street, Suite 1402, Rockville, MD 20850. (301) 610-5300. http://www.ichelp.org.

J

Johns Hopkins Radiosurgery. Weinberg 1469, 600 North Wolfe Street, Baltimore, MD 21287. (410) 614-2886. www.hopkinsmedicine.org/radiosurgery/treatmentoptions/stereotacticradiosurgery.cfm.

Joint Commission (on Accreditation of Health Care Organizations). One Renaissance Blvd. Oakbrook Terrace, IL 60181. (630) 792-5000. Fax: (630) 792-5005.

K

Kaiser Family Foundation. 2400 Sand Hill Road, Menlo Park, CA 94025, Phone: (650) 854-9400. Fax: (650) 854-4800. http://www.kff.org/.

L

League of Intravenous Therapy Education. Empire Building, Suite 3, 3001 Jacks Run Road. White Oak, PA 15131. (412)-678-5025. http://www.lite.org/.

Leukemia & Lymphoma Society. 1311 Mamaroneck Avenue, White Plains, NY 10605. (914) 949-5213. Fax: (914) 949-6691. http://www.leukemia.org.

The Lymphoma Research Foundation of America. 8800 Venice Boulevard, Suite 207, Los Angeles, CA 90034. (800) 500-9976. (310) 204-7040. helpline@lymphoma.org. http://www.lymphoma.org.

M

March of Dimes Birth Defects Foundation. 1275 Mamaroneck Avenue; White Plains, NY. Telephone (914) 428-7100. http://wwwmodimes.org.

Mayo Clinic. 200 First St. S.W., Rochester, MN 55905. (507) 284-2511. http://www.mayoclinic.com.

Medline Plus a service of the National Library of Medicine and the National Institutes of Health, 8600 Rockville Pike, Bethesda, MD 20894. http://www.nlm.nih.gov/medlineplus/.

Midlife Women's Network. 5129 Logan Ave. S., Minneapolis, MN 55419. (800) 886-4354.

Midwives Alliance of North America. 611 Pennsylvania Avenue, SE, #1700, Washington, DC 20003-4303. (888) 923-MANA. http://www.mana.org.

Mitral Valve Repair Center at Mount Sinai Hospital. 1190 Fifth Avenue, New York, NY 10029 (212) 659-6820. http://www.mitralvalverepair.org.

Muscular Dystrophy Association. 3300 E. Sunrise Drive, Tucson, AZ 85718. (800) 572-1717. http://www.mdausa.org.

N

National Abortion Federation. 1660 L Street, NW, Suite 450, Washington, DC 20036. (202) 667-5881. http://www.prochoice.org.

National Accrediting Agency for Clinical Laboratory Sciences. 8410 W Bryn Mawr Ave., Suite 670, Chicago, IL 60631. (773) 714-8880. Fax: (773) 714-8886. Email: info@naacls.org. http://www.naacls.org.

National Adult Day Services Association. 85 South Washington, Suite 316, Seattle, WA 98104. (877) 745-1440. Fax: (206) 461-3218. Email: info@nadsa.org. http://www.nadsa.org.

National Alliance of Breast Cancer Organizations (NABCO). 9 East 37th Street, 10th Floor, New York, NY 10016. (888) 80-NABCO. http://www.nabco.org.

National Amputation Foundation. 40 Church Street, Malverne, NY 11565. (516) 887-3600. www.nationalamputation.org/.

National Association for Continence (NAFC). P.O. Box 1019, Charleston, SC 29402-1019. (800) BLADDER, (843) 377-0900. Fax: (843) 377-0905. Email: memberservices@nafc.org. http://www.nafc.org.

National Association for Home Care & Hospice. 228 7th Street, SE, Washington, DC 20003. (202) 547-7424. Fax: (202) 547-3540. http://www.nahc.org.

National Association for the Deaf. 814 Thayer Ave., Silver Spring, MD 20910. (301) 587-1788, (301) 587-1789 (TDD). http://www.nad.org.

National Association for Women's Health. 300 W. Adams Street, Suite 328, Chicago, IL 60606-5101. (312) 786-1468. http://www.nawh.org

National Association of Emergency Medical Technicians (NAEMT). P. O. Box 1400, Clinton, MS 39060-1400. (800) 34-NAEMT. www.naemt.org.

National Association of Insurance Commissioners, 2301 McGee Street, Suite 800, Kansas City, MO 64108. (816)842-3600. http://www.naic.org/.

National Association of Neonatal Nurses. 4700 West Lake Ave., Glenview, IL 60025-1485. (847) 375-3660 or (800) 451-3795. http://www.nann.org.

National Association to Advance Fat Acceptance (NAAFA). P.O. Box 22510, Oakland, CA 94609. (916) 558-6880. http://www.naafa.org/.

National Blood Data Resource Center (NBDRC). 8101 Glenbrook Road, Bethesda, MD 20814-2749. (301) 215-6506. http://www.nbdrc.org.

National Bone Marrow Transplant Link. 20411 W. 12 Mile Road, Suite 108, Southfield, MI 48076. (800) LINK-BMT (800-546-5268).

National Breast Cancer Coalition. 1101 17th Street, NW, Suite 1300, Washington, DC 20036. (800) 622-2838. Fax: (202) 265-6854. http://www.stopbreastcancer.org.

National Cancer Institute, Public Inquiries Office. Cancer Information Service. 6116 Executive Boulevard, Room 3036A. Bethesda, MD 20892-8322. (800) 4-CANCER (800-422-6237). TTY: (800) 332-8615. http://www.cancer.gov.

National Center for Complementary and Alternative Medicine (NCCAM) Clearinghouse. P.O. Box 7923, Gaithersburg, MD 20898. (888) 644-6226. TTY: (866) 464-3615. Fax: (866) 464-3616. http://www.nccam.nih.gov.

National Center for Health Statistics (NCHS). 3311 Toledo Road, Hyattsville, MD 20782. (800) 232-4636. http://www.cdc.gov/nchs/.

National Center for Infectious Disease, Centers for Disease Control and Prevention. Mailstop C-14, 1600 Clifton Road NE, Atlanta, GA 30333. (800) 232-4636. http://www.cdc.gov/ncidod.

National Center for Policy Analysis. 12770 Coit Rd., Suite 800, Dallas, TX 75251-1339, Phone: (972) 386-6272. Fax: (972) 386-0924 . http://www.ncpa.org.

National Center on Sleep Disorders Research. Two Rockledge Centre, Suite 10038, 6701 Rockledge Drive, MSC 7920, Bethesda, MD 20892-7920. (301) 435-0199. http://www.nhlbi.nih.gov/about/ncsdr/index.htm.

National Cholesterol Education Program: National Heart, Lung, and Blood Institute (NHLBI), National Institutes of Health. PO Box 30105, Bethesda, MD, 20824-0105. (301) 251-1222. http://www.nhlbi.nih.gov/about/ncep/.

National Committee for Quality Assurance. 1100 13th St., NW, Suite 1000, Washington, DC 20005. (202) 955-3500. http://www.ncqa.org.

National Comprehensive Cancer Network. 50 Huntingdon Pike, Suite 200, Rockledge, PA 19046. (215) 728-4788. Fax: (215) 728-3877. Email: information@nccn.org. http://www.nccn.org/.

National Diabetes Information Clearinghouse. 1 Information Way, Bethesda, MD 20892–3560. (800) 860–8747. Fax: (703) 738–4929. Email: ndic@info.niddk.nih.gov. http://diabetes.niddk.nih.gov/about/index.htm.

National Digestive Diseases Information Clearinghouse (NDDIC). 2 Information Way, Bethesda, MD 20892-3570. (800) 891-5389. http://digestive.niddk.nih.gov.

National Digestive Diseases Information Clearinghouse. 2 Information Way, Bethesda, MD 20892–3570. (800) 891–5389. Fax: (703) 738–4929. Email: nddic@info.niddk.nih.gov. http://digestive.niddk.nih.gov/about/index.htm.

The National Down Syndrome Society (NDSS). 666 Broadway, New York, NY 10012. (212) 460-9330 or (800) 221-4602. www.ndss.org.

National Eye Institute. 2020 Vision Place Bethesda, MD 20892-3655. (301) 496-5248. http://www.nei.nih.gov.

National Foundation for Transplants. Corporate Headquarters. 5350 Poplar Ave., Suite 430, Memphis, TN 38119. (800) 489-3863. (901) 684-1697. Fax: (901) 684-1128. http://www.transplants.org.

National Health Service of Great Britain. NHS Direct. Riverside House. 2a Southwark Bridge Road, London, England, SE1 9HA. http://www.nhsdirect.nhs.uk/.

National Heart, Lung and Blood Institute (NHLBI). Building 31, Room 5A48, 31 Center Drive MSC 2486, Bethesda, MD 20892. (301) 592-8573. TTY: (240) 629-3255. Fax: (240) 629-3246. http://www.nhlbi.nih.gov.

National Hospice & Palliative Care Organization (NHPCO). 1700 Diagonal Road, Suite 625, Alexandria, VA 22314. (703) 837-1500. Fax: (703) 837-1233. Email: nhpco_info@nhpco.org. http://www.nhpco.org.

The National Institute for Jewish Hospice (NIJH). 732 University Street, North Woodmere, NY 11581. (800) 446-4448. http://www.nijh.org/.

National Institute of Arthritis and Musculoskeletal and Skin Diseases Information Clearinghouse. 1 AMS Circle, Bethesda, MD 20892-3675. (301) 495-4484 or (877) 226-4267; Fax: (301) 718-6366; TTY: (301) 565-2966. http://www.nih.gov/niams.

National Institute of Diabetes and Digestive and Kidney Diseases (NIDDK). Building 31. Rm 9A06. 31 Center Drive, MSC 2560, Bethesda, MD 20892-2560. (301) 496.3583. http://www2.niddk.nih.gov/.

The National Institute of Neurological Disorders and Stroke (NINDS). National Institutes of Health, Bethesda, MD 20892. http://www.ninds.nih.gov.

National Institute of Occupational Safety and Health (NIOSH). [cited March 13, 2003]. www.cdc.gov/niosh/2000-135.html.

National Institute on Aging. Building 31, Room 5C27, 31 Center Drive, MSC 2292, Bethesda, MD 20892. (301) 496-1752, (800) 222-2225. TTY: (800) 222-4225. Fax: (301) 496-1072. http://www.nia.nih.gov/.

National Institute on Deafness and Other Communication Disorders (NIDCD), National Institutes of Health. 31 Center Drive, MSC 2320, Bethesda, MD 20892-2320. (301) 496-7243. TTY: (301) 402-0252. Fax: (301) 402-0018. Email: nidcdinfo@nidcd.nih.gov. http://www.nidcd.nih.gov.

National Institutes of Health. 9000 Rockville Pike, Bethesda, MD 20892. (301) 496-4000. TTY (301) 402-9612. Email: NIHinfo@od.nih.gov. http://www.nih.gov.

National Jewish Medical and Research Center. Lung-Line. 14090 Jackson Street, Denver, Colorado 80206. http://www.nationaljewish.org.

National Kidney and Urologic Diseases. 3 Information Way, Bethesda, MD 20892-3580. (800) 891-5390. http://kidney.niddk.nih.gov.

National Kidney Foundation. 30 East 33rd Street, New York, NY 10016. (800) 622-9010, (212) 889-2210. Fax: (212) 689-9261. http://www.kidney.org.

National Library of Medicine. 8600 Rockville Pike, Bethesda, MD 20894. (888) 346-3656. http://www.nlm.nih.gov.

National Lymphedema Network. 2211 Post St., Suite 404, San Francisco, CA 94115-3427. (800) 541-3259 or (415) 921-1306. http://www.wenet.net/~lymphnet.

National Marrow Donor Program. Suite 500, 3001 Broadway Street Northeast, Minneapolis, MN 55413-1753. (800) MARROW-2. http://www.marrow.org.

National Organ and Tissue Donation Initiative. http://www.organdonor.gov.

National Organization for Rare Disorders (NORD). 55 Kenosia Avenue, P. O. Box 1968, Danbury, CT 06813-1968. (203) 744-0100. http://www.rarediseases.org.

National Parkinson's Disease Foundation. Bob Hope Parkinson Research Center, 1501 N.W. 9th Avenue, Bob Hope Road, Miami, FL 33136-1494. (305) 547-6666. (800) 327-4545. Fax: (305) 243-4403. http://www.parkinson.org.

National Patient Advocate Foundation. 725 15th St. NW, 10th Floor, Washington, DC 20005, Phone: (202) 347-8009. Fax: (202) 347-5579. Email: action@npaf.org. http://www.npaf.org.

National Patient Safety Foundation (NPSF). 132 MASS MoCA Way, North Adams, MA 01247. (413) 663-8900. http://www.npsf.org/.

National Pressure Ulcer Advisory Panel. 12100 Sunset Hills Road, Suite 130, Reston, VA 20190. (703)464-4849. http://www.npuap.org.

National Prison Hospice Association (NPHA). P. O. Box 4623, Boulder, CO 80306. (303) 447-8051. http://www.npha.org.

National Scoliosis Foundation. 5 Cabot Place, Stoughton, MA 020724. (800) 673-6922. http://www.scoliosis.org

National Stroke Association. 9707 E. Easter Lane, Englewood, CO 80112. (800) Strokes or (303) 649-9299. http://www.stroke.org.

National Transplant Assistance Fund and Catastrophic Injury Program. 150 N. Radnor Chester Road, Suite F-120, Radnor, PA 19087. (800) 642-8399. http://www.transplantfund.org/.

NCCNHR (formerly the National Citizens' Coalition for Nursing Home Reform). 1828 L Street, NW, Suite 801, Washington, DC 20036. (202) 332-2275. www.nccnhr.org.

New England Ophthalmological Society (NEOS). P.O. Box 9165, Boston, MA 02114. (617) 227-6484. http://www.neos-eyes.org/.

North American Society for Head and Neck Pathology. Department of Pathology, H179, P.O. Box 850, Milton S. Hershey Medical Center, Penn State University School of Medicine, Hershey, PA 17033. (717) 531-8246. http://www.headandneckpathology.com/.

North American Society of Pacing and Electrophysiology. 6 Strathmore Rd., Natick, MA 01760-2499. (508) 647-0100. http://www.naspe.org.

North American Spine Society. 22 Calendar Court, 2nd Floor, LaGrange, IL 60525. (877) Spine-Dr. Email: info@spine.org. http://www.spine.org.

O

Obesity Society (formerly the American Obesity Association). 8630 Fenton Street, Suite 814, Silver Spring, MD 20910. (301) 563-6526. http://www.obesity.org.

Office of Cancer Complementary and Alternative Medicine, National Cancer Institute. 6116 Executive Boulevard, Suite 609, MSC 8339, Bethesda, MD 20892. (800) 422-6237. http://www.cancer.gov/cam.

Office of Rare Diseases (NIH). 6100 Executive Boulevard, Room 3A07, MSC 7518 Bethesda, MD 20892-7518. (301) 402-4336. http://www.rarediseases.info.nih.gov/info-diseases.html.

Office of Women's Health. U.S. Food and Drug Administration, 5600 Fishers Lane, Rockville, MD 20857. (301) 827-0350. http://www.fda.gov/womens/default.htm.

Oral Cancer Foundation. 3419 Via Lido, #205, Newport Beach, CA 92663. (949) 646-8000. www.oralcancer.org

Orthopedic Trauma Association. 6300 N. River Road, Suite 727, Rosemont, IL 60018-4226. (847) 698-1631. http://www.ota.org/links.htm.

Our Bodies Ourselves Health Resource Center. 34 Plympton Street, Boston, MA 02118. (617) 451-3666. http://www.ourbodiesourselves.org/.

Overeaters Anonymous (OA). World Service Office, P. O. Box 44020, Rio Rancho, NM 87174-4020. (505) 891-2664. http://www.oa.org(accessed April 18, 2008).

P

Partnership for Caring. 1620 Eye St., NW, Suite 202, Washington, DC 20006. (202) 296-8071. Fax: (202) 296-8352. Toll-free hotline: (800) 989-9455 (option 3). http://www.partnershipforcaring.org/.

Partnership for Organ Donation. Two Oliver Street, Boston, MA 02109. (617) 482-5746. http://www.transweb.org/partnership/.

Periodontal (Gum) Diseases. National Institute of Dental and Craniofacial Research, National Institutes of Health. Bethesda, MD 20892-2190. (301) 496-4261. http://www.nidcrinfo.nih.gov..

Peripheral Vascular Surgery Society (PVSS). 824 Munras Avenue, Suite C, Monterey, CA 93940. (831) 373-0508. http://www.pvss.org.

Physicians and Nurses for Blood Conservation (PNBC). P. O. Box 217, 6-2400 Dundas Street West, Mississauga, ON L5K 2R8. (905) 608-1647. http://www.pnbc.ca.

Pioneer Network. P.O. Box 18648, Rochester, NY 14618. (585) 271-7570. http://www.pioneernetwork.net/.

Planned Parenthood Federation of America. 434 West 33rd Street, New York, NY 10001. (212) 541-7800. (800) 230-PLAN (230-7526). Fax: (212) 245-1845. Or, 1110 Vermont Ave. NW, Suite 300, Washington, DC 20005. (202) 973-4800. Fax: (202) 296-3242. http://www.plannedparenthood.org.

Prevent Blindness America. 211 West Wacker Drive, Suite 1700, Chicago, IL 60606. (800) 331-2020. http://www.preventblindness.org.

Promoting Excellence in End of Life Care, RWJ Foundation National Program Office, c/o The Practical Ethics Center, The University of Montana, 1000 East Beckwith Avenue, Missoula, MT 59812. (406) 243-6601. Fax: (406) 243-6633. Email: excell@selway.umt.edu. http://www.promotingexcellence.org.

Prune Belly Syndrome Network. P. O. Box 2125, Evansville, IN 47728-0125. http://www.prunebelly.org.

R

Radiological Society of North America (RSNA). 820 Jorie Blvd., Oak Brook, IL 60523-2251. (630) 571-2670. http://www.rsna.org/.

Rehydration Project. P. O. Box 1, Samara, 5235, Costa Rica. (506) 656-0504. www.rehydrate.org.

Rothman Institute of Orthopaedics. 925 Chestnut Street, Philadelphia, PA 19107-4216. (215) 955-3458. http://www.rothmaninstitute.com.

Rush Arthritis and Orthopedics Institute. 1725 West Harrison Street, Suite 1055, Chicago, IL 60612. (312) 563-2420. http://www.rush.edu.

S

Second Wind Lung Transplant Association, Inc. 9030 West Lakeview Court, Crystal River, FL 34428. (888) 222-2690. http://www.arthouse.com/secondwind.

Shape Up America! c/o WebFront Solutions Corporation, 15757 Crabbs Branch Way, Rockville, MD 20855. (301) 258-0540. http://www.shapeup.org.

Shrine and Shriner's Hospitals. 2900 Rocky Point Dr., Tampa, FL 33607-1460. (813) 281-0300. http://www.shrinershq.org/.

Simon Foundation for Continence. P.O. Box 835, Wilmette, IL 60091. (800) 23-SIMON (237-4666) or (847) 864-3913. http://www.simonfoundation.org.

The Society for Clinical Vascular Surgery (SCVS). 900 Cummings Center, #221-U, Beverly, MA 01915. (978) 927-8330. http://scvs.vascularweb.org/index.html.

Society for Gastroenterology Nurses and Associates (SGNA). 401 North Michigan Avenue, Chicago, IL 60611-4267. (800) 245-7462. www.sgna.org.

Society for Pediatric Urology (SPU). C/o HealthInfo, 870 East Higgins Road, Suite 142, Schaumburg, IL 60173. http://www.spuonline.org.

Society for Technology in Anesthesia (STA). PMB 300, 223 North Guadalupe, Santa Fe, NM 87501. (505) 983-4923. http://www.anestech.org.

Society for the Advancement of Blood Management (SABM). 350 Engle Street, Englewood, NJ 07631. (866) 894-3916. http://www.sabm.org.

Society for Vascular Surgery. 633 N. St. Clair, 24th Floor, Chicago, IL 60611. (312) 334-2300, (800) 258-7188.

Fax: (312) 334-2320. Email: vascular@vascularsociety.org. http://www.vascularweb.org.

Society of American Gastrointestinal Endoscopic Surgeons (SAGES). 11300 West Olympic Boulevard, Suite 600, Los Angeles, CA 90064. (310) 437-0544. Fax: (310) 437-0585. http://www.sages.org.

Society of Critical Care Medicine (SCCM). 701 Lee Street, Suite 200, Des Plaines, IL 60016. (847) 827-6869; Fax: (847) 827-6869. Email: info@sccm.org. www.sccm.org.

Society of Diagnostic Medical Sonography. 2745 Dallas Parkway, Suite 350, Plano, TX 75093-8730. (214) 473-8057, (800) 229-9506. Fax: (214) 473-8563. http://www.sdms.org/.

Society of Gynecologic Oncologists. 230 West Monroe Street, Suite 710, Chicago, IL 60606. (312) 235-4060. http://www.sgo.org.

Society of Interventional Radiology. 3975 Fair Ridge Drive, Suite 400 North, Fairfax, VA 22033. (800) 488-7284, (703) 691-1805. Fax: (703) 691-1855. http://www.sirweb.org.

Society of Laparoendoscopic Surgeons. 7330 SW 62nd Place, Suite 410, Miami, FL 33143-4825. (305) 665-9959. http://www.sls.org.

Society of NeuroInterventional Surgery (formerly the American Society of Interventional and Therapeutic Neuroradiology, ASITN). 3975 Fair Ridge Drive, Suite 460 South, Fairfax, VA 22033. (703) 691-2272. Fax: (703) 537-0650. Email: info@snisonline.org. http://www.snisonline.org.

Society of Nuclear Medicine (SNM). 1850 Samuel Morse Drive, Reston, VA 20190. (703) 708-9000. www.snm.org.

Society of Surgical Oncology. 85 West Algonquin Rd., Suite 550, Arlington Heights, IL 60005. (847) 427-1400. http://www.surgonc.org.

Society of Thoracic Surgeons. 633 N. Saint Clair St., Suite 2320, Chicago, IL 60611-3658. (312) 202-5800. Fax: (312) 202-5801. Email: sts@sts.org. http://www.sts.org.

Society of Toxicology. 1821 Michael Faraday Drive, Suite 300, Reston, VA 20190. (703) 438-3115. http://www.toxicology.org.

Society of Urologic Nurses and Associates. East Holly Avenue, Box 56, Pitman, NJ 08071-0056. (609) 256-2335. http://suna.inurse.com/.

Southern Thoracic Surgical Association. 633 N. Saint Clair St., Suite 2320, Chicago, IL, 60611-3658. (800) 685-7872. www.stsa.org/.

Spina Bifida Association. 4590 MacArthur Boulevard, NW, Washington , DC 20007. (202) 944-3285, (800) 621-3141. Fax: (202) 944-3295. Email: sbaa@sbaa.org. http://www.spinabifidaassociation.org.

Spine Center. 1911 Arch St., Philadelphia, PA 19103. (215) 665-8300. http://www.thespinecenter.com

SurgeryLinx. MDLinx, Inc. 1025 Vermont Avenue, NW, Suite 810, Washington, DC 20005. (202) 543-6544. http://sgreports.nlm.nih.gov/NN/.

T

Texas Heart Institute. 6770 Bertner Avenue, Houston, TX 77030. (832) 355-4011. Or, PO Box 20345, Houston, TX 77225-0345. http://www.texasheartinstitute.org.

Tissue Adhesive Center, Surgical Therapeutic Advancement Center. P. O. Box 801370, Charlottesville, VA 22908. (434) 243-0315. http://www.healthsystem.virginia.edu/internet/stac/overview/home.cfm.

Transplant Foundation, Inc. 701 SW 27th Ave, Suite 705, Miami, FL 33135. (305) 817-5645 or (866) 900-3172. http://www.transplantfoundation.org/.

Transplant Recipients International Organization (TRIO). International Headquarters: 1000 16th Street, NW, Suite 602, Washington, DC 20036-5705. (800) TRIO-386. http://www.transweb.org/people/recips/resources/support/bkuptrio_main.html.

U

United Cerebral Palsy. 1660 L Street, NW, Suite 700, Washington, DC 20036. (800) 872-5827 or (202)776-0406. TTY: (202) 973-7197. Fax: (202) 776-0414. webmaster@ucp.org. http://www.UCP.org.

United Network for Organ Sharing (UNOS). Post Office Box 2484, Richmond, VA 23218. Or, 700 North 4th Street, Richmond, VA 23219. (804) 782-4800, (804) 782-4817. http://www.unos.org.

United Ostomy Association, Inc. (UOA). 19772 MacArthur Blvd., Suite 200, Irvine, CA 92612-2405. (800) 826-0826. http://www.uoa.org..

United States Administration on Aging. One Massachusetts Ave., Washington, DC 20201. (202) 619-0724. Email: AoAInfo@aoa.hhs.gov. http://www.aoa.gov.

United States Department of Health and Human Services, 200 Independence Avenue, SW, Washington, DC 20201. (877) 696-6775. http://www.hhs.gov.

United States Food and Drug Administration (FDA). 5600 Fishers Lane, Rockville, MD 20857-0001. (888) INFO-FDA. http://www.fda.gov.

United States Living Will Registry. 523 Westfield Ave., P.O. Box 2789, Westfield, NJ 07091-2789. Toll-free: (800) LIV-WILL or (800) 548-9455. http://www.uslivingwillregistry.com/.

United States Pharmacopoeia (USP). 12601 Twinbrook Parkway, Rockville, MD 20852-1790. (800) 227-8772. http://www.usp.org.

United States Renal Data System (USRDS), Coordinating Center. The University of Minnesota, 914 South 8th Street, Suite D-206, Minneapolis, MN 55404. (888) 99USRDS. http://www.usrds.org;.

University of Maryland Medical Center, R. Adams Cowley Shock Trauma Center. 22 South Greene Street,

Baltimore, MD 21201. (410) 328-2757 or (800) 373-4111. www.umm.edu/shocktrauma.

University of Michigan Kellogg Eye Center Department of Ophthalmology and Visual Sciences. 1000 Wall Street, Ann Arbor, MI 48105. (734) 763-1415. http://www.kellogg.umich.edu.

V

Valley Baptist Heart and Vascular Institute. 2101 Pease Street, P.O. Drawer 2588. Harlingen, TX 78550. (956) 389-4848.

Vascular Birthmark Foundation. P.O. Box 106, Latham, NY 12110. (877) VBF-LOOK (daytime) and (877) VBF-4646 (evenings and weekends). www.birthmark.org.

Vascular Disease Foundation. 3333 South Wadsworth Blvd. B104-37, Lakewood, CO 80227. (303) 949-8337, (866) PADINFO (723-4636). http://www.vdf.org.

Vestibular Disorders Association (VEDA). PO Box 4467, Portland, OR 97208-4467. (800) 837-8428. www.vestibular.org.

Visiting Nurse Associations of America (VNAA). 900 19th St, NW, Suite 200, Washington, DC 20006. (202) 384-1420. Fax: (202) 384-1444. Email: vnaa@vnaa.org. http://www.vnaa.org.

Voice Center at Eastern Virginia Medical School. Norfolk, VA 23507. http://www.voice-center.com.

W

The Washington Home Center for Palliative Care Studies(CPCS), 4200 Wisconsin Avenue, NW, 4th Floor, Washington, DC 20016. (202) 895-2625. Fax: (202) 966-5410. Email: info@medicaring.org. http://www.medicaring.org.

WE MOVE, Worldwide Education and Awareness for Movement Disorders. 204 West 84th Street, New York, NY 10024. (800) 437-MOV2. Fax: (212) 875-8389. http://www.wemove.org.

Weight-control Information Network (WIN). 1 WIN Way, Bethesda, MD 20892-3665. (877)946-4627, (202) 828-1025. Fax: (202) 828-1028. http://win.niddk.nih.gov.

Wills Eye. 840 Walnut Street, Philadelphia, PA 19107. (215) 928-3000. http://www.willseye.org.

Wound Care Institute. 1100 N.E. 163rd Street, Suite #101, North Miami Beach, FL 33162. (305) 919-9192. http://woundcare.org.

Wound Healing Society. 13355 Tenth Ave., Suite 108, Minneapolis, MN 55441-5554. [cited April 4, 2003]. http://www.woundheal.org/.

The Wound, Ostomy and Continence Nurses Society. 15000 Commerce Parkway, Suite C, Mt. Laurel, NJ 08054. (888) 224-WOCN (9626). http://www.wocn.org.

Z

Zen Hospice Project. 273 Page Street, San Francisco, CA 94102. (415) 863-2910. http://www.zenhospice.org.

GLOSSARY

A

ABDOMEN. The portion of the body that lies between the thorax and the pelvis. It contains a cavity with many organs.

ABDOMINAL ANEURYSM. Aneurysm that involves the descending aorta from the diaphragm to the point at which it separates into two iliac arteries.

ABDOMINAL AORTIC ANEURYSM. Occurs when an area in the aorta (the main artery of the heart) is weakened and bulges like a balloon. The abdominal section of the aorta supplies blood to the lower body.

ABDOMINAL DISTENSION. Swelling of the abdominal cavity, which creates painful pressure on the internal organs.

ABDOMINAL HERNIA. A defect in the abdominal wall through which the abdominal organs protrude.

ABLATION THERAPY. A procedure used to treat arrhythmias, especially atrial fibrillation.

ABLATION. Removal or destruction of tissue, such as by burning or cutting.

ABO ANTIGEN. Protein molecules located on the surfaces of red blood cells that determine a person's blood type: A, B, or O.

ABO BLOOD GROUPS. A system in which human blood is classified according to the A and B antigens found in red blood cells. Type A blood has the A antigen, type B has the B antigen, AB has both, and O has neither.

ABO BLOOD TYPE. Blood type based on the presence or absence of the A and B antigens on the red blood cells. There are four types: A, B, AB, and O.

ABSCESS. A localized pocket of pus at a site of infection.

ACCESS SITE. The vein tapped for vascular access in hemodialysis treatments. For patients with temporary treatment needs, access to the bloodstream is gained by inserting a catheter into the subclavian vein near the patient's collarbone. Patients in long-term dialysis require stronger, more durable access sites, called fistulas or grafts, that are surgically created.

ACCESSORY ORGAN. A lump of tissue adjacent to an organ that is similar to it, but which serves no important purpose (if it functions at all). While not necessarily harmful, such organs can cause problems if they are confused with a mass, or in rare cases, if they grow too large or become cancerous.

ACETABULAR DYSPLASIA. A type of arthritis resulting in a shallow hip socket.

ACETABULUM. The hollow, cuplike portion of the pelvis into which the femoral head is fitted to make the hip joint.

ACETAMINOPHEN. A common pain reliever (e.g., Tylenol).

ACETIC ACID. Vinegar; very dilute washes of the treated areas with a vinegar solution are suggested by some surgeons after laser skin resurfacing.

ACHALASIA. Failure to relax. The term is often applied to sphincter muscles.

ACID. Any chemical or compound that lowers the pH of a solution below 7.0, meaning that there is a surplus of hydrogen ions dissociated within that solution.

ACIDOSIS. A condition of the blood in which bicarbonate levels are below normal.

ACL RECONSTRUCTION. Repairing a tear of the anterior cruciate ligament (ACL) of the knee using arthroscopy and/or open surgery.

ACOUSTIC WINDOW. Area through which ultrasound waves move freely.

ACQUIRED IMMUNODEFICIENCY SYNDROME (AIDS). A disease syndrome in which the patient's immune cells are destroyed by HIV virus, leaving the patient open to opportunistic infections that a healthy immune system could keep at bay.

ACROMEGALY. A condition in which an overactive pituitary gland pumps out an excess amount of growth hormone.

ACROMIOCLAVICULAR (AC) JOINT. The shoulder joint. Articulation and ligaments between the collarbone and the acromion of the shoulder blade.

ACROMIOCLAVICULAR DISLOCATION. Disruption of the normal articulation between the acromion and the collarbone. The acromioclavicular joint (AC joint) is normally stabilized by several ligaments that can be torn in the process of dislocating the AC joint.

ACROMION. The triangular projection of the spine of the shoulder blade that forms the point of the shoulder and articulates with the collarbone.

ACTINIC KERATOSIS. A crusty, scaly precancerous skin lesion caused by damage from the sun; frequently treated with cryotherapy.

ACTIVATED PARTIAL THROMBOPLASTIN TIME (APTT). A lab test that detects coagulation defects in the intrinsic clotting cascade. Used to regulate heparin dosing.

ACTIVITIES OF DAILY LIVING (ADLS). Self-care activities performed during the course of a normal day such as eating, bathing, dressing, toileting, etc.

ACUITY. Sharpness or clarity of vision.

ACUPUNCTURE. The insertion of tiny needles into the skin at specific spots on the body for curative purposes.

ACUTE HEMOLYTIC TRANSFUSION REACTION (AHTR). A severe transfusion reaction with abrupt onset, most often caused by ABO incompatibility. Symptoms include difficulty breathing, fever and chills, pain, and sometimes shock.

ACUTE MYELOGENOUS LEUKEMIA (AML). Also called acute myelocytic leukemia, a malignant disorder where myeloid blast cells accumulate in the marrow and bloodstream.

ACUTE OTITIS MEDIA. Inflammation of the middle ear with signs of infection lasting less than three months.

ACUTE PAIN. Pain that is usually temporary and results from something specific, such as a surgery, an injury, or an infection.

ACUTE RENAL (KIDNEY) FAILURE. Abrupt loss of kidney function, possibly temporary.

ACUTE TUBULAR NECROSIS. A kidney disease involving damage to the portion of the kidney known as the tubules that causes kidney failure.

ACUTE. Rapid onset of a condition. Also, refers to pain in response to injury or other stimulus that resolves when the injury heals or the stimulus is removed.

ADDICTION. Compulsive, overwhelming involvement with a specific activity. The activity may be smoking, gambling, alcohol, or may involve the use of almost any substance, such as a drug.

ADDISON'S DISEASE. A condition in which the adrenal glands are not functioning properly. Addison's disease can be caused by a problem in the adrenal glands themselves, or in the pituitary gland, which secretes a hormone that affects the adrenal glands.

ADDISONIAN CRISIS. A medical emergency resulting from severe adrenal insufficiency. It can be caused by sudden withdrawal from oral glucocorticoid medications, as well as from damage to the adrenal gland itself. Untreated Addisonian crisis can be fatal.

ADENOCARCINOMA. Cancer that starts in the lining of the small intestine and is the most common type of cancer of the small intestine. These tumors occur most often in the part of the small intestine nearest the stomach and often grow and block the bowel.

ADENOIDS. Clusters of lymphoid tissue located in the upper throat above the roof of the mouth. Some doctors think that removal of the adenoids may lower the rate of recurrent otitis media in high-risk children.

ADENOMA. A benign tumor of an endocrine gland.

ADHESION. A band of fibrous tissue forming an abnormal bond between two adjacent tissues or organs.

ADJUVANT THERAPY. Treatment used to increase the effectiveness of surgery, usually chemotherapy or radiation used to kill any cancer cells that might be remaining.

ADRENAL GLANDS. Two glands located next to the kidneys. The adrenal glands produce the hormones epinephrine and norepinephrine and the corticosteroid (cortisone-like) hormones.

ADRENERGIC. Characteristic of or releasing epinephrine or related substances. The term often refers to the nerve fibers in the sympathetic nervous system that release norepinephrine as a neurotransmitter.

ADSORB. To attract and hold another substance on the surface of a solid material.

ADVANCE DIRECTIVE, OR ADVANCE MEDICAL DIRECTIVE. A general term for two types of documents, living wills and medical powers of attorney, that allow people to give instructions about health care in the event that they cannot speak for themselves.

ADVERSE EVENT. An undesirable and unintended result of a medical treatment or intervention.

AEROBE. Bacteria that require oxygen to live.

AEROBIC BACTERIA. Bacteria that can grow freely in oxygen-rich environments.

AEROBIC EXERCISE. Any type of exercise that is intended to increase the body's oxygen consumption and improve the functioning of the cardiovascular and respiratory systems.

AESTHETIC. Pertaining to beauty. Plastic surgery done to improve the patient's appearance is sometimes called aesthetic surgery.

AFFECT. The external manifestation of a mood or state of mind. Affect is usually observed in facial expression or other body language.

AFFERENT FIBERS. Nerve fibers that conduct nerve impulses from tissues and organs toward the central nervous system.

AGAR. A gelatinous material extracted from red algae that is not digested by bacteria. It is used as a support for growth in plates.

AGENESIS. The absence of an organ or body part due to developmental failure.

AGGLUTINATION. An immunochemical reaction. It is termed positive when two chemicals that are mixed cause clumps to form.

AIDS. Acquired immunodeficiency syndrome. A disease caused by infection with the human immunodeficiency virus (HIV). In people with this disease, the immune system breaks down, opening the door to other infections and some types of cancer.

AIRWAY. The passageway through the mouth, nose, and throat that allows air to enter and leave the lungs; the term can also refer to a tube or other artificial device used to create an air passageway into and out of the lungs when the patient is under general anesthesia or unable to breathe properly.

ALDOSTERONE. A hormone secreted by the adrenal glands that prompts the kidneys to hold onto sodium.

ALGORITHM. A procedure or formula for solving a problem. It is often used to refer to a sequence of steps used to program a computer to solve a specific problem.

ALKALINE. Any chemical or compound that raises the pH of a solution above 7.0, meaning that there is a relative shortage of hydrogen ions dissociated within that solution.

ALKALOID. Any of a group of bitter-tasting alkaline compounds that contain nitrogen and are commonly found in plants. Alkaloids derived from ergot can be used as uterine stimulants.

ALKALOSIS. A condition of the blood and other body fluids in which bicarbonate levels are higher than normal.

ALLELE. Types of genes that occupy the same site on a chromosome.

ALLOGENEIC. Referring to blood donation or bone-marrow transplants between two different, genetically dissimilar people.

ALLOGRAFT. A graft of bone or other tissue taken from a donor.

ALLOPLAST. An implant made of an inert foreign material such as silicone or hydroxyapatite.

ALOPECIA. Hair loss or baldness.

ALPHA-FETOPROTEIN (AFP). A protein normally produced by the liver of a fetus and detectable in maternal blood samples. AFP screening measures the amount of alpha-fetoprotein in the blood. Levels outside the norm may indicate fetal defects.

ALTERNATIVES TO SURGERY . Other treatments for the condition or illness that do not involve surgery; these are usually tried before surgery is an option.

ALTITUDE SICKNESS. A set of symptoms that people who normally live at low altitudes may have when they climb mountains or travel to high altitudes. The symptoms include nosebleed, nausea, and shortness of breath.

ALVEOLAR ARCH. An arch formed by the ridge of the alveolar process of the mandible (jawbone) or maxilla.

ALZHEIMER'S DISEASE. Progressive dementia characterized by worsening memory and other cognitive impairment.

AMBULATE OR AMBULATION. To move from place to place (walk).

AMBULATORY CARE. An outpatient facility; designed for patients who do not require inpatient hospital treatment or care.

AMBULATORY MONITORS. Small portable electrocardiograph machines that record the heart's rhythm, and include the Holter monitor, loop recorder, and trans-telephonic transmitter.

AMBULATORY SURGERY. Surgery done on an outpatient basis; the patient goes home the same day.

AMBULATORY. Referring to a condition that is treatable without admission to a hospital, or to a surgical procedure performed on an outpatient basis.

AMINE. A chemical compound that contains NH_3 (a nitrogen-hydrogen combination) as part of its structure.

AMNIOCENTESIS. A procedure for removing amniotic fluid from the womb using a fine needle.

AMNIOTIC MEMBRANE. A thin membrane that contains the fetus and the protective amniotic fluid surrounding the fetus.

ANAEROBIC. Pertaining to a microorganism (an anaerobe) that either does not use oxygen or actually cannot live in the presence of oxygen.

ANALGESIA. Refers to pain relief without loss of consciousness. An analgesic is a drug that is given to relieve pain. The term also refers to the absence of the ability to feel pain.

ANALYTE. A material or chemical substance subjected to analysis.

ANAPHYLACTIC SHOCK. A potentially fatal allergic reaction to a substance that causes a severe drop in blood pressure, swelling of the respiratory tract with associated breathing problems, rash, and possible convulsions.

ANASTOMOSIS (PLURAL, ANASTOMOSES). The surgical connection of two structures, such as blood vessels or sections of the intestine.

ANDROGENS. A class of chemical compounds (hormones) that stimulates the development of male secondary sexual characteristics.

ANEMIA. A lack of hemoglobin. Hemoglobin is the compound in blood that carries oxygen from the lungs throughout the body and brings waste carbon dioxide from the cells to the lungs, where it is released.

ANENCEPHALY. A hereditary defect resulting in the partial to complete absence of a brain and spinal cord. It is fatal.

ANEROID MONITOR. A monitor that works without fluids, i.e. without mercury.

ANESTHESIA. A combination of drugs administered by a variety of techniques by trained professionals that provide sedation, amnesia, analgesia, and immobility adequate for the accomplishment of a surgical procedure with minimal discomfort, and without injury to the patient.

ANESTHESIOLOGIST. A doctor of medicine (MD) or osteopathy (DO) who has completed advanced training in administering anesthesia and monitoring patients' well-being during surgery. Many anesthesiologists have completed additional training in critical care medicine or pain management.

ANESTHESIOLOGIST. A physician with advanced training in anesthesia (and sometimes other medical specialties) who administers or oversees the administration of anesthesia to the patient and monitors care after surgery.

ANESTHESIOLOGY. The branch of medicine that specializes in the study of anesthetic agents, their effects on patients, and their proper use and administration.

ANESTHETIC. Medicine that causes a loss of feeling, especially pain. Some anesthetics also cause a loss of consciousness.

ANESTHETIST. A nurse trained in anesthesiology who, working as an assistant to a anesthesiologist, administers the anesthesia in surgery and monitors the patient after surgery.

ANEURYSM. A bulge in the wall of a blood vessel caused by the weakening of the vessel wall. Aneurysms can be fatal if the affected blood vessel bursts.

ANGINA. Also called angina pectoris; chest pain or discomfort that occurs when diseased blood vessels restrict blood flow to the heart.

ANGIOEDEMA. An allergic skin disease characterized by patches of circumscribed swelling involving the skin and its subcutaneous layers, the mucous membranes, and sometimes the viscera—also called angioneurotic edema, giant urticaria, Quincke's disease, or Quincke's edema.

ANGIOGRAM. An examination of a part of the body by injecting dye into an artery so that the blood vessels show up on an x ray.

ANGIOGRAPHY. Any of the different methods for investigating the condition of blood vessels, usually via a combination of radiological imaging and injections of chemical tracing and contrasting agents.

ANGIOMATOUS MALFORMATIONS. Tumors in blood vessels.

ANGIOPLASTY. A procedure in which a balloon catheter is used to mechanically dilate the affected area of a diseased artery and enlarge the constricted or narrowed segment; it is an alternative to vascular surgery.

ANGIOTENSIN-CONVERTING ENZYME (ACE) INHIBITOR. A drug that lowers blood pressure by interfering with the breakdown of a protein-like substance involved in blood pressure regulation.

ANGLE (OR ANGLE CLOSURE). The open point in the anterior chamber of the eye at which the iris meets the cornea. Blockage of the angle prevents fluid from leaving the anterior chamber, resulting in closed-angle glaucoma.

ANISMUS. Dysfunctional contraction or spasm of the muscle comprising the anal sphincter.

ANKLE-BRACHIAL INDEX (ABI) TEST. A means of checking the blood pressure in the arms and ankles using a regular blood pressure cuff and a special ultrasound stethoscope (Doppler). The pressure in the ankle is compared to the pressure in the arm.

ANKYLOSING SPONDYLITIS. A form of inflammatory arthritis in which the bones in the spine and pelvis gradually fuse when inflamed connective tissue is replaced by bone.

ANNULUS. A ring-shaped structure.

ANOMALY. A marked deviation from normal structure or function, particularly as the result of congenital defects.

ANOREXIA NERVOSA. An eating disorder marked by refusal to eat, intense fear of obesity, and distortions of body image.

ANTACID. A substance that counteracts or neutralizes acidity, usually of the stomach. Antacids have a rapid onset of action compared to histamine H-2 receptor blockers and proton pump inhibitors, but they have a short duration of action and require frequent dosing.

ANTALGIC. Medication that alleviates pain.

ANTEREOLATERAL. Situated in front and to the side.

ANTERIOR CHAMBER. The front chamber of the eye bound by the cornea in front and the iris in the back. The anterior chamber is filled with aqueous humor. The drainage site for the aqueous fluid is in the anterior chamber.

ANTERIOR CRUCIATE LIGAMENT (ACL). A crossing ligament that attaches the femur to the tibia and stabilizes the knee against forward motion of the tibia.

ANTERIOR MEDIASTINOTOMY. A surgical procedure to look at the organs and tissues between the lungs and between the breastbone and spine for abnormal areas. An incision (cut) is made next to the breastbone and a thin, lighted tube is inserted into the chest. Tissue and lymph node samples may be taken for biopsy.

ANTHRAX. A dangerous pathogen that should contained in a negative pressure room.

ANTIARRHYTHMIC. Medication used to treat abnormal heart rhythms.

ANTIBIOTIC. A chemical substance produced by a microorganism that is able to kill other microorganisms without being toxic to the host. Antibiotics are used to treat diseases in humans, other animals, and plants.

ANTIBODIES. Proteins that are produced normally by specialized white blood cells after stimulation by a foreign substance (antigen) and that act specifically against the antigen in an immune response.

ANTICHOLINERGICS. Drugs that interfere with impulses from the parasympathetic nervous system. They may be given before general anesthesia to reduce airway secretions or the risk of bronchospasm.

ANTICOAGULANT. A medication, also called a "blood thinner," that prevents blood from clotting. This type of medication is used for people at risk of stroke or blood clots.

ANTIDIURETIC HORMONE (ADH). Also called vasopressin. A hormone produced by the hypothalamus and stored in and excreted by the pituitary gland. ADH acts on the kidneys to reduce the flow of urine, increasing total body fluid.

ANTIDIURETIC. A medication or other compound that suppresses the production of urine.

ANTIEMETIC. A drug that prevents emesis, or vomiting.

ANTIGEN. A substance that stimulates the immune system to manufacture antibodies (immunoglobulins). The function of antibodies is to fight off such intruder cells as bacteria or viruses. Antigens stimulate the blood to fight other blood cells that have the wrong antigens. If a person with blood type A is given a transfusion with blood type B, the A antigens will fight the foreign blood cells as though they were an infectious agent.

ANTIHISTAMINE. Medicine that prevents or relieves allergy symptoms.

ANTIMICROBIAL. A compound that prevents the growth of microbes which may include bacteria, fungi, and viruses.

ANTIMYCOTIC. A medicine that can be used to kill yeast and fungus.

ANTIPLATELET DRUG. Drug that inhibits platelets from aggregating to form a plug.

ANTIPYRETIC. A medication that lowers fever.

ANTISEPTIC. Substance preventing or stopping the growth of microorganisms.

ANTITHROMBIC. Preventing clot formation.

ANTITRYPSIN. A substance that inhibits the action of trypsin.

ANTRECTOMY. A surgical procedure for ulcer disease in which the antrum, a portion of the stomach, is removed.

ANTROSTOMY. The operation of opening an antrum for drainage.

ANTRUM. The cavity of a sinus. Also the lower part of the stomach that lies between the pylorus and the body of the stomach. It is also called the gastric antrum or antrum pyloricum.

ANUS. The terminal orifice of the bowel.

ANXIETY. Worry or tension in response to real or imagined stress, danger, or dreaded situations. Physical reactions such as fast pulse, sweating, trembling, fatigue, and weakness may accompany anxiety.

ANXIETY ATTACK. A disorder in which sudden feelings of dread, fear, and apprehension of danger enter a person's mind in an overwhelming manner. Attacks may lead to a state of hyperventilation.

ANXIOLYTICS. Medications given to reduce anxiety; tranquilizers. Benzodiazepines are the anxiolytics most commonly used to premedicate patients before general anesthesia.

AORTA. The main artery that carries blood from the heart to the rest of the body. The aorta is the largest artery in the body.

AORTIC ANEURYSM. Occurs when an area in the aorta (the main artery of the heart) is weakened and bulges like a balloon.

AORTIC DISSECTION. A situation in which a tear in the interior lining of the wall of the aorta causes bleeding between the layers of that major artery.

AORTIC VALVE. The valve between the heart's left ventricle and ascending aorta that prevents regurgitation of blood back into the left ventricle.

APHAKIC. Without a lens. An older form of cataract surgery known as intracapsular extraction left patients' eyes aphakic.

APHERESIS. A procedure in which whole blood is withdrawn from a donor, a specific blood component is separated and collected, and the remainder is reinfused into the patient.

APICOECTOMY. Also called root resectioning. The root tip of a tooth is accessed in the bone and a small amount is shaved away. The diseased tissue is removed and a filling is placed to reseal the canal.

APLASTIC ANEMIA. A disorder in which the body produces inadequate amounts of red blood cells and hemoglobin due to underdeveloped or missing bone marrow.

APNEA. A period of no breathing, sometimes sudden, sometimes prolonged.

APPENDECTOMY. Removal of the appendix.

APPENDIX. A pouch-shaped organ that is attached to the upper part of the large intestine.

APPETITE SUPPRESSANT. A medication given to reduce the desire to eat.

APROTININ. A protein derived from cows' lungs included in some fibrin sealants to prevent the fibrin clot from dissolving.

AQUEOUS HUMOR. The watery fluid produced in the eye that ordinarily leaves the eye through the angle of the anterior chamber.

AREFLEXIA. A condition in which the body's normal reflexes are absent. It is one of the objectives of general anesthesia.

ARGON. A colorless, odorless gas.

ARREST. A sudden stopping of the function of a body organ, such as no breathing (respiratory arrest) or no beating of the heart (cardiac arrest).

ARRHYTHMIA. An abnormal heart rhythm. Examples are a slow, fast, or irregular heart rate.

ARTERIAL BLOOD. Blood from the arteries, the blood vessels that carry oxygen from the lungs to supply the body tissues.

ARTERIAL BLOOD GAS (ABG). A type of blood laboratory test done to check for imbalances in pH or gases that affect pH.

ARTERIAL EMBOLISM. A blood clot arising from another location that blocks an artery.

ARTERIAL LINE. A catheter inserted into an artery and connected to a physiologic monitoring system to allow direct measurement of oxygen, carbon dioxide, and invasive blood pressure.

ARTERIES. Blood vessels that carry blood away from the heart to the cells, tissues, and organs of the body.

ARTERIOGRAM. A diagnostic test that involves viewing the arteries and/or attached organs by injecting a contrast medium, or dye, into the artery and taking an x ray.

ARTERIOLAR BED. An area in which arterioles cluster between arteries and capillaries.

ARTERIOLES. The smallest branches of arteries.

ARTERIOSCLEROSIS. A chronic condition characterized by thickening and hardening of the arteries and the build-up of plaque on the arterial walls. Arteriosclerosis can slow or impair blood circulation.

ARTERIOVENOUS MALFORMATION. An anomaly present since birth in which the arteries and veins in a particular part of the body are caught up in a complex tangle, and in which there is an abnormal pattern of blood flowing from the arteries directly into the veins.

ARTERY. A blood vessel that carries blood from the heart to other parts of the body.

ARTHRITIS. A disease of the joints that arises from wear and tear, age, and, less often, from inflammation.

ARTHRODESIS. Surgery that joins (or fuses) two bones so that the joint can no longer move; it may be done on joints such as the fingers, knees, ankles, or spine.

ARTHROGRAPHY. Visualization of a joint by radiographic means following injection of a contrast dye into the joint space.

ARTHROPLASTY. The surgical reconstruction or replacement of a joint.

ARTHROSCOPE. A pencil-sized fiber-optic instrument fitted with a lens, light source, and camera, used for detailed examination of joints.

ARTHROSCOPY. The introduction of a thin fiber-optic scope (arthroscope) into a joint space to allow direct visualization of internal structures. In some cases, surgical repair can also be performed using the arthroscope.

ARTHROSIS. A disease of a joint.

ARTIFACT. Extra electrical activity typically caused by interference.

ARTIFICIAL SPHINCTER. An implanted device that functions to control the opening and closing of the urethral or anal canal for the expelling of urine or feces, respectively.

ASCITES. An abnormal collection of fluid within the abdomen, often suggests liver disease such as cirrhosis.

ASCITIC FLUID. The fluid that accumulates in the peritoneal cavity in ascites.

ASEPSIS. Freedom from infection or infectious material; also, the absence of viable pathogenic organisms. Asepsis can be accomplished using aseptic techniques, which are the use of surgical practices that restrict microorganisms in the environment and prevent contamination of the surgical wound; they include sterilization of instruments and the wearing of sterile caps, gloves, and masks.

ASPIRATION. The process of removing fluids or gases from the body by suction.

ASSISTED LIVING. A type of facility for people who are not able to live independently but do not require the level of skilled nursing provided by a nursing home.

ASTHMA. An inflammatory respiratory disorder in which the airway becomes obstructed and breathing is difficult.

ASTIGMATISM. A condition in which one or both eyes cannot filter light properly and images appear blurred and indistinct.

ATELECTASIS. Partial or complete collapse of the lung, usually due to a blockage of the air passages with fluid, mucus or infection.

ATHERECTOMY. A non-surgical technique for treating diseased arteries with a rotating device that cuts or shaves away obstructing material inside the artery.

ATHEROMA. A collection of plaque (lesion) blocking a portion of an artery.

ATHEROSCLEROSIS. A condition in which the major arteries throughout the body become obstructed by fatty plaques, causing narrowing, obstruction of blood flow, and ultimately hardening and stiffening of the arterial walls.

ATKINS DIET. A diet that involves eating a high amount of protein and fat with a low amounts of carbohydrates.

ATRESIA. Lack of development. In tricuspid atresia, the triscupid valve has not developed. In pulmonary atresia, the pulmonary valve has not developed.

ATRIA (SINGULAR, ATRIUM). The right and left upper chambers of the heart.

ATRIAL FIBRILLATION. A condition in which the upper chamber of the heart quivers instead of pumping in an organized way.

ATRIAL FLUTTER. A rapid pulsation of the upper chambers of the heart that interferes with normal heart function. Atrial flutter is usually more organized and regular than atrial fibrillation, although it often converts to atrial fibrillation. Atrial flutter occurs most often in people with heart disease and in the first week after heart surgery.

ATRIOVENTRICULAR. Referring to the valves regulating blood flow from the upper chambers of the heart (atria) to the lower chambers (ventricles). There are two such valves, one connecting the right atrium and ventricle and one connecting the left atrium and ventricle.

ATROPHY. Wasting away or degeneration of body tissue. Atrophy of the optic nerve, for example, is one of the defining characteristics of glaucoma.

ATTENTION DEFICIT HYPERACTIVITY DISORDER (ADHD). A disorder involving a developmentally inappropriate degree of inattention and impulsivity. Hyperactivity may or may not be a component. This disorder usually appears in childhood and manifests itself as difficulty at home or school. It sometimes persists into adulthood where it may affect work, relationships, and other social situations.

AUDIOGRAM. A test of hearing at a range of sound frequencies.

AUDIOLOGIST. A health care professional who performs diagnostic testing of impaired hearing.

AUDITORY NERVE. The nerve that carries electrical signals from the cochlea to the brain.

AURICLE. The portion of the external ear that is not contained inside the head. It is also called the pinna.

AUSCULTATION. The act of listening to sounds arising within organs as an aid to diagnosis and treatment.

AUTISM. A childhood disorder that manifests as an inability to communicate with or relate to others, or interact in social situations in a healthy, normal manner. Autism may range from mild to severe and includes repetitive behaviors, the inability to cope with changes from routine activities, and obsessions with specific objects. Autism is sometimes associated with below-normal intelligence or anxiety.

AUTOCLAVE. A heavy vessel that uses pressurized steam for disinfecting and sterilizing surgical instruments.

AUTOGENOUS TISSUE. Tissue or skin taken from any part of a person's body to graft onto another part of the body that needs repairing; laid on as a patch.

AUTOGRAFT. Tissue that is taken from one part of a patient's body and transplanted to another part of the patient's body.

AUTOIMMUNE DISEASE. A disease in which the immune system is overactive and produces antibodies that attack the body's own tissues.

AUTOLOGOUS. From the same person; an autologous breast reconstruction uses the woman's own tissues.

AUTOLOGOUS BLOOD. A patient's own blood, drawn and set aside for use during surgery in case a transfusion is needed.

AUTONOMIC NERVOUS SYSTEM. The part of the nervous system that regulates the activity of heart muscle, smooth muscle, and glands.

AUTOTRANSFUSION. A technique for recovering blood during surgery, separating and concentrating the red blood cells, and reinfusing them in the patient. Also known as blood salvage.

AUXILIARY HOSPITAL SERVICES. A term used broadly to designate such nonmedical services as financial services, birthing classes, support groups, etc. that are instituted in response to consumer demand.

AVASCULAR NECROSIS. A disorder in which bone tissue dies and collapses following the temporary or permanent loss of its blood supply; it is also known as osteonecrosis.

AVULSION. The tearing away of a body part or tissue.

AXILLARY. Pertaining to the armpit.

AXILLARY LYMPH NODE. Lymph nodes under the arm.

AXILLARY VEIN. A blood vessel that takes blood from tissues back to the heart to receive oxygenated blood.

B

B-LYMPHOCYTE. A type of blood cell that is active in immune response.

BACTERIA. Microscopically small one-celled forms of life that cause many diseases and infections.

BACTERICIDAL. An agent that kills bacteria.

BACTERIOSTATIC. An agent that stops the multiplication of bacteria.

BACTERIURIA. The presence of bacteria in the urine.

BACTEROIDES. A family of anaerobic, rod-shaped bacteria. Its organisms are normal inhabitants of the oral, respiratory, intestinal, and urogenital cavities of humans, animals, and insects. Some species are infectious agents.

BALANCED ANESTHESIA. The use of a combination of inhalation and intravenous anesthetics, often with opioids for pain relief and neuromuscular blockers for muscle paralysis.

BALLOON ANGIOPLASTY. A procedure used to open an obstructed blood vessel. A small, balloon-tipped catheter is inserted into the vessel and the balloon is inflated to widen the vessel and push the obstructing material against the vessel's walls. The result is improved blood flow through the vessel.

BAND CELL. An immature neutrophil at the stage just preceding a mature cell. The nucleus of a band cell is unsegmented.

BARIATRIC SURGERY. Weight loss surgery, such as gastric bypass.

BARIATRICS. The branch of medicine that deals with the prevention and treatment of obesity and related disorders.

BARIUM ENEMA. An X-ray test of the bowel performed after giving the patient an enema of a white chalky substance (barium) that outlines the colon and the rectum.

BARIUM SULFATE. A barium compound used during a barium enema to block the passage of x rays during the exam.

BARIUM SWALLOW. Barium is used to coat the throat and the upper digestive tract, a contrast medium that allows the areas to be visualized in x-ray studies.

BAROTRAUMA. Ear pain caused by unequal air pressure on the inside and outside of the ear drum. Barotrauma, which is also called pressure-related ear pain or barotitis media, is the most common reason for myringotomies in adults.

BARRETT'S ESOPHAGUS. A potentially precancerous change in the type of cells that line the esophagus, caused by acid reflux disease.

BARTTER'S SYNDROME. An inherited disorder which affects a number of body processes, including the functioning of the part of the kidney that regulates potassium excretion and absorption. People with Bartter's syndrome have abnormally low blood potassium levels (hypokalemia).

BASAL CELL CARCINOMA. Basal cell carcinoma is the most common malignant tumor, affecting more than 800,000 people annually in the United States.

BASOPHIL. Segmented white blood cell with large dark blue-black granules that releases histamine in allergic reactions.

BELL. The cup-shaped portion of the head of a stethoscope, useful for detecting low-pitched sounds.

BELL'S PALSY. One-sided paralysis of the face that may be due to damage to the facial nerve.

BENIGN PROSTATIC HYPERPLASIA (BPH). Also called benign prostatic enlargement (BPE). Non-cancerous enlargement of the prostate gland as a result of an increase in the number of its constituent cells.

BENIGN TUMOR. An abnormal growth that is not cancerous (malignant), and does not spread to other areas of the body.

BETA BLOCKER. An antihypertensive drug that limits the activity of epinephrine, a hormone that increases blood pressure.

BEVEL. The slanted opening on one side of the tip of a needle.

BEZOAR. A collection of foreign material, usually hair or vegetable fibers or a mixture of both, that may occasionally occur in the stomach or intestines and block the passage of food.

BILATERAL. Occurring on both the right and left sides of the body.

BILATERAL CLEFT LIP. Cleft that occurs on both sides of the lip.

BILE. A fluid produced by the liver and stored in the gallbladder. Bile is important for the appropriate digestion of fats in the intestine.

BILE DUCTS. Tubes carrying bile from the liver to the intestines.

BILIARY ATRESIA. A disease in which the ducts that carry bile out of the liver are missing or damaged is the most frequent reason for transplantation in children. Biliary atresia of the major bile ducts causes cholestasis and jaundice, which does not become apparent until several days after birth; periportal fibrosis develops and leads to cirrhosis, with proliferation of small bile ducts unless these are also atretic; giant cell transformation of hepatic cells also occurs.

BILIARY SYSTEM. The term used to describe the system of ducts that carries the bile flow through the liver and the gallbladder, and ultimately empties into the duodenum. Also called the biliary tract.

BILIRUBIN. A yellow bile pigment found as sodium (soluble) bilirubinate, or as an insoluble calcium salt found in gallstones.

BILIVERDIN. A green bile pigment formed from the oxidation of heme, which is a bilin with a structure almost identical to that of bilirubin.

BINGE EATING DISORDER. An eating disorder in which the person binges but does not try to get rid of the food afterward by vomiting, using laxatives, or exercising.

BIOLOGICAL TISSUE VALVE. A replacement heart valve that is harvested from the patient (autograft), a human cadaver (homograft or allograft), or other animal, such as a pig (heterograft).

BIOMECHANICS. The application of mechanical laws to the structures in the human body, such as measuring the force and direction of stresses on a joint.

BIOPSY. The surgical removal and analysis of a tissue sample for diagnostic purposes. Usually the term refers to the collection and analysis of tissue from a suspected tumor to establish malignancy.

BLADDER. A membranous sac that serves as a reservoir for urine. Contraction of the bladder results in urination.

BLADDER EXSTROPHY. One of many bladder and urinary congenital abnormalities. Occurs when the wall of the bladder fails to close in embryonic development and remains exposed to the abdominal wall.

BLADDER IRRIGATION. To flush or rinse the bladder with a stream of liquid (as in removing a foreign body or medicating).

BLADDER MUCOSA. Mucous coat of the bladder.

BLADDER TUMOR MARKER STUDIES. A test to detect specific substances released by bladder cancer cells into the urine using chemical or immunologic (using antibodies).

BLADDER WASHINGS. A procedure in which bladder washing samples are taken by placing a salt solution into the bladder through a catheter (tube) and then removing the solution for microscopic testing.

BLANK. If an individual has inherited the same HLA antigen from both parents, the HLA typing is designated by the shared HLA antigen followed by a "blank"(-).

BLAST CELLS. Blood cells in early stage of cellular development.

BLAST CRISIS. Stage of chronic myelogenous leukemia where large quantities of immature cells are produced by the marrow, and it is not responsive to treatment.

BLEB. A thin-walled auxiliary drain created on the outside of the eyeball during filtering surgery for glaucoma. It is sometimes called a filtering bleb.

BLEEDING DISORDER. A problem related to the clotting mechanism of the blood.

BLEPHAROPLASTY. Plastic surgery performed on the eyelids.

BLOOD BANK. A laboratory that specializes in blood typing, antibody identification, and transfusion services.

BLOOD PRESSURE. The pressure exerted by arterial blood on the walls of arteries. This depends on the strength of the heart beat, elasticity of the arterial walls, and volume and viscosity (resistance to flow) of blood. The pressure of blood in the arteries is measured in millimeters of mercury by a sphygmomanometer or by an electronic device.

BLOOD SERUM. The fluid portion of the blood.

BLOOD TYPE. Any of various classes into which human blood can be divided according to immunological compatibility based on the presence or absence of certain antigens on the red blood cells. Blood types are sometimes called blood groups.

BLOOD UREA NITROGEN (BUN). Blood urea nitrogen is a chemical waste product of protein metabolism that circulates in the bloodstream. Healthy kidneys remove urea from the bloodstream and it leaves the body in the urine. When the kidneys are not functioning properly, they are unable to filter the urea out of the blood, and blood urea nitrogen levels become elevated.

BODY DYSMORPHIC DISORDER (BDD). A psychiatric condition marked by excessive preoccupation with an imaginary or minor defect in a facial feature or localized part of the body. Many people with BDD seek cosmetic surgery as a treatment for their perceived flaw.

BODY MASS INDEX (BMI). A measurement that has replaced weight as the preferred determinant of obesity. The BMI can be calculated (in American units) as a person's weight in pounds divided by the square of the person's height in inches, multiplied by the conversion factor of 703.

BOLUS. A mass of food ready to be swallowed, or a preparation of medicine to be given by mouth or IV all at once rather than gradually.

BONE DENSITOMETRY TEST. A test that quickly and accurately measures the density of bone.

BONE MARROW. A spongy tissue located within flat bones, including the hip and breast bones and the skull. This tissue contains stem cells, the precursors of platelets, red blood cells, and white blood cells.

BONE MARROW BIOPSY. A test involving the insertion of a thin needle into the breastbone or, more commonly, the hip, in order to aspirate (remove) a sample of the marrow. A small piece of cortical bone may also be obtained for biopsy.

BONE MARROW TRANSPLANT. Healthy marrow is infused into people who have had high-dose chemotherapy for one of the many forms of leukemias, immunodeficiencies, lymphomas, anemias, metabolic disorders, and sometimes solid tumors.

BONE MORPHOGENETIC PROTEINS. A family of substances in human bones and blood that encourage the process of osteoinduction.

BONE SPURS. A sharp or pointed calcified projection.

BONY LABYRINTH. A series of cavities contained in a capsule inside the temporal bone of the skull. The endolymph-filled membranous labyrinth is suspended in a fluid inside the bony labyrinth.

BORBORYGMI. Sounds created by the passage of food, gas or fecal material in the stomach or intestines.

BOTULINUM TOXIN. A toxin produced by the spores and growing cells of *Clostridium botulinum*. It causes muscle paralysis, therefore this toxin can be used to reduce frown lines by temporarily paralyzing the muscles in the face that contract when a person frowns or squints.

BOUGIE. A slender, flexible tube or rod inserted into the urethra in order to dilate it.

BOWEL LUMEN. The space within the intestine.

BRACHIAL. Referring to the arm; the brachial artery is an artery that runs from the shoulder to the elbow.

BRACHYTHERAPY. The use of radiation during angioplasty to prevent the artery from narrowing again (a process called restenosis).

BRADYCARDIA. Relatively slow heart action, usually considered as a rate under 60 beats per minute.

BRAIN DEATH. Irreversible cessation of brain function. Patients with brain death have no potential capacity for survival or for recovery of any brain function.

BRAIN LESION. Physical damage done to a specific part or location of the brain, that may result in specific symptoms or behaviors associated with that brain lesion.

BRCA1 OR BRCA2 GENETIC MUTATION. A genetic mutation that predisposes otherwise healthy women to breast cancer.

BREAST AUGMENTATION. A surgery to increase the size of the breasts.

BREAST BIOPSY. A procedure where suspicious tissue is removed and examined by a pathologist for cancer or other disease. The breast tissue may be obtained by open surgery, or through a needle.

BREATHING RATE. The number of breaths per minute.

BREECH PRESENTATION. The condition in which the baby enters the birth canal with its buttocks or feet first.

BRONCHI. The large air tubes leading from the trachea to the lungs that convey air to and from the lungs.

BRONCHIECTASIS. Persistent and progressive dilation of bronchi or bronchioles as a consequence of inflammatory disease such as lung infections, obstructions, tumors, or congenital abnormality.

BRONCHIOLES. Small airways extending from the bronchi into the lobes of the lungs.

BRONCHITIS. Inflammation of the air passages in the lungs.

BRONCHOALVEOLAR LAVAGE. Washing cells from the air sacs at the end of the bronchioles.

BRONCHODILATOR. A drug that relaxes the bronchial muscles, resulting in expansion of the bronchial air passages.

BRONCHOPLEURAL FISTULA. An abnormal connection between an air passage and the membrane that covers the lungs.

BRONCHOSCOPE. A tubular illuminated instrument used for inspecting or passing instruments into the bronchi.

BRONCHOSCOPY. A medical test that enables the physician to see the breathing passages and the lungs through a hollow, lighted tube.

BRONCHOSPASM. A spasmodic contraction of the muscles that line the two branches of the trachea that lead into the lungs, causing difficulty in breathing. Bronchospasm is a common complication in heavy smokers under anesthesia.

BROTH. A growth mixture for bacteria. Different compounds, such as sugars or amino acids, may be added to increase the growth of certain organisms. Also known as media.

BRUCELLOSIS. An infectious disease transmitted to humans from farm animals, most commonly goats, sheep, cattle, and dogs. It is marked by high fever, pains in the muscles and joints, heavy sweating, headaches, and depression.

BRUIT. A roaring sound created by a partially blocked artery.

BRUNESCENT. Developing a brownish or amber color over time; nuclear cataracts are sometimes called brunescent.

BUCCAL SULCUS. Groove in the upper part of the upper jaw (where there are teeth).

BUCCAL. The interior surface of the cheek.

BUERGER'S DISEASE. An episodic disease that causes inflammation and blockage of the veins and arteries of the limbs. It tends to be present almost exclusively in men under age 40 who smoke, and may require amputation of the hand or foot.

BULIMIA NERVOSA. An eating disorder marked by episodes of binge eating followed by purging, overexercising, or other behaviors intended to prevent weight gain.

BUNION. A swelling or deformity of the big toe, characterized by the formation of a bursa and a sideways displacement of the toe.

BURCH PROCEDURE. A surgical procedure, also called retropubic colposuspension, in which the neck of the bladder is suspended from nearby ligaments with sutures. It is performed to treat urinary incontinence.

BURSA. A sac found in connective tissue that acts to reduce friction between tendon and bone.

BURSITIS. Inflammation of a bursa.

C

CADAVER. A dead body.

CADAVER KIDNEY. A kidney from a brain-dead organ donor used for purposes of kidney transplantation.

CADAVER ORGAN. A pancreas, kidney, or other organ from a brain-dead organ donor.

CADAVER SKIN. Skin donated from another person to treat burns.

CADAVERIC DONOR. An organ donor who has recently died of causes not affecting the organ intended for transplant.

CAESARIAN SECTION. An incision made through the wall of a pregnant woman's abdomen and uterus in order to deliver the fetus. It is commonly abbreviated as C-section.

CALCITONIN. A hormone made by the thyroid gland. Calcitonin is involved in regulating levels of calcium and phophorus in the blood.

CALCIUM CHANNEL BLOCKER. A drug that lowers blood pressure by regulating calcium-related electrical activity in the heart.

CALCULUS. Any type of hard concretion (stone) in the body, but usually found in the gallbladder, pancreas, and kidneys. Calculi (the plural form) are formed by the accumulation of excess mineral salts and other organic material, such as blood or mucous. They can cause problems by lodging in and obstructing the proper flow of fluids, such as bile to the intestines or urine to the bladder.

CALDWELL-LUC PROCEDURE. A surgical procedure in which the surgeon enters the maxillary sinus by making an opening under the upper lip above the teeth.

CALLUS. A localized thickening of the outer layer of skin cells, caused by friction or pressure from shoes or other articles of clothing.

CANCER STAGING. A surgical procedure to remove a lymph node and examine the cells for cancer. It determines the extent of the cancer and how far it has spread.

CANCER SURGERY. Surgery in which the goal is to excise a tumor and its surrounding tissue found to be malignant.

CANCER. The uncontrolled growth of abnormal cells which have mutated from normal tissues.

CANINE TOOTH. In humans, the tooth located in the mouth next to the second incisor. The canine tooth has a pointed crown and the longest root of all the teeth.

CANKER SORE. A blister-like sore on the inside of the mouth that can be painful but is not serious.

CANNULA. A tube inserted into a body cavity.

CAPILLARY. Smallest extremity of the arterial vessel, where oxygen and nutrients are released from the blood into the cells, and cellular waste is collected.

CAPSULAR CONTRACTURE. Thick scar tissue around a breast implant, which may tighten and cause discomfort and/or firmness.

CAPSULE. A general medical term for a structure that encloses another structure or body part. The capsule of the testicle is the membrane that surrounds the glandular tissue.

CAPSULORRHEXIS. The creation of a continuous circular tear in the front portion of the lens capsule during cataract surgery to allow for removal of the lens nucleus.

CAPSULOTOMY. A procedure that is sometimes needed after ECCE to open a lens capsule that has become cloudy.

CARBOHYDRATES. Compounds such as cellulose, sugar, and starch that contain only carbon, hydrogen, and oxygen, and are a major part of the diets of people and other animals.

CARBON DIOXIDE. A heavy, colorless gas that dissolves in water. Abbreviated CO_2, it also produces light that is well absorbed by the skin, so is commonly used for skin resurfacing treatments.

CARCINOMA. A malignant growth that arises from epithelium, found in skin or, more commonly, the lining of body organs.

CARDIAC. Of or relating to the heart.

CARDIAC ANGIOGRAPHY. A procedure used to visualize blood vessels of the heart.

CARDIAC ARREST. A condition in which the heart has no discernable electrical activity to stimulate contraction, therefore no blood is pumped.

CARDIAC ARRHYTHMIA. An irregular heart rate (frequency of heartbeats) or rhythm (the pattern of heartbeats).

CARDIAC CATHETER. Long, thin, flexible tube, which is threaded into the heart through a blood vessel.

CARDIAC CATHETERIZATION. A procedure to pass a catheter to the heart and its vessels for the purpose of diagnosing coronary artery disease, assessing injury or disease of the aorta, or evaluating cardiac function.

CARDIAC DISEASE. Any disease involving the heart.

CARDIAC MARKER. A substance in the blood that rises following a myocardial infarction.

CARDIAC OUTPUT. The liter per minute blood flow generated by contraction of the heart.

CARDIAC PULMONARY BYPASS. A procedure where heart blood is diverted into an inserted pump in order to maintain appropriate blood flow.

CARDIAC REHABILITATION. A structured program of education and activity offered by hospitals and other organizations.

CARDIAC SURGERY. Surgery performed on the heart.

CARDIAC TAMPONADE. A condition in which the sac around the heart is filled with blood and keeps the heart from functioning properly.

CARDIOLOGIST. A physician who specializes in problems of the heart.

CARDIOMYOPATHIES. Diseases of the heart muscle; usually refers to a disease of obscure etiology.

CARDIOPLEGIC ARREST. Halting the electrical activity of the heart by delivery of a high potassium solution to the coronary arteries. The arrested heart provides a superior surgical field for operation.

CARDIOPULMONARY BYPASS. Use of the heart-lung machine to provide systemic circulation, cardiac output, and ventilation of the blood.

CARDIOPULMONARY DISEASE. Illness of the heart and lungs.

CARDIOPULMONARY RESUSCITATION (CPR). An emergency procedure used to restore circulation and prevent brain death to a person who has collapsed, is unconscious, is not breathing, and has no pulse.

CARDIOPULMONARY. Involving both heart and lungs.

CARDIOTHORACIC SURGERY. Surgery involving the chest body cavity known as the thoracic cavity.

CARDIOVASCULAR SYSTEM. The physiological system including the heart and the blood vessels.

CARDIOVERSION. A procedure used to restore the heart's normal rhythm by applying a controlled electric shock to the exterior of the chest.

CARDIOVERTER. A device to apply electric shock to the chest to convert an abnormal heartbeat into a normal heartbeat.

CAROTID ARTERY DISEASE. A condition in which the arteries in the neck that supply blood to the brain become clogged, causing the danger of a stroke.

CAROTID ARTERY. Major artery leading to the brain, blockages of which can cause temporary or permanent strokes.

CAROTID ENDARTERECTOMY. A surgical technique for removing intra-arterial obstructions of the internal carotid artery.

CARPAL BONES. Eight wrist bones arranged in two rows that articulate proximally with the radius and indirectly with the ulna, and distally with the five metacarpal bones.

CARTILAGE. A tough, elastic connective tissue found in the joints, outer ear, nose, larynx, and other parts of the body.

CASE MANAGER. A health-care professional who can provide assistance with a patient's needs beyond the hospital.

CAST. An insoluble gelled protein matrix that takes the form of the renal tubule in which it was deposited. Casts are washed out by normal urine flow.

CASTRATION. Removal or destruction by radiation of both testicles (in a male) or both ovaries (in a female), making the individual incapable of reproducing.

CATARACT. A cloudy or opaque area on or in the lens of the eye.

CATEGORICALLY NEEDY. A term that describes certain groups of Medicaid recipients who qualify for the basic mandatory package of Medicaid benefits. There are categorically needy groups that states participating in Medicaid are required to cover, and other groups that the states have the option to cover.

CATGUT. The oldest type of absorbable suture. In spite of its name, catgut is made from collagen derived from sheep or cattle intestines. Synthetic absorbable sutures have been available since the 1980s.

CATHARTIC. An agent which stimulates defecation.

CATHARTIC COLON. A poorly functioning colon, resulting from the chronic abuse of stimulant cathartics.

CATHETER. A thin, hollow tube inserted into the body at specific points in order to infuse medications, blood components, or nutritional fluids into the body, or to withdraw fluids from the body such as gastric fluid or urine.

CAUDA EQUINA. A bundle of nerve roots in the lower back (lumbar region) of the spinal canal that controls the leg muscles and functioning of the bladder, intestines, and genitals.

CAUDA EQUINA SYNDROME (CES). A group of symptoms characterized by numbness or pain in the legs and/or loss of bladder and bowel control, caused by compression and paralysis of the nerve roots in the cauda equina. CES is a medical emergency.

CAUSALGIA. A severe burning sensation sometimes accompanied by redness and inflammation of the skin.

Causalgia is caused by injury to a nerve outside the spinal cord.

CAUTERIZE. To use heat or chemicals to stop bleeding, prevent the spread of infection, or destroy tissue.

CECUM. The beginning of the large intestine and the place where the appendix attaches to the intestinal tract.

CELLULITE. Dimpled skin that is caused by uneven fat deposits beneath the surface.

CENTRAL LINE. A catheter passed through a vein into large blood vessels of the chest or the heart; used in various medical procedures.

CENTRAL NERVOUS SYSTEM. The brain, spinal cord and the nerves throughout the body.

CENTRAL VENOUS LINE. A catheter inserted into a vein and connected to a physiologic monitoring system to directly measure venous blood pressure.

CEPHALOPELVIC DISPROPORTION (CPD). The condition in which the baby's head is too large to fit through the mother's pelvis.

CEREBRAL ANEURYSM. The dilation, bulging, or ballooning out of part of the wall of a vein or artery in the brain.

CEREBRAL CORTEX. The outer portion of the brain, consisting of layers of nerve cells and their connections. The cerebral cortex is the part of the brain in which thought processes take place.

CEREBRAL PALSY. Group of disorders characterized by loss of movement or loss of other nerve functions. These disorders are caused by injuries to the brain that occur during fetal development or near the time of birth.

CEREBROSPINAL FLUID. A clear fluid that fills the hollow cavity inside the brain and spinal cord. The cerebrospinal fluid has several functions, including providing a cushion for the brain against shock or impact, and removing waste products from the brain.

CEREBROVASCULAR ACCIDENT. Brain hemorrhage, also known as a stroke.

CERVICAL CRYOTHERAPY. Surgery performed after a biopsy has confirmed abnormal cervical cells (dysplasia).

CERVIX. The lower part of the uterus extending into the vagina.

CESAREAN SECTION. A surgical procedure in which incisions are made through a woman's abdomen and uterus to deliver her baby.

CHARCOT'S ARTHROPATHY. Also called neuropathic arthropathy, a condition in which the shoulder joint is destroyed following loss of its nerve supply.

CHEMICAL PEEL. A skin treatment that uses the application of chemicals, such as phenol or trichloroacetic acid (TCA), to remove the uppermost layer of skin.

CHEMICAL TOXICITY. State of physical illness induced by poisoning with toxic chemicals. Chemical toxicities may affect a person's behavior or mental function.

CHEMOPREVENTION. The use of drugs, vitamins, or other substances to reduce the risk of developing cancer or of the cancer returning.

CHEMOTHERAPY. Medical treatment of a disease, particularly cancer, with drugs or other chemicals.

CHEST TUBE. A tube inserted into the chest to drain fluid and air from around the lungs.

CHEST X RAY. A diagnostic procedure in which a small amount of radiation is used to produce an image of the structures of the chest (heart, lungs, and bones) on film.

CHILD LIFE SPECIALIST. A person who has had specific training in the care of children, including understanding growth and development specific to each age range and how to talk to children of different ages.

CHIROPRACTIC. A system of therapy based on the notion that health and disease are related to the interactions between the brain and the nervous system. Treatment involves manipulation and adjustment of the segments of the spinal column. Chiropractic is considered a form of alternative medicine.

CHOLANGITIS. A bacterial infection of the biliary system.

CHOLECYSTECTOMY. Surgical removal of the gallbladder.

CHOLECYSTITIS. Infection and inflammation of the gallbladder, causing severe pain and rigidity in the upper right abdomen.

CHOLELITHIASIS. Also known as gallstones, these hard masses are formed in the gallbladder or passages, and can cause severe upper right abdominal pain radiating to the right shoulder, as a result of blocked bile flow.

CHOLELITHOTOMY. Surgical incision into the gallbladder to remove stones.

CHOLESTASIS. A blockage in the flow of bile.

CHOLESTEATOMA. A destructive and expanding sac that develops in the middle ear or mastoid process.

CHOLESTEROL. An abundant fatty substance in animal tissues. High levels in the diet are a factor in the cause of atherosclerosis.

CHORDAE TENDINEAE. The strands of connective tissue that connect the mitral valve to the papillary muscle of the heart's left ventricle.

CHORDEE. A condition associated with hypospadias in which the penis bends downward during erections.

CHORIOAMNIONITIS. Infection of the amniotic sac.

CHORIONIC VILLUS SAMPLING (CVS). A procedure similar to amniocentesis, except that cells are taken from the chorionic membrane (rather than the amniotic fluid) for testing. These cells, called chorionic villus cells, eventually become the placenta. The samples are collected either through the abdomen, as in amnio, or through the vagina. CVS can be done earlier in the pregnancy than amnio, but carries a somewhat higher risk.

CHORIORETINAL. Relating to the choroid coat of the eye and retina.

CHOROID. The middle of the three tunicae or coats that surround the eyeball; the choroid lies between the retina and the sclera.

CHROMOSOMES. Chromosomes are the strands of genetic material in a cell that occur in nearly identical pairs. Normal human cells contain 23 chromosome pairs—one in each pair inherited from the mother, and one from the father. Every human cell contains the exact same set of chromosomes.

CHRONIC. A condition that is persistent or recurs frequently.

CHRONIC MYELOGENOUS LEUKEMIA (CML). Also called chronic myelocytic leukemia, a malignant disorder that involves abnormal accumulation of white cells in the marrow and bloodstream.

CHRONIC OTITIS MEDIA. Inflammation of the middle ear with signs of infection lasting three months or longer.

CHRONIC PAIN. Pain that lasts more than three months and threatens to disrupt daily life.

CHRONIC RENAL (KIDNEY) FAILURE. Progressive loss of kidney function over several years that can result in permanent kidney failure requiring dialysis.

CILIA. Short hairlike processes that are capable of a lashing movement.

CILIARY BODY. The part of the eye, located behind the iris, that makes the intraocular aqueous fluid.

CIRCULATION. The passage of blood and delivery of oxygen through the veins and arteries of the body.

CIRCUMCISION. The removal of the foreskin of the penis.

CIRRHOSIS. A chronic degenerative disease causing irreversible scarring of the liver.

CLASSIC INCISION. In a cesarean section, an incision made vertically along the uterus.

CLATHRATES. Substances in which a molecule from one compound fills a space within the crystal lattice of another compound. One theory of general anesthesia proposes that water molecules interact with anesthetic molecules to form clathrates that decrease receptor function.

CLAUDICATION. Cramping or pain in a leg caused by poor blood circulation, frequently caused by hardening of the arteries (atherosclerosis). Intermittent claudication occurs only at certain times, usually after exercise, and is relieved by rest.

CLAVICLE. Also called the collar bone, it is a doubly curved long bone that connects the upper limb to the trunk.

CLEAN-CATCH SPECIMEN. A urine specimen that is collected from the middle of the urine stream after the first part of the flow has been discarded.

CLEARANCE. The process of removing a substance or obstruction from the body. Also the rate at which a drug or other substance is removed from the blood by the liver or kidneys.

CLEFT. Split or opening, which can occur in the lip or palate or both.

CLEFT PALATE. A birth defect in which the roof of the mouth is open because the two sides of the palate failed to join together during fetal development.

CLINICAL BREAST EXAM. An examination of the breast and surrounding tissue by a physician, who is feeling for lumps and looking for other signs of abnormality.

CLINICAL NURSE SPECIALISTS. Nurses with advanced training as well as a master's degree.

CLOT. A soft, semi-solid mass that forms when blood gels.

CLOTTING FACTORS. Substances in the blood that act in sequence to stop bleeding by forming a clot.

CO-INSURANCE. The percentage of health care charges that an insurance company pays after the beneficiary pays the deductible. Most co-insurance percentages are 70–90%.

COAGULATION. Blood clotting.

COAGULATION CASCADE. The process of blood clotting. The cascade itself is a series of chemical reactions involving blood proteins and enzymes that occurs wherever there is a break in a blood vessel. The end product of the cascade is a protein called fibrin.

COAGULOPATHY. A defect in the blood clotting mechanism.

COARCTATION OF THE AORTA. A congenital defect in which severe narrowing or constriction of the aorta obstructs the flow of blood.

COATS' DISEASE. Also called exudative retinitis, a chronic abnormality characterized by the deposition of cholesterol on the outer retinal layers.

COCHLEA. The hearing part of the inner ear. This snail-shaped structure contains fluid and thousands of microscopic hair cells tuned to various frequencies.

COGNITION. The mental activity of thinking, learning, and memory.

COLD SORE. A small blister on the lips or face, caused by a virus. Also called a fever blister.

COLECTOMY. The surgical removal of the colon or part of the colon.

COLITIS. Inflammation of the colon, or large bowel.

COLLAGEN. A protein that provides structural support for the skin. Collagen is the main component of connective tissue.

COLLATERAL VESSEL. A side branch or network of side branches of a large blood vessel.

COLLATERALS. Alternate pathways for arterial blood.

COLON. Also called the large intestine, the colon has six major segments: caecum, ascending colon, transverse colon, descending colon, sigmoid colon, and rectum. Its length is approximately 5 ft (1.5 m) in the adult and it is responsible for forming, storing, and expelling waste matter.

COLONOSCOPE. The fiberoptic device used to view the inside of the large intestine, and through which a variety of procedures can be performed, including biopsies and colonic stent placement.

COLONOSCOPY. An examination of the colon performed with a colonoscope.

COLORECTAL. Pertaining to the large intestine and the rectum.

COLORECTAL CANCER. Cancer of the large intestine, or colon, including the rectum.

COLOSTOMY. A temporary or permanent diversion in which the colon opens to the outside of the body through a hole (stoma). Stool is collected outside of the body in a bag attached to the colostomy.

COLPORRHAPY. A surgical procedure in which the vagina is sutured.

COLPOSCOPY. Examination of the cervix through a magnifying device to detect abnormal cells.

COLUMELLA. The strip of skin running from the tip of the nose to the upper lip, separating the nostrils.

COMA. A state of unconsciousness from which a person cannot be aroused, even by strong or painful stimuli.

COMMISSURES. The normal separations between the valve leaflets.

COMMON BILE DUCT. The branching passage through which bile—a necessary digestive enzyme—travels from the liver and gallbladder into the small intestine. Digestive enzymes from the pancreas also enter the intestines through the common bile duct.

COMMON PATHWAY. The pathway that results from the merging of the extrinsic and intrinsic pathways. The common pathway includes the final steps before a clot is formed.

COMORBID. A term applied to a disease or disorder that occurs at the same time as another disease condition. For example, there are a number of health problems that are comorbid with obesity.

COMPATIBLE DONOR. A person whose tissue and blood type are the same as the recipient's.

COMPLETE BLOOD COUNT (CBC). A blood test to check the numbers of red blood cells, white blood cells, and platelets in the blood.

COMPOUND FRACTURE. A fracture in which the broken end or ends of the bone have penetrated through the skin; also known as an open fracture.

COMPULSION. The uncontrollable impulse to perform specific acts. In mental health disorders, compulsions are often repetitive and carried out by the person in order to avoid feelings of anxiety.

COMPUTED TOMOGRAPHY (CT) SCAN. An imaging technique in which cross-sectional x rays of the body are compiled to create a three-dimensional image of the body's internal structures.

CONCEPTION. The union of egg and sperm to form a fetus.

CONCHA. The hollow shell-shaped portion of the external ear.

CONDITIONING. Process of preparing a patient to receive marrow donation, often through the use of chemotherapy and radiation therapy.

CONDUCTIVE HEARING LOSS. A type of medically treatable hearing loss in which the inner ear is usually normal, but there are specific problems in the middle or outer ears that prevent sound from getting to the inner ear in a normal way.

CONDUIT DIVERSION. A surgical procedure that restores urinary and fecal continence by diverting these functions through a constructed conduit leading to an external waste reservoir (ostomy).

CONFIRMATORY TYPING. Repeat tissue typing to confirm the compatibility of the donor and patient before transplant.

CONFIRMATORY TYPING. Repeat tissue typing to confirm the compatibility of the donor and patient before transplant

CONGENITAL DEFECT. A defect present at birth that occurs during the growth and development of the fetus in the womb.

CONGESTIVE HEART FAILURE. A serious condition caused by disease or damage to the heart that weakens the heart's ability to pump a sufficient amount of blood to the body tissues.

CONGREGATE HOUSING. A type of housing arrangement for seniors that offers independent living in separate apartments as well as opportunities to share activities of daily living with other residents. Congregate housing does not usually involve assisted living or skilled nursing care, however.

CONJUNCTIVA. The mucous membrane that covers the eyes and lines the eyelids.

CONJUNCTIVITIS. Inflammation of the conjunctiva, the membrane on the inner part of the eyelids and the covering of the white of the eye.

CONNECTIVE TISSUE. Cells such as fibroblasts, and material such as collagen and reticulin, that unite one part of the body with another.

CONSENT. Permission or agreement.

CONSERVATION SURGERY. Surgery that preserves the aesthetics of the area undergoing an operation.

CONSTIPATION. Difficulty passing a bowel movement. May refer to infrequent passage of stool, or to a hard, dry stool requiring straining and physical effort in order to pass.

CONSTRICT. To squeeze tightly, compress, draw together.

CONSULTATION. Evaluation by an outside expert or specialist, someone other than the primary care provider.

CONTAMINATE. To make an item unsterile or unclean by direct contact.

CONTAMINATION. A breach in the preservation of a clean or sterile object or environment.

CONTINENT. Able to hold the contents of the bladder or bowel until one can use a bathroom. A continent surgical procedure is one that allows the patient to keep waste products inside the body rather than collecting them in an external bag attached to a stoma.

CONTINUOUS POSITIVE AIRWAY PRESSURE (CPAP). A ventilation device that blows a gentle stream of air into the nose during sleep to keep the airway open.

CONTRACEPTION. The prevention of the union of the male's sperm with the female's egg.

CONTRACTURE. An abnormal persistent shortening of a muscle or the overlying skin at a joint, usually caused by the formation of scar tissue following an injury.

CONTRAST AGENT. Also called a contrast medium, this is usually a barium or iodine dye that is injected into the area under investigation. The dye makes the interior body parts more visible on an x-ray film. For myelograms, an iodine based contrast agent is used.

CONVULSION. To shake or effect with spasms; to agitate or disturb violently.

COR PULMONALE. Enlargement of the right ventricle of the heart caused by pulmonary hypertension that may result from emphysema or bronchiectasis; eventually, the condition leads to congestive heart failure.

CORACOID PROCESS. A long curved projection from the scapula overhanging the glenoid cavity; it provides attachment to muscles and ligaments of the shoulder and back region.

CORE NEEDLE BIOPSY (CNB). A procedure using a larger diameter needle to remove a core of tissue from the breast.

CORECTOMY. Another term for iridectomy.

CORN. A horny thickening of the skin on a toe, caused by friction and pressure from poorly fitted shoes or stockings.

CORNEA. Clear, bowl-shaped structure at the front of the eye. It is located in front of the colored part of the eye (iris). The cornea lets light into the eye and partially focuses it.

CORNEAL TOPOGRAPHY. Mapping the cornea's surface with a specialized computer that illustrates corneal elevations.

CORONARY. Of or relating to the heart.

CORONARY ARTERY BYPASS GRAFT SURGERY (CABG). A surgical procedure in which arteries or veins from elsewhere in the patient's body are grafted onto the arteries of the heart as a way to bypass damaged or narrowed heart blood vessels.

CORONARY ARTERY DISEASE. Also called atherosclerosis, it is a buildup of fatty matter and debris in the coronary artery wall that causes narrowing of the artery.

CORONARY BLOOD VESSELS. The arteries and veins that supply blood to the heart muscle.

CORONARY OCCLUSION. Obstruction of an artery that supplies the heart. When the artery is completely blocked, a myocardial infarction (heart attack) results; an incomplete blockage may result in angina.

CORONARY STENT. An artificial support device used to keep a coronary vessel open.

CORONARY VASCULAR DISEASE. Or cardiovascular disease; disease of the heart or blood vessels, such as atherosclerosis (hardening of the arteries).

CORTICOSTEROIDS. A class of drugs that are synthetic versions of the cortisone produced by the body. They rank among the most powerful anti-inflammatory agents.

CORTISOL. A corticosteroid hormone produced by the adrenal gland.

CORTISONE. A steroid compound used to treat autoimmune diseases and inflammatory conditions. It is sometimes injected into a joint to relieve the pain of arthritis.

COSMETIC SURGERY. Surgery that is intended to improve a patient's appearance or correct disfigurement. It is also called aesthetic surgery.

COUCHING. The oldest form of cataract surgery, in which the lens is dislocated and pushed backward into the vitreous body with a lance.

CRANIOCAUDAL. Head to tail, x-ray beam directly overhead the part being examined.

CRANIOFACIAL SURGERY. Surgery of the facial tissue and skull.

CRANIOPHARYNGEAL ACHALASIA. A swallowing disorder of the throat.

CRANIOSYNOSTOSIS. Premature closing of the sutures joining the skull bones.

CRANIOTOMY. A surgical incision into the skull.

CRANIUM. The large, rounded upper part of the skull that encloses the brain.

CREATINE. Creatine is a substance produced by proteins and stored in the muscles. Creatine is a source of energy, allowing muscle contraction to take place. Some creatine is converted to creatinine, and enters the bloodstream, where it is filtered out by healthy kidneys and leaves the body in the urine. When the kidneys are not functioning properly, creatinine levels in the blood become abnormally elevated.

CREATININE. Creatinine is a chemical waste product that is produced by the muscles. Creatinine enters the bloodstream and goes to the kidneys. Healthy kidneys filter out this waste material from the blood. It passes into the urine and out of the body. Unhealthy kidneys, however, are unable to filter out the creatinine from the blood. The creatinine remains circulating in the bloodstream, and levels rise as the muscles continue to produce more and more.

CREATININE CLEARANCE RATE. The clearance of creatinine from the plasma compared to its appearance in the urine. Since there is no reabsorption of creatinine, this measurement can estimate glomerular filtration rate.

CREMASTERIC REFLEX. A reflex in which the cremaster muscle, which covers the testes and the spermatic cord, pulls the testicles back into the scrotum. It is important for a doctor to distinguish between an undescended testicle and a hyperactive cremasteric reflex in small children.

CRICOID CARTILAGE. A ring-shaped piece of cartilage that forms the lower and rear parts of the voice box or larynx; it is sometimes called the annular cartilage because of its shape.

CRICOTHYROID MEMBRANE. The piece of connective tissue that lies between the thyroid and cricoid cartilages.

CRICOTHYROIDOTOMY. An emergency tracheotomy that consists of a cut through the cricothyroid membrane to open the patient's airway as fast as possible.

CRITICAL CARE. The multidisciplinary health-care specialty that provides care to patients with acute, life-threatening illness or injury.

CROHN'S DISEASE. A chronic, inflammatory bowel disease usually affecting the ileum, colon, or both.

CROSS-MATCH. A laboratory test done to confirm that blood from a donor and blood from the recipient are compatible. Serum from each is mixed with red blood cells from the other and observed for hemagglutination.

CROWN. The top part of the tooth. Also, an artificial replacement tooth.

CRYOANESTHESIA. The use of the numbing effects of cold as a surgical anesthetic. For dermabrasion, this involves the spraying of a cold-inducing chemical on the area being treated.

CRYOGEN. A substance with a very low boiling point, such as liquid nitrogen, used in cryotherapy treatment.

CRYOPEXY. Reattachment of a detached retina by freezing the tissue behind the tear with nitrous oxide.

CRYOPROSTATECTOMY. Freezing of the prostate through the use of liquid nitrogen probes guided by transrectal ultrasound of the prostate.

CRYOSURGERY. Freezing and destroying abnormal cells.

CRYOTHERAPY. The therapeutic use of cold to reduce discomfort, or remove abnormal tissue.

CRYPTORCHIDISM. A developmental disorder in which one or both testes fail to descend from the abdomen into the scrotum before birth. It is the most common structural abnormality in the male genital tract.

CRYPTORCHIDISM. A developmental disorder in which one or both testes fail to descend from the abdomen into the scrotum before birth.

CUL-DE-SAC. The closed end of a pouch or tubular cavity; also called a caecum.

CULDOCENTESIS. Removal of material from the pouch of Douglas, a deep peritoneal recess between the uterus and the upper vaginal wall, by means of puncture of the vaginal wall.

CULDOSCOPY. Procedure by which a surgeon performs a colpotomy and inserts a culdoscope, an instrument with a light on the end, through the incision.

CULTURE. A swab of blood, sputum, pus, urine, or other body fluid planted in a special medium, incubated, and allowed to grow for identification of infection-causing organisms.

CULTURE CHANGE. A term that refers to a movement in the United States to make nursing homes more resident-centered and less like hospitals.

CUPID'S BOW. Double curve of the upper lip.

CURETTAGE. Procedure performed with a curette, a spoon-shaped instrument used to scrape tissue.

CURETTE. A scoop-shaped surgical instrument used for removing tissue from body cavities.

CUSHING'S DISEASE. A disease in which too many hormones called glucocorticoids are released into the blood. This causes fat to build up in the face, back, and chest, and the arms and legs to become very thin. Other symptoms include excessive blood sugar levels, weak muscles and bones, a flushed face, and high blood pressure.

CUTANEOUS SQUAMOUS CELL CARCINOMA. Malignant skin tumor of the epidermis or its appendages.

CYANOACRYLATE. The chemical name of liquid surgical adhesive.

CYANOSIS. Blue, gray, or dark purple discoloration of the skin caused by a deficiency of oxygen.

CYCLOCRYOTHERAPY. The use of subfreezing temperatures to treat glaucoma.

CYST. An abnormal sac-like growth in the body that contains liquid or a semisolid material.

CYSTECTOMY. The surgical resection of part or all of the bladder.

CYSTIC ARTERY. An artery that brings oxygenated blood to the gallbladder.

CYSTIC FIBROSIS. A hereditary disease that appears in early childhood, involves functional disorder of digestive glands, and is marked especially by faulty digestion due to a deficiency of pancreatic enzymes, by difficulty in breathing due to mucus accumulation in airways, and by excessive loss of salt in the sweat.

CYSTINE. An amino acid normally reabsorbed by the kidney tubules. Cystinuria is an inherited disease in which cystine and some other amino acids are not reabsorbed by the body in normal amounts. Cystine crystals then form in the kidney, which leads to kidney stones and obstructive renal failure.

CYSTOCELE. Sagging or bulging of the bladder through the front wall of the vagina.

CYSTOPLASTY. Reconstructive surgery of the urinary bladder.

CYSTOSCOPE. Endoscope specially designed for urological use to examine the bladder, lower urinary tract, and prostate gland. The examination is called cystoscopy.

CYSTOTOMY. An incision in the bladder.

CYTOKINE. A protein that regulates the duration and intensity of the body's immune response.

CYTOLOGIST (CYTOLOGY). A medical technologist who specializes in preparing and examining biopsy specimens and cell specimens for changes that may indicate precancerous conditions or a specific stage of cancer.

CYTOMEGALOVIRUS (CMV). Virus that can cause pneumonia in post bone marrow transplant patients.

CYTOPLASM. The part of a cell outside of the nucleus.

CYTOSTATIC. A type of drug that inhibits the process of cell division. Azathioprine is an example of a cytostatic drug.

D

DACRON GRAFT. A synthetic material used in the repair or replacement of blood vessels.

DEBRIDEMENT. The act of removing any foreign material and damaged or contaminated tissue from a wound to expose surrounding healthy tissue.

DEBULKING. The removal of part of a malignant tumor in order to make the remainder more sensitive to radiation or chemotherapy.

DECOMPRESSION. Any surgical procedure done to relieve pressure on a nerve or other part of the body. A laminectomy is sometimes called an open decompression.

DEDICATED. Reserved for a specific purpose. An ambulatory surgical center must have at least one dedicated operating room in order to qualify for accreditation.

DEDUCTIBLE. An amount of money that an insured person is required to pay on each claim made on an insurance policy.

DEEP VEIN THROMBOSIS. The development or presence of a blood clot in a vein deep within the leg. Deep vein thrombosis can lead to pulmonary embolism.

DEFECATION. The act of passing a bowel movement.

DEFIBRILLATION. An electronic process that helps reestablish a normal heart rhythm.

DEFIBRILLATOR. A device that delivers an electric shock to the heart muscle through the chest wall in order to restore a normal heart rate.

DEGENERATIVE ARTHRITIS, OR OSTEOARTHRITIS. A non-inflammatory type of arthritis, usually occurring in older people, characterized by degeneration of cartilage, enlargement of the margins of the bones, and changes in the membranes in the joints.

DEGLOVING. Separating the skin of the penis from the shaft temporarily in order to correct chordee.

DEHISCENCE. Separation or splitting open of the different layers of tissue in a surgical incision. Dehiscence may be partial, involving only a few layers of surface tissue; or complete, reopening all the layers of the incision.

DEHYDRATION. Low overall levels of body fluid. May occur due to increased loss of fluids through sweating, vomiting, or diarrhea.

DELIRIUM. An altered state of consciousness that includes confusion, disorientation, incoherence, agitation, and defective perception (such as hallucinations).

DELTOID MUSCLE. Muscle that covers the prominence of the shoulder.

DELUSION. Conviction of a false belief or wrong judgment despite obvious evidence to the contrary.

DEMENTIA. The progressive loss of cognitive and intellectual function of the brain including impaired memory, judgment, and disorientation, without the impairment of perception or consciousness. It is usually associated with a structural brain disease such as Alzheimer's disease.

DEMYELINATION. The loss of myelin with preservation of the axons or fiber tracts. Central demyelination occurs within the central nervous system, and peripheral demyelination affects the peripheral nervous system as with Guillain-Barré syndrome.

DEOXYHEMOGLOBIN. Hemoglobin with oxygen removed.

DEPARTMENT OF HEALTH AND HUMAN SERVICE (DHHS). It is a federal agency that houses the Centers for Medicare and Medicaid Services, and distributes funds for Medicaid.

DEPRESSANT. A drug or other substance that soothes or lessens tension of the muscles or nerves.

DERMABRASION. A technique for removing the upper layers of skin with planing wheels powered by compressed air.

DERMATOME. A surgical instrument used to cut thin slices of skin for grafts.

DERMIS. The underlayer of skin, containing blood vessels, nerves, hair follicles, and oil and sweat glands.

DESICCATION. Tissue death.

DETOXIFICATION. To remove a poison or toxin, or the effect of such a harmful substance; to free from an intoxicating or addictive substance or from dependence on or addiction to a harmful substance.

DETRUSOR MUSCLE. The medical name for the layer of muscle tissue covering the urinary bladder. When the detrusor muscle contracts, the bladder expels urine.

DEVELOPMENTAL DISORDER. A disorder or disability that occurs because of prenatal or early childhood events that affect cognition, language, motor, or social skills.

DEVIATED SEPTUM. An abnormal configuration of the cartilage that divides the two sides of the nose. It can cause breathing problems if left uncorrected.

DHHS. The Department of Health and Human Service. This federal agency houses the Centers for Medicare and Medicaid Services and distributes funds for Medicaid.

DIABETES MELLITUS. A disease in which a person can't effectively use glucose to meet the needs of the body. It is caused by a lack of the hormone insulin.

DIABETES MELLITUS. A disease in which insufficient insulin is made by the body to metabolize sugars.

DIABETIC NEPHROPATHY. Kidney damage or disease brought on by the long-term effects of diabetes.

DIABETIC RETINOPATHY. Degeneration of the retina related to diabetes; both type 1 and type 2 diabetes can lead to diabetic retinopathy.

DIAGNOSTIC WINDOW. A cardiac marker's timeline for rising, peaking, and returning to normal after a heart attack.

DIALYSATE. A chemical bath used in dialysis to draw fluids and toxins out of the bloodstream and supply electrolytes and other chemicals to the bloodstream.

DIALYSIS. A blood filtration therapy that replaces the function of the kidneys, filtering fluids and waste products out of the bloodstream. There are two types of dialysis treatment: hemodialysis, which uses an artificial kidney, or dialyzer, as a blood filter; and peritoneal dialysis, which uses the patient's abdominal cavity (peritoneum) as a blood filter.

DIALYSIS PRESCRIPTION. The general parameters of dialysis treatment that vary according to each patient's individual needs. Treatment length, type of dialyzer and dialysate used, and rate of ultrafiltration are all part of the dialysis prescription.

DIALYZER. An artificial kidney usually composed of hollow fiber which is used in hemodialysis to eliminate waste products from the blood and remove excess fluids from the bloodstream.

DIAPHRAGM. The large muscle that is located between the abdomen and the chest area. The diaphragm aids in breathing. Also the flat-shaped portion of the head of a stethoscope, useful for detecting high-pitched sounds.

DIAPHYSIS. The shaft of a long bone.

DIASTOLE. Period between contractions of the heart.

DIASTOLIC. Minimum arterial blood pressure during ventricular relaxation or rest.

DIATHERMY. Also called electrocautery, this is a procedure that heats and destroys abnormal cells.

DIETHYLSTILBESTROL (DES). A synthetic form of estrogen that was widely prescribed to women from

1940 to 1970 to prevent complications during pregnancy, and linked to several serious birth defects and disorders of the reproductive system in daughters of women who took DES.

DIETHYLSTILBESTROL (DES). A synthetic hormone that was used in the mid-twentieth century to treat recurrent miscarriages; exposure to DES as a fetus is a risk factor for premature labor.

DIFFERENTIAL. Blood test that determines the percentage of each type of white blood cell in a person's blood.

DIFFUSE ESOPHAGEAL SPASM (DES). An uncommon condition characterized by abnormal simultaneous contractions of the esophagus.

DIFFUSION TENSOR IMAGING (DTI). A refinement of magnetic resonance imaging that allows the doctor to measure the flow of water and track the pathways of white matter in the brain. DTI is able to detect abnormalities in the brain that do not show up on standard MRI scans.

DIGESTIVE TRACT. The stomach, intestines, and other parts of the body through which food passes.

DIGITAL RECTAL EXAM (DRE). Procedure in which the physician inserts a gloved finger into the rectum to examine the rectum and the prostate gland for signs of cancer.

DIGITS. Fingers or toes.

DILATE. To expand or open a valve or blood vessel.

DILATION. The process of enlarging, usually applied to relatively circular openings.

DILATION AND CURETTAGE (D&C). A surgical procedure that expands the cervical canal (dilation) so that the lining of the uterus can be scraped (curettage).

DIMINISHED BREATH SOUNDS. A lack of breath sound due to fluid or air accumulation.

DIMINISHED CHEST EXPANSION. A decrease in the chest expansion due to an inability of the lungs to fully pull air in and push it out.

DIRECTED DONATION. Blood donated by a patient's family member or friend, to be used by the patient.

DISCHARGE PLANNER. A health-care professional who helps patients arrange for health and home care needs after they go home from the hospital.

DISCIPLINE. In health care, a specific area of preparation or training such as social work, nursing, or nutrition.

DISEASE-MODIFYING ANTIRHEUMATIC DRUGS (DMARDS). A group of medications that can be given to slow or stop the progression of rheumatoid arthritis. DMARDs include such drugs as oral or injectable gold, methotrexate, leflunomide, and penicillamine.

DISINFECT. To remove most microorganisms but not highly resistant ones.

DISKECTOMY (OR DISCECTOMY). The surgical removal of a portion of an invertebral disk.

DISSEMINATED INTRAVASCULAR COAGULATION (DIC). A condition in which spontaneous bleeding and clot formation occur throughout the circulatory system. DIC can be caused by transfusion reactions and a number of serious illnesses.

DISSEMINATED INTRAVASCULAR DISSEMINATION. A condition in which the clotting factors in the blood are rapidly used up, resulting in a severe deficit in clotting factors and a very high risk of severe, uncontrollable bleeding.

DIURETIC. A type of medication that increases the amount of urine produced and relieves excess fluid buildup in body tissues. Diuretics may be used in treating high blood pressure, lung disease, premenstrual syndrome, and other conditions.

DIVERTICULA (SINGULAR, DIVERTICULUM). Pouch-like herniations through the muscular wall of an organ such as the stomach, small intestine, or colon.

DIVERTICULITIS. Inflammation or infection of the diverticula of the intestines.

DIVERTICULOSIS. A condition that involves the development of sacs that bulge through the large intestine's muscular walls, but are not inflamed. It may cause bleeding, stomach distress, and excess gas.

DNA. Deoxyribonucleic acid; the substance within the nucleus of all human cells in which the genetic information is stored.

DOCUMENTATION. The process of recording information in the medical chart, or the materials contained in a medical chart.

DOMINANT HAND. The hand that the individual prefers to use for most activities, especially writing.

DONOR. A person who supplies organ(s), tissue or blood to another person for transplantation.

DOPPLER. The Doppler effect refers to the apparent change in frequency of sound-wave echoes returning to a stationary source from a moving target. If the object is moving toward the source, the frequency increases; if the object is moving away, the frequency decreases. The size of this frequency shift can be used to compute the object's speed—be it a car on the road or blood in an artery.

DOPPLER ECHOCARDIOGRAPHY. A testing technique that uses Doppler ultrasound technology to evaluate the pattern and direction of blood flow in the heart.

DORSAL. Referring to a position closer to the back than to the stomach. The laminae in the spinal column are located on the dorsal side of each vertebra.

DOSE LIMITING. Case in which the side effects of a drug prevent an increase in dose.

DOWN SYNDROME. The most prevalent of a class of genetic defects known as trisomies, in which cells contain three copies of certain chromosomes rather than the usual two. Down syndrome, or trisomy 21, usually results from three copies of chromosome 21.

DRAINAGE. The withdrawal or removal of blood and other fluid matter from an incision or wound. An incision that is oozing blood or tissue fluids is said to be draining.

DRESSING. A bandage, gauze pad, or other material placed over a wound or incision to cover and protect it.

DRY EYE. Corneal dryness due to insufficient tear production.

DRY SOCKET. A painful condition following tooth extraction in which a blood clot does not properly fill the empty socket. Dry socket leaves the underlying bone exposed to air and food particles.

DUANE SYNDROME. A hereditary congenital syndrome in which the affected eye shows a limited capacity to move, and is deficient in convergence with the other eye.

DUCTOGRAM. A test used for imaging the breast ducts and diagnosing the cause of abnormal nipple discharges.

DUCTUS ARTERIOSIS. A fetal blood vessel that connects the aorta and pulmonary artery.

DUMPING SYNDROME. A complex physical reaction to food passing too quickly from the stomach into the small intestine, characterized by sweating, nausea, abdominal cramps, dizziness, and other symptoms.

DUODENECTOMY. Excision of the duodenum.

DUODENUM. The first part of the small intestine that connects the stomach above and the jejunum below.

DURA. The strongest and outermost of three membranes that protect the brain, spinal cord, and nerves of the cauda equina.

DURABLE MEDICAL POWER OF ATTORNEY. A legal document that empowers a person to make medical decisions for the patient should the patient be unable to make the decisions.

DYSMENORRHEA. Painful menstruation.

DYSMOTILITY. A lack of normal muscle movement (motility), especially in the esophagus, stomach, or intestines.

DYSPHAGIA. Difficulty and pain in swallowing.

DYSPLASIA. The abnormal form or abnormal development of a body organ or organ system.

DYSPNEA. Difficulty breathing.

DYSTOCIA. Failure to progress in labor, either because the cervix will not dilate (expand) further or (after full dilation) the head does not descend through the mother's pelvis.

E

EALES DISEASE. A disorder marked by recurrent hemorrhages into the retina and vitreous body. It occurs most often in males between the ages of 10 and 25.

EAR MOLDING. A non-surgical method for treating ear deformities shortly after birth with the application of a mold held in place by tape and surgical glue.

EBOLA VIRUS . A dangerous pathogen that should contained in a negative pressure room.

ECG OR EKG. A record of the waves that relate to the electrical impulses produced at each beat of the heart.

ECHOCARDIOGRAPHY. An imaging procedure used to create a picture of the heart's movement, valves, and chambers. The test uses high-frequency sound waves that come from a hand wand placed on the chest. Echocardiogram may be used in combination with Doppler ultrasound to evaluate the blood flow across the heart's valves.

ECLAMPSIA. A serious, life-threatening complication of pregnancy, in which high blood pressure results in a variety of problems, including seizures.

ECTOPIC. Located in an abnormal site or tissue. An ectopic testicle is one that is located in an unusual position outside its normal line of descent into the scrotum.

ECTOPIC BEAT. Abnormal heart beat arising elsewhere than from the sinoatrial node.

ECTOPIC PREGNANCY. A pregnancy that occurs outside of the uterus, most often in the fallopian tubes.

ECTROPION. A complication of blepharoplasty, in which the lower lid is pulled downward, exposing the inner surface.

EDEMA. An abnormal accumulation of fluids in intercellular spaces in the body; causes swelling.

EFFUSION. The escape of fluid from blood vessels or the lymphatic system and its collection in a cavity, in this case, the middle ear.

EGOBRONCHOPHONY. Increased intensity of the spoken voice.

EJACULATION. The act of expelling the sperm through the penis during orgasm. The fluid that is released is called the ejaculate.

EJECTION FRACTION. The fraction of blood in the ventricle that is ejected during each beat. One of the main advantages of the MUGA scan is its ability to measure ejection fraction, one of the most important measures of the heart's performance.

ELECTIVE PROCEDURE. A surgical procedure that is a matter of choice rather than emergency treatment.

ELECTIVE SURGERY. Surgery that would be beneficial to the patient but is not urgent, and is therefore a matter of choice.

ELECTROCARDIOGRAM (ECG OR EKG). A recording of the electrical activity of the heart. An ECG uses externally attached electrodes to detect the electrical signals of the heart.

ELECTROCAUTERY. A technique for sealing a blood vessel with a low-voltage electrified probe.

ELECTROCOAGULATION. The coagulation or destruction of tissue through the application of a high-frequency electrical current.

ELECTRODE. A medium, such as platinum wires, for conducting an electrical current. Used for recording the electrical activity of the body, for example in the heart or the brain.

ELECTRODESICCATION. A method of treating spider veins or drying up tissue by passing a small electric current through a fine needle into the affected area.

ELECTROENCEPHALOGRAM (EEG). A recording of the electrical activity of the nerve cells in the brain. The first such recording was made in 1929 by Hans Berger, an Austrian psychiatrist.

ELECTROLYTE. Ions in the body that participate in metabolic reactions. The major human electrolytes are sodium (Na^+), potassium (K^+), calcium (Ca^{2+}), magnesium (Mg^{2+}), chloride (Cl^-), phosphate (HPO_4^{2-}), bicarbonate (HCO_3^-), and sulfate (SO_4^{2-}).

ELECTROMYOGRAPHY. A test that measures muscle response to nerve stimulation. It is used to evaluate muscle weakness and to determine if the weakness is related to the muscles themselves or to a problem with the nerves that supply the muscles.

ELECTRON. One of the small particles that make up an atom. An electron has the same mass and amount of charge as a positron, but the electron has a negative charge.

ELECTRONYSTAGMOGRAM. A test that involves the graphic recording of eye movements.

ELECTROPHYSIOLOGICAL STUDY. A test that monitors the electrical activity of the heart in order to diagnose arrhythmia. An electrophysiological study measures electrical signals through a cardiac catheter that is inserted into an artery in the leg and guided up into the atrium and ventricle of the heart.

ELECTROSURGICAL DEVICE. A medical device that uses electrical current to cauterize or coagulate tissue during surgical procedures; often used in conjunction with laparoscopy.

ELECTROTHERAPY. The treatment of body tissues by passing electrical currents through them, stimulating the nerves and muscles.

EMASCULATION. Another term for castration of a male.

EMBALMING. Process of treating a dead body with chemicals to preserve it from decay.

EMBOLISM. A blood clot, air bubble, or clot of foreign material that blocks the flow of blood in an artery. When an embolism blocks the blood supply to a tissue or organ, the tissue the artery feeds dies (infarction). Without immediate and appropriate treatment, an embolism can be fatal.

EMBOLIZATION. The purposeful introduction of a substance into a blood vessel to stop blood flow.

EMBOLUS (PLURAL EMBOLI). A gas or air bubble, bit of tissue, blood clot, or foreign object that circulates in the bloodstream until it lodges in a vessel. A large embolus can narrow or block the vessel, which leads to decreased blood flow in the organ supplied by that vessel.

EMESIS BASIN. A basin used to collect sputum or vomit.

EMPHYSEMA. A chronic disease characterized by loss of elasticity and abnormal accumulation of air in lung tissue.

EMPYEMA. An accumulation of pus in the lung cavity, usually as a result of infection.

ENCEPHALITIS. An inflammation or infection of the brain and spinal cord caused by a virus or as a complication of another infection.

ENCEPHALOCELES. Protrusion of the brain through a defect in the skull.

END-STAGE HEART OR LUNG FAILURE. Severe heart or lung disease that does not respond adequately to medical or surgical treatment.

ENDEMIC. Present in a specific population or geographical area at all times. Some diseases that may affect the spleen are endemic to certain parts of Africa or Asia.

ENDOCARDITIS. An infection of the inner membrane lining of the heart.

ENDOCRINE SYSTEM. Group of glands and parts of glands that control metabolic activity. The pituitary, thyroid, adrenals, ovaries, and testes are all part of the endocrine system.

ENDOCRINOLOGIST. A physician who specializes in treating persons with diseases of the thyroid, parathyroid, adrenal glands, and the pancreas.

ENDODONTIC. Pertaining to the inside structures of the tooth, including the dental pulp and tooth root, and the periapical tissue surrounding the root.

ENDODONTIST. A dentist who specializes in the diagnosis and treatment of disorders affecting the inside structures of teeth.

ENDOLYMPH. The watery fluid contained in the membranous labyrinth of the inner ear.

ENDOLYMPHATIC SAC. The pouch at the end of the endolymphatic duct that connects to the membranous labyrinth of the inner ear.

ENDOMETRIAL POLYPS. Growths in the lining of the uterus (endometrium) that may cause bleeding and can develop into cancer.

ENDOMETRIOSIS. A painful disease in which cells from the lining of the uterus (endometrium) become attached to other organs in the pelvic cavity. The condition is hard to diagnose and often causes severe pain as well as infertility.

ENDOMYOCARDIAL BIOPSY. Removal of a small sample of heart tissue to check it for signs of damage caused by organ rejection.

ENDOPHTHALMITIS. An infection on the inside of the eye that may result in vision loss.

ENDORPHINS. Any of a group of proteins with analgesic properties that occur naturally in the brain.

ENDOSCOPE. A narrow, flexible tube with a fiber optic light on it, used to pass into the body for a variety of medical examinations.

ENDOSCOPIC RETROGRADE CHOLANGIOPANCREATOGRAPHY (ERCP). A procedure to x ray the ducts (tubes) that carry bile from the liver to the gallbladder and from the gallbladder to the small intestine.

ENDOSCOPIC ULTRASOUND. An imaging procedure that uses high-frequency sound waves to visualize the esophagus via a lighted telescopic instrument (endoscope) and a monitor.

ENDOSCOPIST. A physician or other medical professional highly trained in the use of the endoscope and related diagnostic and therapeutic procedures.

ENDOSCOPY. The visual inspection of any cavity of the body by means of an endoscope.

ENDOSTEAL IMPLANTS. Dental implants that are placed within the bone.

ENDOTRACHEAL. Located inside the trachea.

ENDOTRACHEAL INTUBATION. A procedure in which a tube is inserted into the trachea in order to administer anesthesia or ventilate the patient.

ENDOTRACHEAL TUBE. A tube inserted through the patient's nose or mouth that functions as an airway and is connected to a ventilator.

EPIGLOTTIS. A cartilaginous lidlike appendage that closes the glottis while food or drink is passing through the pharynx.

ENDOVASCULAR. Within the walls of a blood vessel.

ENDOVASCULAR GRAFTING. A procedure that involves the insertion of a delivery catheter through a groin artery into the abdominal aorta under fluoroscopic guidance.

ENEMA. Insertion of a tube into the rectum to infuse fluid into the bowel and encourage a bowel movement. Ordinary enemas contain tap water, mixtures of soap and water, glycerine and water, or other materials.

ENOPHTHALMOS. A condition in which the eye falls back into the socket and inhibits proper eyelid function.

ENTERAL NUTRITIONAL SUPPORT. Nutrition utilizing an intact gastrointestinal tract, but bypassing another organ such as the stomach or esophagus.

ENTERIC COAT. A coating put on some tablets or capsules to prevent their disintegration in the stomach. The contents of coated tablets or capsules will be released only when the dose reaches the intestine. This may be done to protect the drug from stomach acid, to protect the stomach from drug irritation, or to delay the onset of action of the drug.

ENTERITIS. Inflammation of the mucosal lining of the small intestine.

ENTEROCELE. Sagging or bulging of an area of the intestine into the vagina.

ENTEROSTOMAL THERAPIST. A health care provider who specializes in the care of patients with enterostomies (e.g., ileostomies or colostomies).

ENTITLEMENT. A program that creates a legal obligation by the federal government to any person, business, or government entity that meets the legally defined criteria. Medicaid is an entitlement both for eligible individuals and for the states that decide to participate in it.

ENUCLEATION. Surgical removal of the eyeball.

ENZYME. A protein, produced by cells, that causes chemical changes in other substances.

EOSINOPHIL. Segmented white blood cell with large orange-red granules that increases in response to parasitic infections and allergic reactions.

EPHEDRA. A herb used in traditional Chinese medicine to treat asthma and hay fever. It should never be used for weight management.

EPIDERMIS. The outer layer of skin, consisting of a layer of dead cells that perform a protective function and a second layer of dividing cells.

EPIDIDYMIS. A coiled cordlike structure at the upper border of the testis, in which sperm mature and are stored.

EPIDIDYMITIS. Inflammation of the epididymis.

EPIDURAL. A type of regional anesthetic delivered by injection into the area around the patient's lower spine. An epidural numbs the body below the waist but allows the patient to remain conscious throughout the procedure.

EPIDURAL CATHETER. A thin plastic tube, through which pain medication is delivered, inserted into the patient's back before surgery.

EPIGLOTTIS. A leaf-shaped piece of cartilage lying at the root of the tongue that protects the respiratory tract from aspiration during the swallowing reflex.

EPIKERATOPHAKIA. A procedure in which the donor cornea is attached directly onto the host cornea.

EPILEPSY. The name for a group of syndromes characterized by periodic temporary disturbances of brain function. The symptoms of an epileptic seizure may include loss of consciousness, abnormal movements, falling, emotional reactions, and disturbances of sight or hearing.

EPINEPHRINE. Epinephrine, also called adrenalin, occurs naturally in the body and causes blood vessels to constrict or narrow. As a drug, it is used to reduce bleeding.

EPIPHYSIODESIS. An surgical procedure that partially or totally destroys an epiphysis and may incorporate a bone graft to produce fusion of the epiphysis or premature cessation of its growth; usually performed to equalize leg length.

EPIPHYSIS. A part of a long bone where bone growth occurs from.

EPITHELIAL CELLS. Cells that form a thin surface coating on the outside of a body structure.

EPITHELIUM. The covering of internal and external surfaces of the body, including the lining of vessels and other small cavities. It consists of cells joined by small amounts of cementing substances.

ERBIUM:YAG. A crystal made of erbium, yttrium, aluminum, and garnet that produces light that is well absorbed by the skin, so it is used for skin resurfacing treatments.

ERGOT ALKALOIDS. Compounds derived from a fungus, *Claviceps purpurea*, which grows on rye plants and forms a hard blackish body. Ergot itself is toxic.

EROSION. A gradual breakdown or ulceration of the uppermost layer of tissue lining the esophagus or stomach.

ERUPTION. The emergence of a tooth through the gum tissue.

ERYTHEMA. Redness.

ERYTHROBLASTOSIS FETALIS. A condition in which the incompatability between a mother's Rh-negative blood type and a baby's Rh-positive blood type results in destruction of the baby's red blood cells by maternal antibodies.

ERYTHROPOIETIN. A hormone produced by the kidneys that stimulates the production of red blood cells by bone marrow.

ERYTHROPOIETIN. A hormone secreted chiefly by the kidney (in adults) that stimulates the production of red blood cells.

ESCHAR. A hardened dry crust that forms on skin exposed to burns or corrosive agents.

ESOPHAGEAL SPHINCTER. Muscle at the opening to the stomach that keeps the stomach contents from traveling into the esophagus.

ESOPHAGEAL VARICES . Varicose veins at the lowermost portion of the esophagus. Esophageal varices are easily injured, and bleeding from them is often difficult to stop.

ESOPHAGECTOMY. Surgical removal of the esophagus.

ESOPHAGITIS. Inflammation of the esophagus.

ESOPHAGUS. The muscular tube that connects the mouth to the stomach.

ESRD. End-stage renal disease; chronic or permanent kidney failure.

ESTATE PLANNING. Preparation of a plan of administration and disposition of one's property before or after death, including will, trusts, gifts, and power of attorney.

ESTROGENS. A class of chemical compounds (hormones) that stimulates the development of female secondary sexual characteristics.

ETHMOID SINUSES. Paired labyrinth of air cells between the nose and eyes.

ETHYLENE OXIDE. A colorless gas used to sterilize surgical sutures, bandages, and most other surgical materials or implements.

EUSTACHIAN TUBE. A canal that extends from the middle ear to the pharynx.

EUTHANASIA. To bring about the death of another person who has an incurable disease or condition.

EVENT RECORDER. A small machine, worn by a patient usually for several days or weeks, that is activated by the patient to record his or her EKG when a symptom is detected.

EXCIMER LASER. An instrument that is used to vaporize tissue with a cold, coherent beam of light with a single wavelength in the ultraviolet range.

EXCISION. The surgical removal of a damaged or diseased part of the body.

EXCISIONAL BIOPSY. Procedure in which a surgeon removes all of a lump or suspicious area and an area of healthy tissue around the edges. The tissue is then examined under a microscope to check for cancer cells.

EXOPHTHALMOS. A condition in which the eyes bulge out of their sockets and inhibit proper eyelid function.

EXTRACAPSULAR SURGERY. A cataract surgical procedure in which an incision is made in the cornea to remove the hard center of the lens. The natural lens is then replaced with an intraocular lens (IOL).

EXTRACORPOREAL. Occurring outside the patient's body.

EXTRACORPOREAL CIRCUIT (ECC). The path the hemodialysis patient's blood takes outside of the body. It typically consists of plastic tubing, a hemodialysis machine, and a dialyzer.

EXTRACORPOREAL SHOCK WAVE LITHOTRIPSY (ESWL). The use of focused shock waves, generated outside the body, to fragment kidney stones.

EXTRACTION. The surgical removal of a tooth from its socket in a bone.

EXTRACTION SITE. The empty tooth socket following removal of a tooth.

EXTRAOCULAR MUSCLES. The muscles (lateral rectus, medial rectus, inferior rectus, superior rectus, superior oblique, and inferior oblique) that move the eyeball.

EXTRINSIC PATHWAY. One of three pathways in the coagulation cascade.

EXTRUSION. Pushing out or expulsion. Extrusion of a chin implant is one possible complication of mentoplasty.

EXUDATE. Fluid, cells, or other substances that are slowly discharged by tissue, especially due to injury or inflammation.

EXUDATIVE RD. A type of retinal detachment caused by the accumulation of tissue fluid underneath the retina.

F

FACE LIFT. Plastic surgery performed to remove sagging skin and wrinkles from an individual's face.

FACTOR XIII. A substance found in blood that forms cross-links between strands of fibrin during the process of blood coagulation. Factor XIII is an ingredient in some types of fibrin sealants. It is also known as fibrin stabilizing factor.

FALLOPIAN TUBES. The pair of anatomical tubes that carry the egg from the ovary to the uterus.

FALSE NEGATIVE. Test results showing no problem when one exists.

FALSE POSITIVE. Test results showing a problem when one does not exist.

FASCIA. Fibrous tissue that separates and supports organs and other structures in the body.

FAST TRACK. A protocol for postoperative patients with projected shorter recovery times. Fast-tracking a patient means that they will either bypass PACU completely, or spend a shorter time there with less intensive staff intervention and monitoring.

FATIGUE. Physical or mental weariness.

FECAL INCONTINENCE. The inability to control bowel movement.

FEDERAL POVERTY LEVEL (FPL). The definition of poverty provided by the federal government, used as the reference point to determine Medicaid eligibility for certain groups of beneficiaries. The FPL is adjusted every year to allow for inflation.

FELLOWSHIP TRAINING. Additional specialty training that follows completion of residency training; fellowships are one to two years in length.

FELON. A very painful abscess on the lower surface of the fingertip, resulting from infection in the closed space surrounding the bone in the fingertip. It is also known as whitlow.

FEMALE STERILIZATION. The process of permanently ending a woman's ability to conceive by tying off or cutting apart the fallopian tubes.

FEMORAL. Pertaining to the thigh region.

FEMORAL ARTERY. An artery located in the groin area that is the most frequently accessed site for arterial puncture in angiography.

FEMORAL HEAD. The upper end of the femur.

FEMUR. The medical name for the thighbone. The femur is the largest bone in the human body.

FEVER. An abnormally elevated body temperature, usually defined as being 101 degrees Fahrenheit or more

FIBER. Carbohydrate material in food that cannot be digested.

FIBEROPTICS. In medicine, fiberoptics uses glass or plastic fibers to transmit light through a specially designed tube inserted into organs or body cavities where it transmits a magnified image of the internal body structures.

FIBRILLATION. Independent rapid contraction of cardiac muscle fibers producing no productive contraction, therefore no blood is pumped.

FIBRIN. The protein formed as the end product of the blood clotting process when fibrinogen interacts with thrombin.

FIBRINOGEN. A blood protein made in the liver that is broken up into shorter molecules by the action of thrombin to form fibrin.

FIBROBLAST. A type of cell found in connective tissue involved in collagen production as well as tendon formation and healing.

FIBROID TUMORS. Non-cancerous (benign) growths in the uterus; they occur in 30–40% of women over age 40 and do not need to be removed unless they are causing symptoms that interfere with a woman's normal activities.

FIBROSIS. A condition characterized by the presence of scar tissue, or reticulin and collagen proliferation in tissues to the extent that it replaces normal tissues.

FIBROUS CONNECTIVE TISSUE. Dense tissue found in various parts of the body containing very few living cells.

FIBULA. The bone in the lower leg that is next to and smaller than the tibia. It supports approximately one-sixth of the body weight and produces the outer prominence of the ankle.

FINE NEEDLE BIOPSY. Use of a very thin type of needle to withdraw cells from an organ, a tumor, or other body tissue, in order to examine those cells for abnormalities (such as malignancy).

FINGER STICK. A technique for collecting a very small amount of blood from the fingertip area.

FIRST RESPONDER. A term used to describe the first medically trained responder to arrive on scene of an emergency, accident, natural or human-made disaster, or similar event. First responders may be police officers, fire fighters, emergency medical services personnel, or bystanders with some training in first aid.

FISTULA. An abnormal connection between two organs, or between an organ and the outside of the body.

FIXATIVE. A chemical that preserves tissue without destroying or altering the structure of the cells.

FIXATOR. A device providing rigid immobilization through external skeletal fixation by means of rods (attached to pins which are placed in or through the bone.

FIXED. A term used to describe chemically preserved tissue. Fixed tissue is dead so it does not bleed or sense pain.

FLAP. A piece of tissue used for grafting that has kept its own blood supply.

FLIGHT OF IDEAS. A psychiatric term describing a thought disorder where streams of unrelated words or ideas enter a patient's mind too quickly to be properly vocalized despite the rushed and rapid rate of the patient's speech.

FLOATERS. Spots seen in front of the eyes, caused by clumping of the collagen fibers in the vitreous body.

FLOW METER. Device for measuring the rate of a gas (especially oxygen) or liquid.

FLUORESCEIN DYE. An orange dye used to illuminate the blood vessels of the retina in fluorescein angiography.

FLUOROSCOPE. An imaging device that displays "moving x rays" of the body. Fluoroscopy allows the radiologist to visualize the guide wire and catheter he or she is moving through the patient's artery.

FLUOROSCOPIC ANGIOGRAM. A method of precisely visualizing the brain cardiovascular system and its defects, including aneurysms.

FLUOROSCOPY. A diagnostic imaging procedure that uses x rays and contrast agents to visualize anatomy and motion in real time.

FOLEY CATHETER. A thin tube that is inserted into the urethra (the tube that runs from the bladder to the outside of the body) to allow the drainage of urine.

FOLIC ACID. A water-soluable vitamin belonging to the B-complex group of vitamins.

FOOTPLATE. A flat oval plate of bone that fits into the oval window on the wall of the inner ear; the base of the stapes.

FORAMEN (PLURAL, FORAMINA). The medical term for a natural opening or passage. The foramina of the spinal column are openings between the vertebrae for the spinal nerves to branch off from the spinal cord.

FORCED EXPIRATORY VOLUME (FEV). The volume of air exhaled from the beginning of expiration to a set time (usually 0.5, 1, 2, and 3 seconds).

FORCED VITAL CAPACITY (FVC). The volume of air that can be exhaled forceably after a maximal inspiration.

FORCEPS. An instrument designed to grasp or hold. Forceps usually have a locking mechanism so that they continue to hold tissue when put down by an operator.

FORENSIC. Referring to legal or courtroom proceedings.

FORESKIN. A covering fold of skin over the tip of the penis.

FORMALIN. A clear solution of diluted formaldehyde that is used to preserve liver biopsy specimens until they can be examined in the laboratory.

FRACTIONATED RADIOSURGERY. Radiosurgery in which the radiation is delivered in several smaller doses over a period of time rather than the full amount in a single treatment.

FRACTIONATION. The process of separating the various components of whole blood.

FREE FLAP. A section of tissue is detached from its blood supply, moved to another part of the body, and reattached by microsurgery to a new blood supply.

FREQUENCY. Sound, whether traveling through air or the human body, produces vibrations—molecules bouncing into each other—as the shock wave travels along. The frequency of a sound is the number of vibrations per second. Within the audible range, frequency means pitch: the higher the frequency, the higher a sound's pitch.

FRONTAL BONE. The part of the skull that lies behind the forehead.

FUCHS' DYSTROPHY. A hereditary disease of the inner layer of the cornea.

FUNGAL. Caused by a fungus.

FUNGUS. A member of a group of simple organisms that are related to yeast and molds.

FUSION. A union, joining together; e.g., bone fusion.

G

GADOLINIUM. A very rare metallic element useful for its sensitivity to electromagnetic resonance, among other things. Traces of it can be injected into the body to enhance the MRI pictures.

GAIT. A person's habitual manner or style of walking.

GALLBLADDER. A hollow pear-shaped sac on the under surface of the right lobe of the liver. Bile comes to it from the liver, and passes from it to the intestine to aid in digestion.

GAMETE INTRAFALLOPIAN TUBE TRANSFER (GIFT). A process where eggs are taken from a woman's ovaries, mixed with sperm, and then deposited into the woman's fallopian tube.

GAMMA RAY. A high-energy photon emitted by radioactive substances.

GANGLION. A knot or knot-like mass; it can refer either to groups of nerve cells outside the central nervous system or to cysts that form on the sheath of a tendon.

GANGLIONECTOMY. Surgery to excise a ganglion cyst.

GANGRENE. The death of a considerable mass of tissue, usually associated with loss of blood supply and followed by bacterial infection.

GANTRY. A name for the portion of a CT scanner which houses the X-ray tube and detector array used to capture image information and send it to the computer.

GAS GANGRENE. A severe form of gangrene caused by *Clostridium* infection.

GASTRECTOMY. A surgical procedure in which all or a portion of the stomach is removed.

GASTRIC (OR PEPTIC) ULCER. An ulcer (sore or hole) in the stomach lining, duodenum, or other part of the gastrointestinal system.

GASTRIC GLANDS. Branched tubular glands located in the stomach.

GASTRIC PACING. An experimental form of obesity surgery in which electrodes are implanted in the muscle of the stomach wall. Electrical stimulation paces the timing of stomach contractions so that the patient feels full on less food.

GASTRIC ULCER. An ulcer of the stomach, duodenum, or other part of the gastrointestinal system. Also called a peptic ulcer.

GASTRIN. A hormone produced by cells in the antrum that stimulates the production of gastric acid.

GASTRODUODENOSTOMY. A surgical procedure in which the doctor creates a new connection between the stomach and the duodenum.

GASTROENTEROLOGIST. A physician who specializes in digestive disorders and diseases of the organs of the digestive tract, including the esophagus, stomach, and intestines.

GASTROENTEROLOGY. The branch of medicine that specializes in the diagnosis and treatment of disorders affecting the stomach and intestines.

GASTROESOPHAGEAL REFLUX DISEASE (GERD). A condition in which the contents of the stomach flow backward into the esophagus. There is no known single cause.

GASTROINTESTINAL. Pertaining to the digestive organs and structures, including the stomach and intestines.

GASTROINTESTINAL DISEASES. Diseases that affect the digestive system.

GASTROINTESTINAL TRACT. The path in the body from the mouth, through the stomach, intestines, rectum, and the anus.

GASTROINTESTINAL TUBE. A tube surgically inserted into the stomach for feeding a patient who is unable to eat by mouth.

GASTROJEJUNOSTOMY. A surgical procedure in which the stomach is surgically connected to the jejunum (middle portion of the small intestine).

GASTROSCHISIS. A defect of the abdominal wall caused by rupture of the amniotic membrane or by the delayed closure of the umbilical ring. It is usually accompanied by protrusion of internal organs in the abdomen.

GENDER IDENTITY DISORDER (GID). A mental disorder in which a person strongly identifies with the other sex and feels uncomfortable with his or her biological sex. It occurs more often in males than in females.

GENDER REASSIGNMENT SURGERY. The surgical alteration and reconstruction of a person's sex organs to resemble those of the other sex as closely as possible; it is sometimes called sex reassignment surgery.

GENE. A piece of DNA, located on a chromosome, that determines how such traits as blood type are inherited and expressed.

GENERAL ANESTHESIA. Deep sleep induced by a combination of medicines that allows surgery to be performed.

GENERAL SURGEON. A physician who has special training and expertise in performing a variety of operations.

GENERALIZED INFECTION. An infection that has entered the bloodstream and has general systemic symptoms such as fever, chills, and low blood pressure.

GENETIC. The term refers to genes, the basic units of biological heredity, which are contained on the chromosomes, and contain chemical instructions that direct the development and functioning of an individual.

GENIOPLASTY. Another word for mentoplasty. It comes from the Greek word for "chin."

GENITAL. Sexual organ.

GENITOURINARY RECONSTRUCTION. Surgery that corrects birth defects or the results of disease that involve the genitals and urinary tract, including the kidneys, ureters, bladder, urethra, and the male and female genitals.

GENTIAN VIOLET. An antibacterial, antifungal dye that is commonly applied to the skin during dermabrasion.

GENUINE STRESS INCONTINENCE (GSI). A specific term for a type of incontinence that has to do with the instability of the urethra due to weakened support muscles.

GENUINE URINARY STRESS INCONTINENCE (USI). Stress incontinence due to hypermobility of the urethra.

GERD (GASTROESOPHAGEAL REFLUX DISEASE). A chronic condition in which the lower esophageal sphincter allows gastric acids to reflux into the esophagus, causing heartburn, acid indigestion, and possible injury to the esophageal lining.

GERIATRICIAN. Physician specializing in the care and treatment of older adults.

GERMINOMA. A tumor of germ cells (ovum and sperm cells that participate in production of the developing embryo).

GESTATIONAL AGE. The length of time of growth and development of the young in the mother's womb.

GESTATIONAL DIABETES. A type of diabetes that occurs during pregnancy. Untreated, it can cause severe complications for the mother and the baby. However, it usually does not lead to long-term diabetes in either the mother or the child.

GIGANTISM. A condition in which the individual grows to an abnormally large size. Mental development may or may not be normal.

GINGIVITIS. Inflammation of the gingiva or gums caused by bacterial buildup in plague on the teeth.

GLANS. The cone-shaped tip of the penis.

GLAUCOMA. A group of eye diseases characterized by an increase in intraocular pressure that causes changes in the optic disk and defects in the field of vision.

GLENOHUMERAL JOINT. A ball-and-socket synovial joint between the head of the humerus and the glenoid cavity of the scapula. Also called the glenohumeral articulation or shoulder joint.

GLENOID CAVITY. The hollow cavity in the head of the shoulder blade that receives the head of the humerus to make the glenohumeral or shoulder joint.

GLOMERULONEPHRITIS. A condition in which the filtering structures within the kidneys become damaged, limiting the kidneys' ability to filter waste products from the blood.

GLOTTIS. The vocal part of the larynx, consisting of the vocal cords and the opening between them.

GLUCAGON. A hormone produced in the pancreas that is responsible for elevating blood glucose when it falls below a safe level for the body's organs and tissues.

GLUCOSE-6-PHOSPHATE DEHYDROGENASE (G6PD) DEFICIENCY. An inherited disorder in which the body lacks an enzyme that normally protects red blood cells from toxic chemicals. Certain drugs can cause patients' red blood cells to break down, resulting in anemia. This may also happen when they have a fever or an infection. The condition usually occurs in males. About 10% of black males have it, as do a small percentage of people from the Mediterranean region.

GLUCOSE. The main form of sugar (chemical formula $C_6H_{12}O_6$) used by the body for energy.

GLYCATED HEMOGLOBIN. A test that measures the amount of hemoglobin bound to glucose. It is a measure of how much glucose has been in the blood during a two to three month period beginning approximately one month prior to sample collection.

GLYCOGEN. The form in which glucose is stored in the body.

GLYCOPROTEIN. Any of a group of complex proteins that consist of a carbohydrate combined with a simple protein. Some tumor markers are glycoproteins.

GLYCYLCYCLINES. The name of a new subgroup of tetracyclines derived from minocycline, a semi-synthetic tetracycline. As of 2007, the only drug in this class approved for use is tigecycline.

GOITER. An enlargement of the thyroid gland due to insufficient iodine in the diet.

GONADOTROPINS. Hormones that stimulate the activity of the ovaries in females and testes in males.

GONIOSCOPY. A technique for examining the angle between the iris and the cornea with the use of a special mirrored lens applied to the cornea.

GONORRHEA. A sexually transmitted disease (STD) that causes infection in the genital organs and may cause disease in other parts of the body.

GRAFT. Replacement of a diseased or damaged part of the body with a compatible substitute that can be artificial (metal or other substance) or taken from the body itself, such as a piece of skin, healthy tissue, or bone.

GRAFT VERSUS HOST DISEASE. A life-threatening complication of bone marrow transplants in which the donated marrow causes an immune reaction against the recipient's body.

GRAM STAINING. Use of a purple dye to identify pathogens, usually bacteria.

GRANULE. A small grain or pellet. Medicines that come in granule form are usually mixed with liquids or sprinkled on food before they are taken.

GRANULOCYTES. White blood cells.

GRAVEL. The debris that is formed from a fragmented kidney stone.

GUGLIEMLIMI DETACHABLE COILS. A new method of treating aneurysms that is minimally invasive.

GUIDE WIRE. A wire that is inserted into an artery to guide a catheter to a certain location in the body.

GUIDED IMAGERY. A form of focused relaxation that coaches the patient to visualize calm, peaceful images.

GUILLAIN-BARRÉ SYNDROME. A demyelinating disease involving nerves that affect the extremities and causing weakness and motor and sensory dysfunction.

GUILLOTINE AMPUTATION. An amputation in which the severed part is cut off cleanly by a blade or other sharp-edged object.

GUTTA PERCHA. An inert, latex-like substance used for filling root canals.

GYNECOMASTIA. Overly developed or enlarged breasts in a male.

H

HAIR CELLS. Sensory receptors in the inner ear that transform sound vibrations into messages that travel to the brain.

HAIR FOLLICLE. A tube-like indentation in the skin from which a single hair grows.

HALF-LIFE. The time required for half of the atoms in a radioactive substance to disintegrate.

HALLUCINATION. A false or distorted perception of objects, sounds, or events that seems real. Hallucinations usually result from drugs or mental disorders.

HARMONIC SCALPEL. A scalpel that uses ultrasound technology to seal tissues while it is cutting.

HARVESTING. The process of removing tissues or organs from a donor and preserving them for transplantation.

HCFA. Health Care Financing Administration. A federal agency that provides guidelines for the Medicaid program.

HEAD-UPRIGHT TILT TABLE TEST. A test used to determine the cause of fainting spells. During the test, the patient is tilted at different angles on special table for a period time. During the test, the patient's heart rhythm, blood pressure and other measurements are evaluated with changes in position.

HEALTH CARE AGENT. Also known as the surrogate or patient representative, this is the person who has power of attorney to have the patient's wishes carried out if the patient is incapacitated.

HEALTH CARE FINANCING ADMINISTRATION (HCFA). A federal agency that provides guidelines for the Medicaid program.

HEALTH MAINTENANCE ORGANIZATION (HMO). A broad term that covers a variety of prepaid systems providing health care within a certain geographic area to all persons covered by the HMO's contract.

HEART LUNG MACHINE. A machine that temporarily takes over the function of the heart and lungs during surgical procedures in order to maintaining blood circulation and delivery of oxygen to body tissues while the heart is being operated on.

HEART MONITOR LEADS. Sticky pads placed on the chest to monitor the electrical activity of the heart. The pads are connected to an electrocardiogram machine.

HEART VALVE REPLACEMENT SURGERY. Surgery performed to repair or replace the valves in the heart that control blood flow through the heart and are responsible for the audible heartbeat.

HEARTBURN. A pain in the center of the chest behind the breastbone caused by the contents of the stomach flowing backwards (refluxing) into the lower end of the esophagus and causing irritation.

HELICAL. Having a spiral shape.

HELICOBACTER PYLORI. A spiral-shaped bacterium that was discovered in 1982 to be the underlying cause of most ulcers in the stomach and duodenum.

HEMAGGLUTINATION. The clumping of red blood cells due to blood type incompatibility.

HEMATEMESIS. Vomit that contains blood, usually seen as black specks in the vomitus.

HEMATOCRIT. The proportion of the volume of a blood sample that consists of red blood cells. It is expressed as a percentage.

HEMATOLOGIST. A specialist who treats diseases and disorders of the blood and blood-forming organs.

HEMATOMA. An accumulation of blood, often clotted, in a body tissue or organ, usually caused by a break or tear in a blood vessel.

HEMIFACIAL MICROSOMIA (HFM). A term used to describe a group of complex birth defects characterized by underdevelopment of one side of the face.

HEMOCHROMATOSIS. A genetic disorder known as iron overload disease. Untreated hemochromatosis may cause osteoporosis, arthritis, cirrhosis, heart disease, or diabetes.

HEMODILUTION. A technique in which the fluid content of the blood is increased without increasing the number of red blood cells.

HEMODYNAMIC. Relating to the flow of blood through the circulatory system.

HEMODYNAMICS. Measurement of the movements involved in the circulation of the blood; it usually includes blood pressure and heart rate.

HEMOGLOBIN. The iron-containing protein in the blood that transports oxygen from the lungs to all parts of the body.

HEMOLYSIS. Separation of hemoglobin from the red blood cells.

HEMOPTYSIS. Spitting up of blood derived from the lungs or bronchial tubes as a result of pulmonary or bronchial hemorrhage.

HEMORRHAGE. Major, abnormal blood loss either from a surface wound or from internal trauma.

HEMORRHAGIC STROKE. A disruption of the blood supply to the brain caused by bleeding into the brain.

HEMOSIDERIN. A form of iron that is stored inside tissue cells. The brownish discoloration of skin that sometimes occurs after sclerotherapy is caused by hemosiderin.

HEMOSTASIS. Slowing down or stopping bleeding.

HEMOSTAT. A small surgical clamp used to hold a blood vessel closed.

HEMOSTATIC. Relating to blood clotting and coagulation.

HEMOTHORAX. Blood in the pleural cavity.

HEPARIN. A complex sugar compound used in medicine to prevent the formation of blood clots during hemodialysis, hemoperfusion, and open-heart surgery.

HEPATIC ARTERY. The blood vessel supplying arterial blood to the liver.

HEPATIC DUCT. A duct that carries bile from the liver.

HEPATITIS. Disease of the liver causing inflammation. Symptoms include an enlarged liver, fever, nausea, vomiting, abdominal pain, and dark urine.

HEPATOCELLULAR CARCINOMA. The most common type of liver tumor.

HEPATOCYTE. Liver cell.

HEPATOMA. A liver tumor.

HEREDITARY. Something that is inherited or passed down from parents to offspring. In biology and medicine, the word pertains to inherited genetic characteristics.

HEREDITARY SPHEROCYTOSIS. A hereditary disorder that leads to a chronic form of anemia (too few red blood cells) due to an abnormality in the red blood cell membrane.

HERNIA. The protrusion of an organ or other structure through an opening in the wall that normally contains it.

HERNIATED DISK. A blister-like bulging or protrusion of the contents of the disk out through the fibers that normally hold them in place. Also called ruptured disk, slipped disk, or displaced disk.

HERNIORRHAPHY. The surgical repair of any type of hernia.

HETEROTOPIC BONE. Bone that develops as an excess growth around a joint following joint replacement surgery.

HETEROTROPHIC TRANSPLANTATION. The addition of a donor liver at another site, while the diseased liver is left intact.

HIATAL HERNIA. Protrusion of the stomach upward into the mediastinal cavity through the esophageal hiatus of the diaphragm.

HIGH TIBIAL OSTEOTOMY (HTO). The tibial bone is cut to redistribute weight on the knee for varus alignment deformities or injuries.

HIGH-DENSITY LIPOPROTEIN (HDL). A type of lipoprotein that protects against CAD by removing cholesterol deposits from arteries or preventing their formation.

HIP DYSPLASIA. Abnormal development of the hip joint.

HIPAA. Health Insurance Portability and Accountability Act of 1996.

HIRSUTISM. Excessive or increased growth of facial or body hair in women resembling the male pattern of hair distribution.

HISTOCOMPATIBILITY ANTIGENS. Proteins scattered throughout body tissues that are unique for almost every individual.

HISTOCOMPATIBILITY TESTING. Testing of genotypes of a recipient and potential donor to see if rejection would occur when tissues are transplanted.

HIV INFECTION. An infectious disease that impairs the immune system. It is also known as acquired immune deficiency syndrome or AIDS.

HODGKIN'S DISEASE. A type of cancer involving the lymph nodes and potentially affecting non-lymphatic organs in the later stage.

HOLISTIC. Pertaining to all aspects of the patient, including biological, psychosocial, and cultural factors.

HOLTER MONITOR. A small machine worn by a patient usually for 24 hours, that continuously records the patient's EKG during usual daily activity.

HOME HEALTH AIDE. An employee of a home care agency who provides the same services to a patient in the home as nurses aides perform in hospitals and nursing homes.

HOMEOSTASIS. The process of maintaining balance in the normal vital life functions of a living organism.

HOMOCYSTEINE. An amino acid normally found in small amounts in the blood.

HOODIA. A succulent African plant resembling a cactus said to contain a natural appetite suppressant.

HORMONE. A substance that is produced in one part of the body, then travels through the bloodstream to another part of the body where it has its effect.

HOSPICE. An approach for providing compassionate, palliative care to terminally ill patients and counseling or assistance for their families. The term may also refer to a hospital unit or freestanding facility devoted to the care of terminally ill patients.

HOST. A living organism that harbors or potentially harbors infection.

HUMAN CHORIONIC GONADOTROPIN (HCG). A hormone that is measured to detect early pregnancy.

HUMAN LEUCKOCYTE ANTIGEN (HLA). A group of protein molecules located on bone marrow cells that can provoke an immune response. A donor's and a recipient's HLA types should match as closely as possible to prevent the recipient's immune system from attacking the donor's marrow as a foreign material that does not belong in the body.

HUMAN PAPILLOMAVIRUS (HPV). A family of viruses that cause common warts of the hands and feet, as well as lesions in the genital and vaginal area. More than 50 types of HPV have been identified, some of which are linked to cancerous and precancerous conditions, including cancer of the cervix. A vaccine is now available against some of these viruses.

HUMERUS. The bone of the upper part of the arm.

HYDRAMNIOS. The excessive production of amniotic fluid due to either fetal or maternal conditions.

HYDROCELE. Collection of fluid in the scrotum.

HYDROCEPHALUS. Abnormal dilatation of fluid-containing ventricles in the brain.

HYDROCEPHALUS. The buildup of cerebrospinal fluid in the brain.

HYDROGEL. A gel that contains water, used as a dressing after laser skin resurfacing.

HYDROGEN. The simplest, most common element known in the universe. It is composed of a single electron (negatively charged particle) circling a nucleus consisting of a single proton (positively charged particle). It is the nuclear proton of hydrogen that makes MRI possible by reacting resonantly to radio waves while aligned in a magnetic field.

HYDROGEN IONS. Ions that contain one hydrogen atom with a positive charge. Hydrogen ions cause blood to be acidic.

HYDROSALPINX. A condition in which a fallopian tube becomes blocked and filled with fluid.

HYDROXIDE IONS. Ions that contain one oxygen and one hydrogen atom, with a negative charge. Hydroxide ions cause blood to be alkaline.

HYDROXYAPATITE. A calcium phosphate complex that is the primary mineral component of bone.

HYPERALDOSTERONISM. A disorder of excessive aldosterone secretion.

HYPERCALCEMIA. Excess concentration of calcium in the blood.

HYPERCARBIA. An excess of carbon dioxide in the blood.

HYPERCHLOREMIA. Elevated serum chloride levels.

HYPERCHOLESTEROLEMIA. The presence of excessively high levels of cholesterol in the blood.

HYPERESONANCE ON PERCUSSION. A highly resonating sound when the physician taps gently on a patient's back; this is not a normal finding and should be investigated with an x ray.

HYPERGLYCEMIA. Elevated blood glucose levels.

HYPERHIDROSIS. Excessive sweating. Hyperhidrosis can be caused by heat, overactive thyroid glands, strong emotion, menopause, or infection.

HYPERKALEMIA. An abnormally high concentration of potassium in the blood.

HYPERMOBILE URETHRA. A term that denotes the movement of the urethra that allows for leakage or spillage of urine.

HYPERNATREMIA. Elevated blood sodium levels.

HYPEROPIA. The inability to see near objects as clearly as distant objects, and the need for accommodation to see objects clearly.

HYPEROSMETIC. Hypertonic, containing a higher concentration of salts or other dissolved materials than normal tissues.

HYPEROSMOTIC AGENTS. Causing abnormally rapid osmosis.

HYPERPARATHYROIDISM. A condition in which the parathyroid gland is overactive; usually caused by the presence of an adenoma on one or more of the glands.

HYPERPHOSPHATEMIA. Elevated blood phosphate levels.

HYPERREFLEXIA. A condition in which the detrusor muscle of the bladder contracts too frequently, leading to inability to hold one's urine.

HYPERTENSION. High blood pressure.

HYPERTHYROIDISM. Abnormal overactivity of the thyroid gland. People with hyperthyroidism are hypermetabolic, lose weight, exhibit nervousness, have muscular weakness and fatigue, sweat heavily, and have increased urination and bowel movements. This condition is also called thyrotoxicosis.

HYPERTRIGLYCERIDEMIA. The presence of excessively high levels of TAG in the blood.

HYPERTROPHIC. A type of thick scar that is raised above the surface of the skin, usually caused by increasing or prolonging the inflammation stage of wound healing.

HYPERTROPHY. The overgrowth of muscle.

HYPHEMA. Blood inside the anterior chamber of the eye. Hyphema is one of the risks associated with sclerostomies.

HYPNOSIS. The term is used to refer to a specific verbal technique for refocusing a person's attention in order to change their perceptions, judgment, control of movements, and memory. A hypnotic medication is one that induces sleep.

HYPNOTIC. A medicine that causes sleep.

HYPOALBUMINEMIA . An abnormally low concentration of albumin in the blood.

HYPOCALCEMIA. Low levels of blood calcium.

HYPOCHLOREMIA. Low serum chloride levels.

HYPOCHROMIC. A descriptive term applied to a red blood cell with a decreased concentration of hemoglobin.

HYPODERMIC. Applied or administered beneath the skin. The modern hypodermic needle was invented to deliver medications below the skin surface.

HYPODERMOCLYSIS. A technique for restoring the body's fluid balance by injecting a solution of salt and water into the tissues beneath the skin rather than directly into a vein.

HYPOGLYCEMIA. Low blood glucose levels.

HYPOKALEMIA. Low blood potassium levels.

HYPONATREMIA. Low blood sodium levels.

HYPOPARATHYROIDISM. An endocrine disorder involving a deficiency of secretion of PTH from the parathyroid gland.

HYPOPHARYNX. The last part of the throat or the pharynx.

HYPOPHOSPHATEMIA. Low blood phosphate levels.

HYPOPITUITARISM. A medical condition where the pituitary gland produces lower than normal levels of its hormones.

HYPOSPADIAS. A congenital deformity of the penis where the urinary tract opening is not at the tip of the glans.

HYPOTENSION. Low blood pressure.

HYPOTHERMIA. An abnormally low body temperature, usually defined as being 90 degrees Fahrenheit or less

HYPOTHYROIDISM. Abnormal underfunctioning of the thyroid gland. People with hypothyroidism have a lowered body metabolism, gain weight, and are sluggish.

HYPOTONY. Intraocular fluid pressure that is too low.

HYPOVOLEMIA. An abnormally low amount of blood in the body.

HYPOXEMIA. Oxygen deficiency, defined as an oxygen level less than 60 mm Hg or arterial oxygen saturation of less than 90%. Different values are used for infants and patients with certain lung diseases.

HYPOXIA. Reduction of oxygen supply to tissues below physiological requirements despite adequate perfusion of the tissue by blood.

HYSTERECTOMY. Surgical removal of part or all of the uterus.

I

IATROGENIC. Resulting from the activity of the physician.

ICTAL EEG. An EEG done to determine the type of seizure characteristic of a person's disorder. During this EEG, seizure medicine may be discontinued in an attempt to induce as seizure during the testing period.

IDIOPATHIC. Having an unknown cause or arising spontaneously. Most cases of intussusception in children are idiopathic.

IDIOPATHIC THROMBOCYTOPENIA PURPURA (ITP). A rare autoimmune disorder characterised by an acute shortage of platelets with resultant bruising and spontaneous bleeding.

ILEECTOMY. Excision of the ileum.

ILEOANAL ANASTOMOSIS. A reservoir for fecal waste surgically created out of the small intestine. It retains the sphincter function of the anus and allows the patient to defecate in the normal fashion.

ILEUM. The third and lowest portion of the small intestine, extending from the jejunum to the beginning of the large intestine.

ILEUS. Obstruction in or immobility of the intestines. Symptoms include nausea and vomiting, absent bowel sounds, abdominal pain, and abdominal distension.

ILIAC ARTERY. Large blood vessel in the pelvis that leads into the leg.

ILIZAROV METHOD. A bone fixation technique using an external fixator for lengthening limbs, correcting deformities, and assisting the healing of fractures and infections. The method was designed by the Russian orthopedic surgeon Gavriil Abramovich Ilizarov (1921-1992).

IMMUNE RESPONSE. The body's natural protective reaction against disease and infection.

IMMUNE SYSTEM. Mechanism that protects the body from foreign substances, foreign cells, and pathogens. The thymus, spleen, lymph nodes, white blood cells, including the B cells and T cells, and antibodies are involved in the immune response, which aims to destroy these foreign bodies.

IMMUNOASSAY. A laboratory method for detecting the presence of a substance by using an antibody that reacts with it.

IMMUNOCOMPROMISED. Lacking or deficient in defenses provided by the immune system, usually due to disease state or a side effect of treatment.

IMMUNODEFICIENCY. A disorder in which the immune system is ineffective or disabled due either to acquired or inherited disease.

IMMUNOGLOBULIN. An antibody.

IMMUNOSUPPRESIVE CYTOTOXIC DRUGS. A class of drugs that function by destroying cells and suppressing the immune response.

IMMUNOSUPPRESSION. A disorder or condition where the immune response is reduced or absent.

IMMUNOSUPPRESSIVE MEDICATION. Drugs given to a transplant recipient to prevent his or her immune system from attacking the transplanted organ.

IMMUNOTHERAPY. A method of treating allergies in which small doses of substances that a person is allergic to are injected under the skin.

IMPACTED TOOTH. A tooth that is growing against another tooth, bone, or soft tissue.

IMPACTION GRAFTING. The use of crushed bone from a donor to fill in the central canal of the femur during hip revision surgery, or to fill in the central canal of the tibia during knee revision surgery.

IMPLANTABLE CARDIOVERTER-DEFIBRILLATOR. A device placed in the body to deliver an electrical shock to the heart in response to a serious abnormal rhythm.

IN VITRO FERTILIZATION (IVF). A process in which sperm are incubated with a female egg under carefully controlled conditions, then transferred to the female uterus once fertilization has occurred.

INCARCERATED HERNIA. An inguinal hernia that is trapped in place and cannot slip back into the abdominal cavity, often causing intestinal obstruction.

INCARCERATED INTESTINE. Intestines trapped in the weakened area of the hernia that cannot slip back into the abdominal cavity.

INCARCERATION. The abnormal confinement of a section of the intestine or other body tissues. A femoral hernia may lead to incarceration of part of the intestine.

INCENTIVE SPIROMETER. Device that is used postoperatively to prevent lung collapse and promote maximum inspiration. The patient inhales until a preset volume is reached, then sustains the volume by holding his or her breath for three to five seconds.

INCISION. A cut, usually made by a surgeon during a surgical procedure.

INCISIONAL BIOPSY. A procedure in which a surgeon cuts out a sample of a lump or suspicious area.

INCISIONAL HERNIA. Hernia occuring at the site of a prior surgery.

INCOMPETENT. In a medical context, insufficient. An incompetent sphincter is one that is not closing properly.

INCONTINENCE. The inability to control excretory functions, as defecation (fecal incontinence) or urination (urinary incontinence).

INCUS. The middle of the three bones of the middle ear. It is also known as the "anvil."

INDEMNITY. Protection, as by insurance, against damage or loss.

INDICATED TEST. A test that is given for a specific clinical reason.

INDIRECT COOMBS' TEST. A test used to screen for unexpected antibodies against red blood cells. The patient's serum is mixed with reagent red blood cells, incubated, washed, tested with antihuman globulin, and observed for clumping.

INDUCE. To begin or start.

INFARCTION. An area of dead tissue caused by obstruction of the blood supply to that tissue.

INFECTIOUS DISEASE TEAM. A team of physicians and hospital staff who help control the hospital environment to protect patients against harmful sources of infection.

INFERIOR TURBINATE. Bony projections on each side of the nose.

INFERIOR VENA CAVA. The biggest vein in the body, returning blood to the heart from the lower half of the body.

INFERTILITY. The inability to become pregnant or carry a pregnancy to term.

INFLAMMATION. A process occurring in body tissues, characterized by increased circulation and the accumulation of white blood cells. Inflammation also occurs in such disorders as arthritis and causes harmful effects.

INFLAMMATORY ARTHRITIS. An inflammatory condition that affects joints.

INFLAMMATORY BOWEL DISEASES. Ulcerative colitis or Crohn's disease: chronic conditions characterized by periods of diarrhea, bloating, abdominal cramps, and pain, sometimes accompanied by weight loss and malnutrition because of the inability to absorb nutrients.

INFORMED CONSENT. An educational process between health-care providers and patients intended to instruct the patient about the nature and purpose of the procedure or treatment, the risks and benefits of the procedure, and alternatives, including the option of not proceeding with the test or treatment.

INFRARED. A type of energy wave given off as heat.

INFUSION. Introduction of a substance directly into a vein or tissue by gravity flow.

INGUINAL HERNIA. A weak spot in the lower abdominal muscles of the groin through which body organs, usually the large intestines, can push through as a result of abdominal pressure.

INJECTION. Forcing a fluid into the body by means of a needle and syringe.

INJECTION SNOREPLASTY. A technique for reducing snoring by injecting a chemical that forms scar tissue near the base of the uvula, helping to anchor it and reduce its fluttering or vibrating during sleep.

INNER EAR. The interior section of the ear, where sound vibrations and information about balance are translated into nerve impulses.

INNERVATE. To carry nerve impulses to a particular body part.

INPATIENT SURGERY. Surgery that requires an overnight stay of one or more days in the hospital.

INSIDIOUS. Developing in a stealthy and inconspicuous way. Open-angle glaucoma is an insidious disorder.

INSPECTION. The visual examination of the body using the eyes and a lighted instrument if needed. The sense of smell may also be used.

INSTRUMENTAL ACTIVITIES OF DAILY LIVING (IADLS). Daily tasks that enable a person to live independently.

INSTRUMENTS. Tools or devices that perform such functions as cutting, dissecting, grasping, holding, retracting, or suturing.

INSUFFLATION. Blowing air into the ear as a test for the presence of fluid in the middle ear. Also, inflation of the abdominal cavity using carbon dioxide; performed prior to laparoscopy to give the surgeon space to maneuver surgical equipment.

INSULIN. A hormone produced by the pancreas that is responsible for allowing the body's cells to utilize glucose. The deficiency or absence of insulin is one of the causes of the disease diabetes.

INSULINOMA. A tumor within the pancreas that produces insulin, potentially causing the serum glucose level to drop to dangerously low levels.

INTEGUMENT. A covering; in medicine, the skin as a covering for the body. The skin is also called the integumentary system.

INTENSIVIST. A physician who specializes in caring for patients in intensive care units.

INTERCOSTAL ARTERY. Runs from the aorta.

INTERDISCIPLINARY. Consisting of several interacting disciplines that work together to care for an individual.

INTERLEUKIN-2 (IL-2). A cytokine derived from T helper lymphocytes that causes proliferation of T-lymphocytes and activated B lymphocytes.

INTERMITTENT CATHETERIZATION. Periodic catheterization to facilitate urine flow. The catheter is removed when the bladder is sufficiently empty.

INTERMITTENT CLAUDICATION. Pain that occurs on walking and is relieved on rest.

INTERNSHIP. The first year of residency training

INTERSTITIAL CYSTITIS. A chronic inflammatory condition of the bladder involving symptoms of bladder pain, frequent urination, and burning during urination.

INTERSTITIAL LUNG DISEASE. About 180 diseases fall into this category of breathing disorders. Injury or foreign substances in the lungs (such as asbestos fibers) as well as infections, cancers, or inherited disorders may cause the diseases. They can lead to breathing or heart failure.

INTERSTITIAL RADIATION THERAPY. The process of placing radioactive sources directly into the tumor. These radioactive sources can be temporary (removed after the proper dose is reached) or permanent.

INTERVERTEBRAL DISK. Cylindrical elastic-like gel pads that separate and join each pair of vertebrae in the spine.

INTESTINAL ILEUS. Mechanical or dynamic obstruction of the bowel causing pain, abdominal distention, vomiting, and often fever.

INTESTINAL PERFORATION. A hole in the intestinal wall.

INTESTINE. Commonly called the bowels, divided into the small and large intestine. They extend from the stomach to the anus. The small intestine is about 20 ft (6 m) long. The large intestine is about 5 ft (1.5 m) long.

INTRA-ABDOMINAL PRESSURE. Pressure that occurs within the abdominal cavity. Pressure in this area builds up with coughing, crying, and the pressure exerted when bearing down with a bowel movement.

INTRA-AORTIC BALLOON PUMP. A temporary device inserted into the femoral artery and guided up to the aorta. The small balloon helps strengthen heart contractions by maintaining improved blood pressure.

INTRACRANIAL. Existing or occurring within the cranium; affecting or involving intracranial structures.

INTRACYTOPLASMIC SPERM INJECTION (ICSI). A process used to inject a single sperm into each egg before fertilized eggs are put back into a woman's body; the procedure may be used if the male has a low sperm count.

INTRAOCULAR LENS (IOL) IMPLANT. A small, plastic device (IOL) that is usually implanted in the lens capsule of the eye to correct vision after the lens of the eye is removed. This is the implant used in cataract surgery.

INTRAOCULAR MELANOMA. A rare form of cancer in which malignant cells are found in the part of the eye called the uvea.

INTRAOCULAR PRESSURE (IOP). A measurement of the degree of pressure exerted by the aqueous fluid in the eye. Elevated IOP is usually 21 mm/Hg or higher, but glaucoma can be present when the pressure is lower.

INTRAOPERATIVE. During surgery.

INTRAORAL. Inside the mouth.

INTRATHECAL. Introduced into or occurring in the space under the arachnoid membrane that covers the brain and spinal cord.

INTRAUTERINE DEVICE (IUD). A small flexible device that is inserted into the uterus to prevent pregnancy.

INTRAVENOUS PYELOGRAM (IVP). A type of x ray. After obtaining an x ray of the lower abdomen, a radio-opaque dye is injected into the veins. X rays are then obtained every 15 minutes for the next hour. The dye pinpoints the location of kidney stones. It is also used to determine the anatomy of the urinary system.

INTRAVENOUS SEDATION. A method of injecting a fluid sedative into the blood through the vein.

INTRAVENTRICULAR HEMORRHAGE. Hemorrhage in the ventricles of the brain.

INTRINSIC PATHWAY. One of three pathways in the coagulation cascade.

INTRINSIC SPHINCTER DEFICIENCY. A type of incontinence caused by the inability of the sphincter muscles to keep the bladder closed.

INTUBATION. Placing a tube in the patient's airway to maintain adequate oxygen intake.

INTUSSUSCEPTION. Telescoping of one part of the intestine or the rectum into the neighboring part.

INVASIVE SURGERY. A form of surgery that involves making an incision in the patient's body and inserting instruments or other medical devices into it.

INVASIVENESS. A term that refers to the extent of surgical intrusion into the body or a part of the body. An invasive procedure is one that requires the insertion of a needle, catheter, or surgical instrument.

INVOLUTION. The slow healing and resolution stage of a hemangioma.

IONIZING RADIATION. A type of radiation that can damage living tissue by disrupting and destroying individual cells at the molecular level. All types of nuclear radiation, including x rays, gamma rays, and beta rays, are potentially ionizing. Sound waves physically vibrate the material through which they pass, but do not ionize it.

IRIDECTOMY. Removal of a portion of the iris.

IRIDOPLASTY. Surgery to alter the iris.

IRIDOTOMY. A procedure in which a laser is used to make a small hole in the iris to relieve fluid pressure in the eye.

IRIS (PLURAL, IRIDES). The circular pigmented membrane behind the cornea of the eye that gives the eye its color. The iris surrounds a central opening called the pupil.

ISCHEMIA. A decreased supply of oxygenated blood to a body part or organ, often marked by pain and organ dysfunction, as in ischemic heart disease.

ISLET CELL. The cell type within the pancreas that produces insulin.

ISOENZYME. One of a group of enzymes that brings about the same reactions on the same chemicals, but are different in their physical properties.

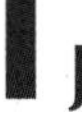

J

JAUNDICE. A condition that results in a yellow tint to the skin, eyes, and body fluids. Bile retention in the liver, gallbladder, and pancreas is the immediate cause, but the underlying cause could be as simple as obstruction of the common bile duct by a gallstone or as serious as pancreatic cancer. Ultrasound can distinguish between these conditions.

JEJUNECTOMY. Excision of all or a part of the jejunum.

JOINT COMMISSION ON ACCREDITATION OF HEALTHCARE ORGANIZATIONS (JCAHO). The accrediting organization that evaluates virtually all U.S. health care organizations and programs. Accreditation is maintained with onsite surveys every three years; laboratories are surveyed every two years.

JUGULAR VEIN. Major vein of the neck that returns blood from the head to the heart.

K

KEGEL EXERCISES. A series of contractions and relaxations of the muscles in the perineal area. These exercises are thought to strengthen the pelvic floor and may help prevent urinary incontinence in women.

KELOID. A raised, irregularly shaped scar that gradually increases in size due to the overproduction of collagen during the healing process. The name comes from a Greek word that means "crablike."

KERATINOCYTES. Dead cells at the outer surface of the epidermis that form a tough protective layer for the skin. The cells underneath divide to replenish the supply.

KERATOCONUS. An eye condition in which the cornea bulges outward, interfering with normal vision; usually both eyes are affected.

KERATOMETER. A device that measures the curvature of the cornea. It is used to determine the correct power for an IOL prior to cataract surgery.

KETOACIDOSIS. A potentially life-threatening condition in which abnormally high blood glucose levels result in the blood becoming too acidic.

KETONES. Substances produced during the breakdown of fatty acids. They are produced in excessive amounts in diabetes and certain other abnormal conditions.

KETOSIS. Abnormally elevated concentration of ketones in body tissues. A complication of diabetes.

KIDNEY STONE. A hard mass that forms in the urinary tract that can cause pain, bleeding, obstruction, and/or infection. Stones are primarily composed of calcium.

KNEE SURGERY. Refers primarily to knee repair, replacement or revision of parts of the knee, both tissue and bond, and includes both arthroscopic and open surgeries.

L

LABIAL. Of or pertaining to the lips.

LACERATION. A type of wound with rough, torn, or ragged edges.

LAMINAE (SINGULAR, LAMINA). The broad plates of bone on the upper surface of the vertebrae that fuse together at the midline to form a bony covering over the spinal canal.

LAMINECTOMY. An operation in which the surgeon cuts through the covering of a vertebra to reach a herniated disk in order to remove it.

LAMINOTOMY. A less invasive alternative to a laminectomy in which a hole is drilled through the lamina.

LANGERHANS' CELLS. Cells in the epidermis that help protect the body against infection.

LAPAROSCOPE. A device consisting of a tube and optical system for observing the inside of the abdomen and its organs.

LAPAROSCOPY. Minimally invasive surgical procedure in which small incisions are made in the abdominal or pelvic cavity and surgical tools are used with a miniature camera for guidance.

LAPAROTOMY. A procedure in which the surgeon opens the abdominal cavity to inspect the patient's internal organs.

LARGE INTESTINE. Also called the colon, this structure has six major divisions: cecum, ascending colon, transverse colon, descending colon, sigmoid colon, and rectum.

LARYNGECTOMY. Surgical removal of the larynx.

LARYNGOPHARYNGECTOMY. Surgical removal of both the larynx and the pharynx.

LARYNGOSCOPE. An endoscope equipped for viewing a patient's larynx through the mouth.

LARYNGOSCOPY. The visualization of the larynx and vocal cords. This may be done directly with a fibreoptic scope (laryngoscope) or indirectly with mirrors.

LARYNGOSPASM. Spasmodic closure of the larynx.

LARYNX. Also known as the voice box, the larynx is composed of cartilage that contains the apparatus for voice production. This includes the vocal cords and the muscles and ligaments that move the cords.

LASER. A device that produces high-intensity, narrowly focused monochromatic light by exciting atoms and causing them to give off their energy in phase.

LASER IN SITU KERATOMILEUSIS (LASIK). A procedure in which the shape of the cornea is changed with an excimer laser in order to correct the patient's vision.

LASER IRIDOTOMY. A procedure, using either the Nd:Yag laser or the argon laser, to penetrate the iris, such that a hole, through which the fluid in the eye can drain, is formed.

LASER SKIN RESURFACING. The use of laser light to remove the uppermost layer of skin. Two types of lasers commonly used in this manner are CO_2 and erbium.

LASER THERAPY. A cancer treatment that uses a laser beam (a narrow beam of intense light) to kill cancer cells.

LATARJET'S NERVE. Terminal branch of the anterior vagal trunk, which runs along the lesser curvature of the stomach.

LATERAL. Of or pertaining to a side (opposite of medial).

LATERAL RELEASE SURGERY. Release of tissues in the knee that keep the kneecap from tracking properly in its groove (sulcus) in the femur; by realigning or tightening tendons, the kneecap can be forced to track properly.

LATISSIMUS DORSI. In Latin, this muscle literally means "widest of the back." This is a large fan-shaped muscle that covers a wide area of the back.

LAVAGE. Washing out.

LAXATIVE. An agent which stimulates defecation.

LE FORT FRACTURE. A term that refers to a system for classifying fractures of the facial bones into three groups according to the region affected.

LEAD. Color-coded wire that connects an electrode to a monitor cable.

LECITHIN. A phospholipid found in high concentrations in surfactant.

LEGG-CALVE-PERTHES DISEASE (LCP). A disorder in which the femoral head deteriorates within the hip joint as a result of insufficient blood supply.

LEGIONNAIRES' DISEASE. A lung disease caused by a bacterium.

LEIOMYOSARCOMA. Leiomyosarcomas are cancers that start growing in the smooth muscle lining of the small intestine.

LENS (THE CRYSTALLINE LENS). A transparent structure in the eye that focuses light onto the retina.

LENS CAPSULE. A clear elastic membrane-like structure that covers the lens of the eye.

LENTICULAR. Lens-shaped; describes a shape of a surgical excision sometimes used to remove hemangiomas.

LEUKEMIA. A type of cancer that affects leukocytes, a particular type of white blood cell. A characteristic symptom is excessive production of immature or otherwise abnormal leukocytes.

LICENSED PRACTICAL NURSE (LPN). A person who is licensed to provide basic nursing care under the supervision of a physician or a registered nurse.

LIFE SUPPORT. Methods of replacing or supporting a failing bodily function, such as using mechanical ventilation to support breathing. In treatable or curable conditions, life support is used temporarily to aid healing until the body can resume normal functioning.

LIGAMENT. A band of fibrous tissue that connects bones to other bones or holds internal organs in place.

LIGAMENTA FLAVA (SINGULAR, LIGAMENTUM FLAVUM). A series of bands of tissue that are attached to the vertebrae in the spinal column. They help to hold the spine straight and to close the spaces between the laminar arches. The Latin name means "yellow band(s)."

LIGATION. Tying off a blood vessel or other structure with cotton, silk, or some other material. Rubber band ligation is one approach to treating internal hemorrhoids.

LIPID. Any organic compound that is greasy, insoluble in water, but soluble in alcohol. Fats, waxes, and oils are examples of lipids.

LIPOMA. A type of benign tumor that develops within adipose or fatty tissue.

LIPOPROTEIN. A chemical combination of a protein and a lipid (fats).

LIPOSHAVING. Involves removing fat that lies closer to the surface of the skin by using a needle-like instrument that contains a sharp-edged shaving device.

LIPOSUCTION. A surgical technique for removing fat from under the skin by vacuum suctioning.

LITHOTRIPSY. A technique for breaking up kidney stones within the urinary tract, followed by flushing out the fragments.

LITTRE'S HERNIA. A Meckel's diverticulum trapped in an inguinal hernia.

LIVING WILL. A document that is usually included in advanced medical directives containing explicit medical procedures that patients' wishes to have or to refuse should they become incapacitated.

LOBECTOMY. Removal of a section of the lung.

LOCAL ANESTHESIA. Anesthesia that numbs a localized area of the body.

LOCALIZED INFECTION. An infection that is limited to a specific part of the body and has local symptoms.

LOCKOUT TIME. The minimum amount of time (usually expressed in minutes) after one dose of pain medication on demand is given before the patient is allowed to receive the next dose on demand.

LONG-TERM CARE (LTC). The type of care one may need if one can no longer perform activities of daily living (ADLs) alone, such as eating, bathing or getting dressed. It also includes the kind of care one would need with a severe cognitive impairment, such as Alzheimer's disease. Care can be received in a variety of settings, including the home, assisted living facilities, adult day care centers, or hospice facilities.

LONG-TERM CARE (LTC) INSURANCE. A type of private health insurance intended to cover the cost of long-term nursing home or home health care.

LOOP ELECTROSURGICAL EXCISION (LEEP). A procedure that can help diagnose and treat cervical abnormalities using a thin wire loop that emits a low-voltage high-frequency radio wave that can excise tissue.

LOOSENESS OF ASSOCIATION. A psychiatric term describing a thought disorder where a patient makes irrelevant connections between seemingly unrelated topics. In a mental health assessment the patient's responses may not seem to correspond to the question asked by the health care provider.

LOUPE. A convex lens used to magnify small objects at very close range. It may be held on the hand, mounted on eyeglasses, or attached to a headband.

LOW TRANSVERSE INCISION. Incision made horizontally across the lower end of the uterus.

LOW-DENSITY LIPOPROTEIN (LDL). A type of lipoprotein that consists of about 50% cholesterol and is associated with an increased risk of CAD.

LOWER EXTREMITY AMPUTATION. To cut a limb from the body.

LUMBAR. Pertaining to the part of the back between the chest and the pelvis.

LUMBAR VERTEBRAE. The vertebrae of the lower back below the level of the ribs.

LUMEN. The channel or cavity inside a tube or hollow organ of the body.

LUMPECTOMY. A less-invasive procedure that just removes the tumor and some surrounding tissue, without removing the entire breast.

LUPUS ERYTHEMATOSUS. A chronic inflammatory disease in which inappropriate immune system reactions cause abnormalities in the blood vessels and connective tissue.

LUXATE. To loosen or dislocate a tooth from its socket.

LYMPH. The almost colorless fluid that bathes body tissues. Lymph is found in the lymphatic vessels and carries lymphocytes that have entered the lymph glands from the blood.

LYMPH NODE BIOPSY. The removal of all or part of a lymph node to view under a microscope for cancer cells.

LYMPH NODES. Small, bean-shaped organs located throughout the lymphatic system. Lymph nodes store special cells that can trap cancer cells and bacteria traveling through the body.

LYMPHANGIOGRAPHY. Injection of dye into lymphatic vessels followed by x rays of the area. It is a difficult procedure, as it requires surgical isolation of the lymph vessels to be injected.

LYMPHATIC SYSTEM. The tissues and organs that produce and store cells that fight infection, together with the network of vessels that carry lymph. The organs and tissues in the lymphatic system include the bone marrow, spleen, thymus gland, and lymph nodes.

LYMPHEDEMA. Swelling caused by an accumulation of fluid from faulty lymph drainage.

LYMPHOCYTES. Type of white blood cells that are part of the immune system. The lymphocytes are composed of three main cell lines: B lymphocytes, T lymphocytes, and natural killer (NK) cells.

LYMPHOMA. A type of cancer that affects lymph cells and tissues, including certain white blood cells (T cells and B cells), lymph nodes, bone marrow, and the spleen. Abnormal cells (lymphocyte/leukocyte) multiply uncontrollably.

LYMPHOPROLIFERATIVE. An increase in the number of lymphocytes. Lymphocytes are a white blood cell (WBC) formed in lymphatic tissue throughout the body—in the lymph nodes, spleen, thymus, tonsils, Peyer patches, and sometimes in bone marrow), and in normal adults, comprising approximately 22–28% of the total number of leukocytes in the circulating blood.

LYMPHOSCINTIGRAPHY. A technique in which a radioactive substance that concentrates in the lymphatic vessels is injected into the affected tissue and mapped using a gamma camera, which images the location of the radioactive tracer.

LYSIS. The process of removing adhesions from an organ. The term comes from a Greek word that means "loosening."

M

MACROCYTIC. A descriptive term applied to a larger than normal red blood cell.

MACROMASTIA. Excessive size of the breasts.

MACROPHAGE. A type of blood cell derived from monocytes that are stimulated by inflammation and stimulate antibody production.

MACROSOMIA. The term used to describe a newborn baby with an abnormally high birth weight.

MACULA. A small, yellowish depressed area on the retina that absorbs the shorter wave lengths of visible light and is responsible for fine detailed vision. This is the part of the retina in which the highest concentration of photoreceptors are found.

MACULAR DEGENERATION. A progressive disease in which the central portion of the retina (the macula) is gradually destroyed.

MAGNETIC FIELD. The three-dimensional area surrounding a magnet, in which its force is active. During MRI, the patient's body is permeated by the force field of a superconducting magnet.

MAGNETIC RESONANCE IMAGING (MRI). A noninvasive diagnostic tool that takes pictures of internal body structures and tissues. Using powerful magnets that force hydrogen atoms in the body to align, the machine sends radio waves toward the lined-up hydrogen atoms, and a computer displays and records the signals that bounce back. Different kinds of tissues (e.g., healthy and diseased) and different kinds of structures (e.g., organs and tumors) send back unique signals.

MALABSORPTION. Defective or inadequate absorption of nutrients from the intestinal tract.

MALABSORPTIVE. A type of bariatric surgery in which a part of the stomach is partitioned off and connected to a lower portion of the small intestine in order to reduce the amount of nutrients that the body absorbs from the food.

MALIGNANT. Cancerous. Cells tend to reproduce without normal controls on growth and form tumors or invade other tissues.

MALIGNANT HYPERTHERMIA. A type of allergic reaction (probably with a genetic basis) that can occur during general anesthesia in which the patient experiences a high fever, the muscles become rigid, and the heart rate and blood pressure fluctuate.

MALIGNANT MESOTHELIOMA. A cancer of the pleura (the membrane lining the chest cavity and covering the lungs) that typically is related to asbestos exposure.

MALIGNANT NEOPLASM. Any malignant cancerous growth or tumor caused by uncontrolled cell division and capable of spreading to other parts of the body than where it formed.

MALIGNANT TUMOR. A cancerous growth that has the potential to spread to other parts of the body.

MALLEUS. One of the three bones of the middle ear. It is also known as the "hammer."

MALOCCLUSION. Malpositioning and defective contact between opposing teeth in the upper and lower jaws.

MALPRACTICE. A doctor or lawyer's failure in his or her professional duties through ignorance, negligence, or criminal intent.

MAMMARY ARTERY. A chest wall artery that descends from the aorta and is commonly used for bypass grafts.

MAMMARY HYPERPLASIA. Increased size of the breast.

MAMMOGRAM. A set of x rays taken of the front and side of the breast used to help diagnose various breast abnormalities.

MAMMOPLASTY. Surgery performed to change the size or shape of breasts.

MANDIBLE. The horseshoe-shaped bone that forms the lower jaw.

MANNITOL. A type of diuretic.

MARFAN SYNDROME. A condition occasionally associated with chest wall deformities, in which the patients have a characteristic tall, thin appearance, and cardiac and great vessel abnormalities.

MASTECTOMY. Removal of all or a portion of breast tissue.

MASTECTOMY, MODIFIED RADICAL. Total mastectomy with axillary lymph node dissection, but with preservation of the pectoral muscles.

MASTECTOMY, RADICAL. Removal of the breast, pectoral muscles, axillary lymph nodes, and associated skin and subcutaneous tissue.

MASTECTOMY, SIMPLE. Removal of only the breast tissue, nipple and a small portion of the overlying skin

MASTOID AIR CELLS. Numerous small intercommunicating cavities in the mastoid process of the temporal bone that empty into the mastoid antrum.

MASTOID ANTRUM. A cavity in the temporal bone of the skull, communicating with the mastoid cells and with the middle ear.

MASTOID PROCESS. A large bony process at the base of the skull behind the ear. It contains air spaces that connect with the cavity of the middle ear.

MASTOIDECTOMY. Hollowing out the mastoid process by curretting, gouging, drilling, or otherwise removing the bony partitions forming the mastoid cells.

MASTOIDITIS. An inflammation of the bone behind the ear (the mastoid bone) caused by an infection spreading from the middle ear to the cavity in the mastoid bone.

MASTOPEXY. Surgical procedure to lift up a breast; may be used on opposite breast to achieve symmetrical appearance with a reconstructed breast.

MATCH. How similar the HLA typing, out of a possible six antigens, is between the donor and the recipient.

MATERNAL BLOOD SCREENING. Maternal blood screening is normally done early in pregnancy to test for a variety of conditions. Abnormal amounts of certain proteins in a pregnant woman's blood raise the probability of fetal defects. Amniocentesis is recommended if such a probability occurs.

MATERNITY. Refers to the mother.

MAXILLA. The facial bone that forms the upper jaw and holds the upper teeth.

MAXILLARY SINUSES. Sinuses located in the cheek under the eye next to the ethmoid sinus.

MAZE PROCEDURE. A surgical procedure used to treat atrial fibrillation. During the procedure, precise incisions are made in the right and left atria to interrupt the conduction of abnormal impulses. When the heart heals, scar tissue forms and the abnormal electrical impulses are blocked from traveling through the heart.

MDR. Multiple drug-resistance

MEAN CORPUSCULAR HEMOGLOBIN (MCH). A calculation of the average weight of hemoglobin in a red blood cell.

MEAN CORPUSCULAR HEMOGLOBIN CONCENTRATION (MCHC). A calculation of the average concentration of hemoglobin in a red blood cell.

MEAN CORPUSCULAR VOLUME (MCV). A measure of the average volume of a red blood cell.

MEATUS. A general term for an opening or passageway in the body.

MECHANICAL VALVE. An artificial device used to replace a patient's heart valve. There are three types: ball valve, disk valve, and bileaflet valve.

MEDIAL (OR LATERAL) NASAL PROMINENCE. The medial (toward the middle) or lateral (toward the sides) are anatomical structures that form and merge the nose of the developing embryo during weeks six to nine in utero.

MEDIASTINOSCOPY. A surgical procedure to look at the organs, tissues, and lymph nodes between the lungs for abnormal areas. An incision (cut) is made at the top of the breastbone and a thin, lighted tube is inserted into the chest. Tissue and lymph node samples may be taken for biopsy.

MEDIASTINUM. The area between the lungs, bounded by the spine, breastbone, and diaphragm, that consists of the heart, thoracic parts of the great vessels, and thoracic parts of the trachea, esophagus, thymus, and lymph nodes.

MEDICAID. Public assistance funded through the state to individuals unable to pay for health care. Medicaid can be accessed only when all prior assets and funds are depleted.

MEDICAL AGENT. A designated representative for the patient who, in advance, is legally empowered to carry out their wishes with respect to medial care.

MEDICAL DIRECTIVES. Legal documents that include a declaration of wishes pertaining to medical treatment (living will) and the stipulation of a proxy decision maker (power of attorney).

MEDICAL ERROR. A preventable adverse event.

MEDICAL SURROGATE. Another name for a medical agent or person legally designated to represent the patient with medical providers.

MEDICALLY NEEDY. A term that describes a group whose coverage is optional with the states because of high medical expenses. These persons meet category requirements of Medicaid (they are children or parents or elderly or disabled) but their income is too high to qualify them for coverage as categorically needy.

MEDICARE. A government program, administered by the Social Security Administration, which provides financial assistance to individuals over the age of 65 for hospital and medical expenses. Medicare does not cover long-term care expenses.

MEDICARE PART A. Hospital insurance provided by Medicare, provided free to persons aged 65 and older.

MEDICARE PART B. Medical insurance provided by Medicare that requires recipients to pay a monthly premium. Part B pays for some medical services Part A does not.

MEDIGAP. A group of 10 standardized private health insurance policies intended to cover the coinsurance and deductible costs not covered by Medicare.

MEDIONECROSIS. Death of the middle layer of tissues in a vessel.

MEDULLARY CAVITY. The marrow cavity in the shaft of a long bone.

MEGACOLON. Abnormally large colon associated with some chronic intestine disorders.

MELANOCYTES. Cells within the epidermis that give skin its color

MELANOMA. A malignant tumor arising from the melanocytic system of the skin and other organs.

MELENA. The passing of blackish-colored stools containing blood pigments or partially digested blood.

MEMBRANOUS LABYRINTH. A complex arrangement of communicating membranous canals and sacs, filled with endolymph and suspended within the cavity of the bony labyrinth.

MENGHINI NEEDLE/JAMSHEDI NEEDLE. Special needles used to obtain a sample of liver tissue by aspiration.

MÉNIÈRE'S DISEASE. Also known as idiopathic endolymphatic hydrops, Ménière's disease is a disorder of the inner ear. It is named for Prosper Ménière (1799–1862), a French physician.

MENINGES. Membranes that cover the brain.

MENINGITIS. An infection of the membranes that cover the brain and spinal cord.

MENISCAL. Pertaining to cartilage.

MENISCUS. The fibrous cartilage within the knee joint that covers the surfaces of the femur and the tibia as they join the patella.

MENTAL DISABILITY. The inability to mentally function due to injury, illness, or toxicity.

MERKEL'S DIVERTICULUM. Tissue faults in the lining of the intestines that are the result of a congenital abnormality originating in the umbilical duct's failure to close. Largely asymptomatic, the diverticula in some cases can become infected or obstructed.

MERPERIDINE. A type of narcotic pain killer that may be used after surgical procedures.

MESENCHYMAL CELLS. Embryonic cells that develop into many structures, including the soft tissues in the lip.

MESENTERY. The membranes, or one of the membranes (consisting of a fold of the peritoneum and enclosed tissues), that connect the intestines and their appendages with the dorsal wall of the abdominal cavity.

METABOLIC ACIDOSIS. A condition in which either too much acid or too little bicarbonate in the body results in a drop in the blood pH (towards acidity).

METABOLIC ALKALOSIS. A condition in which either too little acid or too much bicarbonate in the body results in an elevation in the blood pH (towards alkalinity).

METABOLIC DISTURBANCE. A disturbance in the general function of the body's basic life processes such as energy production. The body's ability to provide the brain with appropriate nourishment can affect the mental status of the individual.

METABOLIC SYNDROME. A combination of medical disorders including diabetes, high blood pressure, and heart disease.

METABOLISM. The sum of all the chemical processes that occur in living organisms; the rate at which the body consumes energy.

METABOLITES. The chemicals produced in the body after nutrients, drugs, enzymes or other materials have been changed (metabolized).

METABOLIZE. The chemical changes that occur in the body, including the changes that occur in the liver, converting molecules to forms that are more easily removed from the body.

METACARPAL BONES. Five cylindrical bones extending from the wrist to the fingers.

METAPHYSIS. The widened end of the shaft of a long tubular bone such as the femur.

METASTASIS. A process in which a malignant tumor transfers cells to a part of the body not directly connected to its primary site. A cancer that has spread from its original site to other parts of the body is said to be metastatic.

METATARSAL JOINT. Having to do with the bones of the foot.

METHICILLIN-RESISTANT *STAPHYLOCOCCUS AUREUS* (MRSA). A strain of Staph. bacteria that is resistant to methicillin and hence poses a greater health threat because it is difficult to control or kill.

METHOTREXATE. A drug that targets rapidly dividing fetal cells, preventing a fetus from developing further.

MICROCYTIC. A descriptive term applied to a smaller than normal red blood cell.

MICRODERMABRASION. A technique for skin resurfacing that uses abrasive crystals passed through a hand piece to even out skin irregularities.

MICROGENIA. An extremely small chin. It is the most common deformity of the chin.

MICROKERATOME. A precision surgical instrument that can slice an extremely thin layer of tissue from the surface of the cornea.

MICROORGANISM. An independent unit of life that is too small to be seen with the naked eye.

MICROSURGERY. Surgery performed under a microscope on nerves and other very small structures with the help of special instruments.

MICROTIA. The partial or complete absence of the auricle of the ear.

MIDDLE EAR. The cavity or space between the eardrum and the inner ear. It includes the eardrum, the three little bones (hammer, anvil, and stirrup) that transmit sound to the inner ear, and the Eustachian tube, which connects the inner ear to the nasopharynx (the back of the nose).

MIDDLE MEATUS. A curved passage in each nasal cavity located below the middle nasal concha and extending along the entire superior border of the inferior nasal concha.

MIDDLE TURBINATE. The lower of two thin bony processes on the ethmoid bone on the lateral wall of each nasal fossa that separates the superior and middle meatus of the nose.

MILIA. Small bumps on the skin that are occur when sweat glands are clogged.

MINIGRAFT OR MICROGRAFT. Transplantation of a small number of hair follicles, as few as one to three hairs, into a transplant site.

MINIMALLY INVASIVE SURGERY. Surgical techniques, especially the use of small instruments and tiny video cameras, that allow surgery to take place without a full operative wound.

MIOTICS. Medications that cause the pupil of the eye to contract.

MISCARRIAGE. The loss of a fetus before it is viable, usually between the third and seventh months of pregnancy. A miscarriage is sometimes called a spontaneous abortion.

MITRAL VALVE. The bicuspid valve that lies between the left atrium and left ventricle of the heart.

MIXED DENTITION. A mix of both "baby teeth" and permanent teeth.

MIXED LYMPHOCYTE CULTURE (MLC). Test that measures level of reactivity between donor and recipient lymphocytes.

MOHS EXCISION. Referring to the excision of one layer of tissue during Mohs surgery. Also called stage.

MONOCHORIONIC PREGNANCY. A pregnancy in which twin fetuses share a placenta.

MONOCYTE. Mononuclear phagocytic white blood cell that removes debris and microorganisms by phagocytosis and processes antigens for recognition by immune lymphocytes.

MONOFILAMENT. A single untwisted strand of suture material.

MONSEL'S SOLUTION. A solution used to stop bleeding.

MORBID. Unwholesome or bad for health. Morbid obesity is a condition in which the patient's weight is a very high risk to his or her health. The NIH (National Institutes of Health) prefers the term "severely obese" to "morbidly obese."

MORBIDITY. A state of disease or illness. Also, a statistic that provides the rate at which an illness or abnormality occurs.

MORBIDLY OBESE. Definition of a person who is 100 lb (45 kg) or more than 50% overweight and has a body mass index above 40.

MORPHINE. A very strong painkiller often used post-surgically.

MORPHOLOGY. Literally, the study of form. In medicine, morphology refers to the size, shape, and structure rather than the function of a given organ. As a diagnostic imaging technique, ultrasound facilitates the recognition of abnormal morphologies as symptoms of underlying conditions.

MORTALITY. The death rate, which reflects the number of deaths per unit of population in any specific region, age group, disease, or other classification, usually expressed as deaths per 1,000, 10,000, or 1,000,000.

MOTILITY. Ability to move freely or spontaneously. Esophageal motility refers to the ability of the muscle fibers in the tissue of the esophagus to contract in order to push food or other material toward the stomach.

MOUTH GUARD. A plastic device that protects the upper teeth from injury during athletic events.

MUCOCILIARY. Involving cilia of the mucous membranes of the respiratory system.

MUCUS. A viscous, slippery secretion that is produced by mucous membranes which it moistens and protects.

MUCOUS MEMBRANE. A membrane rich in mucous glands that lines body passages and cavities communicating directly or indirectly with the exterior of the body (as for example, the alimentary, respiratory, and genitourinary tracts). Mucous membranes functions in protection, support, nutrient absorption, and secretion of mucus, enzymes, and salts.

MULTIFILAMENT. A braided strand of suture material. Multifilament sutures are generally thicker than monofilament and used in such specialties as orthopedic surgery.

MULTIPLE MYELOMA. An uncommon disease that occurs more often in men than in women and is associated with anemia, hemorrhage, recurrent infections and weakness. Ordinarily it is regarded as a malignant neoplasm that originates in bone marrow and involves mainly the skeleton.

MULTIPLE SCLEROSIS. A chronic degenerative neurological disease in which demyelination of the nerves causes progressive weakness and loss of motor function.

MURMUR. The sound made as blood moves through the heart when there is turbulence in the flow of blood through a blood vessel, or if a valve does not completely close.

MUSCULAR DYSTROPHY. A genetic muscle disease that causes progressive muscle weakness along with the breakdown and death of muscle tissue.

MYCOBACTERIUM. Any of a genus of nonmotile, aerobic, acid-fast bacteria that include numerous saprophytes and the pathogens causing tuberculosis and leprosy.

MYELODYSPLASIA. Also called myelodysplastic syndrome, it is a condition in which the bone marrow does not function normally and can affect the various types of blood cells produced in the bone marrow. Often referred to as a preleukemia and may progress and become acute leukemia.

MYELOFIBROSIS. An anemic condition in which bone marrow cells are abnormal or defective and become fibrotic.

MYELOGRAM. A special type of x ray study of the spinal cord, made after a contrast medium has been injected into the space surrounding the cord.

MYELOMA (MULTIPLE MYELOMA). A tumor of plasma cells that originates in bone marrow and usually spreads to more than one bone.

MYELOMENINGOCELES (MMC). A protrusion in the vertebral column containing spinal cord and meninges.

MYOCARDIAL INFARCTION (MI). Commonly known as a heart attack, a myocardial infarction is an episode in which some of the heart's blood supply is severely cut off or restricted, causing the heart muscle to suffer and die from lack of oxygen.

MYOCARDITIS. Inflammation of the muscles of the walls of the heart due to a viral infection.

MYOGLOBIN. A protein that holds oxygen in heart and skeletal muscle. It rises after damage to either of these muscle types.

MYOMA. A tumor consisting of muscle tissue.

MYOPIA. A vision problem in which distant objects appear blurry. Myopia results when the cornea is too steep or the eye is too long and the light doesn't focus properly on the retina. People who are myopic or nearsighted can usually see near objects clearly, but not far objects.

MYOSITIS. Inflammation of muscle tissue.

MYRINGOPLASTY. Surgical restoration of a perforated tympanic membrane by grafting.

MYRINGOTOMY. A procedure that involves making a small incision in the eardrum to release pressure caused by excess fluid accumulation.

N

NARCOTIC. A drug derived from opium or compounds similar to opium. Such drugs are potent pain relievers and can affect mood and behavior. Long-term use of narcotics can lead to dependence and tolerance.

NASAL CANNULA. A piece of flexible plastic tubing with two small clamps that fit into the nostrils and provide supplemental oxygen flow.

NASAL CONCHA. Any of three thin bony plates on the lateral wall of the nasal fossa on each side with or without their covering of mucous membrane.

NASOGASTRIC TUBE. A tube inserted through the nose and throat and into the stomach for direct feeding of the patient.

NATRIURETIC PEPTIDES. Peptides that prompt the kidneys to excrete sodium into the urine and out of the body.

NEARSIGHTEDNESS. A condition in which one or both eyes cannot focus normally, causing objects at a distance to appear blurred and indistinct. Also called myopia.

NECROSIS. Cellular or tissue death; skin necrosis may be caused by multiple, consecutive doses of radiation from fluoroscopic or x-ray procedures.

NECROTIC. Affected with necrosis (cell death).

NEEDLE BIOPSY. The use of a needle to remove tissue from an area that looks suspicious. Tissue removed in a needle biopsy goes to a lab to be checked for cancer cells.

NEO-BLADDER. A term that refers to the creation of a reservoir for urine made from intestinal tissue that allows for evacuation.

NEONATAL JAUNDICE. A disorder in newborns where the liver is too premature to conjugate bilirubin, which builds up in the blood.

NEONATE. A newborn baby.

NEOPLASM. A new growth or tumor.

NEOVASCULAR GLAUCOMA. A form of glaucoma that results from uncontrolled diabetes or hypertension.

NEPHELOMETRY. A method for measuring the light scattering properties of a sample.

NEPHRECTOMY. Surgical removal of a kidney.

NEPHROLITHOTOMY. The removal of renal calculi by an incision through the kidney. The term by itself usually refers to the standard open procedure for the surgical removal of kidney stones.

NEPHROLOGIST. A doctor specializing in kidney disease.

NEPHROSCOPE. An instrument used to view the inside of the kidney during PCNL. A nephroscope has channels for a fiberoptic light, a telescope, and an irrigation system for washing out the affected part of the kidney.

NEPHROTIC SYNDROME. A kidney disorder which causes a cluster of symptoms, including low serum protein, loss of protein in the urine, and body swelling.

NEPHROTOXIC. Destructive to kidney cells. Hemoperfusion can be used to remove nephrotoxic chemicals from the blood.

NEPHROTOXICITY. A building up of poisons in the kidneys.

NEUROBLASTOMA. Solid tumor in children, may be treated by BMT.

NEUROFIBROMATOSIS. A rare hereditary disease that involves the growth of lesions that may affect the spinal cord.

NEUROGENIC BLADDER. A urinary problem of neurological origin in which there is abnormal emptying of the bladder with subsequent retention or incontinence of urine.

NEUROLOGICAL. Pertaining to the nervous system: peripheral nervous system, brain, and spinal cord.

NEUROLOGIST. A physician who specializes in diagnosing and treating disorders of the nervous system.

NEUROMODULATION. Electrical stimulation of a nerve for relief of pain.

NEUROPATHY. Nerve damage.

NEUROSURGERY. Surgery involving the nervous system: peripheral nervous system, brain, and spinal cord. A physician who performs such surgery is called a neurosurgeon.

NEUROTRANSMITTER. Chemicals within the nervous system that transmit information from or between nerve cells.

NEUTRALIZE. The way the body addresses acidity or alkalinity: adding acid to an alkaline environment to arrive at a neutral pH value, or adding bicarbonate to an acidic environment to arrive at a neutral pH value.

NEUTROPHIL. A type of white blood cell. Neutrophils remove and kill bacteria by phagocytosis.

NICOTINE. A poisonous, oily alkaloid in tobacco.

NITROUS OXIDE. A colorless, sweet-smelling gas used by dentists for mild anesthesia. It is sometimes called laughing gas because it makes some people feel giddy or silly.

NOCICEPTOR. A nerve cell that is capable of sensing pain and transmitting a pain signal.

NOMOGRAM. A surgeon's adjustment of the excimer laser to fine-tune results.

NON-INVASIVE. A procedure that does not penetrate the body.

NON-MYELOABLATIVE ALLOGENEIC BONE MARROW TRANSPLANT. Also called "mini" bone marrow transplants. This type of bone marrow transplant involves receiving low-doses of chemotherapy and radiation therapy, followed by the infusion of a donor's bone marrow or peripheral stem cells. The goal is to suppress the patient's own bone marrow with low-dose chemotherapy and radiation therapy to allow the donor's cells to engraft.

NON-PALPABLE. Unable to be detected through the sense of touch. A non-palpable testicle is one that is located in the abdomen or other site where the doctor cannot feel it by pressing gently on the child's body.

NON-UNION. Bone fracture or defect induced by disease, trauma, or surgery that fails to heal within a reasonable time span.

NONABLATIVE. Not requiring removal or destruction of the epidermis. Some techniques for minimizing scars are nonablative.

NONINVASIVE TUMORS. Tumors that have not penetrated the muscle wall and/or spread to other parts of the body.

NONPHARMACOLOGICAL. Referring to therapy that does not involve drugs.

NONPROFIT HOSPITALS. Hospitals that combine a teaching function with providing for uninsured within large, complex networks technically designated as nonprofit institutions. While the institution may be nonprofit, however, its services are allowed to make a profit.

NONSTEROIDAL ANTI-INFLAMMATORY DRUGS (NSAIDS). Drugs that relieve pain and reduce inflammation but are not related chemically to cortisone. Common drugs in this class are aspirin, ibuprofen (Advil, Motrin), naproxen (Aleve, Naprosyn), ketoprofen (Orudis), and several others.

NOREPINEPHRINE. A naturally occurring hormone that acts as a neurotransmitter and affects both alpha- and beta-adrenergic receptors. It is also known as noradrenaline.

NORMAL FLORA. The mixture of bacteria normally found at specific body sites.

NORMOCHROMIC. A descriptive term applied to a red blood cell with a normal concentration of hemoglobin.

NORMOCYTIC. A descriptive term applied to a red blood cell of normal size.

NOSOCOMIAL. Occurring in the hospital or clinical setting.

NOSOCOMIAL INFECTION. An infection acquired in the hospital.

NOTHING BY MOUTH (NPO). NPO refers to the time after which the patient is not allowed to eat or drink prior to a procedure or treatment.

NUCLEAR IMAGING. Method of producing images by detecting radiation from different parts of the body after a radioactive tracer material is administered.

NUCLEUS. The part of a cell that contains the DNA.

NURSE ANESTHETIST. A registered nurse who has obtained advanced training in anesthesia delivery and patient care.

NURSE MANAGER. The nurse responsible for managing the nursing care on the nursing unit and also supervises all of the other personnel who work on the nursing unit.

NURSING UNIT. The floor or section of the hospital where patient rooms are located.

NYHA HEART FAILURE CLASSIFICATION. A classification system for heart failure developed by the New York Heart Association. It includes the following four categories: I, symptoms with more than ordinary activity; II, symptoms with ordinary activity; III, symptoms with minimal activity; IV, symptoms at rest.

NYSTAGMUS. An involuntary, rapid, rhythmic movement of the eyeball, which may be horizontal, vertical, rotatory, or mixed.

O

OBESITY. Excessive weight gain due to accumulation of fat in the body, sometimes defined as a BMI (body mass index) of 30 or higher, or body weight greater than 30% above one's desirable weight on standard height-weight tables.

OBJECTIVE. Not biased by personal opinion; repeatable.

OBSESSION. A recurrent and persistent idea, thought, or impulse that the individual cannot repress.

OBSTETRICS AND GYNECOLOGICAL SURGERY. Surgery involving the reproductive organs or pregnancy.

OBSTRUCTIVE SLEEP APNEA (OSA). A potentially life-threatening condition characterized by episodes of breathing cessation during sleep alternating with snoring or disordered breathing. The low levels of oxygen in the blood of patients with OSA may eventually cause heart problems or stroke.

OBTURATOR. Any structure that occludes an opening. A trocar obturator has a tip used to penetrate the body wall while being held in the cannula of the trocar apparatus.

OCCLUSION. An obstruction or blockage in a blood vessel.

OCCULT. Hidden; concealed from the doctor's direct observation. Some ganglion cysts are occult.

OCULAR HYPERTENSION. A condition in which fluid pressure inside the eye is higher than normal but the optic nerve and visual fields are normal.

OCULAR MELANOMA. A malignant tumor that arises within the structures of the eye. It is the most common eye tumor in adults.

OCULAR ORBIT. Bony cavity containing the eyeball.

OINTMENT. A thick spreadable substance that contains medicine and is meant to be used on the outside of the body.

OLIGOHYDRAMNIOS. Low levels of amniotic fluid during pregnancy.

OLIGURIA. Decreased urine production.

OMBUDSMAN. A patient representative who investigates patient complaints and problems related to hospital service or treatment. He or she may act as a mediator between the patient, the family, and the hospital.

OMPHALOCELE. A hernia that occurs at the navel.

ONCOGENE. A gene that is capable under certain conditions of triggering the conversion of normal cells into cancer cells.

ONCOLOGIST. A physician who specializes in the diagnosis and treatment of tumors.

ONCOLOGY. The branch of medicine that deals with the diagnosis and treatment of cancer.

OOPHORECTOMY. Removal of one or both ovaries in a woman.

OOPHORECTOMY. Surgical removal of the ovaries.

OPEN SURGERY. Surgery using a large incision to lay open area for examination or treatment; in joint surgery, the whole joint is exposed.

OPEN-ANGLE GLAUCOMA. A form of glaucoma in which fluid pressure builds up inside the eye even though the angle of the anterior chamber is open and looks normal when the eye is examined with a gonioscope. Most cases of glaucoma are open-angle.

OPERATIVE NURSE. A nurse specially trained to assist the surgeon and work in all areas of the surgical event to care for the patient.

OPHTHALMOLOGIST. A medical doctor with advanced training in the diagnosis and treatment of eye disease.

OPHTHALMOLOGY. The branch of medicine that deals with the diagnosis and treatment of eye disorders.

OPHTHALMOSCOPE. An instrument for viewing the interior of the eye, particularly the retina. Light is thrown into the eye by a mirror (usually concave) and the interior is then examined with or without the aid of a lens.

OPIOID. A synthetic drug resembling opium or alkaloids of opium.

OPTIC DISC. A visually inactive portion of the retina from which the optic nerve and blood vessels emerge.

OPTIC NERVE. A large nerve found in the posterior part of the eye, through which all the visual nerve fibers leave the eye on their way to the brain.

OPTOMETRIST. A primary health care provider who examines eyes and diagnoses disorders of the eye as well as prescribing eyeglasses, contact lenses, and other vision aids.

ORAL SURGEON. A dentist who specializes in surgical procedures of the mouth, including extractions.

ORAL. Pertaining to the mouth.

ORBICULARIS ORIS. Concentrically shaped muscle that surrounds the upper and lower lips.

ORBIT. The cavity in the skull containing the eyeball; formed from seven bones: frontal, maxillary, sphenoid, lacrimal, zygomatic, ethmoid, and palatine.

ORCHIECTOMY. Surgical removal of one or both testicles in a male; also called an orchidectomy.

ORGAN PROCUREMENT. The process of donor screening, and the evaluation, removal, preservation, and distribution of organs for transplantation.

OROPHARYNX. The part of the throat at the back of the mouth.

ORTHODONTIC TREATMENT. The process of realigning and straightening teeth to correct their appearance and function.

ORTHOGNATHIC SURGERY. Surgery that corrects deformities or malpositioning of the bones in the jaw. The term comes from two Greek words meaning straight and jaw.

ORTHOPEDIC SURGERY. Surgery involving the musculoskeletal system, which includes muscles, tendons, joints, and bones.

ORTHOPEDICS (SOMETIMES SPELLED ORTHOPAEDICS). The branch of surgery that treats deformities or disorders affecting the musculoskeletal system.

ORTHOTIC. A device designed to be inserted into a shoe to help keep the foot in proper alignment, stabilize the heel, support the arch, and distribute body weight more evenly over the foot.

ORTHOTOPIC TRANSPLANTATION. The replacement of a whole diseased liver with a healthy donor liver.

OSMOLALITY. A measurement of urine concentration that depends on the number of particles dissolved in it. Values are expressed as milliosmols per kilogram (mOsm/kg) of water.

OSMOSIS. Passage of a solvent through a membrane from an area of greater concentration to an area of lesser concentration.

OSSICLES. The three small bones of the middle ear: the malleus (hammer), the incus (anvil) and the stapes (stirrup). These bones help carry sound from the eardrum to the inner ear.

OSSICULOPLASTY. Surgical insertion of an implant to replace one or more of the ear ossicles. Also called ossicular replacement.

OSTEOARTHRITIS. Non-inflammatory degenerative joint disease occurring chiefly in older persons, characterized by degeneration of the articular cartilage.

OSTEOBLASTS. Bone cells that build new bone tissue.

OSTEOCLASTS. Bone cells that break down and remove bone tissue.

OSTEOCONDUCTION. Provision of a scaffold for the growth of new bone.

OSTEOCYTES. Bone cells that maintain bone tissue.

OSTEOGENESIS. Growth of new bone.

OSTEOINDUCTION. Acceleration of new bone formation by chemical means. Also refers to the process of building, healing, and remodeling bone in humans.

OSTEOLYSIS. Dissolution and loss of bone resulting from inflammation caused by particles of polyethylene debris from a prosthesis.

OSTEOMALACIA. A disease of adults, characterized by softening of the bone; similar to rickets, which is seen in children.

OSTEONECROSIS. Condition resulting from poor blood supply to an area of a bone and causing bone death.

OSTEOPATHY. A system of therapy that uses standard medical and surgical methods of diagnosis and treatment while emphasizing the importance of proper body alignment and manipulative treatment of musculoskeletal disorders. Osteopathy is considered mainstream primary care medicine rather than an alternative system.

OSTEOPOROSIS. A bone disorder, usually seen in the elderly, in which the bones become increasingly less dense and more brittle.

OSTEOTOMY. The cutting apart of a bone or removal of bone by cutting. An osteotomy is often necessary during hip revision surgery in order to remove the femoral part of the old prosthesis from the femur.

OSTEOTOMY OF THE KNEE. Realignment of the knee, using bone cutting to shift weight bearing from damaged cartilage to healthier cartilage.

OSTIA. A mouth-like opening in a bodily part.

OSTOMY. General term meaning a surgical procedure in which an artificial opening is formed to either allow waste (stool or urine) to pass from the body, or to allow food into the GI tract. An ostomy can be permanent or temporary, as well as single-barreled, double-barreled, or a loop.

OTITIS. Inflammation of the ear, which may be marked by pain, fever, abnormalities of hearing, hearing loss, tinnitus and vertigo.

OTOLARYNGOLOGIST. A surgeon who specializes in treating disorders of the ears, nose, and throat.

OTOLOGY. The branch of medicine that deals with the diagnosis and treatment of ear disorders.

OTOSCLEROSIS. Formation of spongy bone around the footplate of the stapes, resulting in conductive hearing loss.

OTOSCOPY. Examination of the ear with an otoscope, an instrument designed to evaluate the condition of the ear.

OUTPATIENT PROCEDURES. Surgeries that are performed on an outpatient basis, involving less recovery time and fewer expected complications.

OUTPATIENT SURGERY. Also called same-day or ambulatory surgery. The patient arrives for surgery and returns home on the same day. Outpatient surgery can take place in a hospital, surgical center, or outpatient clinic.

OVARIAN CYST. A benign or malignant growth on an ovary. An ovarian cyst can disappear without treatment or become extremely painful and have to be surgically removed.

OVARY. One of the two essential female reproductive organs that produce eggs and sex hormones.

OVEREXPRESSION. Production in abnormally high amounts.

OVULATION. A process in which a mature female egg is released from one of the ovaries (egg-shaped structures located to each side of the uterus) every 28 days.

OXIMETRY. Measuring the degree of oxygen saturation of circulating blood.

OXYGENATION. Saturation with oxygen.

OXYHEMOGLOBIN. Hemoglobin combined with oxygen.

P

PACEMAKER. A surgically implanted electronic device that sends out electrical impulses to regulate a slow or erratic heartbeat.

PACU. The postanesthesia care unit, where the patient is cared for after surgery.

PAIN DISORDER. A psychiatric disorder in which pain in one or more parts of the body is caused or made worse by psychological factors. The lower back is one of the most common sites for pain related to this disorder.

PALATE. The roof of the mouth composed of two anatomical structures, the hard and soft palates.

PALLIATIVE. A type of care that is intended to relieve pain and suffering, but not to cure.

PALPATE. To examine by means of touch.

PALPATION. The examination of the body using the sense of touch. There are two types: light and deep.

PALPEBRAL FISSURE. Eyelid opening.

PALPITATIONS. Forcible pulsation or pounding of the heart that is perceptible to the patient.

PANCREAS. An organ located near the liver and stomach, responsible for various digestive functions. The pancreas produces insulin and glucagon, hormones that are responsible for maintaining safe blood levels of glucose.

PANCREATICODUODENECTOMY. Removal of all or part of the pancreas along with the duodenum. Also known as "Whipple's procedure" or "Whipple's operation."

PANCREATITIS. Inflammation of the pancreas, either acute (sudden and episodic) or chronic, usually caused by excessive alcohol intake or gallbladder disease.

PANIC DISORDER. An disorder in which people have sudden and intense attacks of anxiety in certain situations.

PAP TEST. The common term for the Papanicolaou test, a simple smear method of removing cervical cells to screen for abnormalities that indicate cancer or a precancerous condition.

PARACENTESIS. Surgical puncture of the abdominal cavity for the aspiration of peritoneal fluid.

PARAQUAT. A highly toxic restricted-use pesticide. Death following ingestion usually results from multiple organ failure.

PARASYMPATHETIC NERVOUS SYSTEM. The division of the autonomic (involuntary) nervous system that slows heart rate, increases digestive and glandular activity, and relaxes the sphincter muscles that close off body organs.

PARATHYROID GLANDS. Two pairs of smaller glands that lie close to the lower surface of the thyroid gland. They secrete parathyroid hormone, which regulates the body's use of calcium and phosphorus.

PARATHYROIDECTOMY. A surgical procedure in which one or more parathyroid glands are removed.

PARENCHYMA. The essential elements of an organ, used in anatomical nomenclature as a general term to designate the functional elements of an organ, as distinguished from its framework.

PARENTERAL NUTRITION. The administration of liquid nutrition through an intravenous catheter placed in the patient's vein.

PARENTERAL NUTRITIONAL SUPPORT. Intravenous nutrition that bypasses the intestines and its contribution to digestion.

PARESTHESIA. An abnormal touch sensation, such as a prickling or burning feeling, often in the absence of an external cause.

PARIETAL CELLS. Cells of the gastric glands that secret hydrochloric acid.

PARIETAL PERICARDIUM. External or outer layer of the pericardial cavity.

PARKINSON'S DISEASE. A neurological disease resulting from a deficiency of the neurotransmitter dopamine that is associated with specific recognizable movements, affects, and behavior patterns.

PARONYCHIA. Inflammation of the folds of tissue surrounding the nail.

PARTIAL THROMBOPLASTIN TIME. A test that checks the clotting factors of the intrinsic pathway.

PATELLA. The knee cap; the quadriceps tendon attaches to it above and the patellar tendon below.

PATELLECTOMY. Surgical removal of the patella, or kneecap removal.

PATENCY. The state of being open or unblocked.

PATENT DUCTUS ARTERIOSUS. A congenital defect in which the temporary blood vessel connecting the left pulmonary artery to the aorta in the fetus fails to close in the newborn.

PATERNITY. Refers to the father.

PATHOGEN. A disease-causing organism.

PATHOLOGIST. A doctor who specializes in the diagnosis of disease by studying cells and tissues under a microscope.

PATIENT SELF-DETERMINATION ACT (PSDA). Federal law that ensures that medical providers offer the option of medical directives to patients and include the documents in their medical records.

PATIENT-CONTROLLED ANALGESIA (PCA). An approach to pain management that allows the patient to control the timing of intravenous doses of analgesic drugs.

PEAK EXPIRATORY FLOW RATE. A test used to measure how fast air can be exhaled from the lungs.

PECTORALIS MINOR. A triangular-shaped muscle in front of (anterior) the axilla.

PECTUS CARINATUM. A chest wall deformity characterized by a protrusion of the sternum.

PECTUS EXCAVATUM. A chest wall deformity in which the chest wall takes on a sunken appearance.

PEDIATRIC AGED PATIENT. The pediatric aged patient encompasses several periods during development. The first four weeks after birth are callled the neonatal period. The first year after birth is called infancy, and childhood is from 13 months until puberty (between the ages of 12 and 15 years in girls and 13 and 16 years in boys).

PEDIATRICS. The medical specialty of caring for children.

PEDICLE FLAP. Also called an attached flap; a section of tissue, with its blood supply intact, which is maneuvered to another part of the body.

PELVIC. Located near the pelvis, the skeletal structure comprised of four bones that encloses the pelvic cavity.

PELVIC INFLAMMATORY DISEASE (PID). Inflammation of the female reproductive tract, caused by any of several microorganisms. Symptoms include severe abdominal pain, high fever, and vaginal discharge. Severe cases can result in sterility.

PELVIC ORGANS. The organs inside of the body that are located within the confines of the pelvis. This includes the bladder and rectum in both sexes, and the uterus, ovaries, and fallopian tubes in females.

PERCUSSION. An assessment method in which the surface of the body is struck with the fingertips to obtain sounds that can be heard or vibrations that can be felt. It can determine the position, size, and consistency of an internal organ. It is done over the chest to determine the presence of normal air content in the lungs, and over the abdomen to evaluate air in the loops of the intestine.

PERCUTANEOUS. Through the skin.

PERCUTANEOUS BIOPSY. A biopsy in which the needle is inserted and the sample removed through the skin.

PERCUTANEOUS TRANSLUMINAL CORONARY ANGIOPLASTY (PTCA). A cardiac intervention in which an artery blocked by plaque is dilated, using a balloon catheter to flatten the plaque and open the vessel; it is also called balloon angioplasty.

PERCUTANEOUS. Denoting the passage of substances through unbroken skin; also refers to passage through the skin by needle puncture, including introduction of wires and catheters by the Seldinger technique.

PERCUTANEOUS. Effected or performed through the skin.

PERCUTANEOUS. Performed through the skin. It is derived from two Latin words, *per* (through) and *cutis* (skin).

PERFORATION. The rupture or penetration by injury or infection of the lining of an organ or canal that allows infection to spread into a body cavity, as in peritonitis, the infection of the lining of the stomach or intestines.

PERFUSION SCAN. A lung scan in which a tracer is injected into a vein in the arm. It travels through the bloodstream and into the lungs to show areas of the lungs that are not receiving enough air or that retain too much air.

PERICARDIAL FRICTION RUB. A crackly, grating, low-pitched sound and is heard in both inspiration and expiration.

PERICARDIAL TAMPONADE. The collection of blood in the sac surrounding the heart that causes compression.

PERINEUM. The area between the opening of the vagina and the anus in a woman, or the area between the scrotum and the anus in a man.

PERIODONTITIS. Generalized disease of the gums in which unremoved calculus has separated the gingiva or gum tissue from the teeth and threatens support ligaments of the teeth and bone.

PERIPHERAL ARTERIAL DISEASE (PAD). An occlusive disease of the arteries most often caused by progressive atherosclerosis.

PERIPHERAL ARTERIES. Arteries other than those of the heart and brain, especially those that supply the lower body organs and limbs.

PERIPHERAL ENDARTERECTOMY. The surgical removal of fatty deposits, called plaque, from the walls of arteries other than those of the heart and brain.

PERIPHERAL NERVOUS SYSTEM (PNS). Nerves that are outside of the brain and spinal cord.

PERIPHERAL STEM CELL TRANSPLANT. The process of transplanting peripheral stem cells instead of using bone marrow. The stem cells in the circulating blood that are similar to those in the bone marrow are given to the patient after treatment to help the bone marrow recover and continue producing healthy blood cells. A peripheral stem cell transplant may also be used to supplement a bone marrow transplant.

PERIPHERAL STEM CELLS. Stem cells that are taken directly from the circulating blood and used for transplantation. Stem cells are more concentrated in the bone marrow, but they can also be extracted from the bloodstream.

PERIPHERAL VISION. The outer portion of the visual field.

PERISTALSIS. The wavelike contraction of the muscle fibers in the esophagus and other parts of the digestive tract that pushes food through the system.

PERITONEUM. The smooth membrane that lines the cavity of the abdomen, and surrounds the viscera, forming a closed sac.

PERITONITIS. Inflammation of the membrane lining the abdominal cavity. It causes abdominal pain and tenderness, constipation, vomiting, and fever.

PERIURETHRAL. Surrounding the urethra.

PERSONAL CARE ATTENDANT. An employee hired either through a healthcare facility, home care agency, or private agency to assist a patient in performing ADLs.

PERSONALITY DISORDER. Group of behavioral disorders characterized by maladaptive patterns of behavior, social interactions, or lifestyles that deviate from the healthy normal. Personality disorders are distinct from psychotic disorders.

PH. A measure of the acidity or alkalinity of a solution, relative to a standard solution. A neutral pH value is 7.0. An acidic pH value is below 7.0. An alkaline pH value is above 7.0.

PHACOEMULSIFICATION. A surgical procedure for removal of the crystalline lens in which a needle is inserted through a small incision on the side of the cornea of the eye, allowing the lens contents to fall through the dilated pupil into the anterior chamber where they are broken up by ultrasound and aspirated out of the eye through the incision.

PHACOLYTIC GLAUCOMA. Type of glaucoma causing dissolution of the lens.

PHAGOCYTOSIS. A process by which a white blood cell envelopes and digests debris and microorganisms to remove them from the blood.

PHARMACOLOGIC CARDIOVERSION. The use of medications to restore normal heart rhythm. It is also called chemical cardioversion.

PHARMACOLOGICAL. Referring to therapy that relies on drugs.

PHARMACOLOGIST. Medication specialist who checks patients' blood levels to monitor their response to immunosuppressive medications.

PHARYNX. The cavity at the back of the mouth. It is cone shaped and has an average length of about 3 in (76 mm) and is lined with mucous membrane. The pharynx opens into the esophagus at the lower end.

PHENOTYPE. A trait produced by a gene. For example, the specific HLA antigen(s) inherited for the HLA-A locus is the phenotype for that gene.

PHENYLKETONURIA. (PKU) A genetic disorder in which the body lacks an important enzyme. If untreated, the disorder can lead to brain damage and mental retardation.

PHEOCHROMOCYTOMA. A tumor of specialized cells of the adrenal gland.

PHILTAL DIMPLE. The skin or depression below the nose, extending to the upper lip in the midline.

PHILTRAL UNITS. Consists of several anatomical landmarks: the philtral dimple (the skin or depression below the nose extending to the upper lip in the midline); philtral columns (the skin columns on the right and left side of the philtral dimple); philtral tubercle (in the midline of the upper lip); white roll (a linear tissue prominence that joins the upper lip portion of the philtral dimple and vermilion—the dark pink tissue that makes up the lip); nasal columella (the outer portion of the nose that divides the nostrils).

PHIMOSIS. A tightening of the foreskin that may close the opening of the penis.

PHLEBECTOMY. Surgical removal of a vein or part of a vein.

PHLEBITIS. An inflammation of the walls of a vein.

PHLEBOLOGY. The study of veins, their disorders, and their treatments. A phlebologist is a doctor who specializes in treating spider veins, varicose veins, and associated disorders.

PHLEBOTOMIST. Health care professional trained to obtain samples of blood.

PHOBIA. An intense, abnormal, or illogical fear of something specific such as heights or open spaces.

PHOBIA. An irrational and unfounded fear of a situation, place, or object that causes a state of panic.

PHOTOCOAGULATION . Condensation of material by laser.

PHOTODYNAMIC THERAPY. A cancer treatment that uses a drug that is activated by exposure to light. When the drug is exposed to light, the cancer cells are killed.

PHOTON. A light particle.

PHYSICAL ACTIVITY. Any activity that involves moving the body and results in the burning of calories.

PHYSICAL FITNESS. The combination of muscle strength and cardiovascular health usually attributed to regular exercise and good nutrition.

PHYSIOLOGICAL STATE. The status of the normal vital life functions of a living organism.

PILES. Another name for hemorrhoids.

PILOCARPINE. Drug used to treat glaucoma.

PILONIDAL CYST. A special kind of abscess that occurs in the cleft between the buttocks. Forms frequently in adolescence after long trips that involve sitting.

PINNA. Another name for the auricle; the visible portion of the external ear.

PISTON. The plunger that slides up and down inside the barrel of a syringe.

PITUITARY GLAND. A small, oval-shaped endocrine gland situated at the base of the brain in the fossa (depression) of the sphenoid bone. Its overall role is to regulate growth and metabolism. The gland is divided into the posterior and anterior pituitary, each responsible for the production of its own unique hormones.

PITUITARY TUMORS. Tumors found in the pituitary gland. Most pituitary tumors are benign, meaning that they grow very slowly and do not spread to other parts of the body.

PLACENTA. The organ that develops along with the fetus to connect the fetus to the mother.

PLACENTA PREVIA. The placenta totally or partially covers the cervix, preventing vaginal delivery.

PLACENTAL ABRUPTION. Separation of the placenta from the uterine wall before the baby is born, cutting off blood flow to the baby.

PLANTAR FASCIITIS. An inflammation of the fascia on the bottom of the foot.

PLAQUE. An abnormal deposit on the wall of an artery. Plaque is made of cholesterol, triglyceride, dead cells, lipoproteins and calcium.

PLASMA. The liquid portion of blood, as distinguished from blood cells. Plasma constitutes about 55% of blood volume.

PLASMA CELLS. Cells in the blood and bone marrow that are formed from B lymphocytes, and that produce antibodies.

PLATELET. A disk-shaped structure found in blood that binds to fibrinogen at the site of a wound to begin the clotting process.

PLETHYSMOGRAPHY. A test in which a patient sits inside a booth called a plethysmograph and breathes through a mouthpiece, while pressure and air flow measurements are collected to measure the total lung volume.

PLEURAL CAVITY. The space between the lungs and the chest wall.

PLEURAL SPACE. The small space between the two layers of the membrane that covers the lungs and lines the inner surface of the chest.

PNEUMATIC RETINOPEXY. Reattachment of a detached retina using an injected gas bubble to hold the retina against the back of the eye.

PNEUMOCYSTIS CARINII PNEUMONIA (PCP). A lung infection that affects people with weakened immune systems, such as patients with AIDS or people taking medicines that weaken the immune system.

PNEUMONIA. A disease characterized by inflammation of the lungs. Pneumonia may be caused by bacteria, viruses, or other organisms, or by physical or chemical irritants.

PNEUMOTHORAX. A collection of air or gas in the chest cavity that causes a lung to collapse. Pneumothorax may be caused by an open chest wound that admits air.

PODIATRIST. A physician who specializes in the care and treatment of the foot.

PODIATRY. The surgical specialty that treats disorders of the foot.

POLAND SYNDROME. A condition associated with chest wall deformities in which varying degrees of underdevelopment of one side of the chest and arm may occur.

POLIOMYELITIS. Disorder caused by a viral infection (poliovirus) that can affect the whole body, including muscles and nerves.

POLYCYSTIC KIDNEY DISEASE. A hereditary kidney disease that causes fluid- or blood-filled pouches of tissue called cysts to form on the tubules of the kidneys. These cysts impair normal kidney function.

POLYCYTHEMIA VERA. A disease in which the bone marrow makes too many blood cells.

POLYCYTHEMIA. A condition in which the amount of RBCs are increased in the blood.

POLYDACTYLY. A developmental abnormality characterized by an extra digit on the hand or foot.

POLYGLYCOLIC ACID (PGA). A polyester compound used to make bioabsorbable sutures and staples. It is also used in tissue engineering.

POLYMYALGIA RHEUMATICA. A condition with symptoms of achiness and stiffness, primarily striking older adults.

POLYP. A small growth, usually not cancerous, but often precancerous when it appears in the colon.

POLYSOMNOGRAPHY. A test administered in a sleep laboratory to analyze heart rate, blood circulation, muscle movement, brain waves, and breathing patterns during sleep.

POLYSYNDACTYLY. Condition involving both webbing and the presence of an extra number of fingers or toes.

PORPHYRIAS. A group of disorders involving heme biosynthesis, characterized by excessive excretion of polyphrins. The porphyrias may be either inherited or acquired (usually from the effects of certain chemical agents).

PORPHYRIN. A dark red pigment, sensitive to light, that is found in chlorophyll as well as in a substance in hemoglobin known as heme.

PORTABILITY. A feature that allows employees to transfer health insurance coverage or other benefits from one employer to another when they change jobs.

PORTABLE CHEST X RAY. An x ray procedure taken by equipment that can be brought to the patient. The resulting radiographs may not be as high in quality as stationary x-ray radiographs, but allow a technologist to come to the patient.

PORTAL HYPERTENSION. A condition caused by cirrhosis of the liver. It is characterized by impaired or reversed blood flow from the portal vein to the liver, an enlarged spleen, and dilated veins in the esophagus and stomach.

PORTAL HYPERTENSION. Abnormally high pressure within the veins draining into the liver.

PORTAL VEIN. A large vein that carries blood from the stomach and intestines to the liver.

PORTAL VEIN THROMBOSIS. The development of a blood clot in the vein that brings blood into the liver. Untreated portal vein thrombosis causes portal hypertension.

POSITRON. One of the particles that make up an atom. A positron has the same mass and amount of charge as an electron, but the positron has a positive charge, the electron a negative one.

POSITRON EMISSION TOMOGRAPHY (PET) SCAN. A procedure to find malignant tumor cells in the body. A small amount of radionuclide glucose (sugar) is injected into a vein. The PET scanner rotates around the body and makes a picture of where the glucose is being used in the body. Malignant tumor cells show up brighter in the picture because they are more active and take up more glucose than normal cells.

POSTERIOR CAPSULE OPACIFICATION (PCO). This refers to the opacities that form on the back of the lens capsule after cataract removal or extraction. It is synonymous with a secondary cataract.

POSTERIOR CHAMBER. The posterior part of the eye bound by the lens in front and the retina in back. The posterior chamber is filled with a jellylike substance called the vitreous.

POSTOPERATIVE CARE. Medical care and support required after surgery to promote healing and recovery.

POSTPARTUM. After childbirth or after delivery.

POTASSIUM. A mineral found in whole grains, meat, legumes, and some fruits and vegetables. Potassium is important for many body processes, including proper functioning of nerves and muscles.

PREECLAMPSIA. A condition occurring in pregnancy in which high blood pressure leads to a number of complications, including a decreased ability of the kidneys to appropriately filter wastes from the blood.

PREFERRED PROVIDER ORGANIZATIONS (PPOS). Private health insurance plans that require beneficiaries to select their health care providers from a list approved by the insurance company.

PREGNANCY CATEGORY. A system of classifying drugs according to their established risks for use during pregnancy: category A: controlled human studies have demonstrated no fetal risk; category B: animal studies indicate no fetal risk, and there are no adequate and well-controlled studies in pregnant women; category C: no adequate human or animal studies, or adverse fetal effects in animal studies, but no available human data; category D: evidence of fetal risk, but benefits outweigh risks; category X: evidence of fetal risk, which outweigh any benefits.

PREMATURE. Happening early or occurring before the usual time.

PREMIUM. The amount paid by an insurance policyholder for insurance coverage. Most health insurance policy premiums are payable on a monthly basis.

PREOPERATIVE. Before surgery.

PREPUCE. A fold like the foreskin that covers the clitoris; another name for foreskin.

PRESBYOPIA. A condition affecting people over the age of 40 in which the focusing of near objects fails to work because of age-related hardening of the lens of the eye.

PRESSURE ULCER. Also known as a decubitus ulcer, pressure ulcers are open wounds that form whenever prolonged pressure is applied to skin covering bony outcrops of the body. Patients who are bedridden are at risk of developing pressure ulcers, commonly known as bedsores.

PREVALENCE. The number of cases of a disease or disorder that are present in a given population at a specific time.

PRIMARY CARE PHYSICIAN (PCP). A family practitioner, pediatrician, internist, or gynecologist who takes care of a patient's routine medical needs and refers him or her to a surgeon or other specialist when necessary.

PRIMARY SNORING. Simple snoring; snoring that is not interrupted by episodes of breathing cessation.

PRIMARY TEETH. A child's first set of teeth, sometimes called baby teeth.

PROCTOSIGMOIDOSCOPY. A visual examination of the rectum and sigmoid colon using a sigmoidoscope, also known as sigmoidoscopy.

PROGNOSIS. Expected resolution or outcome of an illness or injury.

PROLAPSE. The falling down or sinking of an internal organ or part of the body. Internal hemorrhoids may prolapse and cause a spasm of the anal sphincter muscle.

PROLAPSED CORD. The umbilical cord is pushed into the vagina ahead of the baby and becomes compressed, cutting off blood flow to the baby.

PROLAPSED UTERUS. A uterus that has slipped out of place, sometimes protruding down through the vagina.

PROLIFERATION. The rapid growth stage of a hemangioma.

PROLOTHERAPY. A technique for stimulating collagen growth in injured tissues by the injection of glycerin or dextrose.

PRONATION. The foot leans toward the inside of the foot, towards the center of the body.

PROPHYLACTIC. Intended to prevent or protect against disease.

PROPRIETARY HOSPITALS. Hospitals owned by private entities, mostly corporations, that are intended to make a profit as well as provide medical services. Most hospitals in health maintenance organizations and health networks are proprietary institutions.

PROSTAGLANDINS. A group of unsaturated fatty acids involved in the contraction of smooth muscle, control of body temperature, and other body functions.

PROSTATE GLAND. A gland in the male that surrounds the neck of the bladder and urethra. The prostate contributes to the seminal fluid.

PROSTATECTOMY. Prostate cancer surgery that includes partial or complete removal of the prostate.

PROSTATITIS. Inflammation of the prostate gland that may be accompanied by discomfort, pain, frequent urination, infrequent urination, and sometimes fever.

PROSTHESIS. A synthetic replacement for a missing part of the body such as a knee or a hip.

PROTEIN. A polypeptide chain, or a chain of amino acids linked together.

PROTHROMBIN. A protein in blood plasma that is converted to thrombin during the clotting process.

PROTHROMBIN TEST. A common test to measure the amount of time it takes for a patient's blood to clot; measurements are in seconds.

PROTOZOAN. A single-celled, usually microscopic organism that is eukaryotic and, therefore, different from bacteria (prokaryotic).

PROXY. A person authorized or empowered to act on behalf of another; also, the document or written authorization appointing that person.

PRUNE BELLY SYNDROME (PBS). A genetic disorder associated with abnormalities of human chromosomes 18 and 21. Male infants with PBS often have cryptorchidism along with other defects of the genitals and urinary tract. PBS is also known as triad syndrome and Eagle-Barrett syndrome.

PSEUDOANEURYSM. A dilation of a blood vessel that resembles an aneurysm.

PSEUDOPHAKIC BULLOUS KERATOPATHY (PBK). Painful swelling of the cornea occasionally occurring after surgery to implant an artificial lens in place of a lens affected by cataract.

PSORIASIS. A skin disease characterized by itchy, scaly, red patches on the skin.

PSYCHIATRIC NURSING. The nursing specialty concerned with the prevention and treatment of mental disorders and their consequences.

PSYCHIATRIST. A medical doctor (MD) who specializes in the treatment of mental health problems and can prescribe medication.

PSYCHOACTIVE. Affecting the mind or behavior.

PSYCHOLOGIST. A health care professional (PsyD or PhD) who is not a medical doctor but can evaluate or provide counseling for patients with mental health issues.

PSYLLIUM. The seeds of the fleawort plant, taken with water to produce a bland, jelly-like bulk which helps to move waste products through the digestive tract and prevent constipation.

PTOSIS. The medical term for drooping of the upper eyelid.

PUBIS. The front portion of the pelvis located in the anterior abdomen.

PUBOCERVICAL FASCIA. Fibrous tissue that separates the vagina and the bladder.

PUBOVAGINAL SLING. A general term for a procedure that places a sling around the urethra without the use of tension between the sling and the urethra. The is often referred to as the Tension-Free Vaginal Tape (TVT) procedure.

PULMONARY. Refers to the respiratory system, or breathing function and system.

PULMONARY ARTERY. The major artery that carries blood from the right ventricle of the heart to the lungs.

PULMONARY DISEASE. Any disease involving the lungs.

PULMONARY EMBOLISM. Potentially life-threatening blockage of a pulmonary artery by fat, air, or a blood clot that originated elsewhere in the body. Symptoms include acute shortness of breath and sudden chest pain.

PULMONARY EMBOLUS. A thrombus that typically detaches from a deep vein of a lower extremity.

PULMONARY FIBROSIS. Chronic inflammation and progressive formation of fibrous tissue in the pulmonary alveolar walls, with steadily progressive shortness of breath, resulting in death from lack of oxygen or heart failure.

PULMONARY FUNCTION TEST. A test that measures the capacity and function of the lungs as well as the blood's ability to carry oxygen. During the test, the patient breathes into a device called a spirometer.

PULMONARY HYPERPLASIA. Underdeveloped lungs.

PULMONARY HYPERTENSION. Abnormally high blood pressure within the pulmonary artery.

PULMONARY HYPOPLASIA. Underdeveloped lungs.

PULMONARY NODULE. A lesion surrounded by normal lung tissue. Nodules may be caused by bacteria, fungi, or a tumor (benign or cancerous).

PULMONARY REHABILITATION. A program that helps patients learn how to breathe easier and improve their quality of life. Pulmonary rehabilitation includes treatment, exercise training, education, and counseling.

PULMONARY VALVE. The heart valve connecting the left atrium and the pulmonary arteries.

PULMONARY VEIN ISOLATION. A surgical procedure used to treat atrial fibrillation. During the procedure, a radio frequency probe, microwave probe, or cryoprobe is inserted and, under direct vision, used to create lesion lines in the heart to interrupt the conduction of abnormal impulses.

PULMONOLOGIST. A physician who specializes in caring for people with lung diseases and breathing problems.

PULP. The soft innermost layer of a tooth, containing blood vessels and nerves.

PULP CHAMBER. The area within the natural crown of a tooth occupied by dental pulp.

PULPITIS. Inflammation of the pulp of a tooth involving the blood vessels and nerves.

PULSE OXIMETRY. A non-invasive test in which a device that clips onto the finger measures the oxygen level in the blood.

PULSUS PARADOXUS. A variation of the systolic pressure with respiration (diminished systolic pressure with inspiration and increased pressure with expiration).

PUNCH GRAFTING. A method of treating a deep scar involving excision of the damaged area, followed by the suturing in of similarly shaped punch of skin that is often taken from behind the ear.

PUPIL. The opening in the center of the iris of the eye that allows light to enter the eye.

PURSE-STRING CLOSURE. A technique used to close circular or irregularly shaped wounds that involves threading the suture through the edges of the wound and pulling it taut, bringing the edges together.

PURULENT. Containing, consisting of or forming pus.

PUS. A fluid that is the product of inflammation and infection containing white blood cells and debris of dead cells and tissue.

PYLORIC SPHINCTER. A broad band of muscle in the pylorus valve at the bottom end of the stomach.

PYLOROPLASTY. Widening of the pyloric canal and any adjacent duodenal structure by means of a longitudinal incision.

PYLORUS. The valve at the bottom end of the stomach that releases food from the stomach into the intestines.

PYREXIA. A temperature of 101°F (38.3°C) or higher in an infant younger than three months or above 102°F (38.9°C) for older children and adults.

Q

QRST COMPLEX. The combined waves of an electrocardiogram for monitoring the heart.

QUADRANTECTOMY. Removal of a quadrant, or about a quarter of the breast.

QUADRICEPS MUSCLES. A set of four muscles on each leg located at the front of the thigh. The quadriceps straighten the knee and are used every time a person takes a step.

QUINOLONES. A group of synthetic antibacterial drugs originally derived from quinine. Nalidixic acid is the first quinolone that was approved for clinical use.

R

RADIAL. Referring to the lower arm. The radial artery is an artery that runs from the elbow, through the wrist, and into the palm of the hand. Also, star-shaped or radiating out from a central point; used to describe the scar-folds that results from a purse-string closure.

RADIAL ARTERY. An artery present in the wrist that is convenient for drawing blood intended for laboratory testing.

RADIATION THERAPY. The use of high-energy radiation from x rays, cobalt, radium, and other sources to kill cancer cells and shrink tumors. Radiation may come from a machine outside the body (external beam radiation therapy) or from materials called radioisotopes. Radioisotopes produce radiation and are placed in or near the tumor or in the area near the cancer cells. This type of radiation treatment is called internal radiation therapy, implant radiation, interstitial radiation, or brachytherapy. Systemic radiation therapy uses a radioactive substance, such as a radio-labeled monoclonal antibody that circulates throughout the body.

RADIO WAVES. Electromagnetic energy of the frequency range corresponding to that used in radio communications, usually 10,000 cycles per second to 300 billion cycles per second. Radio waves are the same as visible light, x rays, and all other types of electromagnetic radiation, but are of a higher frequency.

RADIOFREQUENCY ABLATION. A procedure in which a catheter is guided to an area of heart where abnormal heart rhythms originate. The cells in that area are killed using a mild radiofrequency energy to restore normal heart contractions.

RADIOGRAPH. The actual picture or film produced by an X-ray study.

RADIOGRAPHICALLY DENSE. An abundance of glandular tissue that results in diminished anatomic detail on the mammogram.

RADIOIMAGING. The process of using a radioactively labeled compound to visualize specific types of body tissue.

RADIOIMMUNOASSAY. A method that uses a radioisotope label in an immunoassay.

RADIOLOGIC EXAMS. The use of radiation or other imaging methods to find signs of cancer.

RADIOLOGIST. A medical doctor specially trained in radiology (x ray) interpretation and its use in the diagnosis of diseases and injuries.

RADIOSURGERY. A method of delivering radiation directly to the tumor. This method does not involve surgery and causes little damage to healthy tissue.

RADIOTHERAPY. The treatment of disease with high-energy radiation, such as x rays or gamma rays.

RADIUS. One of the two forearm bones. The largest portion of the radius is at the wrist joint where it articulates with the carpal bones of the hand. Above, the radius articulates with the humerus at the elbow joint.

RANGE OF MOTION. The normal extent of movement (flexion and extension) of a joint.

RAYNAUD'S DISEASE. A disease found mainly in young women that causes decreased circulation to the hands and feet. Its cause is unknown.

REAL-TIME. A type of ultrasound that takes multiple images over time in order to record movement, or the observations obtained while scanning (rather than obtained by looking at films after the procedure).

RECEPTOR. A sensory nerve ending that responds to chemical or other stimuli of various kinds.

RECIPIENT. The person who receives the donated blood marrow.

RECTAL PROLAPSE. Sagging or bulging of the lining of the rectum into the rectum or actually through and out of the anal opening.

RECTOCELE. Sagging or bulging of the rectum through the back wall of the vagina.

RECTUM. The last part of the large intestine (colon) that connects to the anus.

RECTUS MUSCLES. The muscles responsible for movement of the eye.

RECURRENT LARYNGEAL NERVE. A nerve which lies very near the parathyroid glands and serves the larynx or voice box.

RECURRENT ULCER. Stomach ulcers that return after apparently complete healing. These ulcers appear to be caused by helicobacter pylori infections and can generally be successfully treated with a combination of antibiotics and gastric acid reducing compounds, particularly the proton pump inhibitors.

RED BLOOD CELLS. Cells that carry hemoglobin (the molecule that transports oxygen) and help remove wastes from tissues throughout the body.

RED CELL DISTRIBUTION WIDTH (RDW). A measure of the variation in the size of red blood cells.

REDUCTION. The correction of a hernia, fracture, or dislocation.

REFERRAL. The process of directing a patient to a specialist for further diagnostic evaluation or treatment.

REFLEX. An automatic response to a stimulus.

REFLUX. Backflow, also called regurgitation.

REGIONAL ANESTHESIA. Anesthesia that does not makes the patient unconscious; it works by blocking sensation in a region of the body.

REGISTERED NURSE. A graduate nurse who has passed a state nursing board examination and been registered and licensed to practice nursing.

REGULATORY ORGANIZATION. Organization designed to maintain or control quality in health care.

REJECTION. Occurs when the body tries to attack a transplanted organ as a foreign object and produces antibodies to destroy it. Anti-rejection (immunosuppressive) drugs help prevent rejection.

REMISSION. Disappearance of the signs and symptoms of cancer. When this happens, the disease is said to be "in remission." A remission can be temporary or permanent.

RENAL ARTERY ANEURYSM. An aneurysm relating to, involving, or located in the region of the kidneys.

RENAL CELL CARCINOMA. Cancer of the kidney.

REOPERATION. The repeat of a surgical procedure required for a variety of reasons, from surgical failure, replacement of failed component parts, or treatment of progressive disease.

REPERFUSION THERAPY. Restoration of blood flow to an organ or tissue; following a heart attack, quickly opening blocked arteries to reperfuse the heart muscles to minimize damage.

REPLANTATION. The medical term for the reattachment of an amputated digit.

RESECTABLE. Part or all of an organ that can be removed by surgery.

RESECTION. The complete or partial removal of an organ or tissue.

RESIDENCY TRAINING. A five-year period of additional training that follows completion of medical school.

RESIDUAL VOLUME. The volume of air remaining in the lungs, measured after a maximum expiration.

RESISTANT INFECTIONS. Infections that are not cured by standard antibiotic treatment.

RESISTANT ORGANISMS. Organisms that are difficult to eradicate with antibiotics.

RESORBED. Absorbed by the body because of lack of function. This happens to the jawbone after tooth loss.

RESPIRATION. The exchange of gases between red blood cells and the atmosphere.

RESPIRATORY ACIDOSIS. A condition in which abnormal exchange of oxygen and carbon dioxide in the lungs results in too much carbon dioxide being accumulated, and a resultant drop in the blood pH (towards acidity).

RESPIRATORY ALKALOSIS. A condition in which abnormal exchange of oxygen and carbon dioxide in the lungs results in the exhalation of too much carbon dioxide, and a resultant rise in the blood pH (towards alkalinity).

RESPIRATORY DEPRESSION. Decreased rate (number of breaths per minute) and depth (how much air is inhaled with each breath) of breathing.

RESPIRATORY DISTRESS SYNDROME (RDS). Difficulty breathing; found in infants with immature lungs.

RESPIRATORY FAILURE. The sudden inability of the lungs to provide normal oxygen delivery or normal carbon dioxide removal.

RESPIRATORY FUNCTION. The ability of the breathing structures of the body, including the lungs, to function.

RESPIRATORY INFECTIONS. Infections that relate to or affect respiration or breathing.

RESPIRATORY THERAPIST. A health care professional who specializes in assessing, treating, and educating people with lung diseases.

RESPIRATORY THERAPY. The department of any health care facility or agency that provides treatment to patients to maintain or improve their breathing function.

RESTENOSIS. The repeat narrowing of blood vessels that may occur after surgical removal of plaque when preventive measures are not taken.

RESTRAINT. A physical device or a medication designed to restrict a person's movement.

RESTRICTIVE. A type of bariatric surgery that works by limiting the amount of food that the stomach can hold. Vertical banded gastroplasty is a restrictive procedure.

RESUSCITATION. Reviving an unconscious person or restoring breathing.

RETINA. The light-sensing tissue within the eye that sends signals to the brain in order to generate a visual image.

RETINAL DETACHMENT. A serious vision disorder in which the light-detecting layer of cells inside the eye (retina) is separated from its normal support tissue and no longer functions properly.

RETINOBLASTOMA. Malignant (cancerous) tumor of the retina.

RETINOPATHY OF PREMATURITY (ROP). A disorder that occurs in premature infants in which blood vessels in the eye continue to grow in an abnormal pattern after delivery. It can lead to retinal detachment and blindness. ROP is also known as retrolental fibroplasia.

RETRACTOR. An instrument used during surgery to hold an incision open and pull back underlying layers of tissue.

RETROBULBAR HEMATOMA. A rare complication of blepharoplasty, in which a pocket of blood forms behind the eyeball.

RETROGRADE PYELOGRAPHY. A test in which dye is injected through a catheter placed with a cystoscope into the ureter to make the lining of the bladder, ureters, and kidneys easier to see on x rays.

RETROPUBIC URETHROPEXY. A generic term for the Burch procedure and its variants that treat mild stress incontinence by stabilizing the urethra with retropubic surgery.

REVASCULARIZATION. Restoring the body's blood flow after an interruption or blockage has disrupted normal circulation.

REYE'S SYNDROME. A life-threatening disease that affects the liver and the brain and sometimes occurs after a viral infection, such as flu or chickenpox. Children or teenagers who are given aspirin for flu or chickenpox are at increased risk of developing Reye's syndrome.

RH (RHESUS) FACTOR. An antigen present in the red blood cells of 85% of humans. A person with Rh factor is Rh positive (Rh+); a person without it is Rh negative (Rh-). The Rh factor was first identified in the blood of a rhesus monkey.

RH BLOOD TYPE. In general, refers to the blood type based on the presence or absence of the D antigen on the red blood cells. There are, however, other antigens in the Rh system.

RH NEGATIVE. Lacking the Rh factor, which are genetically determined antigens in red blood cells that produce immune responses. If an Rh-negative woman is pregnant with an Rh-positive fetus, her body will produce antibodies against the fetus's blood, causing a disease known as Rh disease. Sensitization to the disease occurs when the women's blood is exposed to the fetus's blood. Rh immune globulin (RhoGAM) is a vaccine that must be given to a woman after an abortion, miscarriage, or prenatal tests in order to prevent sensitization to Rh disease.

RHABDOMYOLYSIS. A condition causing the rapid breakdown of muscle tissue that may be caused by severe injuries or toxic chemicals. It causes the release of muscle tissue breakdown products into the blood in such excess that it may lead to acute renal failure.

RHEUMATIC CARDITIS. Inflammation of the heart muscle associated with acute rheumatic fever.

RHEUMATIC FEVER. An inflammatory disease that arises as a complication of untreated or inadequately treated strep throat infection. Rheumatic fever can seriously damage the heart valves.

RHEUMATOID ARTHRITIS. A condition in which the immune system damages and destroys the synovial lining of the joints. Red, warm, swollen, stiff joints are a common symptom. Over time, other organ systems may also be affected, including the heart, eyes, lungs, and kidneys.

RHINITIS. Inflammation of the membranes inside the nose.

RHINOPLASTY. Surgery performed to change the shape of the nose.

RHYTIDECTOMY. Wrinkle excision. It is an older, alternative term for a face lift.

RHYTIDES. Very fine wrinkles, often of the face.

RICKETTSIA (PLURAL, RICKETTSIAE). A microorganism belonging to a subtype of gram-negative bacteria that multiply only within the cells of a living host. Rickettsiae are usually transmitted to humans and other animals through the bites of ticks, fleas, and lice. They are named for Howard Ricketts (1871–1910), an American doctor.

ROCKY MOUNTAIN SPOTTED FEVER. An infectious disease that is caused by a rickettsia and spread by ticks. Its symptoms include high fever, muscle pain, and spots on the skin.

ROOT CANAL. The space within a tooth that runs from the pulp chamber to the tip of the root.

ROOT CANAL TREATMENT. The process of removing diseased or damaged pulp from a tooth, then filling and sealing the pulp chamber and root canals.

ROSACEA. A disease of the skin marked by constant flushing and acne-like lesions.

ROTABLATION. A nonsurgical technique for treating diseased arteries in which a special catheter with a diamond-coated tip is guided to the point of narrowing in the artery. The catheter tip spins at high speed and grinds away the blockage or plaque on the artery walls.

ROUTINE TEST. A medical test performed on all patients without regard to specific medical conditions.

RUPTURE. The bursting of a blood vessel or organ that has suffered enlargement, bulging, and weakening from unusual pressure.

S

SACRAL NERVE. The nerve in the lower back region of the spine that controls the need to urinate.

SALICYLATES. A group of drugs that includes aspirin and related compounds; used to relieve pain, reduce inflammation, and lower fever.

SALIVARY GLANDS. Three pairs of glands that secrete into the mouth and aid digestion.

SALPINGECTOMY. The surgical removal of a fallopian tube.

SANITIZE. To reduce the number of microorganisms to safe levels.

SAPHENOUS VEIN. A long vein in the thigh or calf commonly used for bypass grafts.

SARCOIDOSIS. A chronic disease with unknown cause that involves formation of nodules in bones, skin, lymph nodes, and lungs.

SARCOMA. A form of cancer that arises in the supportive tissues such as bone, cartilage, fat, or muscle.

SCALING AND ROOT PLANING. A dental procedure to treat gingivitis in which the teeth are scraped inside the gum area and the root of the tooth is planed to dislodge bacterial deposits.

SCAPULA. A large, flat, triangular bone that forms the back portion of the shoulder. It articulates with the clavicle (at the acromion process) and the humerus (at the glenoid). Also called the shoulder blade.

SCAR TISSUE. Scar tissue is the fibrous tissue that replaces normal tissue destroyed by injury or disease.

SCHLEMM'S CANAL. A circular channel located at the point where the sclera of the eye meets the cornea. Schlemm's canal is the primary pathway for aqueous humor to leave the eye.

SCIATICA. Pain in the lower back, buttock, or leg along the course of the sciatic nerve.

SCLERA. The tough, fibrous, white outer protective covering of the eyeball.

SCLEROSANT. An irritating solution that stops bleeding by hardening the blood or vein it is injected into.

SCLEROSE. To harden or undergo hardening. Sclerosing agents are chemicals that are used in sclerotherapy to cause swollen veins to fill with fibrous tissue and close down.

SCLEROTHERAPY. A technique for shrinking hemorrhoids by injecting an irritating chemical into the blood vessels.

SCROTUM. The external pouch containing the male reproductive glands (testes) and part of the spermatic cord.

SEDATION. A condition of calm or relaxation, brought about by the use of a drug or medication.

SEDATIVE. A type of medication given to calm or relax patients before surgery.

SEDENTARY. Characterized by inactivity and lack of exercise. A sedentary lifestyle is a risk factor for high blood cholesterol levels.

SEIZURES. Attacks consisting of sudden and abnormal muscle, sensory, or psychic events resulting from transient dysfunction of the brain.

SENSORINEURAL DEAFNESS. Hearing loss due to the inability to convert sound from vibration to electrical signals. Often involves defects in the function of cochlear hair cells.

SENTINEL LYMPH NODE. The lymph node(s) closest to a cancerous tumor. They are the first nodes that receive lymphatic drainage from the tissues surrounding the tumor.

SEPARATION ANXIETY. A fear of being separated from a parent or loved one; a normal developmental process, occurring at certain points in a young child's life.

SEPSIS. A dangerous physiological state of extensive, systemic bacterial infection.

SEPTAL DEFECTS. Openings in the septum, the muscular wall separating the right and left sides of the heart. Atrial septal defects are openings between the two upper heart chambers and ventricular septal defects are openings between the two lower heart chambers.

SEPTAL MUCOSA. The epithelium in the nasal mucosa.

SEPTIC ARTHRITIS. A pus-forming bacterial infection of a joint.

SEPTICEMIA. Systemic disease associated with the presence and persistence of pathogenic microorganisms or their toxins in the blood.

SEPTUM (PLURAL, SEPTA). The dividing partition in the nose that separates the two nostrils. It is composed of bone and cartilage. Also, an extra fold of tissue down the center of the uterus; this tissue can be removed with a wire electrode and a hysteroscope. Also, the muscular wall that separates the two sides of the heart; an opening in the septum that allows blood to flow from one side to the other is called a septal defect.

SEQUELA (PLURAL, SEQUELAE). An abnormal condition or event resulting from a previous disease or disorder.

SEQUESTRATION. A process in which the spleen withdraws blood cells from the circulation and stores them.

SERIAL X RAYS. A number of x rays performed at set times in the disease progression or treatment intervals. The radiographs will be compared to one another to track changes.

SEROMA. A collection of blood serum or lymphatic fluid in body tissues. It is an occasional complication of vascular surgery.

SERUM (PLURAL, SERA). The clear fluid that separates from blood when the blood is allowed to clot completely. Blood serum can also be defined as blood plasma from which fibrinogen has been removed.

SERUM ALBUMIN. A crystallizable albumin or mixture of albumins that normally constitutes more than half of the protein in blood serum and serves to maintain the osmotic pressure of the blood.

SESTAMIBI. A type of radioimaging pharmaceutical compound that has been deemed medically safe to use in the human body for sestamibi scans.

SETBACK OTOPLASTY. A surgical procedure done to reduce the size or improve the appearance of large or protruding ears; it is also known as pinback otoplasty.

SETON TUBE. An implant placed in the eye that provides an alternative route for aqueous fluid drainage.

SEXUALLY TRANSMITTED DISEASE (STD). A disease that is passed from one person to another through sexual intercourse or other intimate sexual contact.

SHARPS. A general term for needles, lancets, scalpel blades, and other medical devices with points or sharp edges requiring special disposal precautions.

SHINGLES. A disease caused the Herpes zoster virus—the same virus that causes chickenpox. Symptoms of shingles include pain and blisters along one nerve, usually on the face, chest, stomach, or back.

SHOCK. A serious condition in which the body's blood circulation and metabolism is severely impaired by injury, pain, blood loss, or certain diseases. The symptoms of shock include a pale complexion, very low blood pressure, and a weak pulse.

SHORT BOWEL SYNDROME. A condition in which digestion and absorption in the small intestine are impaired.

SHOULDER RESECTION ARTHROPLASTY. Surgery performed to repair a shoulder acromioclavicular (AC) joint. The procedure is most commonly recommended for AC joint problems resulting from osteoarthritis or injury.

SHUNT. A channel through which blood or another body fluid is diverted from its normal path by surgical reconstruction or the insertion of a synthetic tube.

SICKLE CELL DISEASE. Also called sickle cell anemia. An inherited disorder characterized by a genetic flaw in hemoglobin production. (Hemoglobin is the substance within red blood cells that enables them to transport oxygen.) The hemoglobin that is produced has a kink in its structure that forces the red blood cells to take on a sickle shape, inhibiting their circulation and causing pain. This disorder primarily affects people of African descent.

SIGMOID COLON. The last third of the intestinal tract that is attached to the rectum.

SIGMOID SINUS. An S-shaped cavity on the inner side of the skull behind the mastoid process.

SIGMOIDOSCOPY. Endoscopic examination of the lower colon.

SILICOSIS. A progressive disease that results in impairment of lung function and is caused by inhalation of dust containing silica.

SIMPLE OBSTRUCTION. A blockage in the intestine that does not affect the flow of blood to the area.

SIMULATION SCAN. The process of making a mask for the patient and other images in order to plan the radiation treatment.

SINOATRIAL NODE. Specialized tissue in he right atrium that initiates electrical activity in the heart

SINUS. A cavity in a bone of the skull that usually communicates with the nostrils and contains air.

SINUSITIS. Inflammation of the sinuses.

SITZ BATH. A shallow tub or bowl, sometimes mounted above a toilet, that allows the perineum and buttocks to be immersed in circulating water.

SJÖGREN'S SYNDROME. A disease in which the immune system damages and destroys exocrine glands, such as those that produce tears and saliva. Dry eyes and mouth are the usual initial symptoms of this disorder, but other organ systems can also be severely affected over time, including the skin, pancreas, liver, lungs, brain, and kidneys.

SKELETAL TRACTION. Traction in which pins, screws, or wires are surgically connected to bone to which weights or pulleys are attached to exert force.

SKILLED NURSING FACILITY (SNF). A facility equipped to handle individuals with 24-hour nursing needs, postoperative recuperation, or complex medical care demands, as well as chronically-ill individuals who can no longer live independently. These facilities must be licensed by the state in which they operate to meet standards of safety, staffing, and care procedures. Another name for a nursing home.

SKIN FLAP. A piece of skin with underlying tissue that is used in grafting to cover a defect and that receives its blood supply from a source other than the tissue on which it is laid.

SKIN TRACTION. Traction in which weights or other devices are attached to the skin.

SLEEP APNEA SYNDROME. A disorder in which the patient's breathing temporarily stops at intervals during the night due to obstruction of the upper airway. People with sleep apnea syndrome do not get enough oxygen in their blood and often develop heart problems.

SLIDING GENIOPLASTY. A complex plastic surgery procedure in which the patient's jawbone is cut, moved forward or backward, and repositioned with metal plates and screws.

SMALL INTESTINE. The small intestine consists of three sections: duodenum, jejunum and ileum, all of which are involved in the absorption of nutrients. The total length of the small intestine is approximately 22 ft (6.5 m).

SMOKING CESSATION. The act of quitting smoking or withdrawal from nicotine.

SOCIAL WORKER. A health care provider who can provide support to patients and families, including assistance with a patient's psychosocial adjustment needs and referrals for community support.

SOFT TISSUE. Layers of cells that form the skin.

SOMATIZATION DISORDER. A chronic condition in which psychological stresses are converted into physical symptoms that interfere with work and relationships. Lower back pain is a frequent complaint of patients with somatization disorder.

SOMNOPLASTY. A technique that uses radiofrequency signals to heat a thin needle inserted into the tissues of the soft palate. The heat from the needle shrinks the tissues, thus enlarging the patient's airway. Somnoplasty is also known as radiofrequency volumetric tissue reduction (RFVTR).

SONOGRAM. Image, or picture, obtained when using a machine called an ultrasound to look inside the uterus when the mother is pregnant. It is a painless procedure that sends out sound waves to the baby, and as the sound waves bounce off the object—the baby—an image is created on a monitor.

SONOGRAPHER. A technologist or physician who uses an ultrasound unit to takes ultrasound images of patients.

SORBENT. A material used during hemoperfusion to adsorb toxic or waste substances from the blood. Most hemoperfusion systems use resin or activated carbon as sorbents.

SPASM. Sudden, involuntary tensing of a muscle or a group of muscles.

SPECIFIC GRAVITY. The ratio of the weight of a body fluid when compared with water.

SPECULUM. A retractor used to separate the walls of the vagina and aid in visual examination.

SPEECH-LANGUAGE PATHOLOGY. Formerly known as speech therapy, it includes the study and treatment of human communication—its development and disorders.

SPERM GRANULOMA. A collection of fluid that leaks from an improperly sealed or tied vas deferens. The fluid usually disappears on its own, but can be drained, if necessary.

SPERMATIC CORD. A tube-like structure that extends from the testicle to the groin area. It contains blood vessels, nerves, and a duct to carry spermatic fluid.

SPHENOIDAL ELECTRODES. Fine wire electrodes that are implanted under the cheek bones, used to measure temporal seizures.

SPHINCTER. A circular band of muscle fibers that constricts or closes a passageway in the body. The esophagus has sphincters at its upper and lower ends.

SPHINCTER DEFICIENCY. A term related both to urinary and fecal incontinence in which the inability of the sphincter to keep the reservoir closed is a source of severe incontinence.

SPIDER NEVUS (PLURAL, NEVI). A reddish lesion that consists of a central arteriole with smaller branches radiating outward from it. Spider nevi are also called spider angiomas; they are most common in small children and pregnant women.

SPIDER VEINS. Telangiectasias that appear on the surface of the legs, characterized by a reddish central point with smaller veins branching out from it like the legs of a spider.

SPINA BIFIDA. A congenital defect in the spinal column, characterized by the absence of the vertebral arches through which the spinal membranes and spinal cord may protrude.

SPINAL ANESTHESIA. Involves inserting a needle into a region between the vertebrae of the lower back and injecting numbing medications.

SPINAL CANAL. The cavity or hollow space within the spine that contains the spinal cord and the cerebrospinal fluid.

SPINAL FUSION. An operation in which the bones of the spine are permanently joined together using a bone graft obtained usually from the hip.

SPINAL STENOSIS. Narrowing of the canals in the vertebrae or around the nerve roots, causing pressure on the spinal cord and nerves.

SPIRAL CT. Also referred to as helical CT, this method allows for continuous 360-degree X-ray image capture.

SPIROCHETE. A spiral-shaped bacterium. Spirochetes cause such diseases as syphilis and Lyme disease.

SPLEEN. An organ that traps and breaks down red blood cells at the end of their useful life and manufactures some key substances used by the immune system.

SPLENOMEGALY. Enlargement of the spleen.

SPLINT. A thin piece of rigid material that is sometimes used during nasal surgery to hold certain structures in place until healing is underway.

SPONGES. Pieces of absorbent material, usually cotton gauze, used to absorb fluids, protect tissue, or apply pressure and traction.

SPURS. A sharp horny outgrowth of the skin.

SPUTUM. A mucus-rich secretion that is coughed up from the passageways (bronchial tubes) and the lungs.

SPUTUM CYTOLOGY. A lab test in which a microscope is used to check for cancer cells in the sputum.

SQUAMOUS CELL CANCER. A form of skin cancer that usually originates in sun-damaged areas or pre-existing lesions; at first local and superficial, it may later spread to other areas of the body.

SQUAMOUS CELLS. Scaly or plate-like cells.

STABILIZER. A device used to depress the movement of the area around the coronary artery where the anastomosis is made. The stabilizer is used to provide a still, motionless field for suturing.

STAGHORN CALCULUS. A kidney stone that develops a branched shape resembling the antlers of a stag. Staghorn calculi are composed of struvite.

STAGING. The classification of cancers according to the extent of the tumor.

STAHL'S DEFORMITY. A congenital deformity of the ear characterized by a flattened rim and pointed upper edge caused by a fold in the cartilage; it is also known as Vulcan ear or Spock ear.

STAPEDOTOMY. A procedure in which a small hole is cut in the footplate of the stapes.

STAPH INFECTION. Infection with *Staphylococcus* bacteria. These bacteria can infect any part of the body.

STAPHYLOCOCCAL INFECTION. An infection caused by any of several pathogenic species of *Staphylococcus*, commonly characterized by the formation of abscesses in the skin or other organs.

STEATORRHEA. An excess of fat in the stool.

STEM CELLS. Unspecialized cells, or "immature" blood cells, that serve as the precursors of white blood cells, red blood cells, and platelets.

STENOSIS (PLURAL, STENOSES). The narrowing or constriction of an opening or passageway in the body.

STENT. A tube made of metal or plastic that is inserted into a vessel or passage to keep it open and prevent closure.

STEREOTACTIC. Characterized by precise positioning in space. When applied to radiosurgery, stereotactic refers to a system of three-dimensional coordinates for locating the target site.

STERILE. Free from living microorganisms.

STERILIZATION. To make sterile, meaning to deprive of the power of reproducing.

STERNOTOMY. A surgical opening into the thoracic cavity through the sternum (breastbone).

STERNOXIPHOID JUNCTION. The lower junction of the sternum or breastbone.

STERNUM. The breastbone. It connects to ribs one through seven on either side of the chest.

STEROIDS. A component of commonly used immunosuppressive drugs that have negative effects on insulin production.

STETHOSCOPE. A rubber Y-shaped device used to listen to sounds produced by the human body.

STEVENS-JOHNSON SYNDROME. A severe inflammatory reaction that is sometimes triggered by sulfa medications. It is characterized by blisters and eroded areas in the mouth, nose, eyes, and anus; it may also involve the lungs, heart, and digestive tract. Stevens-Johnson syndrome is also known as erythema multiforme.

STIMULANT. A drug or other substance that increases the rate of activity of a body system.

STIMULUS. A factor capable of eliciting a response in a nerve.

STOCKINETTE. A soft elastic material used for bandages and clothing for infants.

STOMA (PLURAL, STOMATA). A surgically created opening in the abdominal wall to allow digestive wastes to pass to the outside of the body.

STOOL. The solid waste that is left after food is digested. Stool forms in the intestines and passes out of the body through the anus.

STRABISMUS. A condition in which the muscles of the eye do not work together, often causing double vision.

STRANGULATED HERNIA. A twisted piece of herniated intestine that can block blood flow to the intestines.

STRANGULATION. A condition in which a vessel, section of the intestine, or other body part is compressed or constricted to the point that blood cannot circulate.

STREP THROAT. A sore throat caused by infection with *Streptococcus* bacteria. Symptoms include sore throat, chills, fever, and swollen lymph nodes in the neck.

STREPTOCOCCAL INFECTION. An infection caused by a pathogenic bacterium of one of several species of the genus *Streptococcus* or their toxins. Almost any organ in the body may be involved.

STRESS INCONTINENCE. Involuntary loss of urine that occurs during physical activity such as coughing, sneezing, laughing, or exercise.

STRESS TEST. A test used to determine how the heart responds to stress. It usually involves walking on a treadmill or riding a stationary bike at increasing levels of difficulty, while the electrocardiogram, heart rate and blood pressure are monitored. If the patient is unable to walk on a treadmill or ride a stationary bike, medications may be used to produce similar results.

STRESS ULCERS. Stomach ulcers that occur in connection with some types of physical injury, including burns and invasive surgical procedures.

STRICTURE. An abnormal narrowing of a body canal or opening. A stricture may also be called a stenosis.

STROKE. An event causing impairment of blood circulation to the brain, causing death of brain tissue and potentially drastically affecting mental functioning.

STROMA . The thickest part of the cornea between Bowman's membrane and Decemet's membrane.

STRUVITE. A crystalline form of magnesium ammonium phosphate. Kidney stones made of struvite form in urine with a pH above 7.2.

SUB-FERTILITY. A decreased ability to become pregnant.

SUBARACHNOID HEMORRHAGE. Bleeding from a ruptured blood vessel in the brain that contaminates the cerebrospinal fluid.

SUBARACHNOID SPACE. A space between membranes that covers and protects the brain.

SUBCAPSULAR. Inside the outer tissue covering of the testicle. A subcapsular orchiectomy is a procedure in which the surgeon removes the inner glandular tissue of the testicle while leaving the outer capsule intact.

SUBCUTANEOUS. Beneath the skin.

SUBCUTANEOUS EMPHYSEMA. A pathologic accumulation of air underneath the skin resulting from improper insufflation technique.

SUBDURAL ELECTRODES. Strip electrodes that are placed under dura mater (the outermost, toughest, and most fibrous of the three membranes [meninges] covering the brain and spinal cord). They are used to locate foci of epileptic seizures prior to epilepsy surgery.

SUBGLOTTIC STENOSIS. An abnormal narrowing of the trachea below the level of the vocal cords.

SUBLINGUAL. Under the tongue.

SUBMENTAL. Underneath the chin.

SUBSTRATE. A substance acted upon by an enzyme.

SUPERIOR VENA CAVA. Large vein that returns blood to the heart from the head, neck, and upper limbs.

SUPINE. Lying horizontally on one's back.

SUPPLEMENTAL SECURITY INCOME (SSI). A federal entitlement program that provides cash assistance to low-income blind, disabled, and elderly people. In most states, people receiving SSI benefits are eligible for Medicaid.

SUPRAVENTRICULAR TACHYCARDIA (SVT). A fast heartbeat that originates above the ventricles.

SURFACTANT. A compound made of fats and proteins that is found in a thin film along the walls of the air sacs of the lungs. Surfactant keeps the surface pressure low so that the sacs can inflate easily and not collapse.

SURGEON. A physician that has completed surgical residency training, passed all examinations and is a Fellow of the American College of Surgeons.

SURGICAL ALTERNATIVES. Surgical options within a range of surgical procedures used to treat a specific condition.

SURGICAL REVISION. The failure of a procedure, which requires surgery be performed to improve the result.

SURGICENTER. Another term for ambulatory surgical center.

SURROGATE. A person who represents the wishes of the patient, chosen by the patient and stipulated by a legal document as power of attorney.

SUTURES. Stiches that are used in surgical procedures to bring two pieces of flesh together or close a wound.

SWAGED NEEDLE. An eyeless surgical needle with the suture material preattached by the manufacturer. Most surgical needles used in the early 2000s are swaged needles.

SWAN-GANZ CATHETER. Also called a pulmonary artery catheter. This type of catheter is inserted into a large vessel in the neck or chest and is used to measure the amount of fluid in the heart and to determine how well the heart is functioning.

SYMPATHETIC NERVOUS SYSTEM. The part of the autonomic nervous system that is concerned with preparing the body to react to situations of stress or emergency; it contains chiefly adrenergic fibers and tends to depress secretion, decrease the tone and contractility of smooth muscle, and increase heart rate.

SYMPATHOMIMETIC DRUGS. Another name for adrenergic drugs.

SYNCHRONIZED ELECTRICAL CARDIOVERSION. The term used to describe cardioversion by the application of a controlled electric shock to the patient's chest.

SYNCOPE. A fainting episode.

SYNDACTYLY. A developmental abnormality in which two or more fingers or toes are joined by webbing between the digits.

SYNDROME. A set of signs or a series of events occurring together that often point to a single disease or condition as the cause.

SYNERGISTIC. Enhancing the effects of another drug. Anesthetics given in combination are often synergistic.

SYNGENEIC. Referring to a bone marrow transplant from one identical twin to the other.

SYNOVIAL FLUID. A fluid that lubricates the joint and helps prevent wear on the bones.

SYNOVITIS. Inflammation of the synovium, the thin membrane lining the joint.

SYSTEMIC CIRCULATION. Circulation supplied by the aorta including all tissue and organ beds, except the alveolar sacs of the lungs used for gas exchange and respiration.

SYSTEMS ANALYSIS. An approach to medical errors and other management issues that looks for problems in the work process rather than singling out individuals as bad or incompetent.

SYSTOLE. Period while the heart is contracting.

SYSTOLIC. Maximum arterial blood pressure during ventricular contraction.

T

T CELLS. Any of several lymphocytes that have specific antigen receptors, and are involved in cell-mediated immunity and the destruction of antigen-bearing cells.

TACHYCARDIA. Rapid heart beat, generally over 100 beats per minute.

TACTILE FREMITUS. A tremor or vibration in any part of the body detected by palpation (palpation is when the clinician gently feels or presses with hands).

TARDIVE DYSKINESIA. A disorder brought on by certain medications that is characterized by uncontrollable muscle spasms.

TAY-SACHS DISEASE. An inherited disease prevalent among the Ashkenazi Jewish population of the United States. Infants with the disease are unable to process a certain type of fat that accumulates in nerve and brain cells, causing mental and physical retardation, and death by age four.

TEACHING HOSPITALS. Hospitals whose primary mission is training medical personnel in collaboration with (or ownership by) a medical school or research center.

TELANGIECTASIA. The medical term for the visible discolorations produced by permanently swollen capillaries and smaller veins.

TEMPLATING. A term that refers to the surgeon's use of x-ray images of an old prosthesis as a template or pattern guide for a new implant.

TEMPORAL ARTERITIS. A condition in which inflammation of the blood vessels that supply the head and neck result in severe, chronic headache, particularly over one temple, as well as fever, weight loss, and severe fatigue.

TEMPORAL LOBE EPILEPSY (TLE). The most common type of epilepsy, with elaborate and multiple sensory, motor, and psychic symptoms. A common feature is the loss of consciousness and amnesia during seizures. Other manifestations may include more complex behaviors like bursts of anger, emotional outbursts, fear, or automatisms.

TENACULUM (PLURAL, TENACULA). A small, sharp-pointed hook set in a handle, used to seize or pick up pieces of tissue during surgical operations.

TENDINITIS. Inflammation of a tendon—a tough band of tissue that connects muscle to bone.

TENDON. A fibrous cord of strong connective tissue that connects muscle to bone.

TESTICLES. The two egg-shaped organs found in the scrotum that produce sperm.

TESTICULAR TORSION. Twisting of the testicle around the spermatic cord, cutting off the blood supply to the testicle. It is considered a urologic emergency.

TESTIS (PLURAL, TESTES). The medical term for a testicle.

TESTOSTERONE. The major male sex hormone, produced in the testes.

TETANUS. A potentially deadly disease produced by a bacterium that may infect crush injuries or penetrating wounds.

TETANY. Inappropriately sustained muscle spasms.

TETRALOGY OF FALLOT. A cyanotic defect in which the blood pumped through the body has too little oxygen. Tetralogy of Fallot includes four defects: a ventricular septal defect, narrowing at or beneath the pulmonary valve, infundibular pulmonary stenosis (obstruction of blood flow out of the right ventricle through the pulmonary valve), and overriding aorta (the aorta crosses the ventricular septal defect into the right ventricle).

THALASSEMIA. A group of inherited disorders that affects hemoglobin production. Because hemoglobin production is impaired, a person with this disorder may suffer mild to severe anemia. Certain types of thalassemia can be fatal.

THORACENTESIS. Removal of fluid from the pleural cavity.

THORACIC. Pertaining to the chest cavity, including the lungs and the area around the lungs.

THORACIC AORTIC ANEURYSM. Occurs when an area in the thoracic section of the aorta (the chest) is weakened and bulges like a balloon. The thoracic section supplies blood to the upper body.

THORACIC VERTEBRAE. The vertebrae in the chest region to which the ribs attach.

THORACOTOMY. A surgical opening into the thoracic cavity.

THORASCOPY. Examination of the chest through a tiny incision using a thin, lighted tube-like instrument (thorascope).

THORAX. The chest area, which runs between the abdomen and neck and is encased in the ribs.

THROMBIN. An enzyme in blood plasma that helps to convert fibrinogen to fibrin during the last stage of the clotting process.

THROMBIN INHIBITOR. One type of anticoagulant medication used to help prevent formation of harmful blood clots in the body by blocking the activity of thrombin.

THROMBOCYTOPENIA. A disorder characterized by a drop in the number of platelets in the blood.

THROMBOCYTOSIS. A vascular condition characterized by high blood platelet counts.

THROMBOEMBOLISM. A blood clot that originates in one area of the body, but travels through the venous system to another area, where it obstructs blood flow. This is particularly problematic when the thromboembolus lodges in the lung.

THROMBOLYSIS. A treatment that opens up blood flow and may prevent permanent damage to the blood vessels.

THROMBOPHLEBITIS. A condition in which blood clots form in veins near surgery site, causing swelling and pain; clots may travel via veins to the heart or lungs causing serious complications.

THROMBOPLASTIN. A protein in blood that converts prothrombin to thrombin.

THROMBOSED. Affected by the formation of a blood clot, or thrombus, along the wall of a blood vessel. Some external hemorrhoids become thrombosed.

THROMBOSIS. The formation or presence of a blood clot within a blood vessel.

THROMBUS. A blood clot that is blocking a blood vessel.

THYMUS. An unpaired organ in the mediastinal cavity that is important in the body's immune response.

THYROID CARTILAGE. The largest cartilage in the human larynx, or voice box. It is sometimes called the Adam's apple.

THYROID DYSFUNCTION. A physical state that involves the failure of the thyroid gland to function properly. Thyroid dysfunction not only affects a person's physical state, but may have secondary effects on their mental state as well.

THYROID GLAND. An endocrine organ in the neck which produces thyroid hormone. Thyroid hormone is involved in important growth and metabolic processes throughout the body.

THYROID STORM. An unusual complication of thyroid function that is sometimes triggered by the stress of thyroid surgery. It is a medical emergency.

TIBIA. The larger of two leg bones that lie beneath the knee. The tibia is sometimes called the shin bone.

TINNITUS. A sensation of noise in the ears, usually a buzzing, ringing, clicking, or roaring sound.

TOCOLYTICS. Drugs administered to stop or delay the onset of labor.

TOLERANCE. A decrease in sensitivity to a drug. When tolerance occurs, a person must take more of the drug to get the same effect.

TONOMETRY. Measurement of the fluid pressure inside the eye.

TONSILLECTOMY. Surgical removal of the tonsils.

TONSILLITIS. Inflammation of a tonsil, a small mass of tissue in the throat.

TONSILS. Oval masses of lymphoid tissue on each side of the throat.

TOPICAL. Applied to the skin surface.

TOTAL LUNG CAPACITY TEST. A test that measures the amount of air in the lungs after a person has breathed in as much as possible.

TOURNIQUET. Any device that is used to compress a blood vessel to stop bleeding or as part of collecting a blood sample. Phlebotomists usually use an elastic band as a tourniquet.

TRABECULAR MESHWORK. Area of fibrous tissue that forms a canal between the iris and cornea, through which aqueous humor flows.

TRABECULOPLASTY. Laser surgery that creates perforations in the trabeculum, to drain built-up aqueous humor and relieve pressure.

TRACHEA. The windpipe; a tough, fibrocartilaginous tube passing from the larynx to the bronchi before the lungs.

TRACHEOBRONCHIAL. Pertaining both to the tracheal and bronchial tubes or to their junction.

TRACHEOSTOMY TUBE. A breathing tube inserted in the neck, used when assisted breathing is needed for a long period of time.

TRACHEOTOMY. The surgical creation of an opening into the windpipe through the neck; it is also called a tracheostomy.

TRANQUILIZER. Medicine that has a calming effect and is used to treat anxiety and mental tension.

TRANSCONJUCTIVAL BLEPHAROPLASTY. A type of blepharoplasty in which the surgeon makes no incision on the surface of the eyelid, but, instead, enters from behind to tease out the fat deposits.

TRANSDUCER. The handheld part of the ultrasound unit that produces the ultrasound waves and receives the ultrasound echos.

TRANSESOPHAGEAL ECHOCARDIOGRAM (TEE). An invasive imaging procedure used to create a picture of the heart's movement, valves, and chambers. The test uses high-frequency sound waves that come from a small transducer passed down the patient's throat. TEE may be used in combination with Doppler ultrasound to evaluate the blood flow across the heart's valves.

TRANSFUSION. The therapeutic introduction of blood or a blood component into a patient's bloodstream.

TRANSILLUMINATION. A technique in which the doctor shines a strong light through body tissues in order to examine an organ or structure.

TRANSPLANTATION. Surgically cutting out hair follicles and replanting them in a different spot on the head.

TRANSPOSITION OF THE GREAT VESSELS. A cyanotic defect in which the blood pumped through the body has too little oxygen because the pulmonary artery receives its blood incorrectly from the left ventricle and the aorta incorrectly receives blood flow from the right ventricle.

TRANSSEXUAL. Person desiring to acquire the external appearance of a member of the opposite gender.

TRANSTRACHEAL JET VENTILATION (TTJV). A technique for ventilating a patient that involves passing oxygen under pressure through a catheter that has been passed through the patient's cricothyroid membrane.

TRANSURETHRAL SURGERY. Surgery in which no external incision is needed. For prostate transurethral surgery, the surgeon reaches the prostate by inserting an instrument through the urethra.

TRANSVERSE PRESENTATION. The baby is laying sideways across the cervix instead of head first.

TRAUMA CENTERS. Specialized hospital facilities that are equipped to deal with emergency life-threatening conditions.

TRAUMA SURGERY. Surgery performed as a result of injury.

TREACHER COLLINS SYNDROME. A disorder that affects facial development and hearing, thought to be caused by a gene mutation on human chromosome 5. Treacher Collins syndrome is sometimes called mandibulofacial dysostosis.

TREMOR. A trembling, quivering, or shaking.

TRENDELENBURG'S TEST. A test that measures the speed at which the lower leg fills with blood after the leg has first been raised above the level of the heart. It is named for Friedrich Trendelenburg (1844–1924), a German surgeon.

TREPHINE. A small surgical instrument that is rotated to cut a circular incision.

TREPONEME. A term used to refer to any member of the genus *Treponema,* which is an anaerobic bacteria consisting of cells, 3–8 μm in length, with acute, regular, or irregular spirals and no obvious protoplasmic structure.

TRIAGE. Prioritizing the needs of patients according to the urgency of their need for care and their likelihood of survival.

TRICHOMONADS. Parasitic protozoa commonly found in the digestive and genital tracts of humans and other animals. Some species cause vaginal infections in women characterized by itching and a frothy discharge.

TRICUSPID VALVE. The right atrioventricular valve of the heart; it has three flaps, whereas the mitral valve has only two.

TRIGLYCERIDE (TAG). A chemical compound that forms about 95% of the fats and oils stored in animal and vegetable cells. TAG levels are sometimes measured as well as cholesterol levels when a patient is screened for heart disease.

TROCAR. A small sharp instrument used to puncture the abdomen at the beginning of the laparoscopic procedure.

TUBAL LIGATION. A surgical sterilization procedure that involves ligating, or blocking and/or tying, the fallopian tubes so eggs can no longer descend from the ovaries to the uterus. Also referred to as getting one's tubes tied.

TUBE FEEDING. Feeding or nutrition through a tube placed into the body through the esophagus, nose, stomach, intestines, or via a surgically constructed artificial orifice called a stoma.

TUBERCULOSIS (TB). An infectious disease that usually affects the lungs, but may also affect other parts of the body. Its symptoms include fever, weight loss, and coughing up blood.

TUMESCENT ANESTHESIA. A type of local anesthesia originally developed for liposuction in which a large volume of diluted anesthetic is injected into the tissues around the vein until they become tumescent (firm and swollen).

TUMOR MARKER. A circulating biochemical compound that indicates the presence of cancer. Tumor markers can be used in diagnosis and in monitoring the effectiveness of treatment.

TUMOR STAGING. The method used by oncologists to determine the risk from a cancerous tumor. A number—ranging from 1A–4B— is assigned to predict the level of invasion by a tumor, and offer a prognosis for morbidity and mortality.

TUNICA (PLURAL, TUNICAE). The medical term for a membrane or piece of tissue that covers or lines a body part. The retina is the innermost of three tunicae that surround the eyeball.

TUNICA VAGINALIS. A sac-like membrane covering the outer surface of the testes.

TURBIDITY. The degree of cloudiness of a urine sample (or other solution).

TURBINATE. Relating to a nasal concha.

TWILIGHT ANESTHESIA. An intravenous mixture of sedatives and other medications that decreases one's awareness of the procedure being performed.

TYMPANIC MEMBRANE. The eardrum. A thin disc of tissue that separates the outer ear from the middle ear.

TYMPANOPLASTY. Procedure to reconstruct the tympanic membrane (eardrum) and/or middle ear bone as the result of infection or trauma.

TYMPANOSTOMY TUBE. Ear tube. A small tube made of metal or plastic that is inserted during myringotomy to ventilate the middle ear.

TYPE 2 DIABETES. Sometimes called adult-onset diabetes, this disease prevents the body from properly using glucose (sugar), but can often be controlled with diet and exercise.

U

ULCER. A lesion or rough spot formed on the surface of an artery.

ULCERATION. Death of tissue cells in a specific area, such as skin.

ULCERATIVE COLITIS. A chronic condition in which recurrent ulcers are found in the colon. It is manifested clinically by abdominal cramping and rectal bleeding.

ULNA. One of the two bones of the forearm. The largest section articulates with the humerus at the elbow joint and the smallest portion of the ulna articulates with the carpal bones in the wrist.

ULTRASOUND,(ULTRASONOGRAM,ULTRASONOGRAPHY). A procedure where high-frequency sound waves that cannot be heard by human ears are bounced off internal organs and tissues. These sound waves produce a pattern of echoes which are then used by the computer to create sonograms, or pictures of areas inside the body.

UMBILICAL CORD BLOOD TRANSPLANT. A procedure in which the blood from a newborn's umbilical cord, which is rich in stem cells, is used as the donor source for bone marrow transplants. Currently, umbilical cord blood transplants are mainly used for sibling bone marrow transplants or to store blood for an anonymous donation. In most cases, umbilical cord blood does not contain enough stem cells to safely use for adult bone marrow transplants.

UMBILICAL RING. An opening through which the umbilical vessels pass to the fetus; it is closed after birth and its site is indicated by the navel.

UMBILICUS. The area where the umbilical cord was attached; also known as the navel or belly button.

UNCINATE PROCESS. A downwardly and backwardly directed process of each lateral mass of the ethmoid bone that joins with the inferior nasal conchae.

UNILATERAL CLEFT LIP. A cleft that occurs on either the right or left side of the lip.

UNITED STATES PHARMACOPOEIA (USP). An authoritative book, updated annually, that contains lists of medicines, dietary supplements, and surgical supplies; defines their doses or other units of measurement; and sets quality standards for their production and proper use. The USP is used by 130 countries around the world in addition to the United States.

UREA. A by-product of protein metabolism that is formed in the liver. Because urea contains ammonia, which is toxic to the body, it must be quickly filtered from the blood by the kidneys and excreted in the urine.

URETER. Either of the paired channels that carry urine from a kidney to the bladder.

URETEROSCOPE. A special type of endoscope that allows a surgeon to remove kidney stones from the lower urinary tract without the need for an incision.

URETHRA. The small tube-like structure that allows urine to empty from the bladder.

URETHRA HYPERMOBILITY. Main factor in stress urinary incontinence, with severity based upon how far the urethra has descended into the pelvic floor through herniation or cystocele.

URETHRAL FASCIAL SLING. A support and compression aid to urethral function using auxillary material made of patient or donor tissue to undergird the urethra.

URETHRITIS. Inflammation of the urinary bladder.

URGENCY. A sudden compelling need to urinate.

URIC ACID. A product of purine breakdown that is excreted by the kidney. High levels of uric acid, caused by various diseases, can cause the formation of kidney stones.

URINALYSIS (PLURAL, URINALYSES). The diagnostic testing of a urine sample.

URINARY CONDUIT DIVERSION. A type of urinary diversion or rerouting that uses a conduit made from an intestinal segment to channel urine to an outside collection pouch.

URINARY CONTINENT DIVERSION. A surgical procedure that restores urinary continence by diverting urinary function around the bladder and into the intestines, thereby allowing for natural evacuation through the rectum or an implanted artificial sphincter.

URINARY INCONTINENCE. Inability to prevent the leakage or discharge of urine. It becomes more common as people age, and is more common in women who have given birth to more than one child.

URINARY RETENTION. The inability to void (urinate) or discharge urine.

URINARY STRESS INCONTINENCE. The involuntary release of urine due to pressure on the abdominal muscles during exercise or laughing or coughing.

URINARY TRACT. The passage through which urine flows from the kidneys out of the body.

URINE. A fluid containing water and dissolved substances excreted by the kidney.

URINE CREATININE LEVEL. A value obtained by testing a 24-hour collection of urine for the amount of creatinine present.

URINE CULTURE. A test which tests urine samples in the lab to see if bacteria are present.

URINE CYTOLOGY. The examination of the urine under a microscope to look for cancerous or precancerous cells.

UROGYNECOLOGIST. A physician that specializes in female medical conditions concerning the urinary and reproductive systems.

UROLITHIASIS. The medical term for the formation of kidney stones. It is also used to refer to disease conditions related to kidney stones.

UROLOGIST. A physician who specializes in problems of the urinary system.

UROLOGY. The branch of medicine that deals with disorders of the urinary tract in both males and females, and with the genital organs in males.

URORADIOLOGIST. A radiologist that specializes in diagnostic imaging of the urinary tract and kidneys.

UTERINE FIBROID. A non-cancerous tumor of the uterus that can range from the size of a pea to the size of a grapefruit. Small fibroids require no treatment, but those causing serious symptoms may need to be removed.

UTERINE PROLAPSE. A condition which the uterus descends into or beyond the vagina.

UTERINE SUSPENSION. Procedure that places a sling under the uterus and holds it in place.

UTERUS. The womb, an organ in females for containing and nourishing the young during development before to birth.

UVEA. The middle of the three tunicae surrounding the eye, comprising the choroid, iris, and ciliary body. The uvea is pigmented and well supplied with blood vessels.

UVEITIS. Inflammation of any part of the uvea.

UVULA. A triangular piece of tissue that hangs from the roof of the mouth above the back of the tongue. Primary snoring is often associated with fluttering or vibrating of the uvula during sleep.

UVULOPALATOPHARYNGOPLASTY (UPPP). An operation to remove the tonsils and other excess tissue at the back of the throat to prevent it from closing the airway during sleep.

V

V/Q SCAN. A test in which both a perfusion scan and ventilation scan are done (separately or together) to show the quantity of air that different areas of the lungs are receiving.

VACUTAINER. A tube with a rubber top from which air has been removed.

VAGINA. A canal in the female body that leads from the cervix to the external orifice opening to the outside of the body.

VAGINAL PROLAPSE. Weakening of the supportive tissues of the uterus and vagina, such that the uterus and cervix bulge into the vaginal canal, or even out through the vaginal opening.

VAGINAL SPECULUM. An instrument that is inserted into the vagina that expands and allows for examination of the vagina and cervix.

VAGOTOMY. A surgical procedure in which the nerves that stimulate stomach acid production and gastric motility (movement) are cut.

VAGUS NERVE. The tenth cranial nerve, running from the head through the neck and chest into the abdomen. Intermittent electrical stimulation of the vagus nerve can help to control epileptic seizures.

VALGUS ALIGNMENT. Alignment of the knee that angles outward due to injury or deformity.

VALGUS. A deformity in which a body part is angled away from the midline of the body.

VALVE. Flaps (leaflets) of tissue in the passageways between the heart's upper and lower chambers.

VAPORIZE. To dissolve solid material or convert it into smoke or gas.

VARICES. Uneven, permanent dilation of veins.

VARICOSE VEIN. A vein that is abnormally enlarged, swollen, and/or dilated, and may be twisted or tortuous.

VARIX (PLURAL, VARICES). The medical term for an enlarged blood vessel.

VARUS ALIGNMENT. Alignment of the knee that angles inward due to injury or deformity.

VARUS. A deformity in which a body part is angled toward the midline of the body.

VAS DEFERENS (PLURAL, VASA DEFERENTIA). The Latin name for the duct that carries sperm from the testicle to the epididymis. In a vasectomy, a portion of each vas deferens is removed to prevent the sperm from entering the seminal fluid.

VASCULAR SURGERY. A branch of medicine that deals with the surgical repair of disorders of or injuries to the blood vessels.

VASCULOGENIC ERECTILE DYSFUNCTION. The inability to attain or sustain an erection satisfactory for coitus, due to atherosclerotic disease of penile arteries, inadequate impedance of venous outflow (venous leaks), or a combination of both.

VASECTOMY. Surgical sterilization of the male, done by removing a portion of the tube that carries sperm to the urethra.

VASOCONSTRICTION. Narrowing of blood vessels, especially as a result of vasomotor action.

VASOEPIDIDYMOSTOMY. A type of vasectomy reversal in which the vas deferens is attached to the epididymis, the structure where sperm matures and is stored.

VASOSPASM. A deadly side effect of aneurysm rupture where the vessels in the brain spontaneously constrict; can cause brain damage or death.

VASOVAGAL REACTION. A collection of symptoms that includes dizziness, fainting, profuse sweating, hyperventilation, and/or low blood pressure that occurs in a small percentage of individuals who donate blood.

VASOVASOSTOMY. A surgical procedure that is done to reverse a vasectomy by reconnecting the ends of the severed vasa deferentia.

VBAC. Vaginal birth after cesarean.

VEIN. A blood vessel that returns oxygen-depleted blood from various parts of the body to the heart.

VENA CAVA. The large vein that drains directly into the heart after gathering incoming blood from the entire body.

VENIPUNCTURE. Puncture of a vein with a needle for the purpose of withdrawing a blood sample for analysis.

VENOUS BLOOD. Blood that carries carbon dioxide from the tissues to the heart and then the lungs to be oxygenated.

VENOUS GRAFT. Transfer of living vein tissue within the same host (from one place of the body to another in the same person).

VENOUS STASIS DISEASE. A condition in which there is pooling of blood in the lower leg veins that may cause swelling and tissue damage, and lead to painful sores or ulcers.

VENOUS SYSTEM. Circulation system that carries blood that has passed through the capillaries of various tissues, except the lungs, and is found in the veins, the right chambers of the heart, and the pulmonary arteries; it is usually dark red as a result of a lower oxygen content.

VENOUS THROMBOSIS. The formation or presence of a blood clot in a vein.

VENOUS VALVES. Folds on the inner lining of the veins that prevent the backflow of blood.

VENTILATE. To assist a patient's breathing by use of a mechanical device or surgical procedure.

VENTILATION SCAN. A lung scan in which a tracer gas is inhaled into the lungs to show the quantity of air that different areas of the lungs are receiving.

VENTILATOR. A machine that helps patients to breathe. It is sometimes called a respirator.

VENTRICLE. A lower pumping chambers of the heart. There are two ventricles, right and left. The right ventricle pumps oxygen-poor blood to the lungs to be re-oxygenated. The left ventricle pumps oxygen-rich blood to the body.

VENTRICULAR FIBRILLATION. An erratic, disorganized firing of impulses from the ventricles, the lower chambers of the heart. The ventricles quiver instead of pumping in an organized way, preventing blood from pumping through the body. Ventricular fibrillation is a medical emergency that must be treated with cardiopulmonary resuscitation (CPR) and defibrillation as soon as possible.

VENTRICULAR TACHYCARDIA. A rapid heart beat, usually over 100 beats per minute. Ventricular tachycardia originates from the lower chambers of the heart (ventricles). The rapid rate prevents the heart from filling adequately with blood, so less blood is able to pump through the body. Ventricular tachycardia can be a serious type of arrhythmia and may be associated with more symptoms.

VERMILION. The dark pink tissue that makes up the lip.

VERTEBRA (PLURAL, VERTEBRAE). The bones of the spinal column. There are 33 along the spine, with five (called L1-L5) making up the lower lumbar region.

VERTEBRAL RECONSTRUCTION. Procedure for reconstruction and support of the vertebrae of the skeletal system.

VERTIGO. An illusory feeling that either one's self or the environment is revolving. It is usually caused either by diseases of the inner ear or disturbances of the central nervous system.

VIDEOSCOPE. A surgical camera.

VIRCHOW'S TRIAD. Three categories of factors that affect a patient's risk of venous thrombosis: alterations in the rate of blood flow; injuries to the tissue lining the walls of the veins; and alterations in the blood's ability to coagulate.

VIRTUAL COLONOSCOPY. Two new techniques that provide views of the colon to screen for colon polyps and cancer. The images are produced by computerized manipulations rather than direct observation through the colonoscope; one technique uses the X-ray images from a CT scan, and the other uses magnetic images from an MRI scan.

VISCERAL PERICARDIUM. Single layer of cells that lines both the internal surface of the heart with the parietal pericardium and the external surface of the heart.

VISUAL FIELD. The total area in which one can see objects in one's peripheral vision while the eyes are focused on a central point.

VISUALIZE. To achieve a complete view of a body structure or area.

VITAL CAPACITY (VC). The volume of air that can be exhaled following a full inspiration.

VITAL SIGNS. Measurements of a patient's essential body functions, usually defined as pulse rate, breathing rate, and body temperature.

VITRECTOMY. Surgical removal of the vitreous body.

VITREOUS BODY. The transparent gel that fills the inner portion of the eyeball between the lens and the retina. It is also called the vitreous humor or crystalline humor.

VOIDING. The medical term for emptying the bladder or urinating.

VOLAR. Pertaining to the palm of the hand or the sole of the foot.

VOLATILE ANESTHETICS. Another name for inhalation anesthetics.

VOLVULUS. An intestinal obstruction caused by a knotting or twisting of the bowel.

VULVA. The external parts of the female genital organs that include the mons pubis, labia majora, labia minora, clitoris, vestibule of the vagina, bulb of the vestibule, and Bartholin's glands.

W

WARFARIN. A drug given to control the formation of blood clots. The PT test can be used to monitor patients being treated with warfarin.

WATCHFUL WAITING. Monitoring a patient's disease state carefully to see if the condition worsens before trying surgery or another therapy. This term is often associated with prostate cancer.

WATERMELON STOMACH. A type of arteriovenous malformation (AVM) that develops in the antrum. The dilated blood vessels in the AVM resemble the stripes of a watermelon. Watermelon stomach is also known as gastric antral vascular ectasia, or GAVE syndrome.

WEGENER'S GRANULOMATOSIS. A rare condition that consists of lesions within the respiratory tract.

WEIGHT TRACTION. Sometimes used interchangeably with skin traction.

WHITE BLOOD CELLS (LEUKOCYTES). Cells of the blood that are responsible for fighting infection.

WITHDRAWAL SYMPTOMS. A group of physical or mental symptoms that may occur when a person suddenly stops using a drug on which he or she has become dependent.

WOLFF-PARKINSON-WHITE SYNDROME. An abnormal, rapid heart rhythm, due to an extra pathway for the electrical impulses to travel from the atria to the ventricles.

X

X RAY. A form of electromagnetic radiation with shorter wavelengths than normal light. X rays can penetrate most structures.

XENOGRAFT. Tissue that is transplanted from one species to another (e.g., pigs to humans).

XTB. Extreme drug-resistant tuberculosis

Z

Z-TRACK INJECTION. A special technique for injecting a drug into muscle tissue so that the drug does not leak (track) into the layers of tissue just beneath the skin.

ZOLLINGER-ELLISON SYNDROME. A condition marked by stomach ulcers, with excess secretion of stomach acid and tumors of the pancreas.

ZYGOMA. The cheek bone in the front of the face below the eye socket, it is connected to the frontal bone of the forehead and the maxilla (upper jaw); sometimes called the zygomaticum, zygomatic bone, or zygomatic arch.

ZYGOTE INTRAFALLOPIAN TUBE TRANSFER (ZIFT). The woman's eggs are fertilized in a laboratory dish and then placed in her fallopian tube.

INDEX

In the index, references to individual volumes are listed before colons; numbers following a colon refer to specific page numbers within that particular volume. **Boldface** references indicate main topical essays. Illustrations are highlighted with an *italicized* page number; and tables are also indicated with the page number followed by a lowercase, italicized *t*.

A

B

C

D

E

F

G

H

I

J

K

L

M

N

O

P

Q

R

S

T

U

V

W

X

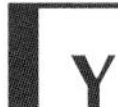

Y

Z